EQUIPMENT THEORY FOR RESPIRATORY CARE, THIRD EDITION

EQUIPMENT THEORY FOR RESPIRATORY CARE, THIRD EDITION

Gary C. White, M.Ed., RRT, CPFT
Director of Clinical Education
Spokane Community College
Spokane, Washington

Delmar Publishers

I (T) P An International Thomson Publishing Company

Albany • Bonn• Boston • Cincinnati • Detroit • London • Madrid • Melbourne
Mexico City • New York • Pacific Grove • Paris • San Francisco • Singapore • Tokyo
Toronto • Washington

NOTICE TO THE READER

Cover Credit: Brucie Rosch

Delmar Staff:
Acquisitions Editor: Dawn Gerrain
Developmental Editor: Debra Flis
Editorial Assistant: Donna Leto
Production Coordinator: John Mickelbank
Art and Design Coordinator: Richard Killar

COPYRIGHT © 1999
By Delmar Publishers

The ITP logo is a trademark under license
Printed in the United States of America

For more information contact:

Delmar Publishers
3 Columbia Circle, Box 15015
Albany, New York 12212-5015

International Thomson Publishing Europe
Berkshire House
168-173 High Holborn
London, WC1V7AA
United Kingdom

Nelson ITP, Australia
102 Dodds Street
South Melbourne,
Victoria, 3205 Australia

Nelson Canada
1120 Birchmont Road
Scarborough, Ontario
M1K 5G4, Canada

International Thomson Publishing France
Tour Maine-Montparnasse
33 Avenue du Maine
75755 Paris Cedex 15, France

International Thomson Editores
Seneca 53
Colonia Polanco
11560 Mexico D. F. Mexico

International Thomson Publishing GmbH
Königswinterer Strasße 418
53227 Bonn
Germany

International Thomson Publishing Asia
60 Albert Street #15-01
Albert Complex
Singapore 189969

International Thomson Publishing Japan
Hirakawa-cho Kyowa Building, 3F
2-2-1 Hirakawa-cho, Chiyoda-ku,
Tokyo 102, Japan

ITE Spain/ Paraninfo
Calle Magallanes, 25
28015-Madrid, Espana

2 3 4 5 6 7 8 9 10   XXX   03 02 01 00 99

Library of Congress Cataloging-in-Publication Data
White, Gary C., 1954–
    Equipment theory for repiratory care / Gary C. White. — 3rd ed.
            p.   cm.
    Includes bibliographical references and index.
    ISBN: 0-7668-0460-7
    1. Respiratory therapy -- Equipment and supplies. 2. Respirators (Medical equipment)   I. Title.
RC735.I5 W48 1998   95-28026
615.8'36—dc21   CIP

Dedication

To my wife, Carolyn,

and

my two sons, "A^2" (Andrew, age twelve, and Austin, age eight), who consistently remind their father just who and what are important. The book is done—and yes, it's March, but there is still plenty of good spring skiing!

CONTENTS

LIST OF EQUIPMENT

PREFACE TO THE THIRD EDITION

CHANGES TO THE THIRD EDITION

The first and second editions of *Equipment Theory for Respiratory Care* have been very well received texts. The features that made the first two editions a success have been retained for the third edition. Many reviewers and fellow educators have requested that the book be expanded to include more equipment and a more comprehensive treatment of the subject. It has been a difficult balance to include more and yet retain the strong features of readability and the student-centered focus of the first two editions.

Many educators have commented that they like the self-assessment quizzes at the end of each chapter; these have continued to be retained. In addition, requests have been made for more clinical scenarios or critical thinking activities.

A new feature has been added to each chapter entitled "Clinical Corner." The purpose of this feature to let is the student to dialog with his or her instructor using these activities as a template or guide. Additionally, they may be used in class for classroom discussion. Answers are not provided in the text; instead, the student should seek out the instructor. Alternatively, an instructor may choose to use these as written assignments.

The troubleshooting sections of the second edition have been well received. Troubleshooting flow charts or algorithms are provided to guide the student through the steps of troubleshooting the equipment. The algorithms include decision making, process and connection nodes in a similar way in which therapy-drive protocols are presented. The goal of these algorithms is to teach the critical thinking process of troubleshooting and to assist the student in the development of a systematic method of problem solving.

FORMAT

This text uses a comprehensive, competency-based approach to describe the equipment employed in the practice of respiratory care. The text emphasizes the physical and engineering principles employed in the operation of this equipment. These principles are then related to a representative sample of equipment; assembly and troubleshooting of the equipment is presented. Selection, assembly and troubleshooting accounts for 25% of the National Board for Respiratory Care (NBRC) written exams.

It is imperative that the student be thoroughly knowledgeable on equipment selection and application to be clinically competent. To assist in the student's understanding of the material, each chapter concludes with a self-assessment quiz using NBRC-type questions. By studying the chapter objectives, reading the text, following the assembly and troubleshooting guides and completing the self-assessment quiz, the student will encounter important concepts and principles in many different ways, thus facilitating their retention.

HIGHLIGHTS

Highlights of this text include the use of a competency-based approach to facilitate the learning of the material. The text headings are keyed to the objectives. This simplifies finding specific areas within each chapter. The physical and engineering principles of operation are illustrated in numerous computer-aided design drawings. Those same principles are applied to a representative sample of equipment. Assembly drawings and a written assembly guide will help the student to correctly prepare the equipment for clinical use. A troubleshooting algorithm provides a logical method for the student to follow when attempting to restore a piece of equipment to operation once its performance has failed or diminished. The "Clinical Corner" feature further helps to bridge the gap from theory to practice. The self-assessment quiz provides students with another opportunity to test their knowledge of the concepts contained within the chapter.

The major priority in the development of the third edition continues to be its readability and student-centered focus. Reading level studies have shown that the reading level of many texts in the field of respiratory care is too high for many of the students studying respiratory care. This text has been made more readable by the elimination of reference citations within the text. Instead, references and suggested readings are listed at the conclusion of each chapter. The use of objectives, format, simplified language, and artwork all help to make this complex subject easier to comprehend.

INSTRUCTIONS TO THE STUDENT

Six steps are listed below that will enable you, the student, to more effectively use this text. If you follow these steps it will be easier for you to understand and apply this seemingly difficult material. Ultimately it will be the application of your knowledge and skill that will enable you to be a good respiratory care practitioner.

1. Read the introduction to the chapter and, though you may not understand all of the terms or concepts, try to visualize what it is you will be learning.
2. Read and study the objectives. The objectives form the core of what will be presented in the chapter. Rephrase the objectives into questions and write them on a piece of paper. As you read the text, answer the questions you have written.
3. Read the text. Relate what you read to the artwork, forming a mental picture of how the equipment works or how the parts fit together to make a whole.
4. In the laboratory or clinical setting, work with the equipment discussed in the chapter you read. Take the equipment apart and assemble it again using the assembly guide. Troubleshoot it by deliberately rendering it inoperational or marginally effective. Follow the troubleshooting algorithms when you are troubleshooting the equipment. Hands-on practice is the fastest way to gain confidence and experience.
5. Dialog with your instructor using the "Clinical Corner" feature.
6. Read the objectives one more time and take the Self-Assessment Quiz to assess your knowledge.
7. Use the Selected Bibliography to expand your knowledge of the subject. Most references may be found in a hospital medical library or respiratory care department.

USE OF THE TROUBLE-SHOOTING ALGORITHMS

At first it may seem that the algorithms are difficult to follow and appear to have little to do with troubleshooting. Visualize the algorithm as a map that will illustrate the potential problems, what needs to be checked, and the steps required to resolve the problem. One step on the algorithm flows to another step until the end is reached.

The symbol shapes denote specific steps or action required by the student, as you progress through an algorithm. The circle-shaped symbol is termed a *terminal symbol* (Figure i-1). This symbol denotes the start or end of an algorithm. The diamond-shaped symbols are *decision symbols*. Within a decision symbol, a question is asked. The answer to the question may only be "yes" or "no." The rectangular-shaped symbols are *process symbols*. These require action on your part. You must perform the steps called out in the process symbol(s) before proceeding. Arrows guide you from one place to another within the troubleshooting algorithm to another or, if the algorithm is split between two pages, it connects one page to another. Simply match the number between the two nodes (i.e., 1 to 1, 2 to 2, etc.).

Gary C. White
1998

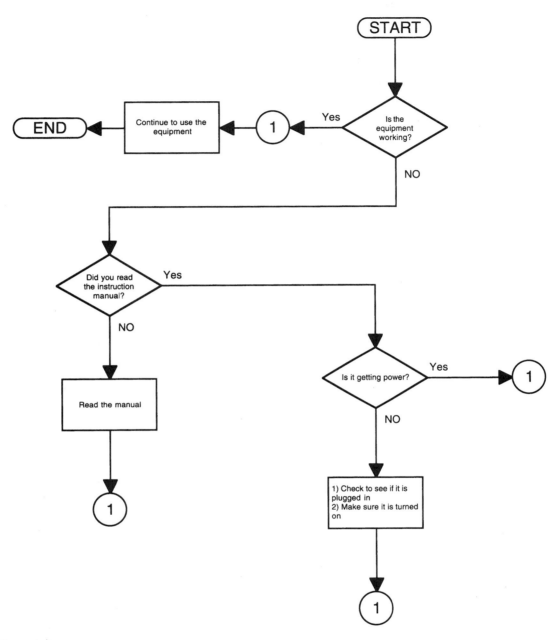

Figure i–1

ACKNOWLEDGMENTS

This type of technical text could not be created without the help and support of respiratory care equipment manufacturers and vendors. The companies listed below all contributed toward the development of this text. Many provided technical manuals, technical drawings and photographs. Others provided equipment or technical advice. I owe a great deal of thanks to these companies, their product managers, marketing managers, engineers, technical support personnel and respiratory care practitioners.

AMBU, Inc.
Aequitron Medical, Inc.
Allied Healthcare Products, Inc.
BEAR Medical Systems
BCI International
Bird Products Corporation
CAIRE, Inc.
Chad Therapeutics, Inc.
DeVilbiss Health Care, Inc.
Hamilton Medical, Inc.
ICN Pharmaceuticals, Inc.
Impact Medical Corporation
Infrasonics, Inc.
J. H. Emerson Company
Laerdal Medical Corporation
Lifecare
Life Support Products, Inc.
Medical Molding Corporation of America
MEDICO, Ogden, Utah
Monaghan Medical
Nellcor, Inc.
Newport Medical Instruments, Inc.
Novametrix Medical Systems
Nonin Medical, Inc.
Ohmeda
Omni-Tech Medical, Inc.
Puritan Bennett Corporation
Respironics, Inc.
Sechrist Industries, Inc.
Siemens Life Support Systems
Utah Welders Supply, Salt Lake City, Utah
Whitmore Medical, Ogden, Utah

In addition to the manufacturers and vendors, other individuals have helped in the creation of this text by reviewing specific content areas. These individuals include Carl G. Wood, Ph.D., Assistant Professor, Automotive and Mechanical Engineering Technology, Weber State University, and Leonard G. Nielsen, MS, MT (ASCP), Associate Professor, Clinical Laboratory Sciences, Weber State University.

I would like to acknowledge the reviewers who read the entire manuscript. Their insight, comments and suggestions helped me to refine the text and produce a better book. They include:

Randall W. Anderson, R.R.T., C.R.T.T., R.C.P.
Respiratory Care Program Coordinator
Spartanburg Technical College
Spartanburg, S.C.

Kerry Jean Connor, M.S., R.R.T.
Director of Clinical Education
Associate Professor of Respiratory Care
Manchester Community-Technical College
Manchester, Conn.

Cynthia Smathers, M.Ed., R.R.T.
Respiratory Care Program Director
Pima Medical Institute
Mesa, Ariz.

Theresa Winschel, R.R.T.
Clinical Coordinator
Hinds Community College–Jackson Branch
Nursing/Allied Health Center
Jackson, Miss.

I would also like to thank Clark Taylor, Instructional Technology, Weber State University. Mr. Taylor provided tremendous help and suggestions toward improving my abilities as a technical photographer.

I owe special thanks to Colton Grigsby. When Colton had finished play time with my son Austin, he introduced me to his mother Becky Grigsby. It was then that I learned of Becky's talent as a technical illustrator. She has demonstrated the ability to accurately render pieces of equipment while communicating concepts and ideas simultaneously. Her art work tremendously enhances the effectiveness of this third edition. Thank you, Becky!

Lastly, I owe thanks to my wife Carolyn, who provided countless hours for me to create yet another book! As my children grow, the demands placed upon my wife, so that I have time to work, also grows. Without her help and support, this third edition would not be possible. Thank you for believing in what I do.

Gary C. White
1998

CHAPTER 1

OXYGEN AND MIXED GAS THERAPY EQUIPMENT

INTRODUCTION

Administering oxygen therapy is involved in most of the tasks performed by a respiratory care practitioner. It is important to understand how oxygen therapy and mixed-gas therapy equipment operate and how to troubleshoot when problems arise.

In this chapter you will study the physics of equipment operation, including gas supply systems and the therapeutic administration devices. Only by thoroughly understanding the equipment and its components can you safely use it and troubleshoot it if it fails to function properly.

OBJECTIVES

After completing this chapter, the student will accomplish the following objectives:

PHYSICS OF THE PRINCIPLES

- Describe the kinetic theory of gases.
- Define the term *gas pressure;* explain what causes it and how it is measured.
- Explain Pascal's law.
- Explain what causes gases to flow from one place to another and how gas flow is measured.
- Explain Bernoulli's principle.
- Describe the principle of viscous shearing and vorticity.
- Explain how ejectors work:
  — in conjunction with venturi tubes
  — with constant area ducts
- Describe choked flow and the conditions under which it occurs.
- Explain the significance of Reynolds' number.
- Apply the following laws to solve for volume, temperature or pressure:
  — Boyle's law
  — Charles' law
  — Dalton's law
  — Gay-Lussac's law
  — Combined or ideal gas law
  — Fick's law
  — Henry's law
  — Graham's law

MEDICAL GAS SUPPLY EQUIPMENT

- Differentiate between the following supply systems; describe their construction and their principles of operation:
  — cylinders
  — liquid reservoirs, including calculation of oxygen duration based on weight
  — piping systems
  — compressors
  — concentrators
- Identify the contents of a medical gas cylinder, using the U.S. and international color code system, for the following gases:
  — oxygen
  — carbon dioxide
  — nitrous oxide
  — cyclopropane
  — helium
  — carbon dioxide and oxygen
  — helium and oxygen
  — air
- Given an oxygen "E" or "H" cylinder, gauge pressure and liter flow, calculate

how long the cylinder will last.
- Identify the markings stamped on the cylinder shoulder.
- List fifteen rules established by the Compressed Gas Association and the National Fire Protection Association for the safe storage and handling of compressed medical gas cylinders.
- Differentiate between the following oxygen regulation devices; describe their construction and principles of operation:
  — direct-acting cylinder valve
  — indirect-acting cylinder valve
  — single-stage reducing valve
  — modified single-stage reducing valve
  — multiple-stage reducing valve
  — regulator
  — oxygen proportioner
  — demand pulse-flow regulators
- Differentiate between the following oxygen flowmeters; describe their construction and principles of operation:
  — Bourdon gauge
  — uncompensated Thorpe tube
  — compensated Thorpe tube

MEDICAL GAS THERAPY EQUIPMENT

- Differentiate between high-flow and low-flow oxygen devices.
- List three characteristics common to oxygen enclosures or environmental devices.

- Differentiate between the following oxygen delivery devices, classifying each as a high-flow or low-flow delivery device, and discuss its principle of operation.
  — nasal cannula
  — reservoir and pendant cannula
  — simple mask
  — partial rebreathing mask (reservoir mask)
  — non-rebreathing mask (reservoir mask)
  — transtracheal catheter
- Describe the operation of high-flow air entrainment devices.
- Differentiate between the following enclosures or environmental devices:
  — isolette
  — head box
  — mist tent (croupette)
- Explain the principle behind hyperbaric oxygen therapy and the equipment utilized for this therapy.
- Differentiate between the equipment utilized for mixed-gas therapy (O_2/He and O_2/CO_2) and that used for oxygen administration.

PHYSICS OF THE PRINCIPLES

BEHAVIOR OF GASES

Gases behave according to the *kinetic theory*. The kinetic theory describes the behavior of ideal gases, and it incorporates five important points. These points are: (1) gases are composed of discrete molecules; (2) the molecules are in random motion; (3) all molecular collisions are elastic, causing no energy transfer between molecules; (4) the molecular activity is directly dependent upon the temperature; and (5) there is no physical attraction between the molecules composing the gas.

Gases are composed of very small, discrete molecules. The distance between molecules is much greater than the actual diameter of the individual molecules. Therefore, gases consist of large amounts of open space between the gas molecules. The volume of the molecules (if they could be gathered together) is very small when compared to the total volume of the molecules and space as a whole.

Gas molecules are in constant, random motion. The molecules travel in a straight line or path. This motion continues until they collide with something else. These collisions can occur with other molecules, the walls of the container holding the gas or other particles. Evidence of these collisions was first described by Robert Brown in 1827. He described the motion of larger particles that moved as a result of the smaller molecules of the gas colliding with them. This random movement can be observed today by watching the behavior of cigarette smoke under a microscope. The random motion of the larger particles is termed *Brownian motion.*

The collisions between molecules are completely elastic. This means that there is no energy transferred as a result of these collisions. Energy is not lost or gained by the molecules as a result of this process. Therefore, the total energy of the gas remains constant.

The kinetic activity or speed of the molecules is largely determined by the temperature. As the temperature of a gas increases, so does the kinetic activity. Conversely, as the temperature of a gas decreases, its kinetic activity decreases.

In ideal gas behavior, the gas molecules do not attract or repel one another. There is no physical attractive force between individual molecules. The molecules move about freely without any significant attractive forces between them.

GAS PRESSURE

Causes

Gas pressure (force per unit area) is caused by the individual gas molecules colliding with one another and the walls of a container. This exerts a force on the container walls. Even gas molecules have mass and a velocity, and thus possess a certain momentum (momentum = mass × velocity). The momentum transferred from these multiple collisions is what creates pressure, or the force on the walls of a container. The temperature of a gas influences the level of kinetic activity and therefore the velocity of the molecules.

Pascal's Law

Blaise Pascal, a seventeenth-century investigator, described how force is transmitted in a fluid. Pascal discovered that a fluid confined in a container will transmit force or pressure uniformly in all directions and that the pressure, or force at the walls of the container, acts perpendicular to that surface.

Since gases behave according to fluid properties, Pascal's law also applies. Pressure at any point in a closed container is equal to the pressure at any other point in the same container. If you take a long, closed tube and pressurize it with a gas, the pressure at one end will be equal to the pressure at the opposite end. Also, the pressure acts equally in all directions, with the force applied perpendicular to all surfaces of the tube.

Measurement of Gas Pressure—Barometers

The atmospheric pressure is measured with an instrument called a barometer. There are two types of barometers, mercury and aneroid.

The *mercury barometer* (Figure 1-1) uses the weight of a column of mercury opposing the force of the atmosphere to measure atmospheric pressure. The barometer consists of a closed column of mercury inverted in a shallow reservoir open to the atmosphere. When the column is inverted in the reservoir, a vacuum is created as gravity pulls the column of mercury down from the top of the closed tube. Atmospheric pressure against the open reservoir balances the gravitational force, pulling the mercury down in the closed tube. The level of the mercury column rises or falls, depending upon the atmospheric pressure exerted against the open reservoir. A calibrated scale adjacent to the mercury column provides a method to measure the height of the column of mercury. For medical and scientific purposes, atmospheric pressure is measured in millimeters of mercury. This measurement is also referred to as *torr* (named after Evangelista Torricelli, the inventor of this barometer).

The *aneroid barometer* (Figure 1-2) consists of an evacuated metal container that has a pressure lower than atmospheric pressure. A spring is attached between the container and a pointer mechanism. This indicates the pressure. As gas pressure increases, the container

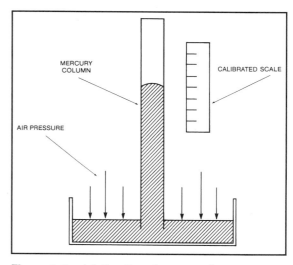

Figure 1-1 *A full section of a mercury barometer. Note how air pressure causes the mercury column to rise in the vertical tube.*

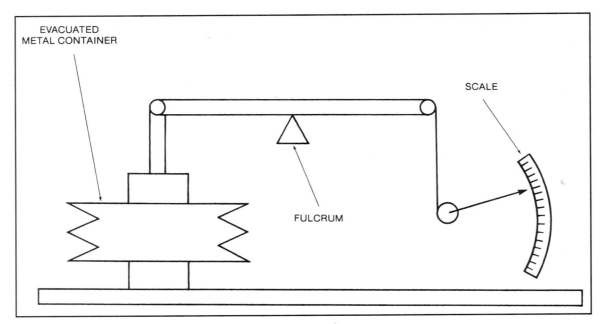

Figure 1-2 *A functional diagram of an aneroid barometer. As air pressure causes the evacuated container to expand or contract, the pointer moves adjacent to the scale.*

is compressed. This causes the pointer to move, indicating an increased pressure. The pointer moves adjacent to a scale calibrated in millimeters of mercury.

Measurement of Gas Pressure— Other Devices

In addition to barometers, mechanical manometers and Bourdon gauges can be used to measure gas pressure.

A mechanical manometer (Figure 1-3) is similar in construction to an aneroid barometer. A diaphragm or evacuated container is exposed to the area where pressure measurement is desired. As gas exerts a force against the diaphragm or container, it causes the pointer's position to change, indicating the pressure. Note that these instruments are calibrated so that atmospheric pressure measures zero on the instrument's scale. The majority of

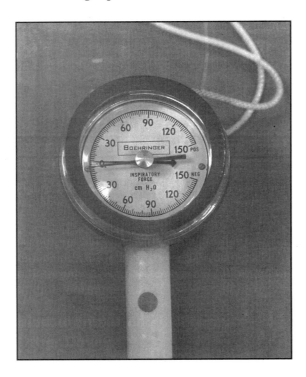

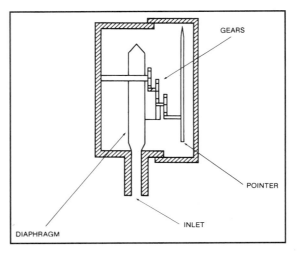

Figure 1-3 *A photograph and functional diagram of an inspiratory force manometer. As pressure causes the evacuated container to expand or contract, the pointer moves adjacent to its scale.*

manometers in respiratory care are calibrated in centimeters of water pressure or Kilopascals (KPa) (le Système International d'Unités [SI], or metric units). Table 1-1 lists standard units of pressure measurement.

A *Bourdon gauge* (Figure 1-4) consists of a hollow coiled metal tube with an elliptical cross section that is exposed to an area where gas pressure measurement is desired. Attached to the coiled tube are a gear mechanism and a pointer. As pressure increases, the tube begins to straighten, causing the gears to turn and the position of the pointer to change. The tube straightens because the pressure causes the cross section of the tube to become rounder. As the cross section changes, the outside of the tube is stretched while the inside becomes compressed. These gauges are commonly found on medical gas cylinders, indicating the pressure inside of the cylinder, and are calibrated in pounds per square inch (psi).

GAS FLOW

Cause

Gas flows from one point to another due to a difference in pressure between the two

TABLE 1-1: Units of Pressure Measurement

UNIT		EQUIVALENT
1 Atm	=	760 mm Hg
		29.921 in Hg
		1034 cm H_2O
		101.325 KPa
		14.7 lb/in²
1 cm H_2O	=	.735 mm Hg
		.0142 lb/in²
1 mmHg	=	1.36 cm H_2O
		.019 lb/in²
1 KPa	=	.133 mm Hg
		.098 cm H_2O
		6.895 lb/in²
1 lb/in²	=	51.7 mm Hg
		70.34 cm H_2O

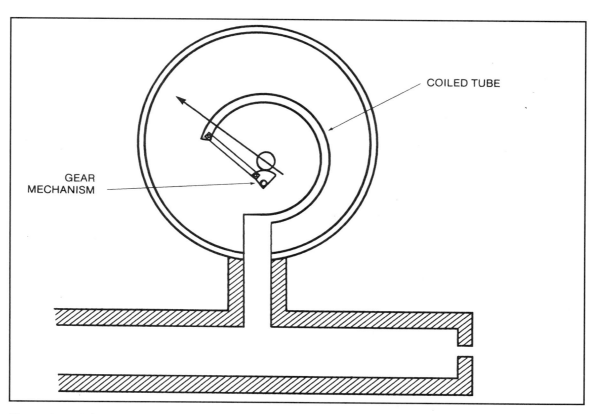

Figure 1-4 *A functional diagram of a Bourdon gauge. As the coiled tube expands, the gear mechanism rotates, causing the pointer to move.*

points. Gas will flow from an area of greater pressure to an area of lower pressure. The area of greater pressure contains gas molecules with greater kinetic activity. As a result of the increased kinetic activity (energy), the molecules push one another, moving from the area of higher energy to the area of lower energy.

The rate of gas flow, or velocity, is dependent on two factors: the difference in pressure (energy) and the size of the opening between the two areas. If the pressure difference is large, gas flow will be faster. If the pressure difference is small, gas flow will be slower. If the opening between the two areas is large, more gas can pass through and the flow will be greater than if the opening is small (Figure 1-5).

Bernoulli's Principle

During the eighteenth century, Daniel Bernoulli studied the flow of gas through tubes. He discovered that as the velocity of a gas increases, the lateral pressure within the tube decreases. This is due to the fact that the total energy content of the gas is constant. The total energy of the gas results from the kinetic energy created by the velocity and pressure energy. As velocity increases, the pressure must decrease for the total energy to remain

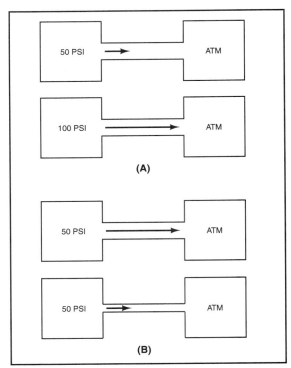

Figure 1-5 *Factors influencing gas flow: (A) two different pressures; (B) two different orifice sizes.*

constant (conservation of energy). As gas flow increases, more of the gas's energy is contained in kinetic energy, causing a further reduction in lateral pressure (Figure 1-6). In this

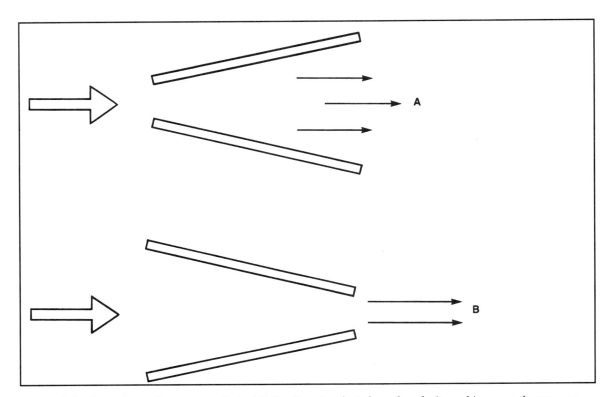

Figure 1-6 *Diverging and converging ducts: (A) the diverging duct slows the velocity and increases the pressure; (B) the converging duct increases the velocity and decreases the pressure.*

application, *Bernoulli's principle* applies to the flow of gas within a tube that changes in area along its length. A cross-sectional change is required to change the velocity. Bernoulli's equation assumes that the fluid is incompressible, that is, that the specific weight (weight per unit volume) is constant. If the fluid were to be compressed, volume would decrease while the weight would remain constant, increasing the specific weight. Keep in mind that gases will remain incompressible at low velocities, generally less than 100 meters per second.

This principle is commonly applied in respiratory care equipment. The reduced pressure within the tube may be used to introduce gases (usually air) or liquids into a low-pressure region of gas flow.

VISCOUS SHEARING, VORTICITY AND EJECTORS

Viscous shearing is another means by which oxygen is mixed with ambient or stationary air. Viscous shearing occurs when a high-velocity jet is injected into a quiescent gas. The high-velocity gas from the jet forms a thin boundary layer, where frictional forces develop between the high-velocity gas and the stationary surrounding air, cleaving it (Figure 1-7). The rapidly flowing gas accelerates the stationary gas, while the stationary gas decreases the velocity of the jet. Shear forces develop along the boundary layer between the two gases. The decelerating, high-velocity jet forms vortices, which envelop the ambient air, along the boundary layer. The viscous shearing effect entrains the room air into the vortices, mixing the oxygen with it. By varying the size of the oxygen jet and the entrainment ports, differing oxygen concentrations can be obtained. Manufacturers have developed specific combinations

of entrainment ports and jet sizes to deliver precise F_iO_2 levels. This principle is applied in High Air Flow with Oxygen Enrichment (*HAFOE*) masks, commonly called "venturi masks."

Venturi's Principle

Venturi expanded Bernoulli's principle by adding a specially shaped tube downstream from the jet. This tube has an increasing radius such that the angle of the walls does not exceed 15 degrees (Figure 1-8A). Note the pressure curve as gas passes through the tube. Pressure is reduced in the center and, due to the Bernoulli effect, progressively increases as the diameter of the tube increases near the outlet (Figure 1-8B). The high velocity of the gas from the nozzle causes ambient air to be mixed with the gas from the nozzle (by viscous shearing and vorticity, described earlier in this chapter), adding to the total quantity of gas flowing through the tube. As the tube expands, gas velocity slows and pressure increases. Venturi tubes are often employed where gas flow can be increased through entrainment of ambient air. Due to the Bernoulli effect, gas velocities through venturi tubes are generally low.

Constant Area Duct

This type of *ducted ejector* is similar to a venturi tube except that instead of restoring lateral pressure, the tube's purpose is to maintain a high velocity following the jet or restriction.

The ejector consists of a straight-walled tube that does not change in diameter downstream from the jet. Gas is entrained at the entrance to the tube (due to viscous shearing and vorticity between the source gas and ambient air) increasing total flow through the device. The tube downstream from the jet shields the flow of gas from entrainment without significantly slowing the velocity of the gas through

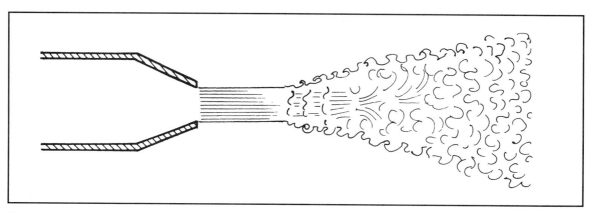

Figure 1-7 *The principle of viscous shearing. Note how the quiescent gas reduces the high velocity of the gas stream through the formation of vortices.*

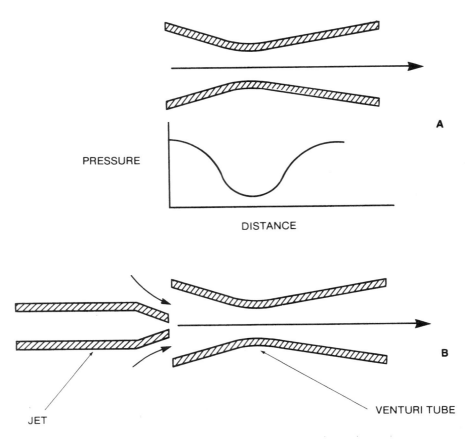

Figure 1-8 *Venturi's principle: (A) an illustration of the pressure gradient through a venturi tube; (B) a functional diagram of a nozzle combined with a venturi tube to form an ejector.*

the device (Figure 1-9). Velocity remains high and pressure remains constant because the diameter of the tube is constant (unlike the venturi tube). An advantage of this device is that an increased pressure downstream from the straight-walled tube has less effect on gas entrainment than with a venturi tube. These devices are employed in nebulizers and oxygen/air entrainment devices where there is moderate resistance downstream from the tube.

Effects of Increased Distal Pressure on Venturi and Constant Area Ducts

An increase in pressure downstream from an ejector will decrease the amount of ambient air entrainment. An increase in pressure may be caused by a kink in the delivery tubing or an obstruction distal to the point of air entrainment. This increase in pressure distal to the jet results in less ambient air entrainment because the total flow through the tube decreases as the back pressure increases. The flow through the jet's nozzle is constant; thus, the entrainment must decrease (Figure 1-10).

CHOKED FLOW OR COMPRESSIBLE FLOW

When a gas is flowing through an orifice or nozzle, the velocity of the gas increases as the pressure upstream (head pressure) of the nozzle increases. When the head reaches pressure 1.893 times the atmospheric pressure for air, the velocity of the gas no longer increases and the flow is choked. This corresponds to sonic flow at the orifice of the jet, which for air at room temperature is approximately 347 meters per second. This velocity corresponds to the speed of sound in air at room temperature. Once the gas reaches sonic velocity, the gas's velocity can no longer increase. Increasing the head pressure will not result in an increased flow when the flow is choked. The behavior of *choked flow* may be predicted using the choked flow equation, but this is beyond the scope of this text.

Choked flow is used in nebulizers when the head pressure driving the jet exceeds 26 psi, making the gas velocity out of the nozzle's exit sonic. Liquids are drawn into the gas flow from the reservoir via the capillary tube

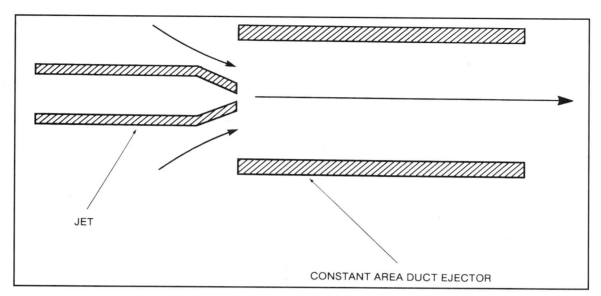

Figure 1-9 *A functional diagram of a constant-area duct ejector.*

at the boundary layer by shear forces and vorticity.

When these high-velocity jets are used in ventilators, the gas flow downstream from the nozzle at a distance of approximately three times the diameter of the nozzle exit ceases to be well behaved or laminar. At this point a shear layer develops and ambient gas may be entrained by vorticity. When used in this application, these jets are sometimes referred to as injectors, although the term *ejector* is technically more correct. If designed properly, the flow output from an ejector will exceed the flow provided by the nozzle alone.

Reynolds' Number

Reynolds' number is used to determine if gas flow through a tube is laminar or turbulent. *Laminar gas flow* is a smooth, uniform flow that requires less energy (pressure) to sustain. Turbulent gas flow is more erratic and irregular, requiring more energy to sustain. Figure 1-11 compares turbulent and laminar gas flow. The Reynolds number formula is as follows:

$$\text{Reynolds' Number} = \frac{\text{Velocity} \times \text{Density} \times \text{Diameter}}{\text{Viscosity}}$$

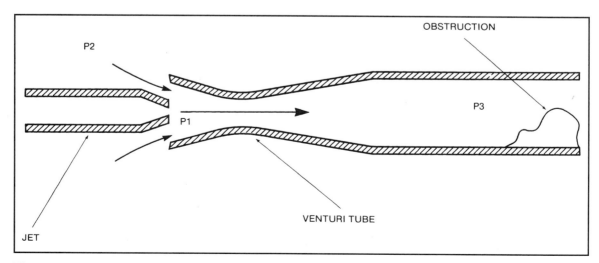

Figure 1-10 *An obstruction can result in decreased air entrainment through a venturi tube. P1 is less than P2 (atmospheric), and the obstruction causes P3 to be greater than P2. Note that the obstruction increases pressure distal to the entrainment ports, thus decreasing gas entrainment.*

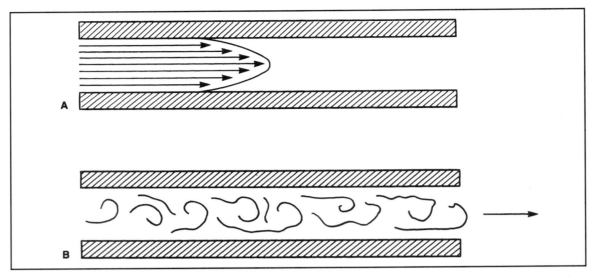

Figure 1-11 *(A) Laminar and (B) turbulent gas flow.*

Note that if you include the correct units in the calculation of Reynolds' number, the units cancel one another, resulting in a number that is dimensionless. As a general rule, if the Reynolds number is greater than 2000, flow will be turbulent. If the Reynolds number is less than 2000, flow will be laminar.

Poiseuille's Law

Poiseuille described the resistance to the flow of gas or liquid through a tube when the flow is laminar. He determined that it is directly related to volumetric flow, length of the tube and viscosity of the gas, and inversely related to the radius of the tube to the fourth power. This law is generally expressed in the following formula:

$$\dot{V} = \frac{\Delta P \times \pi \times r^4}{8 \times 1 \times \mu}$$

$\dot{V}$ = volumetric flow rate (velocity $\times$ area)

ΔP = pressure gradient

π = 3.1415

r = radius of the tube

μ = viscosity of the gas

l = length of the tube

Resistance is equal to the change in pressure divided by the volumetric flow rate.

$$R = \frac{\Delta P}{\dot{V}}$$

Solving Poiseuille's law for resistance:

$$R = \frac{8 \times 1 \times \mu}{\pi \times r^4}$$

This formula is often simplified for clinical applications to the following:

$$\Delta P = \dot{V} \times R$$
$$\dot{V} = \frac{\Delta P}{R}$$

ΔP = pressure gradient

$\dot{V}$ = volumetric flow rate

R = resistance

Simply stated, as the radius of a tube decreases by one-half, resistance increases sixteen times. As gas velocity increases, resistance to gas flow also increases. Increasing the length of a tube also will increase resistance to flow. These relationships will become very important when studying mechanical ventilation of the lungs. For example, if secretions within the airways increase, the effective radius of the airway decreases and resistance to gas flow increases dramatically. This will require higher pressures within the airway to maintain a constant flow.

For turbulent flow, the relationship between flow rate, pressure gradient, and the radius of the tube is more complex. This is because the flow is affected by the shape of the tube, viscous forces that dissipate energy, and the Reynold's number. Generally, the volumetric flow rate is proportional to the radius to the 2.7th power, expressed as the following:

$$\dot{V} \approx r^{2.7}$$

The effect of radius on volumetric flow rate is not as great for turbulent flow as it is for laminar flow, but the effect is still quite pronounced. If the radius decreases by one-half, the volumetric flow rate is decreased by a factor of sixteen for laminar flow, and by a factor of between six and seven for turbulent flow. Generally, the flow of gas through most respiratory care equipment is turbulent rather than laminar. Laminar flow occurs physiologically within the lungs after several branches in the bronchial system.

GAS LAWS

An understanding of the gas laws is important in the practice of respiratory care. During mechanical ventilation, volumes, pressures, flows and the temperature of the gas delivered to a patient are routinely manipulated to better match changes in the patient's condition. It is important to be able to predict how these changes will affect gas delivery to the patient.

When performing mathematical calculations, it is important to use consistent units in all equations. For example, one can not mix cmH_2O and psi and expect correct results. It will be necessary to convert temperatures, and sometimes pressures, depending on the circumstances under which the gas laws are applied.

When converting temperature scales, you will need to apply the formulas listed in Table 1-2.

The two new temperature scales introduced are called the *absolute* temperature scales. Both scales are referenced to absolute zero. Therefore, neither scale will have negative numbers since the lowest temperature is zero.

Boyle's Law

Boyle's law relates the volume of a gas to its pressure. With temperature remaining constant, the volume of a gas varies inversely with the pressure. Boyle's law is described in the following formula:

$P_1V_1 = P_2V_2$

P_1 = original pressure
V_1 = original volume
P_2 = new pressure
V_2 = new volume

This formula is commonly rearranged as follows to solve for the original pressure (P_1) or the new pressure (P_2).

$$P_1 = \frac{P_2V_2}{V_1}$$

$$P_2 = \frac{P_1V_1}{V_2}$$

TABLE 1-2: Temperature Conversion

Degrees Fahrenheit to Degrees Celsius

$\frac{5}{9}$ (Fahrenheit Temperature − 32) = Degrees Celsius

Degrees Celsius to Degrees Farenheit

$\frac{9}{5}$ (Celsius Temperature) + 32 = Degrees Farenheit

Degrees Celsius to Degrees Kelvin

Celsius Temperature + 273 = Degrees Kelvin
30 C + 273 = 303 K

Degrees Fahrenheit to Degrees Rankine

Fahrenheit Temperature + 460 = Degrees Rankine
70 F + 460 = 530 R

For example:

Given the following, V_1 = 500 ml, P_1 = 700 mmHg and P_2 = 300 mmHg, find the new volume.

$$\frac{P_1 \times V_1}{P_2} = V_2$$

$$\frac{700 \text{ mmHg} \times 500 \text{ ml}}{300 \text{ mmHg}} = 1,167 \text{ ml}$$

This law is often applied in calculating tubing compliance during mechanical ventilation of the lungs.

Charles' Law

Charles' law states that if pressure remains constant, the volume of a gas varies directly with the temperature (in degrees Kelvin). As the temperature increases, the volume of the gas also will increase. As the temperature of the gas decreases, volume will decrease. Charles' law is summarized in the following formula:

$$\frac{V_1}{T_1} = \frac{V_2}{T_2}$$

Before beginning this calculation, the temperature must first be converted to Kelvin, or absolute, temperature. To convert from Celsius to

Kelvin, add 273 degrees. For example, given an original volume of 400 ml, an original temperature of 20 degrees Celsius and a new temperature of 40 degrees Celsius, find the new volume.

$$V_2 = \frac{T_2 V_1}{T_1}$$

Converting Celsius to Kelvin:

$20° + 273° = 293\ K$

$40° + 273° = 313\ K$

$$V_2 = \frac{313°K \times 400\ ml}{293\ K}$$

$= 427.3\ ml$

An easy way to demonstrate this law is to attach an inflated balloon to a small narrow-necked chemistry flask, then heat the flask with a Bunsen burner. As the gas warms, it expands, causing the balloon to become larger.

Dalton's Law

Dalton's law is sometimes referred to as the law of partial pressures. Dalton described how the pressure of a gas composed of a mixture of gases is equal to the sum of the partial pressures of all the discrete gases. That is, the total is equal to the sum of the parts. Furthermore, he stated that the partial pressure each gas exerts would be the same as if the gas occupied the total volume alone. Lastly, the partial pressure of each gas is proportional to its volumetric percentage.

For example:

Gas mixture D is composed of 15 mmHg gas A, 25 mmHg gas B and 200 mmHg gas C. What is the total pressure?

Gas A =	15 mmHg
Gas B =	25 mmHg
Gas C = +	200 mmHg
Total Pressure =	240 mmHg

What is the percentage of each gas in the mixture?

Gas A percentage =

$15\ mmHg / 240\ mmHg = 6.3\%$

Gas B percentage =

$25\ mmHg / 240\ mmHg = 10.4\%$

Gas C percentage =

$200\ mmHg / 240\ mmHg = 83.3\%$

Another example of this law's use is the calculation of the partial pressures of the various gases in the atmosphere. Air is composed of nitrogen, oxygen, argon and other gases sometimes referred to as trace gases.

Nitrogen	78.08%
Oxygen	20.95%
Argon	.93%
Carbon Dioxide	.03%
Trace Gases	.01%

At an atmospheric pressure of 640 mmHg (Denver, Colorado), what is the partial pressure of oxygen and how does that compare to the partial pressure of oxygen in Seattle, Washington (atmospheric pressure of 760 mmHg)?

Denver, Colorado:

$640\ mmHg \times .2095 = 134.08\ mmHg$

Seattle, Washington:

$760\ mmHg \times .2095 = 159.22\ mmHg$

There is a partial pressure difference of 25.14 mmHg for oxygen between the two cities due to a difference in atmospheric pressure.

Gay-Lussac's Law

Gay-Lussac described the relationship between pressure and temperature of a gas. He found that as temperature increases pressure will increase as long as volume is constant. This relationship is described in the following formula:

$$\frac{P_1}{T_1} = \frac{P_2}{T_2}$$

For example:

A gas at 30° C and 700 mmHg is compressed to 900 mmHg. What is the new temperature?

$$\frac{P_2 \times T_1}{P_1} = T_2$$

$30°\ C + 273° = 303\ K$

$$\frac{900\ mmHg \times 303\ K}{700\ mmHg} = 389.6\ K$$

$389\ K - 273° = 117°\ C$

This law can be illustrated when a bicycle tire is inflated using a manual tire pump. As the air is compressed in the pump, its temperature increases. After the tire is inflated, the tire pump is noticeably warmer. In respiratory care equipment, air compressors have external fins that conduct and dissipate the heat generated when the ambient air is compressed.

Combined Gas Law

The *combined gas law,* or general gas law, is a combination of Boyle's, Charles' and Gay-Lussac's laws. It is useful in determining pressure, volume or temperature changes. The law is summarized in the following formula:

$$\frac{P_1 \times V_1}{T_1} = \frac{P_2 \times V_2}{T_2}$$

For example:

A gas at a pressure of 200 mmHg, 300° K, occupying 6 liters has its temperature increased to 400° K while occupying the same volume. Find the new pressure.

$$\frac{P_1 \times V_1 \times T_2}{T_1 \times V_2} = P_2$$

$$\frac{200 \text{ mmHg} \times 6 \text{ liters} \times 400 \text{ K}}{300 \text{ K} \times 6 \text{ liters}} = 267 \text{ mmHg}$$

GAS DIFFUSION

Besides pressure, volume and temperature relationships, it is important to understand gas diffusion. Gas diffusion is important physiologically in that gases constantly move from the atmosphere into our bodies, and then from our cells into our blood, by means of diffusion. There are three important laws of gas diffusion: Fick's, Henry's and Graham's laws.

Fick's Law

Fick's law describes how a gas diffuses into another gas. Fick's law states that the rate of diffusion of a gas into another gas is proportional to its concentration. That is, as the concentration gradient between the gases increases, the rate of diffusion will increase. Given two gases, where Gas A has a higher concentration than Gas B, Gas A will diffuse more rapidly than Gas B due to its greater concentration.

Henry's Law

Henry's law describes how gases diffuse into and out of liquids. Henry's law states that the rate of a gas's diffusion into a liquid is proportional to the partial pressure of that gas at a given temperature. Applying Henry's law, observe what happens when you open a bottle of soda pop. Once the cap is removed, bubbles can be seen moving toward the surface of the liquid and bursting once they reach the surface. The partial pressure of carbon dioxide is greater in the liquid than in the atmosphere. Therefore, carbon dioxide gas diffuses from the dissolved state (liquid) to a gaseous state and escapes into the atmosphere.

Graham's Law

Gas diffusion in the blood is more complex than what occurs as described in Henry's law. Other factors, such as the gram molecular weight and solubility of the gases, must be accounted for when understanding diffusion across the alveolar capillary membrane.

Graham's law states that the rate of gas diffusion through a liquid is proportional to the solubility of a gas and inversely proportional to the gram molecular weight. Comparing oxygen and carbon dioxide, oxygen's solubility is .023, while carbon dioxide's solubility is .510.

$$Solubility\ of\ CO_2 = \frac{.510}{.023}$$

$$= \frac{22}{1}$$

This relationship shows that carbon dioxide is over 20 times more soluble in the blood than oxygen. Once the gases are dissolved, they must diffuse through the blood. In determining the rate of diffusion, you must now account for the gram molecular weight.

$$Solubility = \frac{(Sol\ coef\ CO_2)\ (\sqrt{gmw}\ O_2)}{(Sol\ coef\ O_2)\ (\sqrt{gmw}\ CO_2)}$$

$$= \frac{(.510)\ (\sqrt{32})}{(.023)\ (\sqrt{44})}$$

$$= \frac{19}{1}$$

This relationship shows that carbon dioxide is 19 times more diffusible in the blood than oxygen. This relationship is true, assuming that the partial pressures for the two gases are equal. Normally in the alveolus, the partial pressure of oxygen is greater than that for carbon dioxide, resulting in a slightly greater rate of diffusion for oxygen.

MEDICAL GAS SUPPLY EQUIPMENT

COMPRESSORS

Medical *compressors* provide oil-free compressed air to power equipment and also to mix with pure oxygen to provide lower oxygen concentrations. The compressed air must be oil free for two primary reasons: (1) oil particles, when inhaled, are not healthy, (2) oil droplets, when mixed with oxygen, may result in spontaneous combustion. (Spontaneous combustion is the ignition of a substance without the addition of heat.) There are three types of compressors: piston, diaphragm and centrifugal.

Piston Compressor

A piston compressor utilizes a piston driven by an electric motor (Figure 1-12). Carbon or *Teflon®* piston rings seal the piston against the cylinder wall, eliminating the need for oil. The compressed air is fed into a storage reservoir providing a large supply of air to meet high flow demands. A filter at the outlet removes any particles from the compressed air. The pressure is then reduced to 50 psi by

ASSEMBLY AND TROUBLESHOOTING

Assembly—Piston Compressor

To prepare a piston compressor for use, complete the following instructions.

1. Connect the power cord to the correct electrical outlet—115 volts, alternating current (VAC).

2. Attach equipment requiring compressed air to the threaded outlet.

3. Check inlet filter for obstruction and, if required, clean or replace it.

4. Turn on the compressor with the on/off switch.

5. Verify correct outlet pressure (50 psi) with the gauge provided.

Troubleshooting

Troubleshooting compressors is very easy. Unfortunately, if the unit fails to operate, little can be done other than to take the compressor to an authorized repair center. When troubleshooting this equipment, please follow the suggested troubleshooting algorithm (ALG 1-1).

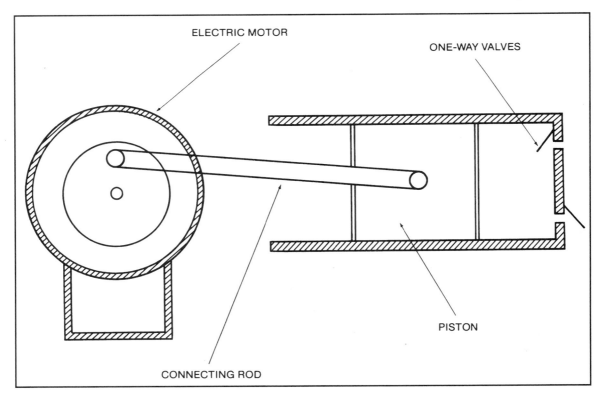

Figure 1-12 *A functional diagram of a piston compressor.*

ASSEMBLY AND TROUBLESHOOTING

Assembly—Diaphragm Compressor

To prepare a diaphragm compressor for use, complete the following instructions.

1. Connect the power cord to the correct electrical outlet (115 VAC).

2. Attach equipment requiring compressed air to the threaded outlet.

3. Check inlet filter for obstruction and, if required, clean or replace it.

4. Turn on the compressor with the on/off switch.

Troubleshooting

Troubleshooting diaphragm compressors is very easy. Unfortunately, if the unit fails to operate, little can be done other than to take the compressor to an authorized repair center. When troubleshooting this equipment, please follow the suggested troubleshooting algorithm (ALG 1-1).

means of a reducing valve before the air is fed into a piping system.

Diaphragm Compressor

Diaphragm compressors utilize a flexible diaphragm driven by an electric motor to compress the air. Diaphragm compressors are typically employed to power small nebulizers. They are not capable of providing the large amounts of compressed air needed

for large equipment. Figure 1-13 depicts a typical diaphragm compressor suitable for home use.

Centrifugal Compressor

The centrifugal compressor utilizes an electrically powered impeller mounted eccentrically within the compressor housing. As the impeller rotates, it compresses the air. Centrifugal force and the decreasing size of the

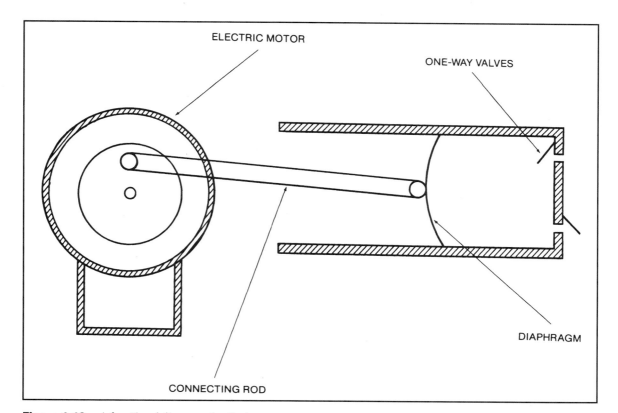

Figure 1-13 *A functional diagram of a diaphragm compressor.*

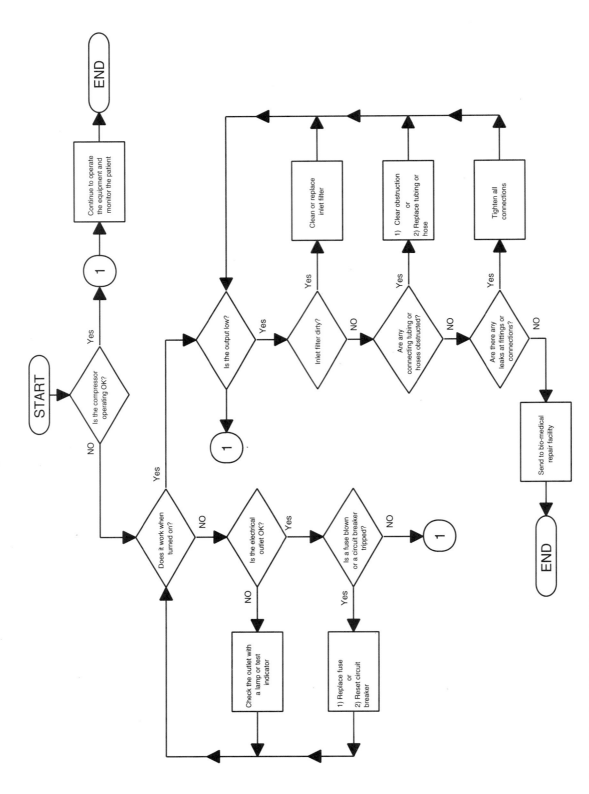

ALG 1-1 *An algorithm describing how to troubleshoot a compressor.*

chamber compress the gas as the impeller turns (Figure 1-14). These compressors are incorporated in some adult mechanical ventilators such as the Bennett MA-1.

A larger version of this type of compressor is used to provide a compressed air source for hospitals and other institutions. These rotary compressors use similar principles of operation, except that a working fluid (usually water) is used between the impeller and the compressor housing. The working fluid allows tolerances to be greater between the impeller and the compressor housing, reducing wear and eliminating the need for lubrication. A water separator and particle filters purify the air prior to delivery to the hospital piping system.

Water traps should be used with all ventilators powered by compressed gases. Water can become condensed as air or oxygen is pressurized. A contemporary ventilator's pneumatic, electronic control and monitoring system can be damaged by water that may be contained in the high pressure supply lines. To avoid this potential problem, the use of water traps is recommended by most manufacturers.

CONCENTRATORS

Oxygen concentrators are electrically powered devices that separate the oxygen from the atmosphere and deliver it under pressure for medical use. There are two types of oxygen concentrating devices, molecular sieve and membrane types.

The molecular sieve concentrator is more effective than the membrane type. Inlet air to a compressor is passed through a particle filter to remove large particles from the air. Then the gas is passed through a *bacteria filter* that removes particles as small as .3 microns. The filtered air is then compressed by a compressor to approximately 20 psi, and conducted to molecular sieves containing Zeolite. The compressed gas alternately charges one sieve and then the other. The Zeolite in the sieve adsorbs some of the nitrogen and passes the oxygen contained in the ambient air, thus increasing the oxygen concentration.

The process of *adsorption* is a surface phenomenon in which the gas molecules are forced under pressure into the pores of the Zeolite. As the nitrogen oxygen mixture (air) flows through the pores of the Zeolite, the ni-

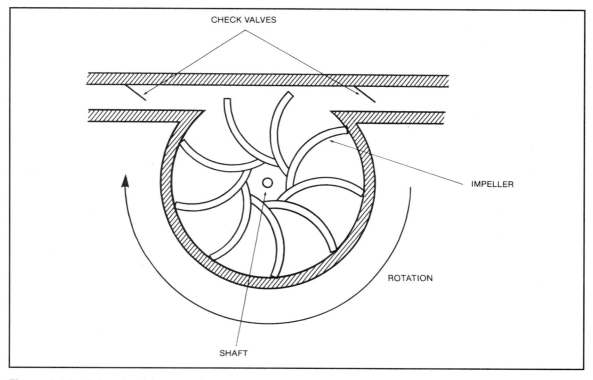

Figure 1-14 *A functional diagram of a centrifugal compressor.*

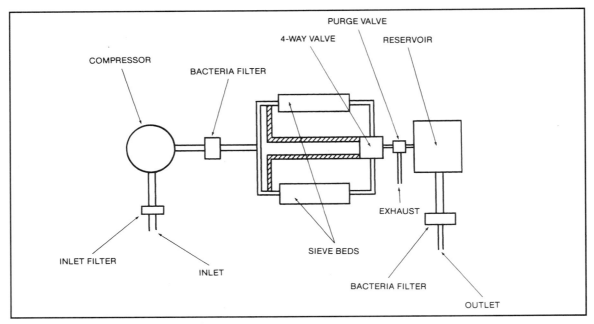

Figure 1-15 *A functional diagram of an oxygen concentrator.*

trogen molecules stick or adhere to the surface and the oxygen molecules pass through. When the sieve is depressurized, the nitrogen is released to the atmosphere and exhausted, separating it from the oxygen-enriched gas.

Oxygen concentrators use some of the oxygen-rich gas flowing from one sieve to purge the other sieve. This is done prior to pressurization to improve oxygen percentage levels. The purge cycle helps to rid the canister of nitrogen before it is again pressurized with room air.

Oxygen concentration will vary between 50% and 90% depending on the flow rate out of the concentrator. If the flow rate is set for 2 liters (L) per minute or less, the oxygen concentration will be 90%. If flow is increased to 10 liters per minute, the oxygen concentration drops to 50%. Figure 1-15 shows a schematic of a typical oxygen concentrator and its component parts.

The membrane type, commonly called an enricher, uses a semipermeable polymer membrane to remove the nitrogen from the air. An air compressor forces the air through the one-micron-thick membrane, allowing the smaller oxygen molecules to pass. A membrane enricher can provide a concentration of 40% oxygen at flow rates between 1 and 10 liters per minute.

DeVilbiss MC84 Oxygen Concentrator

The MC84 oxygen concentrator is designed to deliver high concentrations of oxy-

gen for the patient requiring oxygen therapy (Figure 1-16). Concentrators compress room air and separate the nitrogen from the oxygen by using molecular sieve technology. The MC84 provides 94% oxygen ± 3% at 1 L/min,

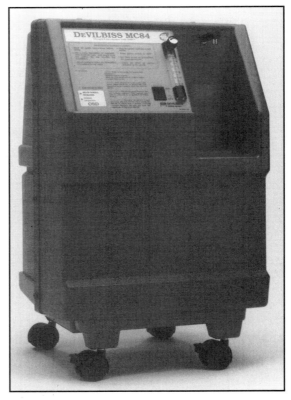

Figure 1-16 *A photograph of the DeVilbiss DeVO/ MC84 oxygen concentrator. (Courtesy DeVilbiss Health Care, Inc., Somerset, PA)*

95% oxygen ± 3% at 2 – 4 L/min, and 93% oxygen ± 3% at 5 L/min. The oxygen concentrator offers the homecare patient the convenience of continuous oxygen therapy without the need for compressed gaseous cylinders or liquid oxygen systems.

ASSEMBLY AND TROUBLESHOOTING

Assembly—DeVilbiss MC84

1. Position the oxygen concentrator in the room where your patient will spend the majority of his/her time. Be sure to choose a location away from heaters, radiators, and hot-air registers. Place the unit so that the back and sides are at least 6 inches away from any objects to assure adequate air flow through the unit.

2. Located on the back of the MC84 is a gross particle filter. You can remove the filter by rotating the knob 1/4 turn counterclockwise and pulling the filter assembly away from the unit. Inspect the gross particle filter for lint or other debris. The oxygen patient is instructed to wash this filter *at least* once a week. The filter may be washed in a solution of warm water and dishwashing detergent and then rinsed thoroughly with warm tap water and toweled dry. The filter should be completely dry before it is reinstalled. The gross particle filter may also be cleaned daily by using a vacuum cleaner attachment without removing the filter from the concentrator. The filter must still be washed weekly.

3. If humidification has been prescribed:
   a. Fill the humidifier reservoir with distilled water to the "fill" line and then thread the humidifier directly onto the fixed oxygen Diameter Index Safety System (DISS) outlet so that the humidifier is suspended.
   b. Attach the desired length of oxygen delivery tubing (not to exceed 50 feet, or 15 meters) to the humidifier outlet. If condensation occurs when using longer lengths of oxygen tubing, condensation may be reduced by using a removable humidifier stand.

4. If humidification has *not* been prescribed:
   a. Thread a green "Christmas Tree" fitting onto the fixed oxygen DISS outlet fitting and attach the desired length of oxygen delivery tubing (not to exceed 50 feet, or 15 meters).

5. Connect the cannula, transtracheal cannula, or mask to the oxygen delivery tubing.

6. Check to be certain that the power switch is in the "OFF" position. Select an electrical outlet (120 v, 60 Hz) that is not connected by a wall switch and is independent of other appliances. The MC84 is equipped with a two-prong plug and is double-insulated to guard against electric shock.

7. Depress the power switch to the "ON" position. An audible/visual safety alarm will briefly sound. If the red "SERVICE REQUIRED" light illuminates during operation, the audible alarm will also sound and the unit will automatically turn itself off. Press the power switch to the "OFF" position. Then turn the unit on again. If the red indicator light stays on, call your dealership or medical supply company to have the unit serviced by an authorized technician.

8. The MC84 is also equipped with an oxygen-sensing device (OSD) which monitors the oxygen concentration leaving the concentrator. There are two OSD indicator lights on the front panel: the green indicator light denotes normal oxygen concentration (85% oxygen and above), and the yellow indicator light denotes below-normal oxygen concentration (75–84.99% oxygen). If the yellow light is illuminated, the unit may still be operated, but service is required. If the yellow light is illuminated and it is ac-

companied by an audible alarm every 5 seconds, turn the unit off, use an alternate oxygen source (cylinder backup), and contact the dealer or medical supply company for replacement.

9. Adjust the flowmeter to the prescribed oxygen setting by turning the flowmeter knob counterclockwise to increase the flow of oxygen.

Troubleshooting

Follow the suggested troubleshooting algorithm (ALG 1-2) to assist you in troubleshooting this concentrator.

If the "On/Off" switch is in the "ON" position, the unit is not operating, the power light is off, and an audible alarm is sounding:

1. Check to be certain that the power cord is plugged into a 120 v, 60 Hz electrical outlet.

2. The electrical outlet may not have power. Test the outlet with a household lamp or radio. If the power is not on at the outlet, use another outlet.

3. The circuit breaker on the MC84 has tripped. Press the black reset button on the rear cover. If the breaker trips again, contact your dealer for service.

If the MC84 is not operating, the "On/Off" switch is in the "ON" position, and the red "SERVICE REQUIRED" alert is illuminated:

1. The motor thermal protection circuit has opened.
   a. If the unit fails to restart in 45 minutes, contact your dealer for service.

2. The air intake or exhaust is blocked.
   a. Check and service the gross particle filter if required.
   b. Check for objects blocking discharge air from the bottom right side of the unit.

If the unit is operating but you are unable to obtain the desired flow of enriched gas:

1. Blocked oxygen delivery device or connecting tubing.
   a. Remove the delivery device (cannula, catheter, or transtracheal catheter) from the extension tubing. If flow is restored, clean or replace the delivery device.
   b. Disconnect the extension tubing from the humidifier. If flow is restored, check the tubing for kinks or obstructions, or replace the tubing as required.

2. Blocked or defective humidifier.
   a. Remove the humidifier from the outlet of the MC84. If flow is restored, clean or replace the humidifier.

3. Use of excessive length of connecting tubing. Use a maximum of 50 feet, or 15 meters, of tubing.

Troubleshooting the oxyge- sensing device (OSD).

If both the green and yellow OSD lamps are illuminated or both lamps are off:

1. The OSD has malfunctioned: contact your dealer or medical equipment supply company for service.

If the yellow indicator light is illuminated and no audible alarm is heard:

1. The oxygen concentration is between 75 and 84.9%. The unit may continue to be operated, but service is required.
   a. Check to ensure that the flow meter is set correctly.
   b. Check the air intake and exhaust outlets.

If the yellow indicator light is illuminated and an audible alarm is heard every 5 seconds:

1. Utilize a backup source of oxygen (cylinder).

2. Contact your dealer or medical supply company for service.

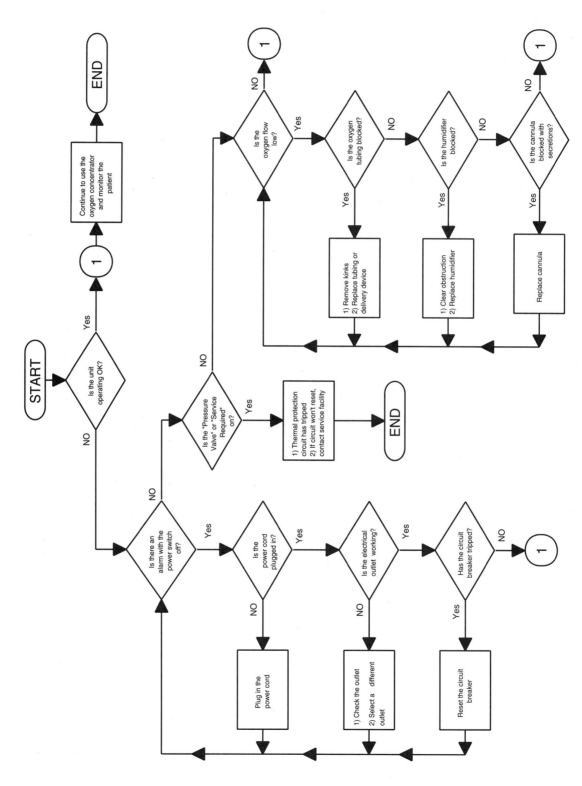

ALG 1-2 *An algorithm describing how to troubleshoot the DeVilbiss DeVO/MC84 oxygen concentrator.*

Puritan Bennett Companion 492a

The Puritan Bennett Companion 492a oxygen concentrator operates using two molecular sieves to separate oxygen from room air (Figure 1-17). The unit is capable of providing 95% oxygen concentration ± 3% at flows between 1 and 3 L/min. If the oxygen flow is 4 L/min, oxygen concentrations are 92% ± 3%. During normal operation the Companion 492a will consume an average of 330 watts electrical power. Ideally, the concentrator should be the only item connected to the electrical outlet and on that electrical circuit.

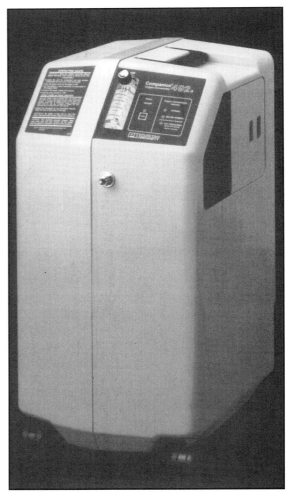

Figure 1-17 *A photograph of the Puritan Bennett Companion 492a oxygen concentrator. (Courtesy Puritan Bennett Corporation, Lenexa, KS)*

ASSEMBLY AND TROUBLESHOOTING

Assembly—Puritan Bennett Companion 492a

1. Place the Companion 492a concentrator in the room where your patient will spend the majority of his/her time. Be sure to choose a location away from heaters, radiators and hot-air registers. Place the unit such that the right and left sides have a minimum clearance of at least 6 inches away from any walls or drapes to ensure adequate air flow through the unit.

2. On the right side, at the upper left-hand corner, is a gross particle filter. Remove the filter by pulling it away from the side of the unit. (It is secured by Velcro strips.) Inspect the filter for lint or other debris. If required, wash the filter in warm detergent, rinse it in water and allow it to dry. Alternatively, you may use a vacuum cleaner and vacuum the debris from the filter using a wand attachment.

3. Attach a humidifier to one of the two humidifier adapters. (One is extra long for smaller humidifiers.)

4. Connect the oxygen delivery device to the humidifier outlet (cannula, transtracheal cannula, or catheter). Additional oxygen connecting tubing may be used to increase your pa-

tient's mobility. Up to 50 feet of additional tubing may be connected.

5. Check to be certain that the "On/Off" switch is in the "OFF" position. Connect the electrical power cord on the back of the Companion 492a to a 110 v, 60 Hz electrical outlet.

6. Turn the unit on by depressing the "On/Off" rocker switch to the "ON" position. Once the unit is on, you can hear the compressor operating.

7. Adjust the oxygen flow to the prescribed setting.

Troubleshooting

Follow the suggested troubleshooting algorithm (ALG 1-3), to assist you in troubleshooting this concentrator.

If the "On/Off" switch is in the "ON" position and an audible alarm is sounding, the system pressure has dropped below 5 psi:

1. Check to be certain that the power cord is plugged into a 110 v, 60 Hz electrical outlet.

2. The inlet bacteria filter may be clogged, preventing adequate gas flow to the compressor.
   a. Contact your dealer for service.

3. The compressor may not be operating or operating properly, preventing adequate pressurization.
   a. Contact your dealer for service.

If the Companion 492a is not operating, the "On/Off" switch is in the "ON" position, an audible alarm can be heard, and the front panel power indicator is off:

1. The unit is not receiving electrical power. Even though the Companion 492a is not receiving power, the alarm will still operate from a 9-volt battery.
   a. Check to ensure that the power cord is plugged in.
   b. The electrical outlet may not be functioning. Test the outlet with a household lamp or radio. If it is inoperative, move the Companion 492a to another outlet.
   c. The circuit breaker has tripped. Open the filter compartment on the right side of the unit and push the circuit breaker to reset it. If it trips again, contact your dealer for service.

If the unit is operating but you are unable to obtain the desired flow of enriched gas:

1. Blocked oxygen delivery device or connecting tubing.
   a. Remove the delivery device (cannula, catheter, or transtracheal catheter) from the extension tubing. If flow is restored, clean or replace the delivery device.
   b. Disconnect the extension tubing from the humidifier. If flow is restored, check the tubing for kinks or obstructions, or replace the tubing as required.

2. Blocked or defective humidifier.
   a. Remove the humidifier from the outlet of the Companion 492a. If flow is restored, clean or replace the humidifier.

LIQUID RESERVOIR SYSTEMS

Bulk Supply Systems

Bulk supply systems are used to supply large amounts of medical gas to a hospital or other institution. It is more economical to operate a bulk system than to use many small cylinders. The construction of a bulk liquid storage reservoir is very similar to an enlarged steel thermos. An outer steel shell encloses several layers of insulation in a near vacuum. The inner wall contains the liquid gas (see Figure 1-18). Standards of bulk reservoir construction have been established by the American Society of Mechanical Engineers. Liquid oxygen is stored in the reservoir at a temperature of −183° Celsius. Liquid oxygen continuously vaporizes, creating pressure. Pressure relief valves are incorporated into the reservoir to release pressure. The release

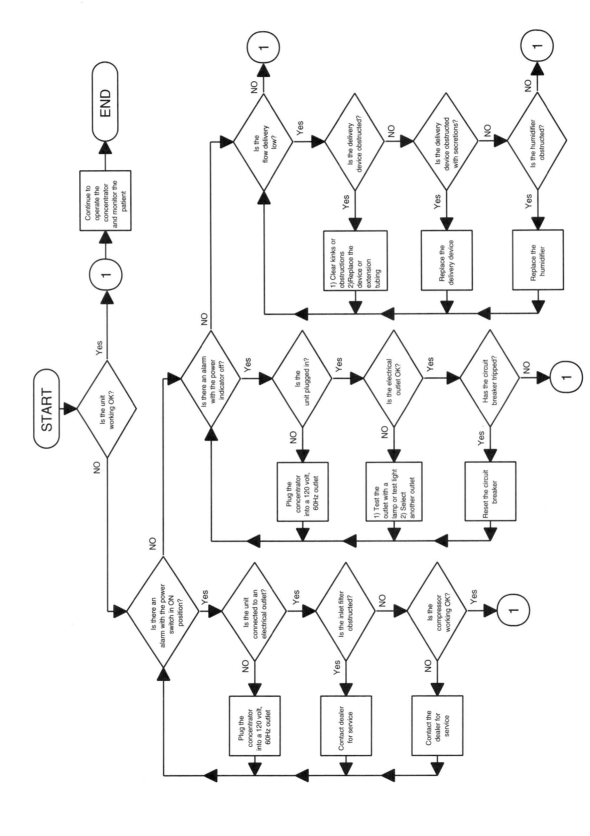

ALG 1-3 *An algorithm describing how to troubleshoot the Puritan Bennett Companion 492a oxygen concentrator.*

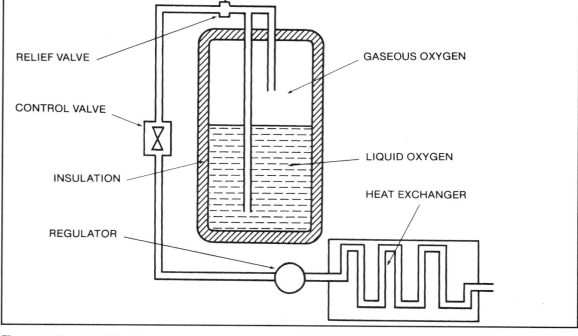

Figure 1-18 *A bulk liquid oxygen storage and supply system. Note the insulated container, control valve and heat exchanger. The heat exchanger converts the liquid to a gas by warming it.*

of pressure, as the gas expands, cools the reservoir (Gay-Lussac's law).

It is important to size the reservoir properly, so that the use of gas exceeds the rate of vaporization. If too much gas is lost to the atmosphere by vaporization, it may not be economical to operate the bulk system. An advantage of storing oxygen in liquid form is that one cubic foot of liquid oxygen expands to 861 heat exchanger cubic feet of gaseous oxygen (1:861 ratio). The liquid oxygen is fed into a heat exchanger like a radiator; it warms the liquid to a gas (Figure 1-18). Once the liquid has vaporized to a gas, pressure will have increased. The pressure is reduced to 50 psi by passing through a reducing valve. After the pressure has been reduced to 50 psi, the gas is then fed into the piping system.

Portable Reservoirs

Smaller liquid reservoirs have been designed for home and ambulatory use (Figure 1-19). The principles of construction are similar to the large bulk systems described earlier, only smaller in scale.

The larger reservoirs designed for stationary use in the home vary in capacity from 20 to 43 liquid liters. Although the capacity may

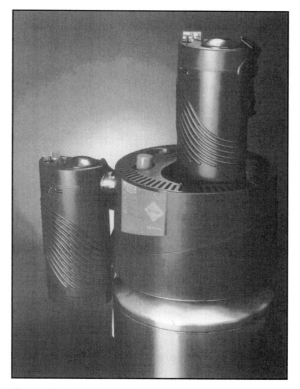

Figure 1-19 *A contemporary portable liquid home oxygen system. The larger reservoir is for use in the home. The smaller portable reservoir may be filled from the larger one for trips away from home lasting up to eight hours at flow rates less than 2 liters per minute. (Courtesy CAIRE, Inc., Bloomington, MN)*

ASSEMBLY AND TROUBLESHOOTING

Assembly—Portable Liquid Oxygen Systems

Little is required for proper assembly of portable liquid reservoirs. The following guide will help you in the assembly and preparation of the reservoir for use.

1. Ensure that the reservoir is filled by checking the weight gauge provided.
   a. Should the reservoir require filling, contact your local vendor.

2. Attach a flowmeter and humidifier to the threaded outlet of the reservoir.

3. Attach the oxygen therapy equipment to the outlet of the humidifier.

4. Turn on the flowmeter to the ordered setting and observe for proper flow.

When transfilling the ambulatory reservoirs, follow the manufacturer's instructions carefully. Since connections and attachment vary, specific instructions are not included here. **When transfilling the portable reservoir, exercise caution. The extreme cold temperatures of the fittings may result in cryogenic burns!**

Troubleshooting

When troubleshooting this equipment, please follow the suggested troubleshooting algorithm (ALG 1-4).

1. If gas fails to flow from the oxygen therapy device:
   a. Check to ensure the reservoir is full using the weight gauge or other gauge provided by the manufacturer.
   b. Check all connections for tightness. Check for leaks by feeling and by listening for escaping gas.
   c. Make certain that the humidifier is assembled correctly and that it is not obstructed. Check to ensure that all threaded connections are tight.
   d. Check oxygen tubing for kinks or obstruction.
   e. If (a) through (d) are satisfactory, contact your local vendor.

seem small, remember that one liquid liter of oxygen is equal to 861 gaseous liters. This makes the capacity in gaseous liters range from 16,400 to 35,200 liters. Physical size ranges of these reservoirs are diameters of 12–15 inches and heights of 27–38 inches and weights that vary, when full, between 84 and 160 lbs.

The smaller portable reservoirs are designed to be easily carried on the shoulder or placed into a small cart for ambulation. The liquid capacities of these portable units range from .6 liters to 1.23 liters, giving them a gaseous capacity of 500 to 1058 liters. Weights of these units when full vary from 5.3 to 9.0 lbs.

Oxygen conservation devices such as pulse demand flow regulators (described later in this chapter), when used in conjunction with the liquid reservoirs, can dramatically extend the duration of oxygen supply. These devices, when coupled with liquid supply systems and cylinders, can result in oxygen savings of 3–7 times when compared to conventional continuous oxygen flow delivery.

Portable Oxygen Duration

It may be necessary to calculate the duration of oxygen flow from these portable liquid reservoirs. These calculations are all based upon the weight of the units. All portable systems incorporate some form of spring scale to estimate the contents remaining. Many are calibrated in fourths and some use LED displays to further subdivide the contents into smaller increments. However, these scales are only estimates and do not accurately reflect the contents remaining in the reservoirs.

Sometimes it may be necessary to accurately calculate the number of liters or duration in time remaining in a portable liquid system. These calculations are also based upon weight. However, since the accuracy of spring scales varies, all calculations shown incorporate a scale factor (.80) to allow for variation in scales. It is also required that you know the empty weight of the reservoir you are working with. This can be found in the owner's manual or service manual.

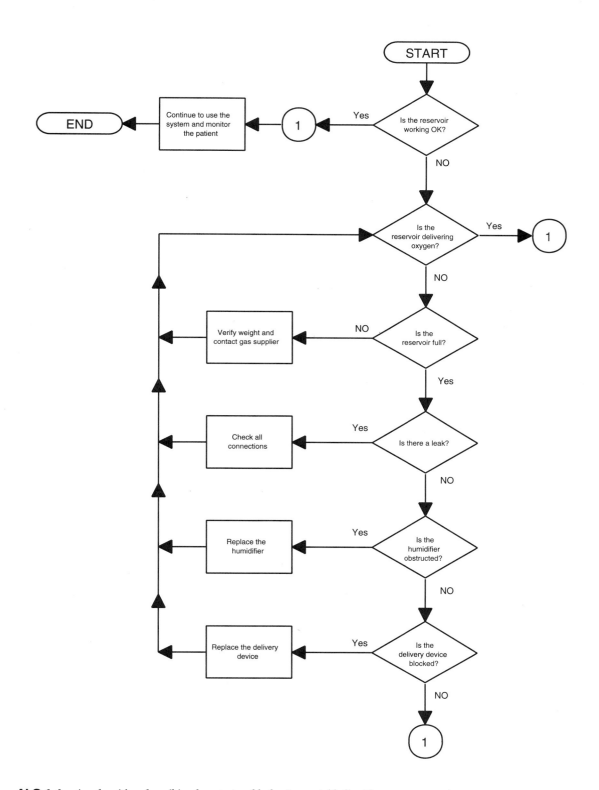

ALG 1-4 *An algorithm describing how to troubleshoot a portable liquid oxygen reservoir.*

Derivation of the formula:

(1) Density of O_2 at its boiling point = 1141 kg/m³

(2) 1141.0 kg/m³ (2.2 lb/kg) = 2510.2 lb/m³

(3) 2510.2 lbs/m³ (.001 m³/L) = 2.5102 lbs/L

(4) 1 liter (liquid) = 860.6 liters (gaseous)

$$\frac{860.6 \text{ liters (gas)}}{2.5102 \text{ lbs/L (liquid)}} = \frac{342.8 \text{ L(gas)}}{\text{lbs(liquid)}}$$

RESULT: There are 342.8 L gaseous oxygen per lb of liquid oxygen.

For example:

You are working with a patient in her home who is using a large portable reservoir at 2 L/min. She wants to know how long her reservoir will last before it needs to be re-filled. The indicator says it is 1/2 full, but she is still concerned. What is the duration of the reservoir?

Empty Weight = 60 lbs (from service manual)
Current Weight = 145 lbs
Scale Factor = .80

(145 lbs − 60 lbs [liquid]) × 342.8 L (gas)/lb (liquid) × .80 = 23,310 L (gas)

$$\frac{23,310 \text{ L (gas)}}{2 \text{ L/min}} = 11,655 \text{ minutes}$$

$$\frac{11,655 \text{ minutes}}{60 \text{ min/hr}} = 194 \text{ hours, or 8 days}$$

Notice in the calculation that the capacity in liters was multiplied by .80. This scale factor gives you a reserve or cushion of 20% to allow for accuracy variation in the spring scale used to weigh the liquid reservoir.

PIPING SYSTEMS

Piping systems provide a safe, convenient way to distribute medical gases throughout an institution. The initial cost of these systems is quite high; however, over time they may be more cost effective than cylinders, depending on the quantity of medical gases used.

CONSTRUCTION OF PIPING SYSTEMS

The National Fire Protection Association has established standards for the construction and operation of medical gas piping systems.

Supply

Oxygen may be supplied from a *manifold* of two or more cylinders, a bulk liquid reservoir or both. A manifold consists of two or more cylinders connected together using high-pressure steel or copper tubing. When two or more cylinders are interconnected, the total volume of gas available is greater than a single cylinder alone. Part C of Figure 1-20 depicts a schematic of an oxygen supply system using two cylinder manifolds. Figure 1-20 illustrates the three primary types of supply systems. The supply system is designed to meet the institution's needs, and requires periodic filling from an oxygen vendor. Liquid gas can be delivered whenever the reservoir requires filling, or on a regularly scheduled basis. It is transported to the institution by truck or by rail.

A reserve supply is required to provide up to 24 hours of oxygen in the event that the main supply becomes depleted. The reserve supply can consist of a smaller liquid reservoir or a manifold of cylinders. When pressure in the main supply drops, a valve automatically activates the reserve supply.

The pressure is reduced by means of a regulator or reducing valve before the gas enters the piping system.

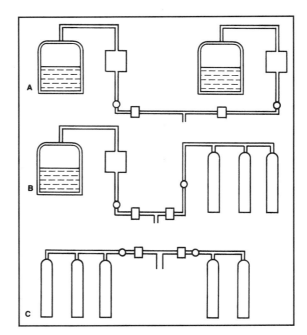

Figure 1-20 *Bulk oxygen supply systems which are typical for most medical care facilities. (A) Liquid primary and liquid reserve, (B) Liquid primary and cylinder reserve and (C) Cylinder primary and cylinder reserve.*

Piping System Construction

A piping system conducts the gas through copper pipes to points of use. This piping system is similar in design to the water system in your home or apartment; however, it must conform to stricter standards of construction. These systems are made from seamless K- or L-type copper tubing. The tubing must meet specific standards regarding its ability to withstand pressure without rupturing. All joints are sweat soldered using silver solder.

Sweat soldering is accomplished by applying heat to the joint using a torch. The solder is melted, flows into the joint, and seals it. Flux may be used to clean the joint and allow the solder to adhere to the metal better.

After soldering, joints are carefully checked for leaks. The pipes are independently supported to the building structure at specified intervals. This means that nothing else may be attached to the building's structure at the same point where the medical gas piping system is attached. Following construction, the system is cleaned of any flux or debris and pressure tested. The system is pressurized to 1.5 times its working pressure with dry, oil-free air or with nitrogen. Each joint is then checked for leaks. The system is allowed to stand for 24 hours at this pressure and must remain leak free during this time in order to pass final inspection.

Following the pressure test, both the oxygen and air supply lines are charged with gas. The oxygen piping system is supplied by a bulk oxygen system, while a medical air compressor supplies gas for the air piping system. The outlets are then tested for purity. Oxygen and air lines are checked with analyzers to ensure that they are delivering the correct gas. Once the purity test has been completed, the system may be used for patient care.

Safety Features

Safety features in a medical gas piping system include alarms, zone valves, riser valves and pressure sensors.

Alarms are included in a piping system. These alert personnel to pressure drops in the system caused by leaks or depletion of the gas supply. The alarm must be placed in an area that is attended 24 hours a day. For this reason, the hospital telephone switchboard is a common location for medical gas alarm panels.

Zone valves are shutoff valves placed at strategic positions so that gas supply to different areas may be cut off in the event of a fire. Zone valves also are placed at the base of risers (pipes conducting gas from one floor to another), as shown in Figure 1-21. In some acute care facilities, Respiratory Care Practitioners (RCPs), are required to identify and turn off the appropriate zone valves in the event of a fire. If a zone valve is turned off, the RCP is also responsible to ensure that patients requiring oxygen receive it from cylinders or another source during transport from the scene of a fire and also when returning the patients to their rooms.

Pressure sensors are placed throughout the piping system to monitor pressure. Line pressure in most hospital systems is 50 psi.

Station Outlets

Medical gas outlets, located at the points of desired use, are termed station outlets. Special fittings are incorporated into these outlets, preventing the connection of equipment designed for a different gas. Examples of these fittings include Diameter Indexed Safety Fittings and quick-connect fittings.

The Diameter Indexed Safety System (DISS) was designed by the Compressed Gas Association. This system utilizes differing thread pitch, connection diameter, and internal and external threading to prevent the attachment of equipment designed for dissimilar gases or gas mixtures (Figure 1-22). It is designed for pressures less than 200 psi, which by definition is termed low pressure. Check valves, incorporated into station outlets, prevent gas loss when not in use.

Quick-connect fittings vary from one manufacturer to another. These fittings are designed to be rapidly connected or disconnected without the use of threads. Figure 1-23 shows an example of one manufacturer's quick-connect outlet.

CYLINDERS

Oxygen cylinders provide a convenient method of providing oxygen delivery to a patient. The smaller cylinder sizes are portable, facilitating their use in an emergency, ambulatory, or transport setting. Oxygen cylinders are safe and effective when handled correctly.

Cylinder Construction

The construction of oxygen cylinders is strictly regulated by the Department of Transportation (DOT). Medical gas cylinders are seamless, either made from high strength chrome molybdenum steel or a high strength

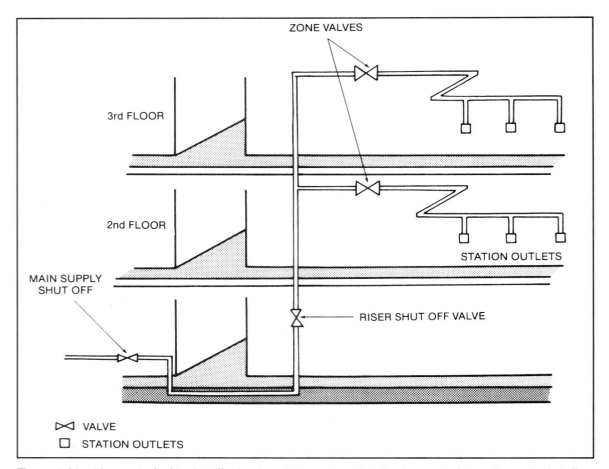

Figure 1-21 *Placement of safety shutoff valves in a piping system. Note the placement of the main supply shutoff, riser valves and zone valves.*

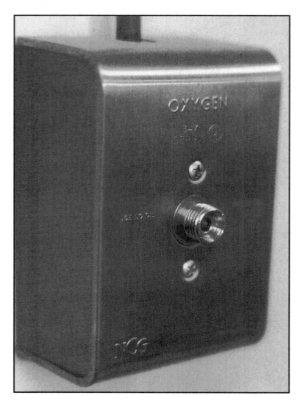

Figure 1-22 *A DISS oxygen fitting.*

aluminum alloy. Steel cylinders are spun into shape while the steel is still hot. Following shaping, the steel is heat treated to retain its tensile strength. Recently, the aluminum alloy cylinders have gained popularity due to their lighter weight. High strength steel cylinders are stamped with the marking "DOT 3AA." "DOT" refers to the Department of Transportation and "3AA" indicates heat treated high strength steel. The designation "3AL" denotes aluminum construction. Typically, cylinders are filled to a pressure 10% greater than the working pressure indicated on its shoulder, providing the cylinder has passed the required hydrostatic testing.

Cylinder Markings

The DOT requires that cylinder data be stamped on the shoulder of the cylinder (Figures 1-24 and 1-25).

Hydrostatic Testing

Every five years a cylinder is subjected to a hydrostatic test to measure its elasticity. The cylinder is filled to a pressure equal to 5/3 its

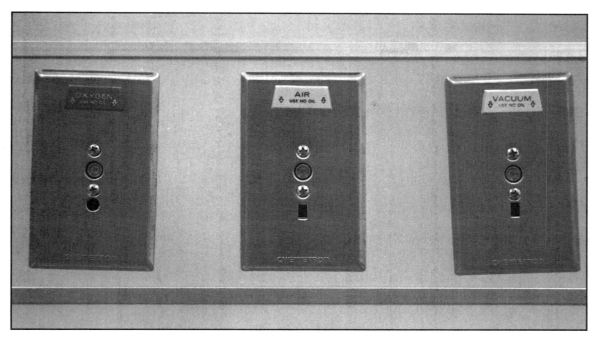

Figure 1-23 *Three quick-connect fittings. Left to right are oxygen, air and vacuum.*

working pressure and cylinder expansion is measured. If the expansion is within tolerance, the cylinder is returned to service. If the cylinder fails the test, it is removed from service and destroyed. The inspector's mark and the date of the test, followed by a "+" sign (steel cylinders only), are then stamped into the shoulder of the cylinder. If a star follows the inspection date, the cylinder may go for ten years before another hydrostatic test is performed (steel cylinders only).

Cylinder Sizes

Medical gas cylinders are manufactured in many sizes (Figure 1-26, p. 34). The most common sizes encountered in the hospital environment are the "H" and the "E" cylinders. The "H" cylinder contains 244 cubic feet of oxygen and weighs approximately 135 pounds. The "E" cylinder contains 22 cubic feet of oxygen and weighs approximately 16 pounds. Since the "E" cylinder is smaller and lighter, it is

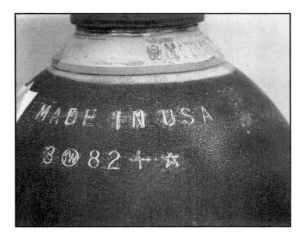

Figure 1-24 *Cylinder markings indicate the cylinder has passed inspection. The inspection was performed in March 1982. The inspector's mark is between the month and year. The "+" sign indicates the cylinder complies with the hydrostatic test. The star marking indicates the cylinder may go ten years before being tested again.*

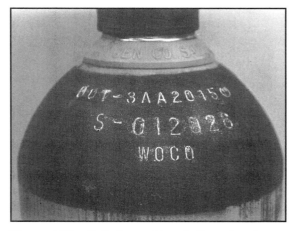

Figure 1-25 *Cylinder markings indicate that the cylinder is made from high tensile strength heat-treated steel (DOT 3AA) and has a service pressure of 2015 psi (2015). The serial number is below the DOT numbers and the owner's stamp is below the serial number.*

ASSEMBLY AND TROUBLESHOOTING

Assembly—Oxygen Cylinders

To prepare a cylinder for use, complete the following instructions.

1. Transport the cylinder to the point of use using a cylinder cart. Be sure that the protective valve cap is in place when transporting the cylinder.

2. Position the cylinder upright and attach it using chains provided at the point of use, or use a cylinder stand to prevent it from tipping over.

3. Remove the protective cap ("H" cylinder). The smaller "E" cylinders have a piece of shrink-wrap plastic tape protecting the cylinder valve and outlet. Remove the protective tape prior to attaching a regulator or reducing valve.

4. Announce to personnel or patients in the area that a loud noise will occur.

5. Position the cylinder such that the cylinder valve opening is pointing away from any people in the room. "Crack" the cylinder by quickly opening and closing the valve to eliminate debris from the cylinder valve opening.

6. Attach an appropriate regulator to the cylinder and attach the oxygen therapy equipment to the regulator.

7. Slowly turn on the cylinder valve.

8. Read the pressure gauge and determine if the contents of the cylinder are adequate for the duration of therapy.

Troubleshooting

Troubleshooting a cylinder is quite simple since this oxygen supply system has so few moving parts. The following is a suggested troubleshooting algorithm (ALG 1-5).

1. Check for leaks at the connection between the cylinder and regulator. If leaks are present, tighten the connection.

a. A leak can be detected by a hissing sound. The amplitude or volume of the sound indicates the severity of the leak.

b. Subtle leaks may be detected by feeling for gas flow with your hands around the connections.

c. If you suspect a leak but can't detect it:
   [1.] Use a solution of mild detergent and water and brush the solution around the fittings. Leaks will cause bubbles to form, indicating their presence.

d. If a leak is detected, turn off the cylinder valve bleeding all pressure from the regulator and retighten all connections.

2. Check for leaks between the regulator and the oxygen therapy equipment and tighten as appropriate.

a. A leak can be detected by a hissing sound. The amplitude or volume of the sound indicates the severity of the leak.

b. Subtle leaks may be detected by feeling for gas flow with your hands around the connections.

c. If you suspect a leak but can't detect it:
   [1.] Use a solution of mild detergent and water and brush the solution around the fittings. Leaks will cause bubbles to form, indicating their presence.

d. If a leak is detected, turn off the cylinder valve bleeding all pressure from the regulator and retighten all connections.

3. If gas fails to flow from the cylinder, check the pressure gauge to ensure that the cylinder has pressure.

a. If the cylinder contains pressure, check the regulator outlet for obstructions.

b. If the above is satisfied, replace the regulator with another and try again.

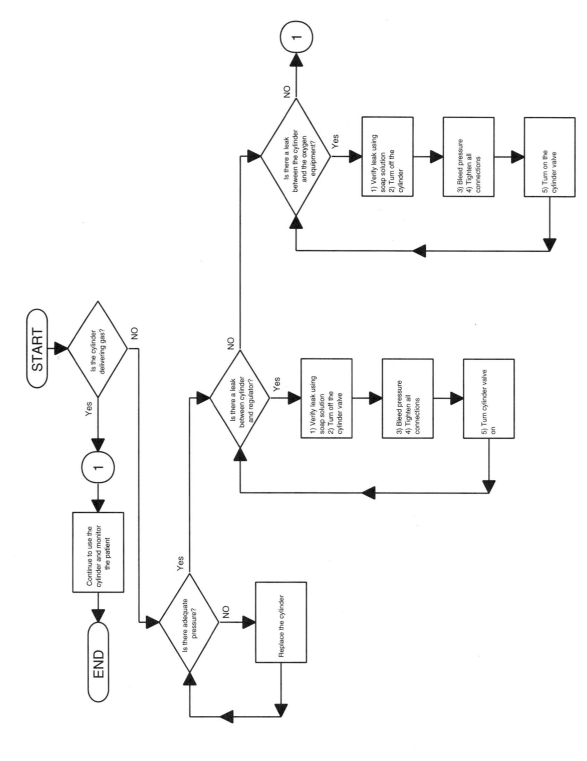

ALG 1-5 *An algorithm describing how to troubleshoot medical gas cylinders.*

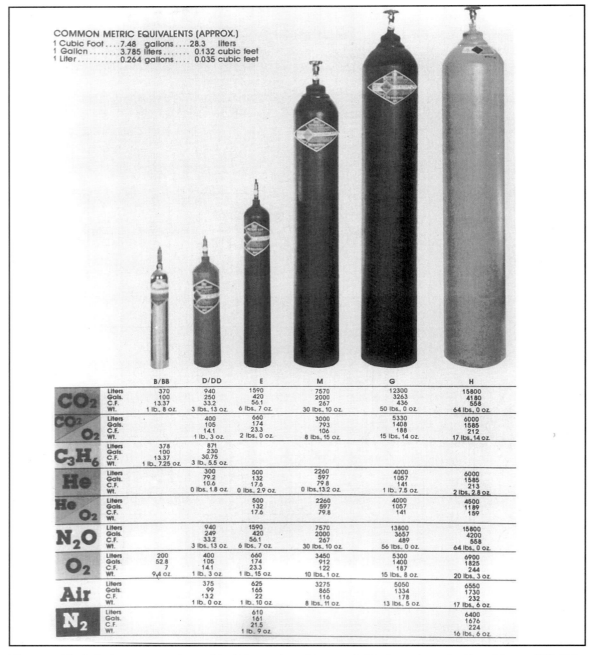

Figure 1-26 *Cylinders are manufactured in different sizes. (Courtesy BOC Gases, formerly Airco, Murray Hill, NJ)*

usually used for ambulation of patients (with a cart) and for transporting patients from one place to another within the hospital.

Color Coding

The Compressed Gas Association has developed a color code for the different medical gases and gas mixtures. This code was published by the Department of Commerce through the recommendation of the Bureau of Standards. An international color code also exists for medical gases. The only difference between the two color codes is the color for cylinders containing oxygen (see Table 1-3).

The international color is white, while the United States still uses green. In addition to the color code, each cylinder is required to have a label indicating the cylinder's contents.

TABLE 1-3 Cylinder Color Coding

GAS	COLOR CODE	
	UNITED STATES	INTERNATIONAL
Oxygen	Green	White
Carbon dioxide	Gray	Gray
Nitrous oxide	Light blue	Light blue
Cyclopropane	Orange	Orange
Helium	Brown	Brown
Carbon dioxide and oxygen	Gray and green	Gray and white
Helium and oxygen	Brown and green	Brown and white
Air	Yellow	White and black

Labeling of cylinder contents is required by the United States Pharmacopeia (USP), a division of the Food and Drug Administration (FDA). The USP controls the purity standards of compressed gases for medical use.

If the label and the color code do not match, the cylinder should not be used and should be returned to the vendor. The most reliable indicator of what is contained in the cylinder is the label.

SAFETY RULES FOR CYLINDER USE

Common sense and the practice of certain safety precautions will ensure safety for both you and your patient. Remember at all times that a medical gas cylinder contains gas pressurized up to 2200 psi. If the cylinder or cylinder valve were to rupture, disastrous consequences could result. Rules and precautions, recommended by the Compressed Gas Association and published in their pamphlet "Characteristics and Safe Handling of Medical Gases, 1971," are summarized in Table 1-4.

DURATION OF GAS FLOW

In order to calculate how long a cylinder will last at a given liter flow, it is important to remember four key facts. (1) When full, an "H" cylinder contains 244 cubic feet of oxygen. (2) When full, an "E" cylinder contains 22 cubic feet of oxygen. (3) Full cylinders contain 2200 psi pressure. (4) One cubic foot of oxygen equals 28.3 liters. Once these facts

have been committed to memory, the duration of any "H" or "E" cylinder may be calculated.

Tank Factors

It is common practice to use tank factors in the calculation of cylinder duration. By knowing the four key facts listed above, these factors may be derived. Table 1-5 illustrates how these factors are derived.

Once these factors have been derived, it is easy to convert from gauge pressure (psi) directly to liters. To accomplish this, multiply the gauge pressure by the tank factor for that cylinder. For example:

You are asked to help move a patient from the Emergency Room to the Intensive Care Unit, which usually takes about twenty minutes. You are manually ventilating the patient using a resuscitation bag at a liter flow of 15 liters per minute. Will the department's "E" cylinder containing 1000 psi have enough gas for the transport?

Step 1:
"E" tank factor

$$= \frac{22 \text{ cu. ft.} \times 28.3 \text{ liters/cu. ft.}}{2200 \text{ psi}}$$

$$= .28 \text{ liters/psi}$$

Step 2:
Content of cylinder

$$= \text{tank factor} \times \text{gauge pressure}$$

$$= .28 \text{ liters/psi} \times 1000 \text{ psi}$$

$$= 280 \text{ liters}$$

TABLE 1-4 Safety Rules for Cylinder Use

Moving Cylinders
1. Always leave protective valve caps in place when moving a cylinder.
2. Do not lift a cylinder by its cap.
3. Do not drop a cylinder, strike two cylinders against one another, or strike other surfaces.
4. Do not drag or slide cylinders; use a cart.
5. Use a cart whenever loading or unloading cylinders.

Storing Cylinders
1. Comply with local and state regulations for cylinder storage as well as with those established by the National Fire Protection Association.
2. Post the names of gases stored.
3. Keep full and empty cylinders separate. Place the full cylinders in a convenient spot to minimize handling of cylinders.
4. Keep storage areas dry, cool, and well ventilated. Storage rooms should be fire-resistant.
5. Do not store cylinders close to flammable substances such as gasoline, grease, or petroleum products.
6. Protect the cylinders from being damaged by cuts or abrasions. Do not store them in areas where they may be damaged by moving or falling objects. Keep cylinder valve caps on at all times.
7. Cylinders may be stored in the open; however, keep them on a platform so they are above the ground. In some parts of the country, shading may be required due to high temperatures. If ice and snow accumulate, thaw at room temperature or use water cooler than 125° F.
8. Protect cylinders from potential tampering by untrained, unauthorized individuals.

Withdrawing Cylinder Contents
1. Allow cylinders to be handled by experienced, trained individuals only.
2. The user of the cylinder is responsible for verifying the cylinder contents before use. If the contents are in doubt, do not use the cylinder. Return it to the supplier.
3. Leave the protective valve cap in place until you are ready to attach a regulator or other equipment.
4. Follow safety precautions. Make sure the cylinder is well supported and protected from falling over.
5. Always crack the cylinder valve prior to attaching a regulator or reducing valve. (Refer to previous "Assembly and Troubleshooting" section.)
6. Use appropriate reducing valves or regulators when attaching equipment designed for lower operating pressures than those contained in the cylinder.
7. Do not force any threaded connections. Verify that the threads you are using are designed for the same gas or gas mixture in accordance with the American Standard Safety System.
8. Connect a cylinder to a manifold designed for high pressure cylinders only.
9. Use equipment only with cylinders containing the gases for which the equipment was designed.
10. Open cylinder valves slowly. Never use a wrench or hammer to force a cylinder valve open. Treat cylinders and cylinder valves with care.
11. Do not use compressed gases to dust off yourself or your clothing.
12. Keep all connections tight to prevent leakage.
13. Before removing a regulator, turn off the valve and bleed the pressure.
14. Never use a flame to detect leaks with flammable gases.
15. Do not store flammable gases with oxygen. Keep all flammable anesthetic gases stored in a separate area.

Reprinted by permission from Gary C. White, Basic Clinical Lab Competencies for Respiratory Care, 3rd Edition, Delmar Publishers, Inc., 1998.

TABLE 1-5 Tank Factor Calculation

$$\text{Tank Factor} = \frac{\text{Size (cu. ft.)} \times 28.3 \text{ liters/cu. ft.}}{\text{Pressure when full}}$$

$$\text{"H" cylinder} = \frac{244 \text{ cu. ft.} \times 28.3 \text{ liters/cu. ft.}}{2200 \text{ psi}}$$

$$= 3.14 \text{ liters/psi}$$

$$\text{"E" cylinder} = \frac{22 \text{ cu. ft.} \times 28.3 \text{ liters/cu. ft.}}{2200 \text{ psi}}$$

$$= .28 \text{ liters/psi}$$

Step 3:

$$\text{Duration in minutes} = \frac{\text{cylinder contents}}{\text{liter flow}}$$

$$= \frac{280 \text{ liters}}{15 \text{ liters/minute}}$$

$$= 18 \text{ minutes}$$

Answer: No, the cylinder will not last!

Note: It is common to arrive at an answer of hours expressed as a decimal form—for example, 6.3 hours. Each tenth of an hour is 6 minutes, so 6.3 hours equals 6 hours and 18 minutes.

It is common clinical practice to leave 500 psi remaining in the cylinder prior to changing it, providing that a maximum duration is not desired (airborne or ground transport). By leaving 500 psi in the cylinder, water, other gases and foreign material can not enter the cylinder, helping to extend its useful life.

To calculate the cylinder duration, leaving 500 psi in a cylinder, follow the example outlined below.

You are asked to set a patient up on an oxygen mask at 12 L/min in the x-ray department. The facility is in an older part of the institution and does not have piped oxygen. You move an "H" cylinder to the area to supply oxygen for your patient. The cylinder gauge reads 1250 psi. How long will the cylinder last if you leave 500 psi remaining in the cylinder?

Step 1:
"H" tank factor

$$= \frac{244 \text{ cu. ft.} \times 28.3 \text{ liters/cu. ft.}}{2200 \text{ psi}}$$

$$= 3.14 \text{ L/psi}$$

Step 2:
Content of cylinder

$$= \text{tank factor} \times (\text{gauge pressure} - 500 \text{ psi})$$

$$= .28 \text{ L/psi} (1250 \text{ psi} - 500 \text{ psi})$$

$$= 2355 \text{ L}$$

Step 3:

$$\text{Duration in minutes} = \frac{\text{cylinder contents}}{\text{liter flow}}$$

$$= \frac{2355 \text{ L}}{12 \text{ L/min}}$$

$$= 196 \text{ minutes}$$

$$= 3 \text{ hours } 12 \text{ minutes}$$

This type of problem and others like it are very common in clinical practice. Your patient's safety may depend on your ability to remember how to perform these simple calculations.

OXYGEN REGULATION DEVICES

Cylinders that contain highly pressurized gas would be dangerous to use without specialized equipment to regulate gas flow and allow safe attachment of other equipment. It is important to understand the operation of cylinder valves and reducing valves to safely use cylinders.

Direct Acting Cylinder Valve

As its name implies, the *direct acting cylinder valve* operates by opening and closing the valve seat directly. As the valve stem or wheel is turned, the valve plunger moves up or down, acting directly on the valve seat. As the valve seat is opened, gas moves from the area of high pressure (within the cylinder) to the area of lower pressure (out of the cylinder). Figure 1-27 shows the component parts of the cylinder valve. The valve plunger is threaded, so as the stem is turned, it opens or closes. The direct acting cylinder valve is a type of needle valve.

Diaphragm Cylinder Valve

In this type of cylinder valve, a diaphragm opens or closes the valve seat. As the valve stem is turned, the threaded plunger moves up or down, allowing the diaphragm to open or close the valve seat. Gas pressure then displaces the diaphragm, allowing gas to flow out of the cylinder. These valves are usually employed with cylinders having a lower working pressure of 1500 psi or less (Figure 1-28).

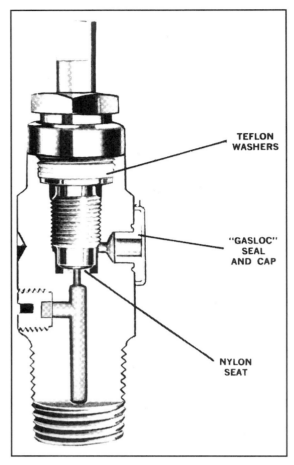

Figure 1-27 *A full section of a direct acting cylinder valve. (Courtesy BOC Gases, formerly Airco, Murray Hill, NJ)*

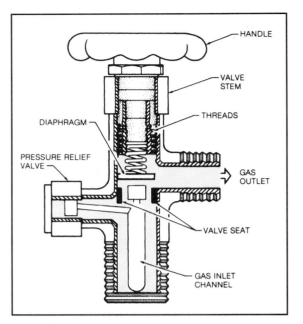

Figure 1-28 *A functional diagram of an indirect acting cylinder valve.*

Cylinder Valve Safety Features

Several safety features are incorporated into cylinder valves.

Since cylinders contain many different gases, the Compressed Gas Association has designed a system to prevent the interchange of dissimilar gases. In other words, the safety system is designed to prevent the attachment of an oxygen regulator to a nitrous oxide medical gas cylinder. The two types of valve outlet safety systems are the American Standard and the Pin Index Safety System (PISS).

The American Standard Safety System (ASSS) is incorporated into the valves for the larger cylinders (sizes "M", "G", "H"). This system uses differing thread pitches, internal left- and right-hand threads, and external threading to prevent the attachment of equipment not designed for the gas contained in the cylinder. Figure 1-29 shows acetylene and oxygen American Standard fittings. Note how one

is internally threaded and the other is externally threaded.

The smaller cylinder valves (sizes "AA"–"E") use a yoke type connection between the cylinder valve and the reducing valve. The Pin Index Safety System incorporates pins in the reducing valve yoke and holes on the cylinder valve at specified positions to prevent the attachment of equipment not designed for the gas contained in the cylinder. Figure 1-30 illustrates how this safety system works using the different pin positions.

In addition to the indexing safety systems, pressure release devices are built into the cylinder valves. These pressure relief devices will open if pressure or temperature rises beyond safe limits. The two types of pressure relief devices are the frangible disk and the fusible plug. These devices may be used singly or in combination with one another.

The frangible disk pressure relief consists of a thin metal disk that contains the pressure within the valve. If the pressure within the cylinder rises abnormally, the disk will burst or fracture, releasing pressure before the cylinder walls rupture.

The fusible plug pressure relief is made from an alloy that will melt when the ambient temperature exceeds 208–220° Fahrenheit. When the plug melts or distorts, pressure will be released, preventing rupture of the cylinder.

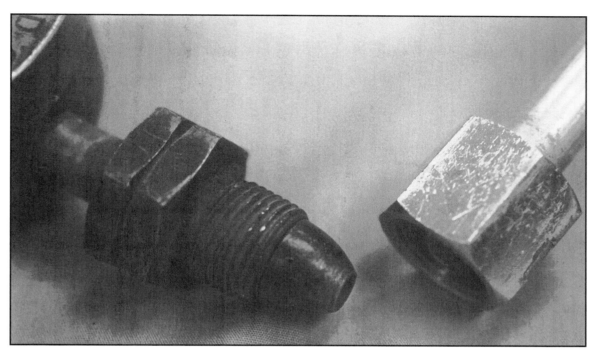

Figure 1-29 *Differing threads and pitches for cylinder valve connections. Note the threads on the left are external (acetylene), and the threads on the right are internal (oxygen).*

REDUCING VALVES

Single Stage Reducing Valve

A single stage reducing valve reduces the pressure from the cylinder to a working pressure in one step or stage. All reducing valves operate by using two opposing forces, spring tension and gas pressure separated by a flexible diaphragm. Figure 1-31 illustrates the component parts of a single-stage reducing valve and its operation. Gas pressure in the cylinder displaces the diaphragm upward. When gas pressure and spring tension are equal, the diaphragm is flat, closing the poppet valve. As the pressure within the chamber drops, spring tension forces the diaphragm down, opening the poppet valve. This cycle repeats itself with the diaphragm oscillating back and forth, opening and closing the poppet valve. Spring tension determines the outlet pressure from the reducing valve. The tension may be fixed or adjustable depending on the reducing valve's

OXYGEN	2-5
AIR	1-5
He/O_2 (80% and under)	2-4
CO_2/O_2 (7% or under)	2-6
NITROUS OXIDE	3-5

Figure 1-30 *Pin index positions for medical gases.*

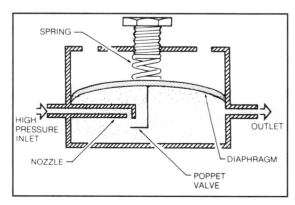

Figure 1-31 *Functional diagram of a single stage reducing valve.*

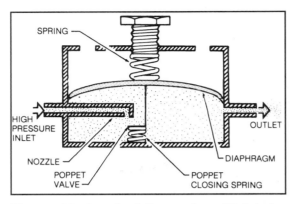

Figure 1-32 *Functional diagram of a modified single stage reducing valve. Note the addition of a poppet closing spring.*

construction. If the tension is adjustable, there is usually a screw provided that will allow adjustment of the tension against the diaphragm.

Modified Single Stage Reducing Valve

The modified single stage reducing valve is similar to the single stage reducing valve. The difference between the two is that the modified single stage reducing valve has a poppet closing spring in addition to the spring above the diaphragm. Figure 1-32 illustrates the component parts of this reducing valve. The poppet closing spring allows the poppet valve to open and close faster, providing greater flow rates.

Multistage Reducing Valves

Multistage reducing valves are simply two or more single stage reducing valves in series

with one another. Figure 1-33 shows the component parts of this reducing valve. The first stage reduces the cylinder to an intermediate pressure of approximately 200 psi. The second stage then reduces the pressure to the desired working pressure, usually 50 psi. Each stage operates independently from the other.

The addition of the additional stage allows more precise regulation of pressure and a greater flow rate than is possible with a single stage reducing valve. Common applications of multistage reducing valves include powering of mechanical ventilators. These applications require high flows and a stable pressure source.

Reducing Valve Safety Features

Several safety features are incorporated into the design of reducing valves. These include pressure relief valves, or pop-off valves, and indexing of the inlet and outlet.

Each stage of a reducing valve is required to have a safety relief valve in the event that excess pressure develops within the stage. The safety relief will exhaust excessive pressure before the reducing valve housing bursts.

The inlet of the reducing valve is indexed with either American Standard indexing or the Pin Index Safety System indexing. Both of these systems were developed by the Compressed Gas Association and discussed earlier in this chapter.

The outlet of the reducing valve uses Diameter Indexed Safety System threads. This safety system was also discussed earlier in this chapter.

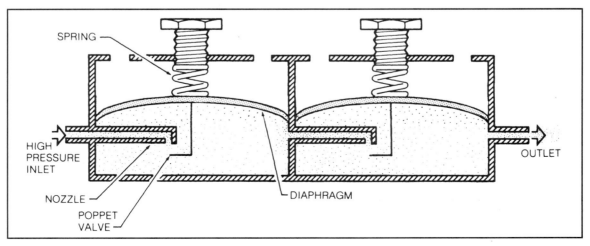

Figure 1-33 *Functional diagram of a two stage reducing valve. Note how two single stage regulators are connected in series to form a two stage regulator.*

ASSEMBLY AND TROUBLESHOOTING

Assembly—Oxygen Reducing Valves

Follow the suggested guidelines when assembling a reducing valve for use.

1. Select a reducing valve appropriate for the intended use. If high flow rates are desired (80-120 liters/min.), use a two stage or modified single stage reducing valve.

2. Remove the protective valve cap ("H" cylinder) or protective tape ("E" cylinder) and "crack" the tank by opening and closing the valve quickly to expel any foreign material. Perform this task with the valve pointing away from yourself and other people.

3. Attach the reducing valve to an appropriate cylinder valve (American Standard fitting or Pin Index fitting).

4. Attach the oxygen equipment to the reducing valve.

5. Turn on the cylinder valve.

Troubleshooting

Troubleshooting a cylinder and reducing valve primarily involves checking for leaks. The following is a suggested troubleshooting algorithm (ALG 1-6).

1. Check for leaks at the connection to the cylinder. If leaks are present, tighten the connection.

2. Check for leaks between the reducing valve and the oxygen therapy equipment and tighten as appropriate.

3. If gas fails to flow from the cylinder, check the pressure gauge to ensure that the cylinder has pressure.
   a. If the cylinder contains pressure, check the reducing valve outlet for obstructions.
   b. If the above is satisfied, replace the reducing valve with another and try again.

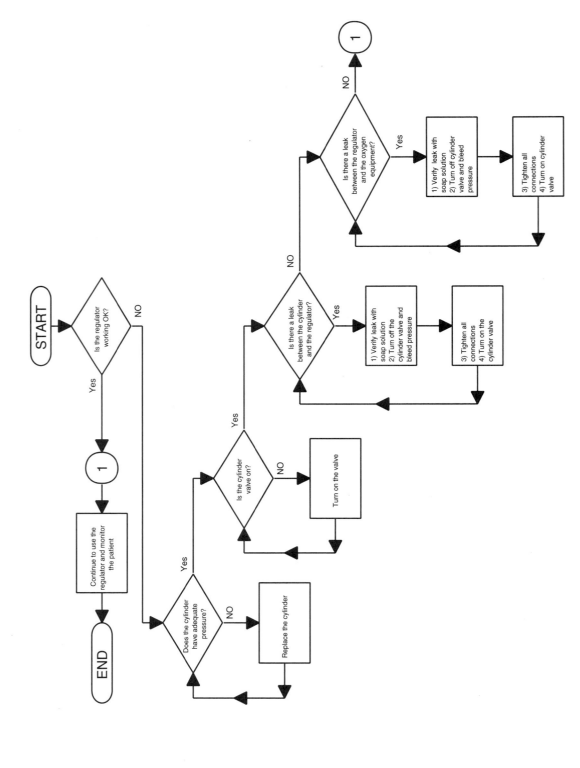

ALG 1-6 *An algorithm describing how to troubleshoot medical gas regulators and reducing valves.*

REGULATORS

When a flowmeter and a reducing valve are joined together into a common unit, it is termed a *regulator*. Regulators are more convenient than separate reducing valves and flowmeters. Only one high pressure connection is required (between the cylinder and the regulator) and they are more compact in size. A regulator consists of a reducing valve with a Bourdon-type flowmeter, or a reducing valve with a Thorpe tube flowmeter. Both of these flowmeters are discussed later in this chapter.

PROPORTIONERS (AIR-OXYGEN BLENDERS)

Blenders are devices that mix air and oxygen to precise concentrations. These devices provide a stable 50 psi source of mixed gas. Common applications of blenders include, but are not limited to, powering ventilators, Continuous Positive Airway Pressure (CPAP) systems, and controlled oxygen therapy. Blenders are very compact and convenient to use, requiring a 50 psi source of oxygen and air.

Principle of Operation

Air and oxygen entering the blender are first directed into two chambers on opposite sides of a diaphragm that balances the air and oxygen pressures (regulator section). If the incoming pressures are unequal, the regulator portion of the blender balances the pressures so that they are equal (Figure 1-34). It is important that the pressures are equal, because if one gas entered the proportioning valve at a greater pressure, more of that gas would be delivered, altering the percentage from what is desired.

Gas exiting from the regulator section then passes through a proportioning valve. The oxygen percentage control adjusts the proportions of air and oxygen. If 80% oxygen is desired, turning the control opens the oxygen side more while proportionally closing the air side.

Most manufacturers incorporate a built-in alarm system into the blender. If gas pressure from the supply lines (air or oxygen) drops within the regulation section, an audible alarm will sound.

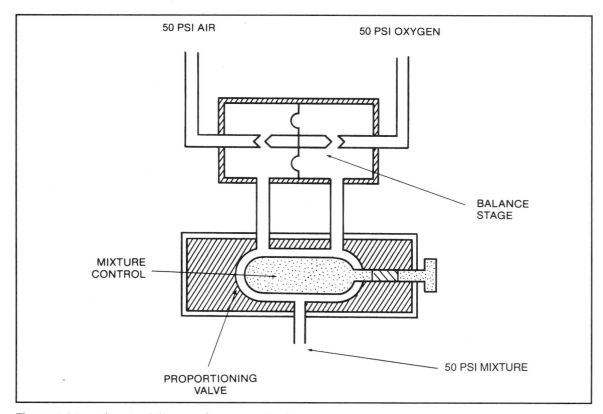

Figure 1-34 *A functional diagram of an oxygen blender.*

ASSEMBLY AND TROUBLESHOOTING

Assembly—Oxygen Blenders

To prepare a blender for use, follow the instructions listed below.

1. Ensure a supply of compressed oxygen and air at 50 psi. The supply devices may include an oxygen piping system or cylinders with appropriate regulators.

2. Connect a 50 psi hose to the air supply and to the air inlet fitting on the blender.

3. Connect a 50 psi hose to the oxygen supply and to the oxygen inlet on the blender.

4. Read the pressure gauges on the blender to verify line pressure (if provided).

5. Check the pressure alarm by disconnecting the air or oxygen source.

6. Adjust the blender to the desired F_iO_2 (fraction of inspired oxygen).

7. Attach the oxygen therapy device or other medical equipment to the outlet of the blender.
    a. If the outlet does not have a one-way check valve, attach the equipment to the blender before attaching the oxygen and air supply lines.

8. Verify oxygen concentration with an oxygen analyzer.

Troubleshooting

Troubleshooting a blender consists of checking for leaks and verifying oxygen concentration. The following is a suggested algorithm (ALG 1-7).

1. Sources of leaks:
    a. Between the gas source (piping system or regulator) and the high pressure hoses.
    b. Between the high pressure hoses and the blender.
    c. Between the blender and the oxygen equipment.

2. Verify the oxygen concentration using an oxygen analyzer. If there is a tremendous discrepancy (greater than ± 2%), calibrate the analyzer and repeat verification. If the discrepancy still exists, replace the blender and have the defective unit repaired by your local vendor or authorized biomedical repair facility.

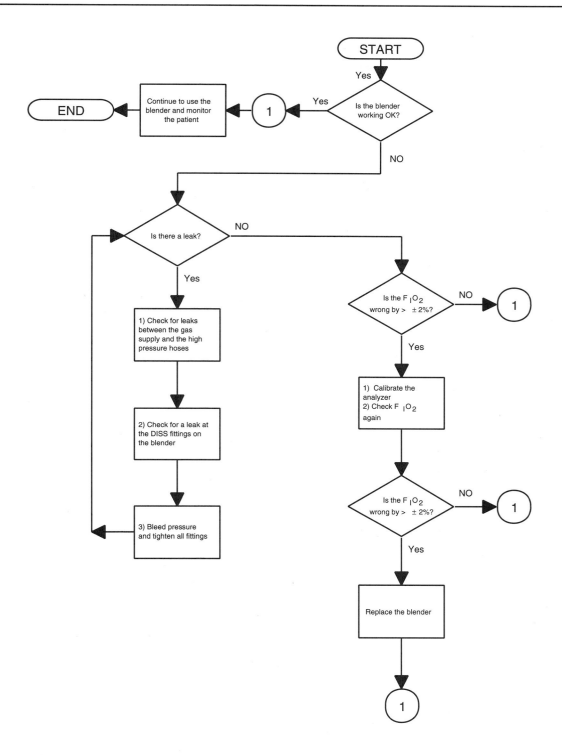

ALG 1-7 *An algorithm describing how to troubleshoot an oxygen blender.*

OXYGEN FLOWMETERS

Bourdon Gauge (Fixed Orifice Flowmeter)

A *Bourdon gauge flowmeter* consists of a Bourdon gauge and an adjustable reducing valve (Figure 1-35). Gas flows through the adjustable reducing valve, past the Bourdon gauge, and then passes through a fixed orifice distal to the Bourdon gauge. The adjustable reducing valve can vary the pressure between the reducing valve outlet and the fixed orifice. As pressure increases, flow out of the device also increases. The increase in pressure between the reducing valve outlet and the fixed orifice causes the coiled tube in the Bourdon gauge to straighten. The gauge, however, is recalibrated to indicate flow rather than pressure as the coiled tube straightens (employing Poiseuille's law).

This flowmeter is accurate as long as the outlet is at ambient pressure. Any increase in pressure distal to the fixed orifice will cause this flowmeter to read inaccurately. This can be caused by obstructions to flow or attachment of equipment that causes back pressure to develop. It is possible to obstruct the outlet

and the Bourdon gauge will indicate a flow higher than is being delivered.

The Bourdon gauge flowmeter is lightweight and very compact. Another advantage of this device is that it will operate in any position. The flowmeter will operate in unusual positions because none of the moving parts is gravity dependent. Therefore, it is popular in emergency and transport settings (ambulance, intra-hospital transport, airborne transport).

Any oxygen connecting tubing, or tubing to oxygen administration devices, must be carefully checked for kinks or obstructions. In a noisy, bumpy environment (ambulance or airborne transport), physically touch and follow the tubing with your hands to verify that the tubing has not been obstructed. Stretchers, equipment or other care providers' feet placed on the tubing could obstruct oxygen flow. You can't tell by monitoring the gauge if oxygen is flowing or not!

Uncompensated Thorpe Tube Flowmeter

The components of an uncompensated *Thorpe tube flowmeter* include a "V"-shaped ta-

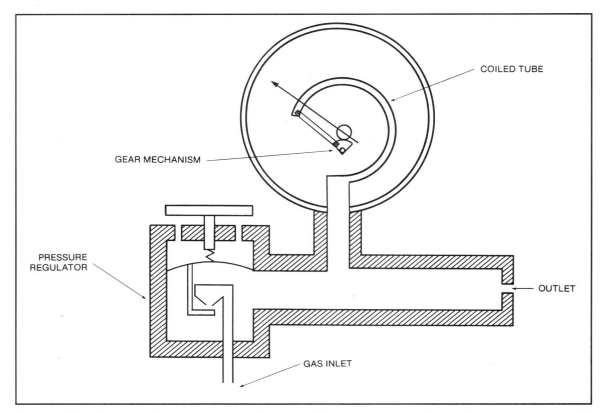

Figure 1-35 *A functional diagram of a Bourdon flowmeter. This is also known as a fixed orifice flowmeter.*

pered tube (Thorpe tube), a float, and a needle valve (Figure 1-36). Note how the needle valve is positioned proximal to the Thorpe tube.

The Thorpe tube becomes a variable orifice. The Thorpe tube gradually increases in diameter from its base to the top of the tube. The flowmeter is calibrated with the pressure inside of the tube equal to ambient pressure.

The float provides a means of indicating the flow rate. As the needle valve is opened, gas pressure pushes the ball up in the Thorpe tube, overcoming gravity. At equilibrium, gas pressure equals gravitational attraction and the float is stable. As the float moves up in the Thorpe tube, the tube becomes larger and more and more gas flows around it.

The needle valve provides a means of adjusting gas flow into the Thorpe tube. As the needle valve is progressively opened, more gas flows into the tube.

The term "uncompensated Thorpe tube flowmeter" refers to the fact that it is uncompensated for back pressure. If pressure is applied distally to the Thorpe tube, for example from a kinked connecting tube or other obstruction, the Thorpe tube becomes pressurized. As the pressure in the Thorpe tube increases, the pressure gradient between the bottom and the top of the float decreases, causing the float to fall. The flow indication may actually be lower than the delivered flow.

Compensated Thorpe Tube Flowmeter

A compensated Thorpe tube flowmeter is similar in design to an uncompensated one with one exception. A compensated Thorpe tube's needle valve is distal to the Thorpe tube (Figure 1-37). Since the needle valve is placed distal to the Thorpe tube, pressure within the tube is equal to line pressure or 50 psi when connected to a gas source.

Back pressure applied distally to the needle valve has no effect on its performance. Additional pressure or restriction causes the flowmeter to behave as if the needle valve is closed further, restricting flow. If enough pressure is applied to stop the flow, eventually the pressure proximal and distal to the needle valve will equal 50 psi, the float will no longer be suspended, and gas flow will cease.

When working with Thorpe tube flowmeters, it is often necessary to know if it is compensated or uncompensated. There are three ways to identify a compensated flowmeter: (1) The label will state, "Calibrated at 760 mmHg, 70° F, 50 psig inlet and outlet pressure." (2) With the needle valve closed, the float will rapidly jump up the Thorpe tube when the flowmeter is connected to an oxygen source. (3) Check the position of the needle valve; if it is downstream from the Thorpe tube, it is compensated.

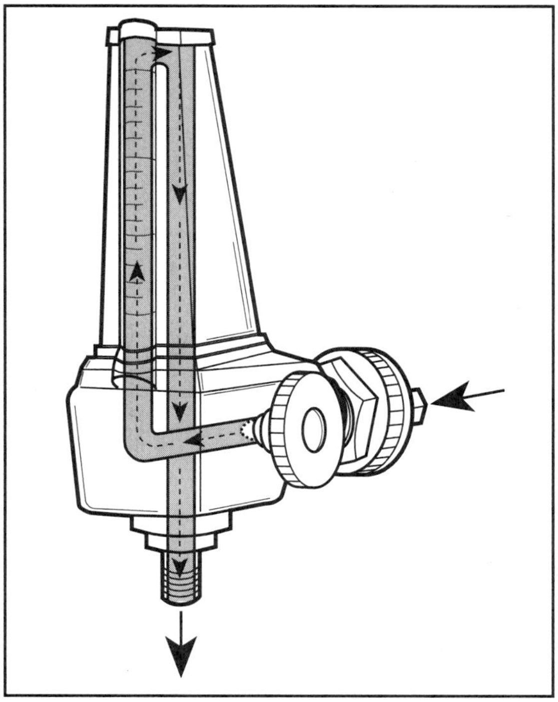

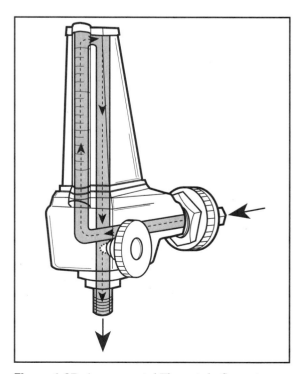

Figure 1-36 *An uncompensated Thorpe tube flowmeter.*

Figure 1-37 *A compensated Thorpe tube flowmeter.*

ASSEMBLY AND TROUBLESHOOTING

Assembly—Oxygen Flowmeters

Flowmeters are very easy to assemble for use. Complete the following instructions to prepare a flowmeter.

1. Attach the flowmeter to an appropriate 50 psi gas source using DISS or quick-connect fittings.

2. Attach the appropriate therapy equipment to the DISS fitting on the flowmeter outlet.

3. When using a Bourdon flowmeter, carefully check all supply tubing for kinks or obstructions.

4. Adjust the flow to the desired setting.

5. A Thorpe tube flowmeter can be identified when it is connected to a 50 psi gas source. The float on a Thorpe tube flowmeter will quickly rise and fall when the tube is pressurized to the 50 psi line pressure.

Troubleshooting

Troubleshooting a flowmeter primarily consists of checking for leaks. Periodically, a flowmeter should be checked against a calibration standard for accuracy (calibration flowmeter or volume displacement spirometer). When troubleshooting this equipment, please follow the suggested troubleshooting algorithm (ALG 1-8).

1. Sources of leaks:
   a. Connection between flowmeter and 50 psi gas source.
   b. Connection between flowmeter and the therapy equipment.

2. If the flowmeter fails to deliver expected flow or behaves erratically, check it against a calibration standard and if necessary have it repaired.

Ranges of Flowmeters

Several manufacturers offer flowmeters with expanded calibration scales that extend beyond the range of the typical 0 to 15 L/min flowmeter's calibrated range.

A high-range flowmeter is calibrated from 0 to 75 L/min in 5 L/min units (Figure 1-38, Part A). The high-range flowmeter is useful in Continuous Positive Airway Pressure (CPAP) and high-flow oxygen delivery systems with high-flow clinical applications. Low-range flowmeters have scales calibrated between 0 and 3 L/min in quarter-L/min intervals (Part B of Figure 1-38) and are useful in pediatrics and chronic obstructive lung disease patients.

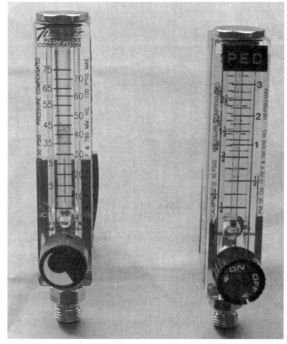

A   *B*

Figure 1-38 *(A) A photograph of a high-range flowmeter, calibrated from zero to seventy five liters per minute. (B) A photograph of a low-range (pediatric) flowmeter, calibrated from zero to three liters per minute.*

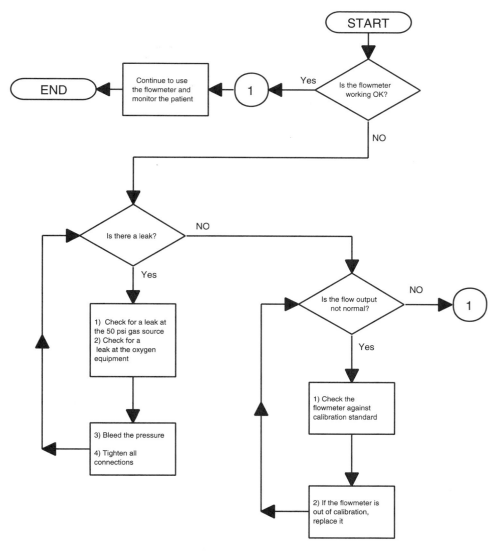

ALG 1-8 *An algorithm describing how to troubleshoot medical gas flowmeters.*

MEDICAL GAS THERAPY EQUIPMENT

HIGH- AND LOW-FLOW OXYGEN DELIVERY SYSTEMS

The *term high-flow oxygen delivery system* does not refer to the liter flow of oxygen powering the device. Rather it refers to the fact that the device delivers all of the patient's inspiratory flow needs. With a high flow system, all of the inspired gas the patient breathes is delivered by the oxygen device.

These oxygen delivery systems most commonly employ viscous shearing or vorticity to mix ambient air with oxygen. (Viscous shear-

ing was discussed earlier in this chapter.) Oxygen powering the device mixes with room air delivering a high flow of mixed gas at a precise F_IO_2 (fraction of inspired oxygen, expressed as a decimal). The total flow delivered to the patient is greater than the flow set on the oxygen flowmeter. Total flows and air/oxygen entrainment ratios will be discussed later in this chapter.

Low-flow oxygen delivery devices provide part of a patient's inspiratory gas flow needs. The remainder of the gas the patient inhales comes from room air. Since the gas delivered from the oxygen device mixes with unknown and varying amounts of room air, the amount of F_IO_2 delivered varies.

The variation in the F_IO_2 is dependent upon

the patient's tidal volume (depth of breathing) and respiratory rate. If the tidal volume is large, more room air will be inspired in proportion to the oxygen delivered from the device. As the respiratory rate increases, room air entrainment also increases. If the proportion of room air increases, the delivered F_IO_2 will decrease.

HIGH-FLOW OXYGEN DELIVERY SYSTEMS

Venturi Masks/High Air Flow with Oxygen Entrainment (HAFOE)

The venturi or HAFOE mask utilizes the viscous shearing effect of two different gases to entrain room air (Figure 1-39). The term "venturi" is really incorrectly applied to describe the operation of these devices. The high-flow gas from the jet forms a boundary layer, cleaving the relatively stationary room air. This viscous shearing effect entrains the room air, mixing the oxygen with it. By varying the size of the oxygen jet and the entrainment ports, differing oxygen concentrations may be obtained. The ratio of air entrainment to oxygen flow may be calculated using the following formula.

$$\frac{Liters\ of\ Air\ Entrained}{Liters\ of\ Oxygen} = \frac{1.0 - F_IO_2}{F_IO_2 - .21}$$
$$F_IO_2 = Desired\ Oxygen\ Concentration$$

It is important to remember that F_IO_2 is expressed as a decimal and not as a percentage when solving this equation.

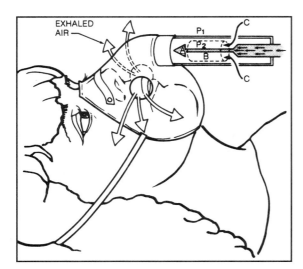

Figure 1-39 *A pictorial representation of a venturi mask. Note the room air entrainment lateral to the oxygen jet. (A) High-velocity jet. (B) Region of viscous shearing. (C) Room air entrainment.*

For example:
You are using an entrainment device set at an F_IO_2 of .40. What is the air-to-oxygen entrainment ratio?

$$\frac{Liters\ of\ Air\ Entrained}{Liters\ of\ Oxygen} = \frac{1.0 - F_IO_2}{F_IO_2 - .21}$$

$$\frac{Liters\ of\ Air\ Entrained}{Liters\ of\ Oxygen} = \frac{1.0 - .40}{.40 - .21}$$

$$\frac{Liters\ of\ Air\ Entrained}{Liters\ of\ Oxygen} = \frac{3}{1}$$

Often you will be required to calculate the total flow rate from an entrainment device. To calculate the total flow (air and oxygen) being delivered to the patient, you must know: (1) the air-to-oxygen entrainment ratio and (2) the liter flow of oxygen entering the device.

Total Flow
        = Liters of Air Entrained + Liters of Oxygen

For example:
An entrainment mask is set at 24%. The oxygen flow to the mask is 3 L/min. What is the total flow (air and oxygen) to the patient?
Step 1: What is the air-to-oxygen entrainment ratio?

$$\frac{Liters\ of\ Air\ Entrained}{Liters\ of\ Oxygen} = \frac{1.0 - F_IO_2}{F_IO_2 - .21}$$

$$\frac{Liters\ of\ Air\ Entrained}{Liters\ of\ Oxygen} = \frac{1.0 - .24}{.24 - .21}$$

$$\frac{Liters\ of\ Air\ Entrained}{Liters\ of\ Oxygen} = \frac{25}{1}$$

This means that for every liter of oxygen entering the mask, there are 25 liters of air being entrained.
Step 2: What is the total flow?

Total Flow = Liters of Air + Liters of Oxygen
Total Flow = $(3 \times 25) + 3$
Total Flow = 78 Liters per Minute

Manufacturers have developed specific combinations of entrainment ports and jet sizes to deliver precise F_IO_2 levels. These combinations depend on the ratio of air entrainment in proportion to oxygen flow to determine the oxygen concentration. These ratios are summarized in Table 1-6.

High-flow systems are designed to flood the patient's face with a high flow of gas containing a constant F_IO_2. The theory behind the use of this system is that if enough flow is provided, the patient will not entrain any room

ASSEMBLY AND TROUBLESHOOTING

Assembly—High-Flow Oxygen Delivery Devices

Correct assembly and troubleshooting of high-flow oxygen delivery systems is important for correct operation and patient safety. The following is a suggested assembly guide.

1. Obtain an appropriate oxygen source (cylinder, piping system, liquid reservoir, or concentrator) with a flowmeter calibrated for an appropriate flow range.

2. Attach the flowmeter to the 50 psi oxygen source.

3. Attach a humidifier to the flowmeter. **Note:** If you are using a venturi mask, do not use a humidifier. Water droplets and particles may alter the performance from the desired F_IO_2.

4. Attach the oxygen connecting tube to the humidifier.

5. Adjust the flow so that the entrainment device exceeds the patient's inspiratory needs or, when using an anesthesia bag-mask, adjust the flow so the reservoir bag does not deflate during inspiration.

6. Placement of the oxygen therapy device:
   a. Place the mask on the bridge of the patient's nose, adjusting the strap so it is snug but not tight.
   b. If the mask is a reservoir type, ensure that the reservoir is free to expand without pressure from bed covers or other objects.
   c. When using an anesthesia bag-mask, check for proper operation of the one-way valves and correct assembly.
   d. Adjust the head strap so it is snug but not too tight.
   e. Verify oxygen concentration of the venturi mask system.

Troubleshooting

Troubleshooting high-flow oxygen masks consists of checking for leaks and proper flow from the mask. The following is a suggested algorithm (ALG 1-9).

1. Check the following sources for leaks:
   a. Check the connection between the flowmeter and the 50 psi gas source.
   b. Check the connection between the flowmeter and the humidifier.
   c. Check the connection between the connecting tube and the humidifier.

2. If gas fails to flow from the mask:
   a. Verify that the oxygen flowmeter is turned on and an adequate supply of gas exists.
   b. Check the oxygen connecting tube for kinks or obstructions.
   c. Verify that the humidifier is operating properly.

---

air. The success of the concept depends on the oxygen percentage (air-to-oxygen entrainment ratio) and the patient's inspiratory flow demands. If the patient's inspiratory flow demands exceed the flow from the mask, room air will be entrained and the F_IO_2 will become variable and not fixed.

For example:

A patient is ordered a 35% venturi mask. He is breathing at a rate of 20 breaths per minute with a minute volume of 8 liters at an Inspiratory-to-Expiratory ratio (I:E)

of 1:2. Is the device providing adequate flow if the flowmeter is set at 6 liters per minute?

1. Calculate the patient's inspiratory flow demands.

Tidal volume

= minute volume/frequency

= 8 liters/20 breaths per minute

= .4L (400 mL)

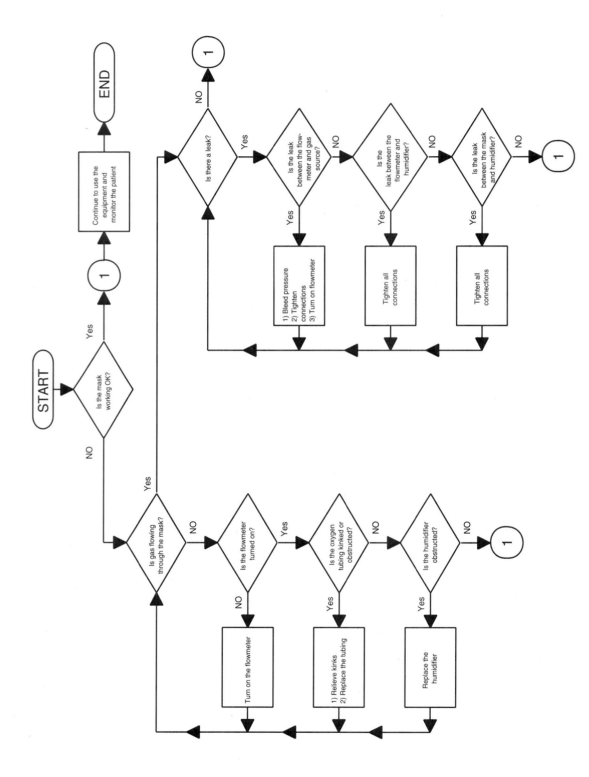

ALG 1-9 *An algorithm describing how to troubleshoot oxygen non-rebreathing masks.*

TABLE 1-6 Air to Oxygen Entrainment Ratios

ROOM AIR-TO-OXYGEN RATIO	OXYGEN CONCENTRATION
25:1	24%
10:1	28%
8:1	30%
5:1	35%
3:1	40%
1.7:1	50%
1:1	60%
0:1	100%

Reprinted by permission from Gary C. White, Basic Clinical Lab Competencies for Respiratory Care, 3rd Ed., Delmar Publishers, Inc., 1998.

Total ventilatory cycle

$$= 60 \text{ seconds}/20 \text{ bpm}$$
$$= 3 \text{ seconds}$$

Inspiratory time is 1 second at an I:E ratio of 1:2.

Inspiratory flow demand
$$= .4 \text{ liters}/\text{second}$$
$$= .4 \text{ liters}/\text{second} \times 60 \text{ seconds}/\text{minute}$$
$$= 24 \text{ liters}/\text{minute}$$

2. Calculate flow through the device and compare. Air-to-oxygen entrainment ratio at 35% = 5:1.

Total flow at 6 liters/min
$$= 30 \text{ liters air} + 6 \text{ liters oxygen}$$
$$= 36 \text{ liters per minute}$$

3. Conclusion: The device exceeds the patient's inspiratory flow needs by 12 liters/minute.

Anesthesia Bag-Mask Systems

Anesthesia bags can be combined with ventilation masks and valves to construct a true non-rebreathing system (Figure 1-40). One one-way valve prevents exhaled gas from mixing with the oxygen delivered to the bag and the other one-way valve prevents the entrainment of room air during inspiration. If the fit is tight and the flow is adequate, this device can provide up to 100% oxygen delivery. The oxygen flow is adjusted so that the reservoir bag never collapses during inspiration. This device also may be used to administer mixed gas therapy such as He/O_2 or O_2/CO_2.

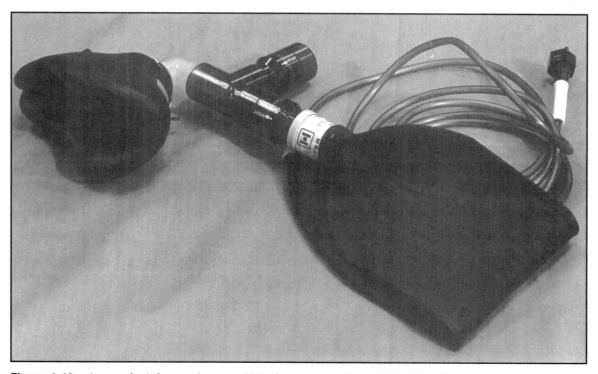

Figure 1-40 *An anesthesia bag-mask system. Note the one-way valves and their flow direction.*

LOW-FLOW OXYGEN DELIVERY DEVICES

Nasal Cannula and Catheter

The nasal cannula is an example of a low-flow oxygen delivery device. The cannula rests on the patient's upper lip, with the curve of the prongs directed posteriorly into the nasal passages. Oxygen at a flow between 1 to 6 liters per minute enters the patient's nose, filling the anatomic reservoir (Figures 1-41 and 1-42).

The anatomic reservoir consists of the nasopharynx and oropharynx (Figure 1-43). In the adult its volume is approximately 50 milliliters. As a patient breathes, there is a slight pause between exhalation and inspiration. During this pause, the anatomic reservoir fills with oxygen. Therefore, the first 50 milliliters of each breath is pure oxygen, and the remainder consists of oxygen mixed with room air. As discussed earlier, the F_IO_2 varies depending on the patient's tidal volume and respiratory rate. Table 1-7 indicates the approximate F_IO_2 delivery with these devices.

The nasal catheter operates on a similar principle to that of the nasal cannula. The catheter is positioned by passing it through the nose and the turbinates with the tip rest-

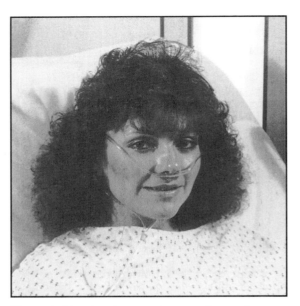

Figure 1-42 *A patient wearing a nasal cannula.*

ing at the level of the uvula in the oropharynx (Figure 1-44). Oxygen entering the device flows directly into the oropharynx. The F_IO_2 delivery is similar to that of the nasal cannula.

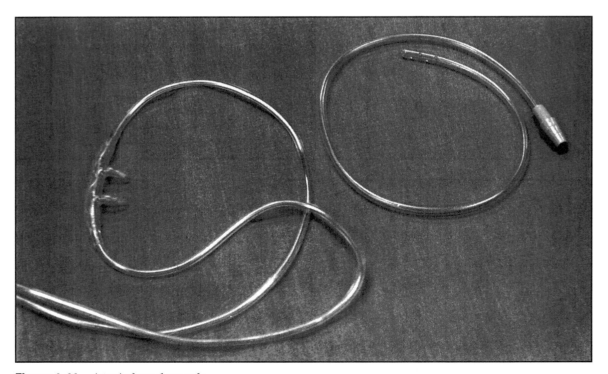

Figure 1-41 *A typical nasal cannula.*

ASSEMBLY AND TROUBLESHOOTING

Assembly—Nasal Cannula

Nasal cannulas are one of the most common oxygen administration devices. Although a nasal catheter is used less frequently, it is also important to understand its use. It is essential to understand how to assemble and troubleshoot these devices. The following is a suggested assembly guide.

1. Obtain an appropriate oxygen source (cylinder, piping system, liquid reservoir, or concentrator) with a flowmeter calibrated for an appropriate flow range.

2. Attach the flowmeter to the 50 psi oxygen source.

3. Attach a humidifier to the flowmeter.

4. Attach the oxygen connecting tube to the flowmeter.

5. Adjust the flow to the ordered level prior to placing the device on the patient.

6. Placement of the oxygen therapy device:
   a. Nasal catheter
      [1.] Lubricate the catheter with sterile water-soluble lubricant.
      [2.] Estimate the length of the catheter by measuring from the pinna of the ear to the tip of the nose.
      [3.] Pass the catheter gently down one nare until the tip is visible behind the uvula.
      [4.] If the patient gags following placement of the nasal catheter, it has been placed too far down the airway. Withdraw the catheter a centimeter or two.
      [5.] You may find that it is helpful to use a tongue depressor to depress the tongue and a flashlight, or otoscope, to visualize the nasal catheter and its placement.
   b. Nasal cannula
      [1.] Place the cannula resting on the upper lip with the prongs pointed down into the nasal passages.
      [2.] Secure the strap around the head so it is snug but not tight, or adjust the lariat strap beneath the chin as shown in Figure 1-42.
   c. Reservoir cannula
      [1.] Place the reservoir so it rests on the upper lip and adjust the strap so it is comfortable.
   d. Pendant cannula
      [1.] Place the pendant reservoir on the patient's chest. Rest the prongs of the cannula on the upper lip and direct them into the nasal passages.
      [2.] Adjust the strap so the cannula is comfortable.

Troubleshooting

Troubleshooting cannulas and catheters primarily consists of checking for flow from the device and checking for leaks. The following is a suggested troubleshooting algorithm (ALG 1-10).

1. Check the following sources for leaks:
   a. The connection between the flowmeter and the 50 psi gas source may not be tight.
   b. The connection between the flowmeter and the humidifier may be loose.
   c. The connection between the cannula and the humidifier may not be snug.

2. If gas fails to flow from the cannula or catheter:
   a. Verify that the oxygen flowmeter is turned on and an adequate supply of gas exists.
   b. Check the oxygen connecting tube for kinks or obstructions.
   c. Verify that the humidifier is operating correctly.
   d. Check the cannula or catheter for obstruction caused by dried secretions. If obstructed, replace the cannula or catheter.

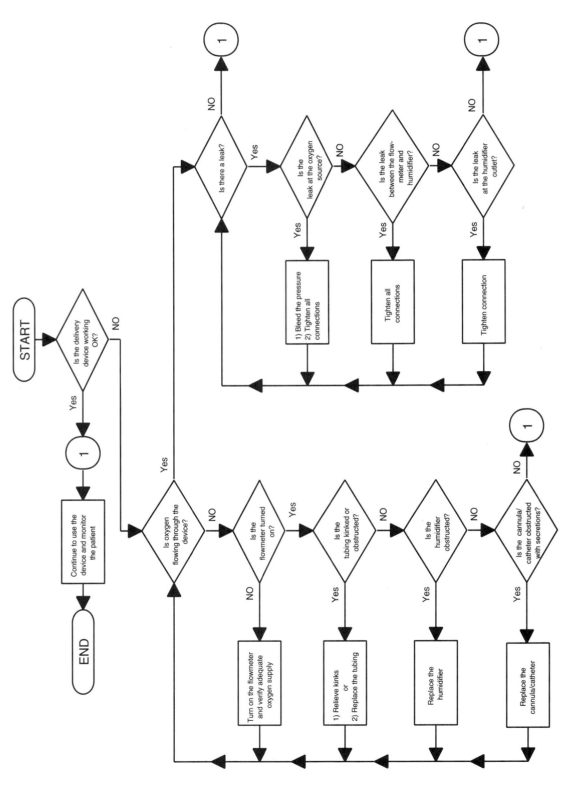

ALG 1-10 *An algorithm describing how to troubleshoot a cannula.*

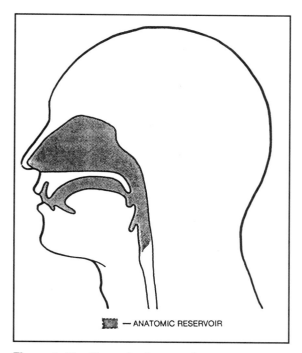

Figure 1-43 *The anatomic reservoir.*

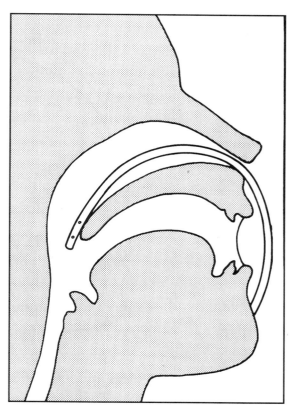

Figure 1-44 *A pictorial representation indicating the correct placement of the nasal catheter. Note that the tip of the catheter is immediately posterior to the uvula and has not been advanced past it.*

TABLE 1-7 Nasal Cannula Oxygen Concentrations

100% O_2 FLOW IN LITERS	APPROXIMATE F_IO_2
1 L	.24
2 L	.28
3 L	.32
4 L	.36
5 L	.40
6 L	.44

Adapted from Gary C. White, Basic Clinical Lab Competencies for Respiratory Care, *3rd Ed., Delmar Publishers, Inc., 1998.*

Reservoir and Pendant Cannulas

The reservoir cannula and the pendant cannula are two contemporary devices designed to maintain F_IO_2 levels at lower flow rates. By providing a small reservoir, oxygen flow may be reduced without affecting the oxygen delivery. This is a particular advantage during ambulation or exercise. The performance of these devices, however, is variable. Figure 1-45 shows a pendant cannula (Part A) and a reservoir cannula (Part B) and their application.

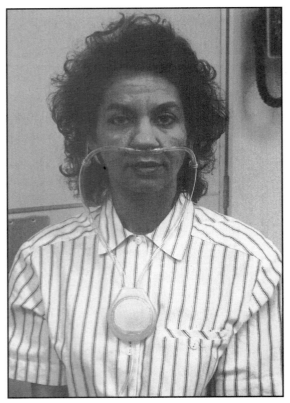 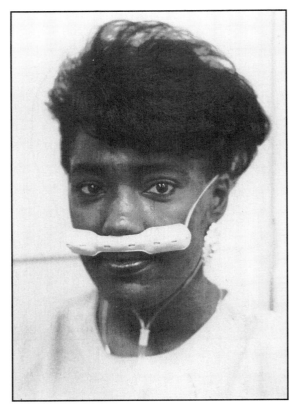

Figure 1-45 *(A) A pendant oxygen cannula applied to a patient. (B) A reservoir oxygen cannula applied to a patient.*

DEMAND PULSE FLOW OXYGEN DELIVERY DEVICES

Demand pulse flow oxygen delivery devices are oxygen delivery devices which are designed to deliver oxygen only during the inspiratory phase. During a normal ventilatory cycle, when using continuous flow oxygen, oxygen delivered during the last part of inspiration (dead space volume) and the oxygen delivered during exhalation are not usable. Dead space volume is the portion of oxygen delivered which does not participate in gas exchange at the alveoli (Figure 1-46). Demand pulse flow oxygen delivery devices are able to sense the start of the inspiratory phase, and deliver oxygen only during inspiration (Figure 1-47). By delivering oxygen only during that part of the ventilatory cycle that is usable (oxygen that can participate in gas exchange), oxygen is conserved when these devices are compared to continuous flow oxygen delivery devices. Since these devices deliver a minimal flow of dry gas, humidification requirements are eliminated. These devices are most commonly used in the home setting, where oxygen conservation can result in substantial cost savings.

When initially setting up an oxygen system on ambulatory patients, it is helpful to perform an exercise oximetry study with both continuous flow and demand pulse flow oxygen systems to insure adequate oxygen saturation. Not all patients will be able to maintain adequate oxygen saturations during demand pulse flow delivery. Therefore, it is important to adjust the demand pulse oxygen delivery flow rate to meet the patient's needs during exercise, as documented by oximetry. Some patients with severe pulmonary disease may not tolerate demand pulse flow oxygen delivery systems at all. In these patients, continuous flow oxygen systems are required to maintain adequate oxygen saturations.

Transtracheal Systems DOC 2000 Demand Oxygen Controller

The Transtracheal Systems DOC 2000 demand oxygen controller is a pulse demand oxygen delivery device that conserves oxygen by delivering it only during inspiration (Fig-

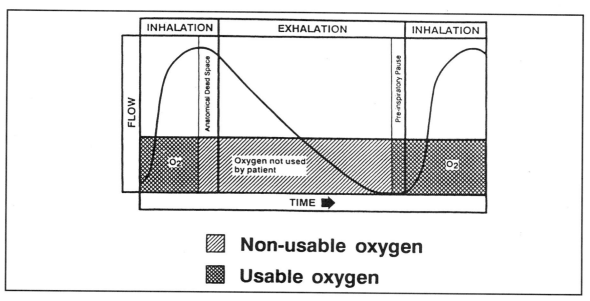

Figure 1-46 *A graph illustrating usable and nonusable oxygen during continuous flow delivery. (Courtesy Puritan Bennett Corporation, Lenexa, KS)*

ure 1-48). The unit is electronically controlled and may be powered by a rechargeable Ni-Cad battery or a 120 v, 60Hz power adapter, which also functions to recharge the Ni-Cad battery. When the Ni-Cad battery is fully charged, the DOC 2000 can operate between 8 and 10 hours before requiring a recharge.

Inspiratory Detection

The DOC 2000 detects inspiration using a sensitive pressure transducer. During inspira-

tion, a subambient pressure is created in the patient's nares as the lungs expand. When the pressure transducer senses the drop in pressure, a valve opens, delivering oxygen to the patient.

Oxygen Flow Control

The operation of the DOC 2000 is based upon switching the patient between the oxygen source (valve 2) and the pressure sensor (valve 1). When valve 2 is not energized, oxy-

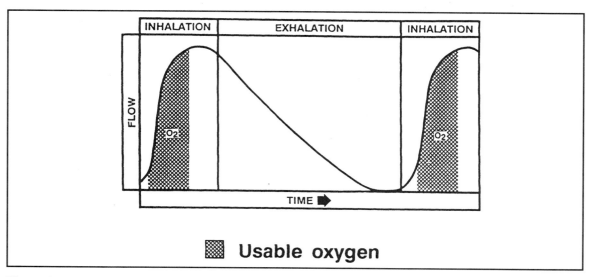

Figure 1-47 *A graph illustrating usable and nonusable oxygen during pulsed demand flow delivery. (Courtesy Puritan Bennett Corporation, Lenexa, KS)*

ASSEMBLY AND TROUBLESHOOTING

Assembly

1. Connect the DOC 2000 to an oxygen source.
   a. An oxygen cylinder requires the use of a regulator to reduce the cylinder pressure and to set the oxygen delivery to the prescribed flow. The DOC 2000 is attached to the outlet of the regulator.
   b. A liquid system requires the use of a flowmeter, which is used to set the desired flow rate. The DOC 2000 is attached to the outlet of the flowmeter.
   c. A portable liquid reservoir may also be used by threading a barbed hose fitting adapter into the inlet port of the DOC 2000 and attaching the other end to the outlet of the portable reservoir set at the appropriate flow rate.

2. Connect the delivery tubing of the nasal cannula or transtracheal catheter to the barbed outlet of the DOC 2000. Delivery tubing should never exceed 35 feet in length.

3. Depress the "On/Off" button on the top of the unit to turn the unit on. The unit will perform a self calibration (about 1 second) and then will operate normally.

Troubleshooting

When troubleshooting the DOC 2000, please follow the suggested troubleshooting algorithm (ALG 1-11).

1. The unit fails to deliver oxygen flow.
   a. Check tubing and cannula or transtracheal catheter for obstructions or kinks.
   b. Make certain that the oxygen flowmeter is on and that there is a sufficient quantity of oxygen (pressure for cylinders or weight for liquid systems).
   c. The patient may not be generating a sufficient inspiratory effort to activate the inspiratory detection circuit. Patients with advanced lung disease may not be candidates for pulsed oxygen delivery and may require continuous flow.

2. The green LED remains illuminated after the unit is turned on.
   a. Disconnect the cannula/transtracheal catheter from the DOC 2000 and turn the unit off for at least 30 seconds. Turn the unit back on and allow it to self-calibrate. Reconnect the delivery device, which should function normally.
   b. If the unit fails to recalibrate, discontinue using that unit and replace it. Send the defective unit to the manufacturer or an appropriate biomedical repair facility.

3. The yellow LED is illuminated and an audible alarm is heard.
   a. The battery requires recharging. Discontinue battery operation and connect the unit to its AC adapter/charger.

4. The red LED is illuminated and an audible alarm is heard.
   a. An inspiratory effort has not been detected for the past 50 seconds.
   b. Check the patient to be certain that the patient is OK.
   c. Check the delivery tubing for obstructions or kinks.

gen flows from the source directly to the patient (Figure 1-49). Simultaneously, when valve 2 is not energized, valve 1 is energized, which connects the transducer (U11) to the normally closed atmospheric port. Each time the pressure transducer is referenced to ambient pressure, it recalibrates itself, which maintains a consistent sensitivity threshold.

During exhalation, valve 2 is energized, which closes it and stops the flow of oxygen. Valve 1 is not energized, which connects the pressure transducer to the patient through

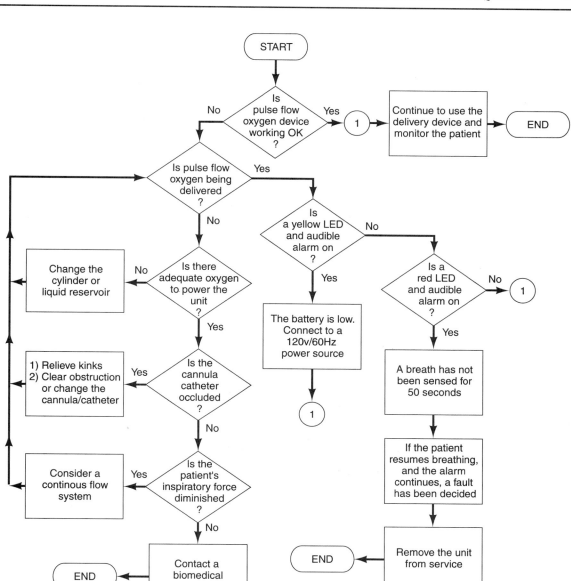

ALG 1-11 *An algorithm describing how to troubleshoot the Transtracheal Systems DOC 2000 demand oxygen controller.*

the normally open port of valve 1 (Figure 1-49). Once a pressure drop is detected, valve 2 opens and valve 1 closes, beginning the inspiratory cycle once again.

Monitoring System

The DOC 2000 uses a green light-emitting diode (LED) for two functions. When the unit is first turned on, the LED illuminates and stays on for approximately 1 second, indicating that power is on and that the unit is self-

calibrating. Once the patient is connect to the DOC 2000, the green LED will illuminate during inspiration. This tells the operator/user that inspiration has been detected and that oxygen flow is initiated.

A yellow LED and audible alarm alerts the operator/user of a low battery level. In the event this alarm system is activated, discontinue battery operation and connect the unit to its AC power pack/charging unit. The Ni-Cad battery can be recharged in approximately 13 hours.

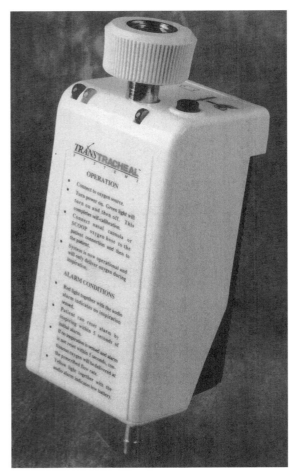

Figure 1-48 *A photograph of the DOC 2000 demand oxygen controller. (Courtesy Transtracheal Systems, Englewood, CO)*

The DOC 2000 also incorporates a system default signal indicator/alarm detector. A red LED illuminates if the unit does not sense an inspiratory effort within approximately 45 seconds. When this occurs, the red LED illuminates and a continuous audible alarm sounds. If an inspiratory effort is detected within 8 to 10 seconds, the unit will reset itself. If no inspiratory effort is detected within approximately 50 seconds, valve 2 opens, delivering the prescribed oxygen flow continuously.

DeVilbiss OMS 20 and EX2000D

DeVilbiss Health Care, Inc., markets two electronically controlled demand pulse flow oxygen delivery devices (Parts A and B of Figure 1-50). The OMS 20 is designed to be used with 20 psi liquid oxygen systems. The OMS 20 may be operated from an internal battery for up to 23 hours or by an optional 115 v, 60 Hz power adapter. The unit senses the patient's inspiratory efforts and delivers a pulse of oxygen during early inspiration. Pulsed oxygen delivery may be provided at flows of between 0.25 and 6 liters per minute.

The EX2000D is designed for use on small oxygen cylinders having a yoke type cylinder valve. The EX2000D is powered by a standard alkaline "C" cell battery. Once the battery is installed, the unit is slipped over the cylinder yoke, and the T-handle is hand-tightened until it seals against the cylinder valve, much like a standard regulator is secured. A selector switch on the right of the unit allows the operator to select between continuous flow and pulsed dose oxygen delivery.

Inspiratory Detection

The DeVilbiss units use a very sensitive pressure transducer to detect the patient's inspiration. As the patient inhales through his/her nasal cannula, the subambient pressure created in the patient's lungs is transmitted to the DeVilbiss unit through the cannula. A subambient pressure (Trigger Level – .02 cm H_2O) causes an electrical signal to be sent from the pressure transducer (sensor) to the solenoid valve. Once inspiration is detected by the transducer, an electrical signal opens the solenoid valve, delivering a pulse of oxygen.

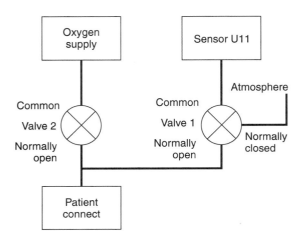

Figure 1-49 *A schematic diagram of the DOC 2000 demand oxygen controller. (Courtesy Transtracheal Systems, Englewood, CO)*

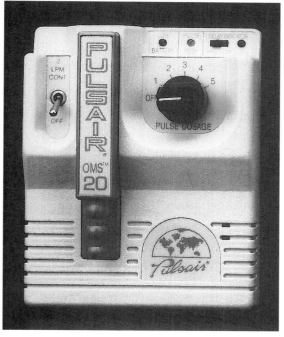

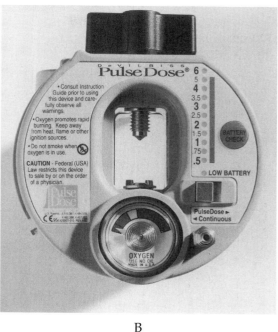

A   B

Figure 1-50 (A) *A photograph of the DeVilbiss OMS 20.* (B) *A photograph of the DeVilbiss EX2000D pulse flow oxygen system. (Courtesy DeVilbiss Health Care, Inc. Somerset, PA)*

Oxygen Flow Control

Oxygen flow (OMS 20) is determined by the setting on the Pulse Dosage switch. The Pulse Dosage switch is a rotary switch which determines how long the solenoid valve remains open. As the flow rate setting is increased by turning the Pulse Dosage switch, the time the solenoid valve remains open is also increased. This is a time based variable circuit with a constant flow rate. The volume of oxygen delivered to the patient is solely determined by the amount of time the solenoid valve remains open. Therefore, when the respiratory rate increases, the patient actually receives more oxygen. This would be referred to as a "rate response" type of oxygen delivery.

Liter flow on the EX2000D is adjusted by connecting the unit to a cylinder and by attaching a short length of tubing between the EX2000D and an external flowmeter used for calibration purposes. An Allen wrench is inserted into the fitting on the bottom of the EX2000D, and flow is adjusted until the desired flow is displayed on the external flowmeter. Once the desired flow is set, the wrench is removed, along with the calibration flowmeter and connecting tubing.

Monitoring Systems

The DeVilbiss OMS 20 and EX2000D have several monitoring features built into the units. These features include low battery detection, pulse delivery indication and a detection delay indicator.

The low battery indicator will light and an audible alarm will sound when the battery power becomes low. When this condition is detected, it is important to recharge the internal battery using the 120 v, 60 Hz adapter supplied with the unit.

During inspiration, a green LED will illuminate when a pulse is delivered. The sensor circuit sends an electrical signal to illuminate the LED simultaneously with the signal sent to the solenoid valve. Whenever the solenoid valve is opened, the green Pulse Dose LED is also illuminated for the duration of the valve's open time.

A detection delay system is also incorporated into the design of the DeVilbiss units. If an inspiratory effort is not detected within a specified time interval (the time interval is adjustable from 6 to 60 seconds), a red LED will illuminate and a continuous audible alarm will sound. This feature may be turned "ON" or "OFF" by using the two-position Delay Detector switch.

ASSEMBLY AND TROUBLESHOOTING

Assembly—DeVilbiss OMS 20/EX2000D

1. Connect the DeVilbiss to an appropriate oxygen source.
   a. The OMS 20 is designed for liquid oxygen systems with a pressure range of 18 to 28 psi. Use of the unit with higher-pressure sources will damage it.
   b. The EX2000D is designed to be mated to a small cylinder with a yoke-type cylinder valve much like a standard regulator is mated to that type of valve. The unit is aligned with the pin index safety system and the T-handle is tightened to secure it to the valve.

2. Set the continuous flow toggle valve switch to the "OFF" position.

3. Set the Pulse Dosage switch to the "OFF" position.

4. Connect the patient's delivery device (nasal cannula, catheter or transtracheal catheter) to the DeVilbiss unit. **Note: The manufacturer recommends not using more than 35 feet of oxygen delivery tubing.** Use of longer lengths of tubing may adversely affect oxygen delivery and inspiratory detection. Also, do not use a humidification device!

5. Set the Pulse Dosage switch to the prescribed flow rate setting.
   a. It is important to perform this step prior to attaching the delivery device to the patient. Once the Pulse Dose switch is turned from "OFF" to the desired setting, the pressure transducer is referenced to ambient pressure. If the delivery device is attached to the patient when this step is performed, an incorrect pressure reference may result, causing problems with inspiratory detection and oxygen delivery.

6. Attach the oxygen cannula to the patient's nose.

7. Observe the unit for correct operation by the Pulse Dose LED illuminating with each breath.

Troubleshooting

When troubleshooting this equipment, please follow the suggested troubleshooting algorithm (ALG 1-12).

If the DeVilbiss fails to deliver demand pulsed oxygen flow:

1. Verify that the oxygen source has an adequate supply.
   a. Check the pressure gauge on the oxygen cylinder.
   b. Check the weight of the liquid system.

2. Check to ensure that the Toggle Valve switch is in the "OFF" position and not the "Continuous Flow" position.

3. Battery not charged.
   a. Check the battery condition and recharge it as required.

4. Verify that the Pulse Dosage switch is set on one of the five settings and is not turned "OFF."

5. Check the oxygen delivery device or connecting tubing for obstructions.
   a. Relieve any kinks in the tubing.
   b. If mucous or other obstructions are present, replace the tubing.
   c. Note that these devices are not designed to be used with humidifiers.

6. The Trigger Sensitivity may need adjustment.
   To adjust the Trigger Sensitivity, insert a small precision screwdriver into the hole labeled "SENS ADJUST" on the back of the unit.
   a. Rotate the screwdriver clockwise slowly just until the unit senses a patient effort (green LED is illuminated).
   b. Adjusting the sensitivity such that it is too sensitive may result in oxygen delivery during inspiration or erratic delivery with patient movement.

If the red Low Battery LED is illuminated and an intermittent beeping sound is heard:

1. The battery is becoming discharged and needs to be recharged.
   a. Connect the unit to a 115 v, 60 Hz, electrical outlet using the provided adapter. Allow at least 8 hours for a full charge.

If the red Detection Delay LED is illuminated and a continuous beep is heard:

1. The DeVilbiss unit failed to detect a breath within the detection delay time window.
   a. Adjust the detection delay to a longer time interval (if the interval is less than 60 seconds).
   Insert a precision screwdriver into the opening labeled "DELAY IND" on the rear of the unit. Rotate the adjustment screw clockwise to increase the time interval.
   b. If the delay detection alarm is more prevalent during sleeping hours, sleep apnea may be present. Have the patient consult his/her physician for evaluation.

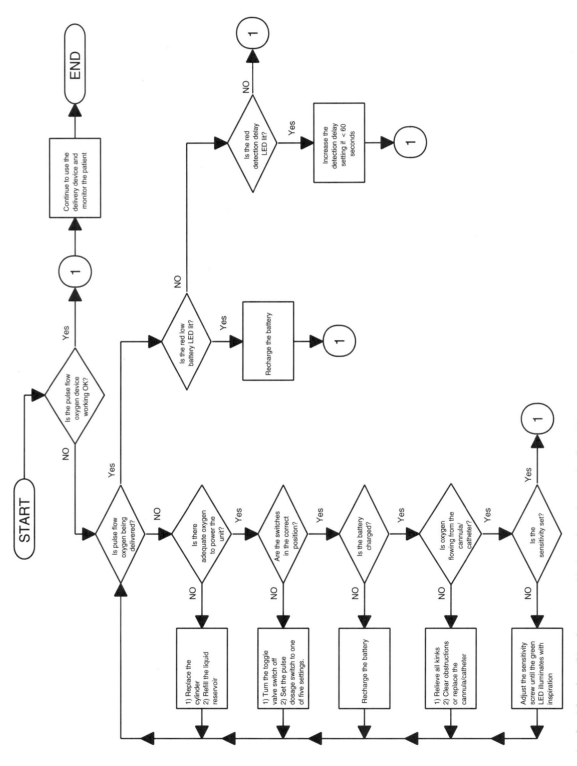

ALG 1-12 *An algorithm describing how to troubleshoot the Pulsair pulse flow delivery systems.*

Chad Therapeutics Oxymatic 301 and Oxymatic 2400

Chad Therapeutics, Inc. has designed and is marketing two electronic demand flow pulse delivery oxygen conserving devices (Figure 1-51). The model 301 is designed for portable operation (intermittent), and the model 2400 is designed for continuous use, although it may also be used with portable oxygen systems. Both units electronically sense the end of expiration and the beginning of inspiration and deliver a pulse of oxygen within .2 seconds following the start of inspiration. Both units are powered by common alkaline "C" size batteries. The battery life averages 3 to 4 weeks of use.

Inspiratory Detection

During inspiration, a subambient pressure is created in the lungs as the lungs expand. During exhalation, chest wall recoil creates a pressure in the lungs which is greater than ambient pressure. These very small pressure changes are communicated to the Oxymatic units through the patient's nasal cannula.

The Oxymatic units have an internal flexible diaphragm that changes position in response to the pressure changes in the patient's lungs. The neutral position (position between exhalation and inspiration) is electronically detected. When diaphragm motion away from the neutral position is detected, inspiration is detected. An electronic signal is transmitted to the solenoid valve, opening it and delivering a 35 mL pulse of oxygen within 0.2 seconds of the start of inspiration.

Oxygen Flow Control

The Oxymatic units deliver a constant 35 mL pulse of oxygen when the solenoid valve opens. The units control oxygen flow delivery by altering how frequently these constant volume pulses are delivered.

Clinical trials have shown that when the Oxymatic units deliver 35 mL pulse of oxygen every breath, this is equivalent to a continuous oxygen flow of 4 L/min (determined by oxygen saturation). When a pulse is delivered three out of every four breaths (75% of the time), this is equivalent to a continuous flow of 3 L/min. When a pulse is delivered every other breath (50% of the time), this is equivalent to 2 L/min continuous flow. When oxygen is delivered one out of every four breaths (25% of the time), this is equivalent to 1 L/min continuous flow.

Because of the unique pulse delivery (alternate breath delivery below 4 L/min), some patients may be uncomfortable initially when using these units. It is important to explain how these units work and that even though the patient may not feel oxygen

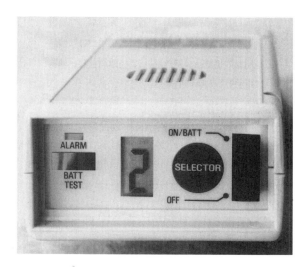

Figure 1-51 *Photographs of (A) the Chad Therapeutics Oxymatic 301 and (B) Oxymatic 2400 pulse flow oxygen delivery systems. (Courtesy of Chad Therapeutics, Inc., Chatsworth, CA)*

ASSEMBLY AND TROUBLESHOOTING

Assembly—Chad Therapeutics Oxymatic

1. Install a fresh alkaline "C" size battery by removing the battery cover and slipping the new battery into place. Observe the correct polarity when installing the battery ("+" and "−").

2. Connect a nasal cannula to the Oxymatic using the special cannula connector provided by the manufacturer.

3. Connect the Oxymatic to an appropriate oxygen source which is regulated to between 20 and 25 psi. This connection should be made using the tubing and female "bayonet" connector provided by the manufacturer. Rotate the fitting clockwise to lock it into place.

4. Turn on the oxygen supply by opening the cylinder valve or setting your liquid system to its maximum flow setting.

5. Set the flow rate on the Oxymatic unit:
   a. Oxymatic 201-A
      Rotate the thumbwheel on the top of the unit until the desired flow (1-4) is displayed.
   b. Oxymatic 2400
      [1.] Position the black rocker switch into the "ON" position.
      [2.] Depress the "SELECTOR" button until the desired flow rate appears in the "Setting Indicator" window. An LED will indicate the flow rate setting (1-4).

6. Attach the nasal cannula to your patient's face, observing the correct procedure discussed previously in this chapter.

Troubleshooting

When troubleshooting this equipment, please follow the suggested troubleshooting algorithm (ALG 1-13).

If the Oxymatic unit does not pulse delivering oxygen:

1. The battery has been fully discharged. Replace the battery as required.

2. The battery has been installed incorrectly with the polarity reversed. Reinstall the battery observing the correct polarity ("+" and "−").

3. The oxygen supply has been exhausted. Replace the cylinder or refill the liquid system as required.

4. The Oxymatic unit may not be sensing inspiration.
   a. Check the cannula for correct placement.
   b. Check the cannula for any kinks or obstructions.

If the Oxymatic delivers continuous flow and does not pulse:

1. The regulated pressure is too high. Ensure that the regulated oxygen pressure is between 20 and 25 psi.

If the battery fails to last the usual three to four weeks of operation.

1. An incorrect battery has been used. Use only Alkaline batteries.

If the apnea alarm sounds and the red LED alarm flashes.

1. The patient is apneic. Check the patient.

2. The unit may be failing to detect inspiration.
   a. Check the cannula for correct position and application.
   b. Check the cannula for kinks or obstructions.

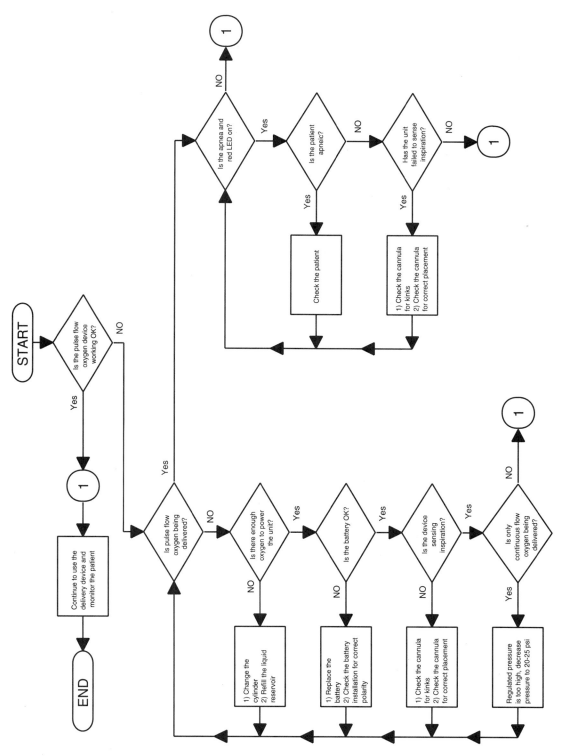

ALG 1-13 *An algorithm describing how to troubleshoot the Chad Therapeutics pulse flow delivery systems.*

flow on each breath, it is equivalent to what they have been receiving. As noted earlier in this section, it is important to conduct an oximetry trial to determine the oxygen needs of a patient who is using a conserving device.

Monitoring Systems: Oxymatic 301

The monitor on the Oxymatic 301 is a battery test indicator. To use the battery tester, move the thumbwheel selector on the top of the unit to the "Battery Test" position. Observe the indicator to assess the battery's condition. If the indicator is red, replace the battery before use. If the indicator is amber, you should have a replacement battery available to use. If the indicator is green, the battery has sufficient electrical energy to operate the unit. The Oxymatic 301 uses a common alkaline "C" size battery.

Monitoring Systems: Oxymatic 2400

The Oxymatic 2400 has a battery test feature, a low battery warning indicator and an apnea alarm. All of these conditions can be monitored on the top of the unit.

The battery test can be performed by moving the black rocker switch to the "ON/BATT" position while the unit is on. The "BATT TEST" display will indicate the battery's condition. If the display is dark green, the battery is in good condition. With use, the color of the green indicator becomes progressively lighter. When the display is amber in color, approximately 48 hours of battery life remains. If the indicator is red, 24 hours of life remains and the battery should be changed.

The low battery warning is a blinking LED display in the Indicator Setting window that resembles a battery. When the battery life falls to around 24 hours of continuous use, the low battery warning will flash intermittently. When this condition is observed, the battery should be changed as soon as possible.

Apnea detection is built into the Oxymatic 2400. If the unit fails to sense inspiration over a period of 40 seconds, the alarm system is activated. An audible and visual alarm will alert the user to this condition. A flashing red light labeled "ALARM" on the top of the unit will flash intermittently along with the audible alarm. Besides apnea, kinks in the patient's tubing or patient disconnects can also cause this alarm.

Transtracheal Catheter

A transtracheal catheter is a small catheter surgically inserted into the trachea at the second cartilage ring. By supplying oxygen flow directly into the trachea, this device can maintain F_IO_2 levels at a lower oxygen flow than with a nasal cannula. These devices are used primarily for patients who require continuous long-term oxygen therapy. The transtracheal catheter may use up to 59% less oxygen than conventional oxygen cannulas. This is because adequate PaO_2 levels (arterial oxygen tensions) may be achieved at oxygen flows as low as 1/4 liter per minute. Figure 1-52 shows

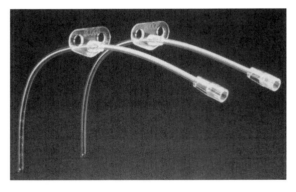

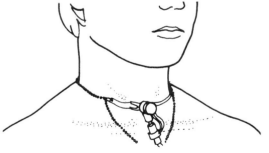

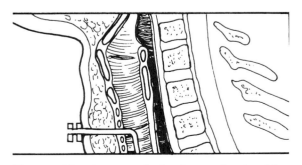

Figure 1-52 *A transtracheal catheter and a pictorial representation showing its correct placement.*

a transtracheal oxygen catheter and its placement.

Hazards involving the use of these devices include infection, subcutaneous emphysema and hemoptysis. Lower costs and cosmetic advantages must be carefully weighed against these potential hazards.

Simple Oxygen Mask

A simple oxygen mask is a lightweight mask applied to a patient's face. Figures 1-53 and 1-54 show a typical simple mask and how it is applied. The principle behind a simple mask is to add reservoir space (the mask) in addition to the anatomic reservoir. During the pause between exhalation and inspiration, the mask and anatomic reservoir fill with pure oxygen. During the first part of inspiration, pure oxygen is inhaled. During the later part, oxygen and room air are mixed in the mask and inhaled. As with nasal cannula use, F_IO_2 delivery varies depending upon tidal volume and respiratory rate. Typical oxygen delivery is between 35% and 55% oxygen at 6–12 L/min.

Since the patient also exhales into the mask, the mask may collect exhaled carbon dioxide. This is not desired. Therefore, it is important to maintain enough oxygen flow into the mask to flush the exhaled carbon dioxide, usually 6-12 liters per minute or greater, and monitor the patient.

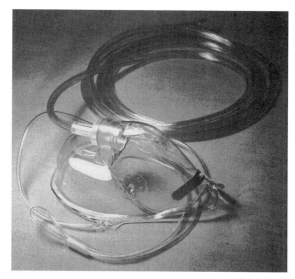

Figure 1-53 *A simple oxygen mask.*

delivered by this mask typically contains up to 60% oxygen. Oxygen flow is adjusted so that the reservoir bag is not allowed to fully collapse during inspiration.

The non-rebreathing mask is similar to the partial rebreathing mask except that one-way valves have been added to the mask's exhalation port(s) and between the mask and reservoir bag (Figure 1-56). The one-way valve between the mask and reservoir helps to prevent exhaled gas from mixing with the oxygen in the reservoir bag. The one-way valve on the

Partial Rebreathing and Non-Rebreathing Masks

The partial rebreathing and non-rebreathing masks are sometimes referred to as reservoir masks. A reservoir bag is added to the mask to provide an additional reservoir for oxygen.

The partial rebreathing mask (Figure 1-55) has a reservoir bag attached that is open to the mask. As the name implies, the patient rebreathes part of his exhaled gas. When the patient exhales, approximately the first third of expiration is from the anatomic dead space that has not participated in gas exchange and is rich in oxygen. It is this portion that fills the reservoir bag. The remaining exhaled gas exits through the exhalation ports. As the patient pauses between expiration and inspiration, additional oxygen flows into the mask and reservoir bag. When the patient inhales, a mixture of oxygen and air is inhaled. The oxygen

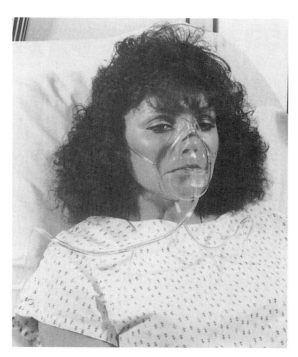

Figure 1-54 *A patient correctly wearing a simple oxygen mask.*

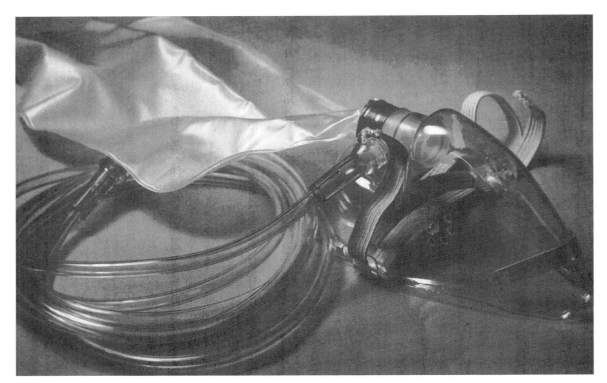

Figure 1-55 *A disposable partial rebreathing mask.*

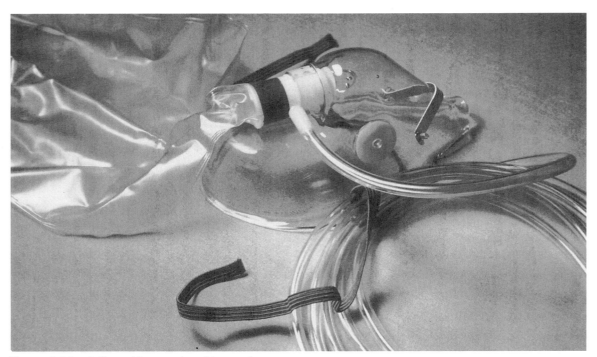

Figure 1-56 *A disposable non-rebreathing mask.*

exhalation port(s) closes during inspiration to prevent room air from entering the mask. Many manufacturers include only a single one-way valve on the side of the mask. In the event oxygen flow were to be interrupted, the patient may still inhale through the side port without the one-way valve.

The performance of the disposable non-rebreathing mask can vary considerably. The fit of the mask, operation of one-way valves, and oxygen flow may all contribute to decrease the F_IO_2 delivery. The disposable non-rebreathing masks can typically deliver oxygen concentrations of up to 70%.

ASSEMBLY AND TROUBLESHOOTING

Assembly—Oxygen Masks

Oxygen masks are quite common in clinical practice. Therefore, it is important to understand how to assemble and troubleshoot these oxygen administration devices correctly. The following is a suggested assembly guide.

1. Obtain an appropriate oxygen source (cylinder, piping system, liquid reservoir, or concentrator) with a flowmeter calibrated for an appropriate flow range.

2. Attach the flowmeter to the 50 psi oxygen source.

3. Adjust the flow to the ordered level or, when using a partial rebreathing or non-rebreathing mask, adjust the flow so the reservoir bag does not deflate during inspiration.

4. Placement of the oxygen therapy device:
   a. Place the mask on the bridge of the patient's nose first, adjusting the strap so it is snug but not too tight.
   b. If the mask is a reservoir type, ensure that the reservoir is free to expand without pressure from bed

covers or other objects.
   c. When using a non-rebreathing mask, check for proper operation of the one-way valves.

Troubleshooting

Troubleshooting oxygen masks consists of checking for leaks and proper flow from the mask. The following is a suggested troubleshooting algorithm (ALG 1-14).

1. Check the following sources for leaks:
   a. Check the connection between the flowmeter and the 50 psi gas source.
   b. Check the connection between the flowmeter and the humidifier.
   c. Check the connection between the connecting tube and the humidifier.

2. If gas fails to flow from the mask:
   a. Verify that the oxygen flowmeter is turned on and an adequate supply of gas exists.
   b. Check the oxygen connecting tube for kinks or obstructions.

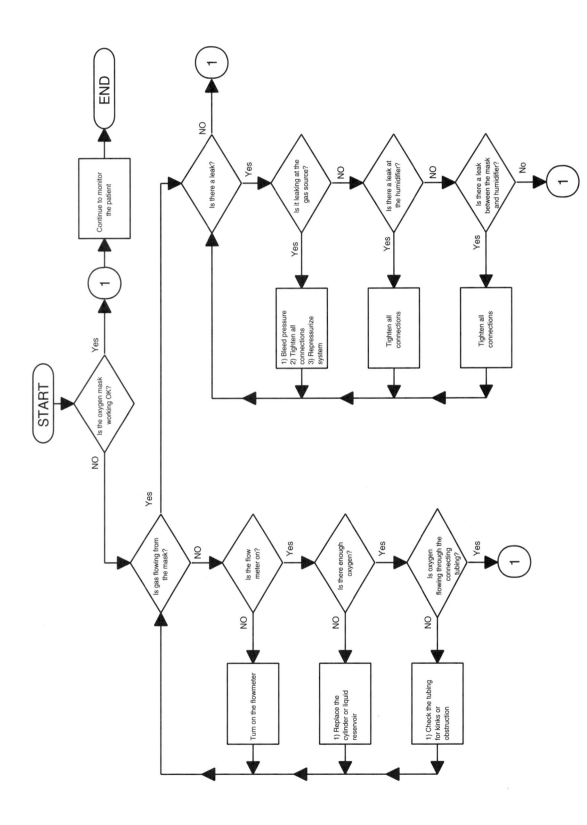

ALG 1-14 *An algorithm describing how to troubleshoot an oxygen mask.*

OXYGEN ENCLOSURES OR ENVIRONMENTAL DEVICES

Incubators

The incubator is a transparent box used to regulate an infant's environmental temperature. It also may be used to control the F_1O_2 (Figure 1-57). Due to the large volume of the incubator and the frequent nursing care an infant requires, it is difficult to maintain a consistent oxygen concentration. Therefore, these devices are rarely used for oxygen regulation, but rather are used to control the thermal environment.

Head Box

The head box is a transparent box designed to enclose an infant's head (Figure 1-58). Frequently, head boxes are used inside an isolette, with the isolette controlling the thermal environment and the head box providing the consistent F_1O_2. Flow is adjusted into the head box so that the infant will not entrain any room air around its neck. The gas entering the head box is premixed (usually using a blender) and then humidified and heated. Nebulizers are not recommended since noise levels may become excessive. Since the head box encloses the infant's head, the isolette may be opened for nursing care to other portions of the body without affecting the F_1O_2.

When delivering oxygen to an infant in a head box, it is important to analyze the F_1O_2. Using a calibrated oxygen analyzer (refer to Chapter 5 for the assembly, calibration and troubleshooting of oxygen analyzers), measure the oxygen concentration at the infant's face near the bottom of the head box. A variation of oxygen concentrations can occur between the bottom and top of the head box. If a variation is found, repeated measurements at various locations can determine how that particular hood "mixes" gases and what settings work best. Pulse oximetry and transcutaneous monitoring are also helpful to assure that the F_1O_2 delivered is adequate to maintain the patient's oxygen requirements.

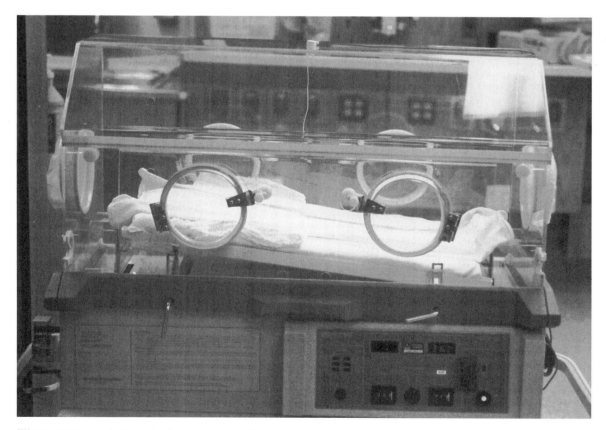

Figure 1-57 *A photograph of a contemporary incubator.*

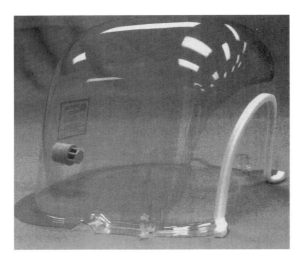

Figure 1-58 *A photograph of a head box.*

ASSEMBLY AND TROUBLESHOOTING

Assembly—Oxygen Hood/Head Box

Infants requiring a hood need close supervision and attention. Careful assembly and troubleshooting is important for optimal therapy. The following is a suggested assembly guide.

1. Choose a proper sized hood for the infant. Select one that covers the head without being too large.

2. Ensure a proper gas source for the blender or mixing device. Attach a flowmeter calibrated in the appropriate flow range.

3. Confirm correct blender assembly and operation as discussed earlier in the chapter.

4. Select an appropriate heated humidifier to meet inspiratory flow needs. Examples may include the Bear VH-820, Bird Humidifier, Conchapack, Fisher and Paykel MR450 or equivalent.

5. Connect large bore tubing to the outlet of the humidifier and to the head box. Provide a means of temperature monitoring at the inlet of the head box.

6. Verify oxygen concentration and flow using an oxygen analyzer and observing for flow.

Troubleshooting

Troubleshooting oxygen hoods primarily involves checking for leaks, ensuring flow, and monitoring temperature. When troubleshooting this equipment, please follow the suggested troubleshooting algorithm (ALG 1-15).

1. Sources for leaks:
   a. Between the gas source (piping system or regulator) and the high pressure hoses.
   b. Between the high pressure hoses and the blender.
   c. The connection between the blender and the humidifier.

2. Verify the oxygen concentration using an oxygen analyzer. If there is a tremendous discrepancy, calibrate the analyzer and repeat verification. If the discrepancy still exists, replace the blender and have the defective unit repaired by your local vendor or authorized biomedical repair facility.

3. Temperature monitoring:
   a. Many of the new humidifiers have provisions for servo control. A sensor automatically adjusts the temperature to the desired level. Even with servo control, it is important to monitor inlet temperatures.

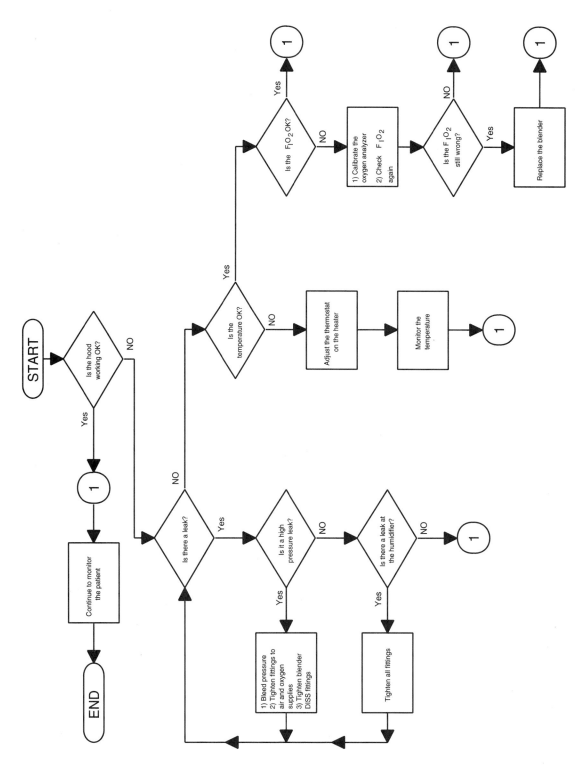

ALG 1-15 *An algorithm describing how to troubleshoot an oxygen hood.*

Mist Tents

Mist tents (croupettes) are plastic tents that are large enough to enclose a small child (Figure 1-59). The primary application of these tents is for aerosol therapy. However, the oxygen environment also may be controlled using these devices. The child's activity, opening and closing the tent for nursing care, and difficulty in sealing the tent all contribute to variations in the F_IO_2. These tents are usually powered by a high-output aerosol device. If additional oxygen is required, the oxygen may be bled in from a flowmeter or another nebulizer.

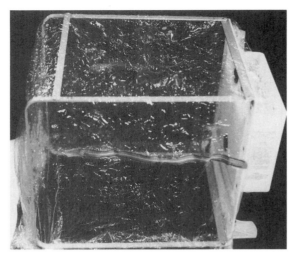

Figure 1-59 *A photograph of a croupette.*

ASSEMBLY AND TROUBLESHOOTING

Assembly—Croupette

Assembly of croupettes and mist tents will vary with manufacturers. The following is a suggested assembly guide.

1. Ensure a source of 50 psi gas to power the unit and an oxygen flowmeter.

2. Attach the canopy frame to the bed per manufacturer's instructions.

3. Attach the canopy to the frame following the manufacturer's instructions.

4. Fill the nebulizer with sterile distilled water.

5. Add ice to the reservoir as required or connect the cooling unit to an appropriately rated 110 volt electrical outlet.

6. Adjust the oxygen flow to between 12 and 15 liters per minute.

7. Place the infant into the canopy and tuck the edges under the mattress.

8. After 20 to 30 minutes, verify oxygen concentration and adjust as appropriate.

Troubleshooting

Troubleshooting croupettes consists of checking for leaks and verifying oxygen concentrations. When troubleshooting this equipment, please follow the suggested troubleshooting algorithm (ALG 1-16).

1. Sources for leaks:
   a. Check the connection between the flowmeter and oxygen connecting tube.
   b. Check the canopy seal between the mattress and the canopy.
   c. See if the canopy zippers are open.

2. Factors that affect oxygen concentration:
   a. Opening and closing the canopy frequently.
   b. Child's toys obstructing inlets or circulation outlets.

3. Fire hazards:
   a. Croupette canopies contain a large volume of oxygen, therefore children's toys should be limited to nonbattery operated toys and ones that do not generate sparks!

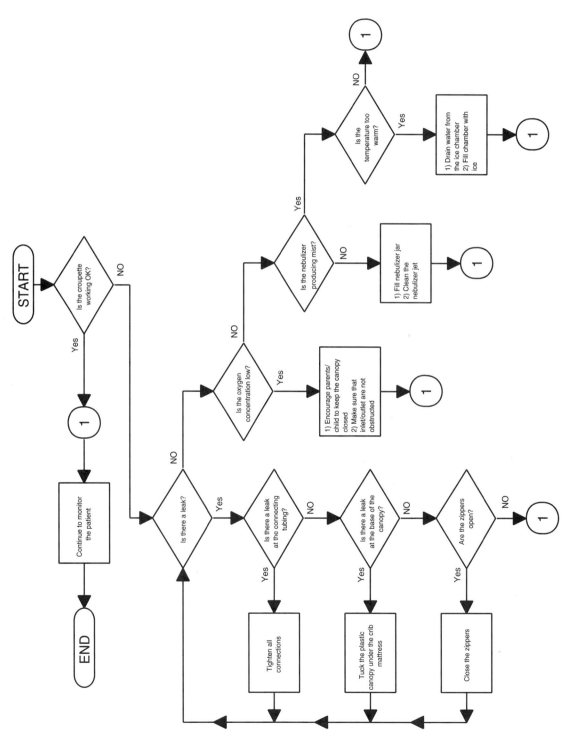

ALG 1-16 *An algorithm describing how to troubleshoot a croupette.*

HYPERBARIC OXYGEN THERAPY

Hyperbaric oxygen therapy, as defined by the Undersea Hyperbaric Medical Society (UHMS), is the exposure of a patient or patients to a pressure greater than one atmosphere absolute while breathing 100% oxygen either continuously or intermittently. This therapy was once confined to decompression sickness (caisson disease), but now has been utilized in the treatment of other disorders. The physiological effects of hyperbaric oxygen therapy include the mechanical effects as well as the oxygenation effects.

Physiological Effects of Hyperbaric Oxygen Therapy

The mechanical effects of hyperbaric oxygen therapy are related to the increased pressures. Any trapped gas bubbles, when exposed to the increased pressure during hyperbaric treatment, will decrease in size (Boyle's law). At a constant temperature (body temperature), the increased pressure causes the volume of the trapped gas bubbles to decrease. This effect is utilized in the treatment of decompression sickness and gas embolisms.

The oxygenation effects of hyperbaric oxygen therapy include the supersaturation of plasma, vasoconstriction, gas washout (gases other than oxygen), increased effectiveness of white blood cells and neovascularization tissue by improved collagen synthesis.

The supersaturation of the plasma occurs due to the increased partial pressure of oxygen under the hyperbaric conditions. PaO_2 levels can reach 1500 mmHg during therapy. This increase in plasma saturation improves oxygen transport even to areas with minimal perfusion.

Vasoconstriction during hyperbaric oxygen therapy has also been documented. It is not known how this occurs, but it is important in the management of localized "compartmented" disorders.

Increased elimination of other gases during hyperbaric treatment is possible due to the high driving force (partial pressure) of oxygen. Other gases, such as nitrogen and carbon monoxide, can be more quickly eliminated from the body by use of hyperbaric therapy than is possible at ambient pressures.

White blood cells have an increased ability to fight infections when exposed to hyperbaric oxygen therapy. It is thought that the increase in available oxygen results in increased oxida-

tive mechanisms which help the cells to perform their function better. Additionally, hyperbaric oxygen therapy is lethal to anaerobic microorganisms.

Neovascularization to poorly perfused tissues occurs as a result of hyperbaric oxygen therapy. The periodic increased oxygenation promotes the formation of fibroblasts, osteoblasts and granulocytes and collagen formation. This promotes capillary budding into areas that were previously not perfused, improving circulation. This effect has been helpful in the management of radiation necrosis of bone tissue, necrotizing fasciitis, gas gangrene and other difficult-to-manage wounds and disorders.

The accepted conditions that may benefit from hyperbaric oxygen therapy include:

- Gas gangrene
- Radiation necrosis
- Carbon monoxide / cyanide poisoning
- Ischemic tissue transplants
- Necrotizing soft tissue infections
- Decompression sickness
- Refractory osteomyelitis
- Refractory anaerobic infections
- Severe acute anemia or hemorrhage (blood loss anemia)
- Crush injury / Traumatic ischemia
- Ischemic tissue transplants
- Enhanced healing of problematic wounds

Equipment for Hyperbaric Oxygen Therapy

To delivery hyperbaric oxygen therapy, a specialized chamber is required. The two types of chambers are the multiplace and monoplace chambers.

The multiplace chamber is a large vessel that can accommodate more than one patient at a time. The chamber is pressurized with room air and the patient breathes oxygen via a non-rebreathing mask or other device. Additionally, these chambers allow for a health care provider to be with the patient during the therapy. The advantages of the multiplace chamber are that more than one patient can be treated simultaneously, and that the health care provider can treat any emergent conditions that may arise during treatment. The disadvantages of the multiplace chambers are that they are very large, and very expensive to purchase and maintain.

The monoplace chamber is a small chamber capable of treating only one patient at a

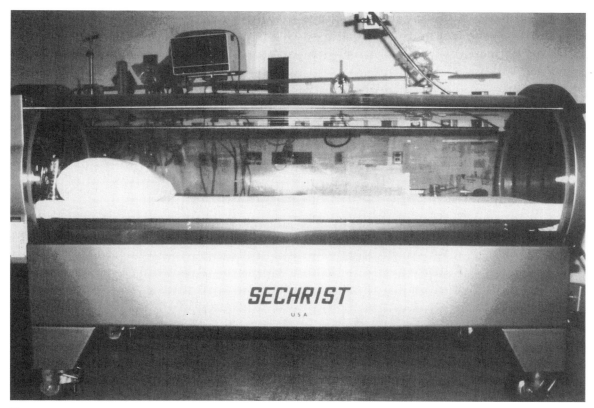

Figure 1-60 *A photograph of a monoplace hyperbaric chamber.*

time (Figure 1-60). Typically, these chambers are pressurized with oxygen, although air may also be used. They are much smaller and can be placed more conveniently than the multiplace chambers. The disadvantage of the monoplace chambers is that the health care provider must depressurize the chamber to treat any emergent problems that may arise during therapy.

Contraindications/Hazards

The only absolute contraindication for hyperbaric oxygen therapy is an untreated pneumothorax which occurred during therapy. During decompression, the gas in the pneumothorax will greatly expand (Boyle's law). It is important to provide a path for the gas to escape by the placement of a chest tube or needle thoracentesis.

Patients with upper respiratory infections may have difficulty clearing their ears during pressurization and decompression. Decongestants may help alleviate the problem. It may be required in some cases to delay treatment (if not emergent), until the upper respiratory infection subsides.

Patients with predisposed pulmonary disease, who air trap, may have difficulty with hyperbaric treatment. A slower decompression rate may assist these patients in eliminating gas as it expands due to decreased pressures.

Some patients may be unable to equalize pressures in their middle ears. Tympanic membrane rupture is possible during hyperbaric oxygen therapy. Some patients may require the placement of bilateral tympanotomy tubes for this type of therapy.

MIXED GAS THERAPY

He/O_2 Therapy

Helium/oxygen mixtures have been administered for some time in the treatment of obstructive airway diseases. The rationale is that a gas of lesser density can more easily bypass the obstruction and therefore be inspired with less effort and resistance. Gas mixtures are available in 20/80% and 30/70% oxygen-to-helium mixtures. The densities of the mixtures compared to oxygen are 1.8 (20/80%) and 1.6 (30/70%) times less dense, respectively.

A tight-fitting anesthesia bag-mask system is usually employed for therapy (see Figure 1-40). Gas flow is adjusted so that the reservoir bag never collapses. Typically, precise gas flow is not required. The purpose of the tight-fitting mask is to ensure that the lighter gas will not escape from the mask and avoid being inhaled.

If accurate flows are ordered, one can use the density difference to calculate what an oxygen flowmeter should read. The oxygen flowmeter setting is equal to the desired flow (ordered flow) divided by the density difference from oxygen (1.8 or 1.6). Alternatively, specially calibrated flowmeters can be purchased to be used with the specific gas mixtures.

Carbon Dioxide/Oxygen Therapy

CO_2/O_2 therapy has been used for many years for treatment of various disorders. The scientific rationale for such therapy, however, is questionable. This therapy is typically administered using a disposable, non-rebreathing mask. Gas mixtures are available in 5/95% and 7/93% carbon dioxide–to-oxygen mixtures. Therapy should be limited to between five and fifteen minutes at a time.

When administering this gas mixture, it is important to monitor the patient's heart rate, respiratory rate and blood pressure carefully. Alterations in these readings or a change in mental state would warrant discontinuation of therapy.

CLINICAL CORNER

Medical Gas Supply Equipment

1. You are on-call for a home care company that employs you as a respiratory care practitioner. A patient who was just set up at home on a liquid oxygen system calls with a complaint. Over the phone, Mr. Smith says: "My new oxygen bottle is hissing. I am worried it might explode." What should you tell your new client, and what would you recommend that he do?

2. You are preparing to transport a patient from the intensive care unit (ICU) to the floor. In order to do so, you set up an "E" cylinder to provide oxygen to his cannula. When you turn on the cylinder valve, you hear a leak. Describe the steps you would take to correct the problem.

3. You are setting up a new patient at home with an oxygen concentrator. The patient requests that she be allowed enough freedom of movement to reach the bathroom, the kitchen and her bedroom (the location of the concentrator). Describe how you would evaluate the concentrator's placement and any limitations you might impose regarding maximum lengths of extension tubing.

4. Describe a clinical situation in which you might select a single-stage reducing valve and another in which you

might select a two-stage reducing valve.

5. You are evaluating a patient for a pulsed-demand regulator for his portable oxygen system. Describe how you would appropriately evaluate him, state which of the devices discussed in the text is best for a given patient and explain why.

6. You are using a Bourdon gauge flowmeter for a helicopter transport. What safety precautions should you be aware of when using this type of regulator?

Medical Gas Therapy Equipment

1. Describe two clinical situations, one in which you would select a low-flow device and another in which you would select a high-flow device. Be specific regarding pathology, blood gases and respiratory assessment.

2. You adjust a patient's venturi mask from 40% to 50%. However, you observe that the patient is still desaturating, despite the higher oxygen concentration. Describe what you should evaluate to determine whether the mask is meeting the patient's needs.

3. You are called to set up a head box in the nursery for a newborn who is desaturating. What equipment should you take with you (assume that the unit has piped oxygen) and how would you set up the system?

Self-Assessment Quiz

1. "Gases being composed of discrete molecules in random motion" best describes:
   a. The ideal gas law.
   b. The kinetic theory of gases.
   c. Dalton's law.
   d. Charles' law.
   e. Bernoulli's principle.

2. The kinetic activity of gases is largely dependent upon:
   a. Their concentration.
   b. The pressure.
   c. The temperature.
   d. The type of gas.

3. Chambers A and B are connected by high-pressure tubing and separated by a valve. If chamber A contains 500 psi of gas and chamber B contains 50 psi of gas, what will occur when the valve is opened?
   a. The pressures in the chambers will remain equal.
   b. Chamber A will be pressurized by chamber B.
   c. Gas will flow from chamber A to chamber B until pressures equalize.
   d. The pressure in chamber B will increase to a level greater than in chamber A.
   e. Nothing will occur.

4. Pascal's law best describes:
   a. The relationship between volume and pressure of a gas.
   b. The relationship between pressure and temperature of a gas.
   c. The relationship between temperature and volume of a gas.
   d. The equal distribution of pressure transmitted by a fluid.

5. A device used clinically to measure small pressures is termed a:
   a. Mercury barometer.
   b. Aneroid barometer.
   c. Manometer.
   d. Thermometer.
   e. Reducing valve.

6. A Bourdon gauge:
   I. Uses a coiled tube.
   II. Uses a sealed diaphragm.
   III. Measures pressure.
   IV. Measures flow.
   a. I and II
   b. I and IV
   c. II and III
   d. II and IV

7. The statement, "As temperature increases, pressure also increases," best describes:
   a. Gay-Lussac's law.
   b. Dalton's law.
   c. Henry's law.
   d. Charles' law.
   e. Fick's law.

8. Bernoulli's theorem best describes:
   a. The relationship between temperature and pressure of a gas.
   b. The relationship between volume and pressure of a gas.
   c. An energy balance or conservation between velocity and pressure.
   d. The relationship between pressure of a gas and its ability to dissolve into a liquid.

9. An air entrainment mask operates by mixing source gas (oxygen) and room air. This device operates using:

a. Viscous shearing and vorticity.
b. Bernoulli's theorem.
c. Venturi's principle.
d. Poiseuille's law.

10. You are analyzing the F_iO_2 of a patient's HAFOE device, which reads 0.85. The entrainment port is set at 40%. Why would the analyzed oxygen concentration differ so much from the setting?
    a. The analyzer is malfunctioning.
    b. The patient's respiratory rate is affecting oxygen delivery.
    c. More room air is being entrained.
    d. There may be an obstruction distal to the entrainment port.

11. A gas's velocity is said to be choked when:
    a. Velocity can no longer increase.
    b. A maximum temperature is reached.
    c. Pressure is at a maximum.
    d. The concentration is at a maximum.

12. A patient with reactive airway disease is experiencing bronchospasm. The patient's work of breathing has dramatically increased in the last few minutes. This is an example of:
    I. Poiseuille's law.
    II. The Bernoulli theorem.
    III. Increased airway resistance.
    IV. Decreased lateral pressure.
    a. I and III
    b. I and IV
    c. II and III
    d. II and IV

13. You measure the volume of gas exiting a delivery device at 22 degrees Celsius to be 1.50 liters. The gas passes through a heater, warming it to 37 degrees Celsius. What is the actual volume delivered to the patient?
    a. 1.56 liters.
    b. 2.00 liters.
    c. 2.50 liters.
    d. 3.12 liters.

14. "The rate of gas diffusion into or out of a liquid is directly proportional to the partial pressure of the gas" best describes:
    a. Charles' law.
    b. Fick's law.
    c. Henry's law.
    d. Gay-Lussac's law.

15. Given the following gas mixture:
    Gas A = 20%
    Gas B = 50%
    Gas C = 30%
    Total pressure equals 600 mmHg.
    Find the partial pressure of Gas A.
    a. 10 mmHg.
    b. 20 mmHg.
    c. 80 mmHg.
    d. 60 mmHg.
    e. 120 mmHg.

16. Which of the following is constructed in a similar way to a thermos bottle?
    a. Oxygen cylinder.
    b. Oxygen concentrator.
    c. Liquid oxygen reservoir.
    d. Oxygen piping system.
    e. Air compressor.

17. Safety features incorporated into regulators or reducing valves include:
    I. DISS outlet.
    II. PISS inlet.
    III. American Standard inlet.
    IV. Pressure relief valve(s).
    a. I only
    b. I and II only
    c. II and III only
    d. I, II and III only
    e. I, II, III, and IV

18. Which of the following is (are) true for an "H" size oxygen cylinder?
    I. When full, it contains 2,200 psi.
    II. It contains 22 cubic feet of gas.
    III. It will have "3AA" stamped on the shoulder.
    IV. It contains 244 cubic feet of gas.
    a. I only
    b. I and II only
    c. I and III only
    d. I, III, and IV only
    e. I, II, and III only

19. The marking "3AA" indicates:
    a. The cylinder type.
    b. The contents of the cylinder.
    c. The cylinder serial number.
    d. The cylinder size.
    e. The manufacturer's code.

20. A device that mixes air and oxygen is termed a (an):
    a. Concentrator.
    b. Oxygen enricher.
    c. Oxygen proportioner.
    d. Compressor.
    e. Reducing valve.

21. When troubleshooting an oxygen concentrator, you find that the device is operating yet you are unable to obtain the desired flow of oxygen-enriched gas. Possible problems include:
    I. A tripped circuit breaker.
    II. Obstructed delivery tubing.
    III. Obstructed humidifier.
    IV. A dirty filter.
    a. I
    b. I and II
    c. II and III
    d. I and IV

22. When making a call on a home care patient, you weigh her liquid reservoir, which registers 80 lbs. You know the manufacturer's weight to be 60 lbs, and that your patient uses 3 L/min oxygen. How much gas does her reservoir contain, and can she wait for 5 hours before your company's delivery truck arrives when she has
    I. 12,340 L oxygen remaining?
    II. 5,484 L oxygen remaining?
    III. 30 hours' duration remaining?
    IV. 84 hours' duration remaining?
    a. I and III
    b. I and IV
    c. II and III
    d. II and IV

23. An advantage of using a demand pulse flow oxygen delivery system in the home care environment is:
    I. Less oxygen is used.
    II. It is less expensive for the patient.
    III. A humidifier is not required.
    a. I
    b. II
    c. I and II
    d. I, II and III

24. Back pressure will affect the accuracy of which of the following flowmeters?
    I. Compensated Thorpe tube.
    II. Uncompensated Thorpe tube.
    III. Bourdon flowmeter.
    a. I only
    b. I and II only
    c. I and III only
    d. II and III only
    e. I, II, and III only

25. Which of the following are low-flow oxygen delivery devices?
    I. Venturi mask.
    II. Nasal cannula.
    III. Anesthesia bag-mask.
    IV. Disposable non-rebreathing mask.
    a. I and II only
    b. II and III only
    c. II and IV only
    d. I and III only
    e. I and IV only

26. A venturi mask set at 24% oxygen with an oxygen flow of 4 L/min provides a total flow of:
    a. 40 L/min.
    b. 55 L/min.
    c. 88 L/min.
    d. 95 L/min.
    e. 104 L/min.

27. When checking on a patient wearing a partial rebreathing mask, you note that the bag deflates markedly during inspiration. You should:
    a. Not be concerned.
    b. Increase the oxygen flow.
    c. Leave the oxygen flow the same.
    d. Change the patient to a simple oxygen mask.

28. You must set up a patient in the emergency room on an oxygen delivery device administering a high F_IO_2 as quickly as possible. The best oxygen delivery device to use would be:
    a. A simple mask.
    b. A partial rebreathing mask.
    c. A disposable non-rebreathing mask.
    d. A venturi mask.

29. You must select an oxygen delivery device for a patient who is sensitive to small changes in F_IO_2. The patient requires moderate oxygen concentrations. However, if the patient's oxygen concentration varies much, she might rapidly desaturate. The best delivery device for this patient would be:
    a. A simple mask.
    b. A partial rebreathing mask.
    c. A disposable non-rebreathing mask.
    d. A venturi mask.

30. Hyperbaric oxygen therapy utilizes which gas law to achieve its effect?
    a. Boyle's law.
    b. Charles' law.
    c. Henry's law.
    d. Dalton's law.
    e. Gay-Lussac's law.

Selected Bibliography

Aloan, Claire A., *Respiratory Care of the Newborn*, J. B. Lippincott Company, 1987.

Beckham, Richard, et al., "Sound Levels inside Incubators and Oxygen Hoods Used with Nebulizers and Humidifiers," *Respiratory Care*, Vol. 27, No. 1, pp. 33–40, 1982.

Chad Therapeutics, *Product Information and Instructions for Use, Model 301 Oxymatic Electronic Oxygen Conserver*, Chad Therapeutics, Chatsworth, CA, 1993.

Chad Therapeutics, *Product Information and Instructions for Use, Model 2400 Oxymatic, Electronic Oxygen Conserver System*, Chad Therapeutics, Chatsworth, CA, 1993.

Chigier, Norman, *Energy, Combustion, and Environment*, McGraw-Hill Book Company, 1981.

Compressed Gas Association, *Handbook of Compressed Gases*, Van Nostrand Reinhold Company, 1981.

DeVilbiss Health Care, *DeVO/MC29 and DeVO/MC44 Patient Guide*, DeVilbiss Health Care, Inc., Somerset, PA, 1988.

DeVilbiss Health Care, *DeVilbiss DeVO/MC44-90 Oxygen Concentrator Service Manual*, DeVilbiss Health Care, Inc., Somerset, PA, 1987.

Grenard, Steve, *The Hazards of Respiratory Therapy Equipment*, Lenn Educational Medical Services, Inc., 1973.

Gonzales, Susan C., "Efficacy of the Oxymizer Pendant in Reducing Oxygen Requirements of Hypoxemic Patients," *Respiratory Care*, Vol. 31, No. 8, pp. 681–88, 1986.

Kerby, Gerald R., et al., "Clinical Efficacy and Cost Benefit of Pulse Flow Oxygen in Hospitalized Patients," *Chest*, Vol. 97, No. 2, pp. 369–72, 1990.

McPherson, Stephen, *Respiratory Therapy Equipment*, C. V. Mosby Company, 1985.

Miller, Franklin, Jr., *College Physics*, Harcourt Brace Jovanovich, 1972.

Pierson, David J., et al., *Foundations of Respiratory Care*, Churchill Livingstone, Inc., 1992.

Pulsair, *Oxygen Management Systems 20/50 Liquid Oxygen and High Pressure Oxygen, Service and Repair Manual*, Pulsair, Inc., Ft. Pierce, FL, 1990.

Puritan Bennett Corporation, *Companion 5 Oxygen Saver Operating Instructions*, Puritan Bennett Corporation, Lenexa, KS, 1989.

Puritan Bennett Corporation, *Puritan Bennett Companion 5 Oxygen Saver, Service Manual*, Puritan Bennett Corporation, Lenexa, KS, 1989.

Sacci, Robert, "Air Entrainment Masks: Jet Mixing Is How They Work; The Bernoulli and Venturi Principles Are How They Don't," *Respiratory Care*, Vol. 24, No. 10, pp. 928–31, 1979.

Shapiro, Barry A., *Clinical Application of Respiratory Care*, Year Book Medical Publishers, 1985.

Tiep, Brian L., et al., "Pulsed Nasal and Transtracheal Oxygen Delivery," *Chest*, Vol. 97, No. 2, pp. 364–68, 1990.

Ward, Jeffrey J., "Equipment for Mixed Gas and Oxygen Therapy," in T. A. Barnes et al. (eds.), *Respiratory Care Practice*, Year Book Medical Publishers, 1988.

CHAPTER 2

HUMIDITY AND AEROSOL THERAPY EQUIPMENT

——— INTRODUCTION ———

Many respiratory care procedures involve the administration of humidity or aerosol. Normally, humidification of inspired gases is physiologically accomplished in our upper airways. Medical gases are anhydrous (free of water) and must be humidified to prevent undesirable pathological consequences such as retained secretions, mucous plugging, and irritation.

Many pieces of equipment are used in respiratory care to humidify gases and produce aerosols. Each operates using several fundamental principles. In this chapter you will learn the physics of humidity, the principles of humidification and aerosol generation, and the equipment used to humidify gases and aerosolize liquids.

——— OBJECTIVES ———

After completing this chapter, the student will accomplish the following objective: be able to achieve a score of 80% or better on a written self-assessment quiz.

PHYSICS OF HUMIDITY AND AEROSOL THERAPY

- Define and differentiate between humidity and aerosol.
- Explain how humidity is measured.
- Define the term *evaporation*.
- Explain how a temperature increase can increase a gas's capacity for humidity.
- Define the term *humidity deficit,* and explain how humidity therapy may reduce it.
- Describe the physical characteristics of aerosols.
- Describe four factors that influence an aerosol particle's deposition in the pulmonary system.
- Explain how choked flow is applied to generate an aerosol.

HUMIDITY THERAPY EQUIPMENT

- Explain three ways a humidifier can be designed to increase its efficiency.
- Explain the principles of operation of the following types of humidifiers:
  — Pass-Over
  — Bubble and Bubble Jet
  — Misty Ox Laminar Diffuser Humidifier
  — Wick
  — Diffusion Grid (Cascade Type)
  — Heat and Moisture Exchangers

AEROSOL THERAPY EQUIPMENT

- Differentiate between a mainstream and a sidestream nebulizer.
- Explain the principles of operation of small volume nebulizers, their assembly, and how to troubleshoot them.
- Explain the principle of operation, assembly, and troubleshooting of large volume jet nebulizers.
- Explain the operation and application of metered dose inhalers (MDIs) and spacer devices.

- Explain the functional characteristics and application of the following aerosol delivery devices:
  — Aerosol mask
  — Trach mask
  — Face tent
  — Brigg's adapter
  — Drainage bag
- Explain the principle of operation of an ultrasonic nebulizer.

- Explain the assembly and troubleshooting of the following ultrasonic nebulizers.
  — DeVilbiss Model 65
  — DeVilbiss Ultra-Neb 99
  — Timeter Compu-neb
  — Small volume ultrasonic nebulizers for medication delivery.
- Describe the characteristics of a pediatric mist tent and its assembly and troubleshooting.

PHYSICS OF HUMIDITY AND AEROSOL THERAPY

HUMIDITY AND AEROSOLS

Humidity

Humidity is water that is in the gaseous state. Water vapor is composed of individual water molecules contained in a gas. Water vapor or humidity behaves in a similar way to gas molecules—it exerts a pressure and is in constant random motion. In order to calculate the partial pressure of a gas containing humidity, the partial pressure of water vapor must be accounted for when adding the partial pressures. For example, when calculating the partial pressures of ambient air that is fully saturated with water vapor, the partial pressure of the water vapor must be accounted for (Dalton's law of partial pressures).

Barometric pressure
$$= 760 \text{ mmHg}$$
Partial pressure of H_2O at 24° Celsius
$$= 23.8 \text{ mmHg}$$
760 mmHg – 23.8 mmHg
$$= 736.2 \text{ mmHg}$$
(partial pressure of gases)
Partial pres. of O_2
$$= 736.2 \times .2095 = 154.23$$
Partial pres. of N_2
$$= 736.2 \times .7808 = 574.83$$
Partial pres. of Ar
$$= 736.2 \times .0093 = \quad 6.85$$
Partial pres. of CO_2
$$= 736.2 \times .0003 = .22$$
Inert gases
$$= 736.2 \times .0001 = .07$$

Aerosols

An *aerosol* by definition is particulate matter suspended in a gas. The particulate matter can be liquid or solid. An example of an aerosolized solid is Cromolyn sodium, a medication that can be delivered in powdered form and inhaled while suspended. Liquids are aerosolized in clinical practice both for bland aerosol therapy (primarily for the hydration of the pulmonary tract) and for administration of medications directly to the pulmonary system.

MEASUREMENT OF HUMIDITY

Humidity can be quantified several ways, including actual content in grams or milligrams of water, partial pressure of water vapor, and relative humidity.

Water Content or Absolute Humidity

Desiccants are compounds that absorb water. By drying a desiccant so that it is anhydrous (without any water content) and weighing it, then passing a gas through it so that the water is removed from the gas, one can determine the actual water content of the gas. The difference in weight before and after passing the gas through the desiccant would equal the water content of the gas. As you recall from basic physics or chemistry classes, one gram of water equals one milliliter of water. The process of measuring water content has been done for gases at various temperatures, a sample of which is shown in Table 2-1. Notice that as temperature increases, the ability of a gas to hold water also increases. The actual water content when a gas is fully saturated is termed *maximum absolute humidity* or *capacity*.

Partial Pressure

Water vapor behaves like a gas. The random motion of water molecules exerts a pressure in a way similar to gas exerting pressure (see Chapter 1, Dalton's law). Therefore, it is possible to measure the partial pressure water vapor exerts at various contents and pressures (Table 2-1). As the temperature of a gas increases, kinetic activity increases, so the pressure also increases.

The magnitude of the pressure exerted by water vapor is independent of the barometric pressure. Its magnitude is solely dependent upon temperature and relative humidity. Therefore, at a given temperature and relative humidity, the partial pressure of water vapor is a constant regardless of the barometric pressure. The partial pressure of water vapor must always be accounted for (subtracted), when calculating the partial pressures of other gases in a mixture.

Relative Humidity

Relative humidity is humidity expressed as a percentage of a gas's capacity (water content when fully saturated). The capacity may be determined by using tables such as Table 2-1. Relative humidity is derived by dividing the actual water content of a gas by its capacity at that temperature, as shown in the following equation.

$$\text{Relative humidity} = \frac{\text{Actual humidity}}{\text{Capacity}}$$

Example: You are administering a humidified gas containing 23 mg/L water. The temperature of the gas is 30° Celsius. What is the relative humidity of the gas you are administering?

$$\begin{aligned}\text{Relative humidity} &= \frac{\text{Actual humidity}}{\text{Capacity}} \\ &= \frac{23 \text{ mg/L}}{30.35 \text{ mg/L}} \\ &= .757 \text{ or } 75.7\%\end{aligned}$$

Example: The local radio announcer states that it is 30° Celsius and the relative humidity is 45%. What is the actual humidity?

$$\begin{aligned}\text{Relative humidity} &= \frac{\text{Actual humidity}}{\text{Capacity}} \\ \text{Actual humidity} &= \text{Relative humidity} \\ &\quad \times \text{Capacity} \\ &= .45 \times 30.35 \text{ mg/L} \\ &= 13.66 \text{ mg/L}\end{aligned}$$

Note: 30.35 mg is the capacity at 30° C (from Table 2-1).

EVAPORATION

Evaporation is the process of water moving from a liquid to a gaseous state. Molecules in a liquid, like those in a gas, are in random motion. The kinetic energy of molecules in a liquid, however, is less than the kinetic energy of molecules in a gas. There are also variations in the energy levels of molecules within a liquid.

TABLE 2-1 Water Content and Pressures at Different Temperatures

TEMPERATURE (° CELSIUS)	WATER CONTENT (MG/L) CAPACITY	PARTIAL PRESSURE (TORR)
0	4.85	4.58
5	6.80	6.54
10	9.40	9.20
15	12.83	12.79
20	17.30	17.51
25	23.04	23.69
30	30.35	31.71
35	39.60	42.02
37	43.90	47.00
40	51.10	55.13
45	65.60	71.66
50	83.20	92.30

Adapted from Table 17-2, Burton, Hodgkin, and Gee, Respiratory Care: A Guide to Clinical Practice, *J. B. Lippincott, 1984. Reprinted with permission.*

Those molecules with sufficient kinetic energy will overcome the attractive forces between molecules in the liquid and escape as vapor. When those molecules with sufficient energy escape from the liquid, the overall energy level of the liquid declines, and the temperature decreases (evaporative heat loss). When this occurs at room temperature, heat from the ambient air transfers to the liquid, restoring the energy level and the process is repeated until the liquid is gone.

As the temperature of a liquid is increased, the kinetic activity of its molecules is also increased. Therefore, more molecules will have sufficient energy to escape as vapor.

HUMIDITY DEFICIT

Humidity deficit is a physiological term that refers to the difference between the inspired gas's water content and the water content of a gas at body temperature and pressure. At body temperature and pressure saturated (BTPS), inspired gas is at 37° Celsius, contains 43.9 mg/L of water, exerts a partial pressure of 47 mmHg, and is fully saturated. These conditions at BTPS are termed body humidity. Humidity deficit then is the difference between body humidity and the actual humidity of the inspired gas as illustrated in the following formula.

Humidity deficit
= Body humidity – Actual humidity

Example: You are administering a gas at 25° Celsius with a relative humidity of 50%. What is the humidity deficit?

(a) Fully saturated, a gas at 25° C contains 23.04 mg/L.
Relative humidity × Capacity
= Actual humidity
.50 × 23.04 mg/L = 11.52 mg/L
(b) Humidity deficit
= Body humidity – Actual humidity
= 43.9 mg/L – 11.52 mg/L = 32.38 mg/L

Humidity deficit becomes clinically significant when it is large and is sustained for a prolonged period of time. Pathological changes occur in the pulmonary system causing retention of secretions, airway plugging, or obstruction and infection with pathogenic bacteria.

Since medical gases are anhydrous, it is important to humidify the gases before they are administered. Proper humidification of inspired gases will reduce the humidity deficit and prevent any adverse pathological changes from occurring.

PHYSICAL CHARACTERISTICS OF AEROSOLS

As discussed earlier, aerosols are particles suspended in a gas. Clinically liquids are aerosolized more frequently than solids. Therefore, the majority of this discussion will focus on the aerosolization of liquids.

Particle Size and Mass

As the size of an aerosol particle increases, so does its mass. If the radius of a sphere doubles, the volume will increase approximately eight times ($V = 4 \times k \times r^3$). As volume increases, mass will increase proportionally. Therefore, an increase or reduction in the size of a particle will dramatically change its mass. As the mass of the aerosol particle decreases, gravity will have less effect on it and it will remain suspended longer.

PHYSICAL NATURE OF PARTICLES

A discussion of the physical nature of aerosol particles is important in understanding how they behave clinically. Physical factors include its tonicity, its electric charge, and whether a particle is hygroscopic. As you will learn later, physical features influence a particle's ability to remain suspended and how deeply it penetrates the pulmonary system.

Hygroscopic

If an aerosol is *hygroscopic,* it has a tendency to absorb water. As the particle absorbs water, it increases in size and mass. When inhaled, hygroscopic aerosols will deposit in the pulmonary system sooner than non-hygroscopic aerosols. This is because the particles will coalesce or combine, forming larger particles with greater mass, which will no longer remain in suspension.

Tonicity

Tonicity refers to the concentration of solutes in a solution relative to their concentration in body fluids. A hypertonic solution will gain water from body fluids, due to its greater concentration of solutes. An isotonic solution will remain stable (neutral toward water absorption), since solute concentrations are similar to body fluids. A hypotonic solution will lose water, since its solute concentrations are less than that of body fluids.

Hypertonic solutions (> .9% NaCl) absorb water. When aerosolized they become hygroscopic, increasing in size as discussed earlier.

Isotonic solutions (.9% NaCl), when aerosolized, are neutral in their affinity to water. Therefore, particle sizes tend to remain stable.

Hypotonic solutions (< .9% NaCl) release water and, when aerosolized, decrease in size. As their size decreases, so does their mass.

Electrical Charge

Due to the methods employed to aerosolize liquids, the aerosol particles become electrically charged. Electrical charge seems to have little effect physiologically; however, it may have significant effect on the function of surrounding electrical equipment.

FACTORS INFLUENCING AEROSOL DEPOSITION IN THE AIRWAYS

Many factors influence an aerosol's ability to deposit into the pulmonary system. These factors include: (1) particle size and gravitational effects, (2) inertia, (3) temperature and humidity and (4) the patient's respiratory pattern (Table 2-2).

Particle Size and Gravity

As particle size and mass increase, gravitational forces act on the particle to a greater degree, tending to remove it from suspension. Ideally, all particles should be small enough that effects of gravity are minimal. However, when particles become too small, they remain suspended and never deposit in the pulmonary system. Particle sizes between 1 and 5

TABLE 2-2 Factors that Influence Aerosol Stability and Penetration into the Airways

---

Particle size and mass

Hygroscopic properties

Tonicity

Inertia

Temperature and humidity of the delivery gas

Patient's respiratory pattern

---

microns are clinically optimal for peripheral deposition in the respiratory bronchioles.

Inertia

Inertia is also related to particle size and mass. As Newton stated, inertia equals mass times velocity. A particle with greater mass, when placed in motion, will have a greater inertia than a particle with a smaller mass. Newton also stated that once an object is placed in motion, it tends to stay in motion unless acted upon by an outside force. An aerosol particle with a large mass will tend to travel in a straight line even if the gas suspending it changes direction. Larger particles will be removed from suspension in the upper airways, and not penetrate further into the pulmonary system. Smaller particles with less mass will travel further into the lungs.

Temperature and Humidity

As the temperature of the *carrier gas* (the gas conducting the suspended aerosol particles) increases with humidity held constant, the aerosol particles will have a tendency to evaporate into the carrier gas. If the aerosol is introduced into a humid carrier gas, the particles will coalesce (combine), forming larger particles.

Respiratory Pattern

A significant factor influencing pulmonary deposition of aerosols is the patient's respiratory pattern. A slow deep inspiration followed by a brief pause before exhalation will increase aerosol deposition into the lungs. An example of this desired effect can be illustrated by the administration of bronchodilators. Maximal penetration and deposition is desired to reduce bronchospasm. Good patient instruction and monitoring can influence the effectiveness of aerosol therapy to a large degree. If a patient is properly instructed, the patient can inhale slowly to a larger than normal tidal volume, and hold his/her breath at end inspiration. By modifying the breathing pattern in this way, aerosol penetration and deposition can be maximized.

APPLICATION OF CHOKED FLOW

Choked flow is applied in many aerosol generators to produce an aerosol. As described in Chapter 1, choked flow occurs when a gas's velocity through a nozzle can no longer be increased by increasing the head pressure. When the flow is choked, the flow at the nozzle exit is sonic. Liquids may be entrained into the gas flow by placing a capillary tube into the boundary layer near the nozzle exit.

Liquid is drawn from the reservoir, up the capillary tube and into the gas stream by a combination of shear forces, vorticity and a pressure differential (Figure 2-1). The shear forces are the greatest within a distance of three times the diameter of the nozzle's opening. The effect of vorticity is most pronounced once the boundary layer becomes turbulent, and vortices form. The pressure differential is created by the removal of fluid from the capillary tube at the top by shear forces and vorticity. Since the base of the tube is occluded (immersed in water), the removal of fluid (mass) at the top results in a region of low pressure within the capillary tube. The greater pressure at the base of the capillary tube (atmospheric pressure) forces water up the tube, filling the void (conservation of mass). Once the liquid reaches the top of the capillary tube, it is continuously entrained into the high velocity gas by shear forces and vorticity. Once entrained, the liquid is instantly broken up into an aerosol with a wide range of particle sizes.

The *baffle* distal to the jet and capillary tube stabilizes the aerosol particle size by *inertial impaction*. A baffle may consist of a ball or a wall downstream from the nozzle exit. As discussed earlier, the aerosol particles with a large volume have a large mass. As the gas flow changes direction around the baffle, the large particles resist changes in direction and impact against the baffle. Only smaller particles with small masses are able to follow the gas flow around the baffle and remain suspended. The difference between an atomizer and a nebulizer is that an *atomizer* does not have a baffle to stabilize particle size. A *nebulizer* has a baffle and is therefore able to better control the particle size.

HUMIDITY THERAPY EQUIPMENT

FACTORS INFLUENCING HUMIDIFIER EFFICIENCY

There are three factors that can be applied in the design of *humidifiers* to increase their efficiency. These are temperature, surface area for gas-to-liquid contact, and the time that the gas is exposed to the liquid. Manufacturers utilize these factors to improve the clinical efficiency of their humidifiers.

Temperature

By increasing the temperature of the liquid, the molecules' kinetic activity increases. As the molecules gain energy, more of them will have enough energy to escape as a vapor, increasing the humidity output.

Furthermore, as the temperature of the solution is increased, the temperature of the gas is also increased as it passes over the solution. A warm gas has a greater capacity for water vapor than a cold gas.

Surface Area

Surface area for gas-to-water contact is also an important factor in determining humidity. Increasing the surface area for contact will increase the humidity.

Time for Contact

The time that the gas is allowed to interface with the solution also influences humidity. If the time for contact can be increased, humidity also will be increased. Slowing the flow of gas may not be desired since many clinical applications require high flows, in excess of 50 liters per minute.

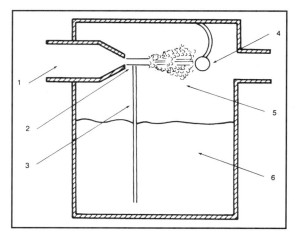

Figure 2-1 *A functional diagram of a pneumatic nebulizer. (1) The high pressure nozzle. (2) Area of maximum shear force. (3) Capillary tube. (4) Baffle. (5) Area of vorticity (approximately three nozzle diameters from the nozzle exit). (6) Reservoir.*

HUMIDIFIERS

Room Humidifier

Contemporary room humidifiers employed in clinical practice are, in reality, aerosol generators. The majority of these devices operate using centrifugal force. The aerosol exiting the device evaporates in the ambient air, increasing the humidity of the room.

Centrifugal force is applied using a spinning disk (Figure 2-2). As an electric motor spins the disk, water is drawn up through the

---

ASSEMBLY AND TROUBLESHOOTING

Assembly—Room Humidifiers

Room humidifiers are quite simple and have few moving parts. The following is a suggested assembly guide.

1. Remove the motor housing from the humidifier and fill the reservoir with water to the correct level indicated on the side of the unit.

2. Replace the motor housing with the hollow shaft immersed in the water reservoir.

3. Connect the power cord to a suitable 110 volt outlet and turn on the humidifier.

4. Observe for aerosol output.

Troubleshooting

Since these humidifiers are simple in their operation, troubleshooting them is quite easy. However, if the unit fails to operate, little can be done by the respiratory care practitioner to correct malfunctions. When troubleshooting this equipment, please follow the suggested troubleshooting algorithm (ALG 2-1).

1. If the humidifier fails to produce adequate aerosol and the motor functions properly:
   a. First disconnect the power.
   b. Check the outlet for obstructions.
   c. Be certain the reservoir is filled properly.
   d. Check the breaker combs for integrity. If the breaker combs are broken or absent, replace the unit or take it to an authorized repair center.

2. If the motor fails to operate:
   a. Check the integrity of the electrical outlet by using another electrical device to test it.
   b. If the electrical outlet is good and the motor still fails to operate, replace the unit or take it to an authorized repair center.

3. Clean the humidifier daily and change the water at least twice each day.

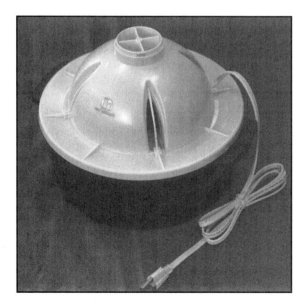 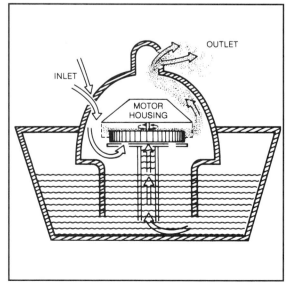

Figure 2-2 *A photograph and a functional diagram of a centrifugal room humidifier.*

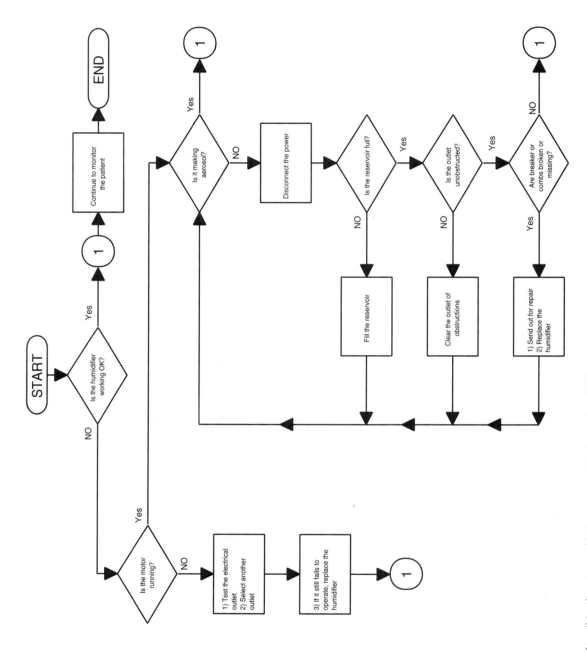

ALG 2-1 *An algorithm describing how to troubleshoot a centrifugal room humidifier.*

hollow shaft by capillary action. When the water encounters the spinning disk, it is thrown outward by centrifugal force. The breaker combs surrounding the spinning disk shatter the water particles, producing an aerosol. The evaporating aerosol causes the humidity of the room to increase.

Large amounts of air pass through this type of humidifier, making it a potential source of nosocomial infections. The large water reservoir is also a source for bacterial growth or contamination. When these devices are used, it is important to keep them clean and change the water in the reservoir frequently.

Pass-Over Humidifier

The pass-over humidifier is the simplest of all the humidifiers. Gas flow passes over a reservoir of water. Water evaporates into the gas, increasing the humidity of the gas. Efficiency of these humidifiers can be increased by heating the water, increasing the rate of evaporation. Figure 2-3 shows this type of humidifier, which is used in the Emerson 3-PV adult ventilator.

ASSEMBLY AND TROUBLESHOOTING

The simplicity of these humidifiers facilitates assembly and troubleshooting.

Assembly—Pass-Over Humidifier

1. Separate the top and bottom portions of the humidifier and fill it to the correct level with sterile distilled water.

2. Reconnect the top and bottom portions of the humidifier.

3. Ensure that the heating element is connected properly.

Troubleshooting

When troubleshooting this equipment, please follow the suggested algorithm (ALG 2-2).

1. If humidity output is inadequate:
   a. Check for obstructions at the outlet of the humidifier.
   b. Be certain the reservoir is filled properly.
   c. Check the heating element for proper operation. If it is not operating properly, check power connections and any fuses or circuit breakers on the ventilator.

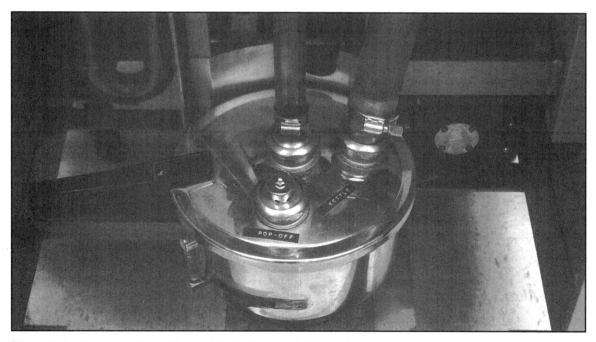

Figure 2-3 *A pass-over humidifier used in the Emerson 3-PV ventilator.*

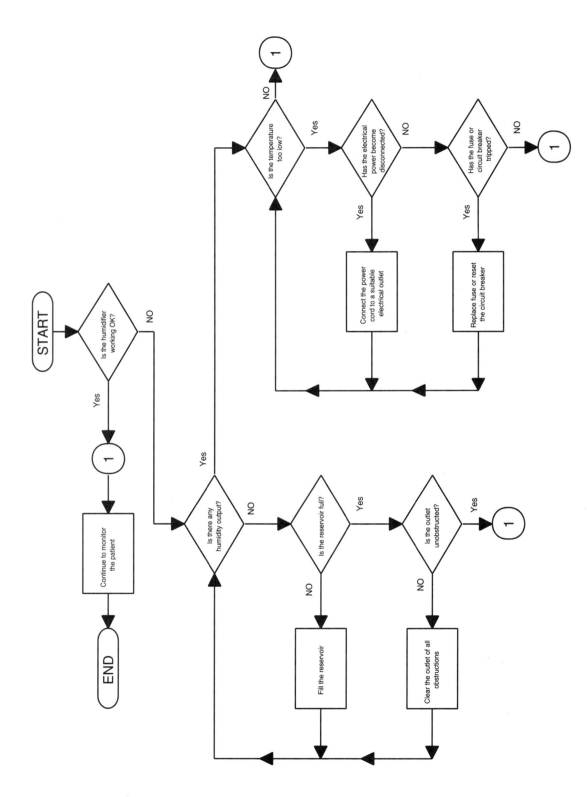

ALG 2-2 *An algorithm describing how to troubleshoot a pass-over humidifier.*

Bubble Humidifier

The majority of the disposable humidifiers used for oxygen therapy are bubble humidifiers. Efficiency and output vary, depending on many factors. These factors include liter flow through the humidifier, ambient temperature, and time of operation. The output of these devices may vary from 33 to 40% relative humidity at 37° Celsius.

These humidifiers operate by bubbling gas up through a reservoir of water (Figure 2-4). Gas enters the humidifier through the DISS fit-

ASSEMBLY AND TROUBLESHOOTING

Bubble humidifiers are the most common humidifiers utilized in respiratory care. There are numerous models and manufacturers producing these devices. Disposable humidifiers are available both prefilled with sterile water and unfilled. Construction of these humidifiers varies, as does their assembly. Follow the manufacturer's instructions when assembling these units for clinical use. The following assembly guide will apply to the majority of the humidifiers in use today.

Assembly—Bubble Humidifiers

1. Disposable humidifiers are packaged aseptically in a plastic wrap. Open the package and remove the parts, maintaining aseptic technique.

2. Most humidifiers come in two parts (see Figure 2-6). The top portion consists of the DISS oxygen fitting, pressure relief, and oxygen nipple outlet. The bottom part is the water reservoir.

Prefilled:

   a. Attach the top portion to the bottom following the manufacturer's recommendations.
   b. When the parts are attached, gently squeeze the sides of the reservoir, listening for gas escaping through the outlet. By doing this you can be assured that the reservoir has been properly pierced by the top part of the humidifier.
   c. Attach the humidifier to the DISS fitting on a flowmeter.
   d. Attach the oxygen therapy equipment to the outlet of the humidifier.
   e. Adjust the flowmeter to the desired oxygen flow rate.

   f. Check for oxygen flow and bubbles in the reservoir.
   g. Check the safety relief valve by obstructing the oxygen connecting tube. Pinch it or aseptically obstruct the humidifier outlet.

Non-prefilled:

   a. Aseptically fill the reservoir to the indicated level using sterile distilled water.
   b. Attach the top portion to the reservoir, following the manufacturer's instructions.
   c. Attach the humidifier to the DISS fitting on a flowmeter.
   d. Attach the oxygen therapy equipment to the nipple outlet of the humidifier.
   e. Adjust the flowmeter to the desired oxygen flow rate.
   f. Check the safety relief valve by obstructing the oxygen connecting tube. Pinch it or aseptically obstruct the humidifier outlet.

Troubleshooting

When troubleshooting this equipment, please follow the suggested troubleshooting algorithm (ALG 2-3).

If oxygen fails to flow from the humidifier:

1. Check to ensure that the flowmeter is turned on.

2. If the humidifier is prefilled, ensure that the reservoir has been pierced and that gas can flow through it.

3. Check the outlet for obstructions.

4. Check the oxygen containing tubing for obstructions or kinks.

5. If (1) through (4) are satisfactory, replace the humidifier.

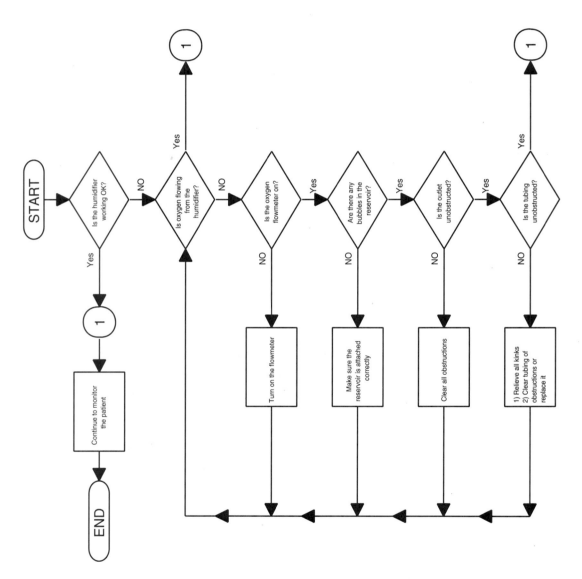

ALG 2-3 *An algorithm describing how to troubleshoot a bubble humidifier.*

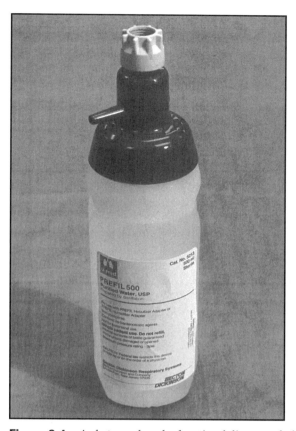

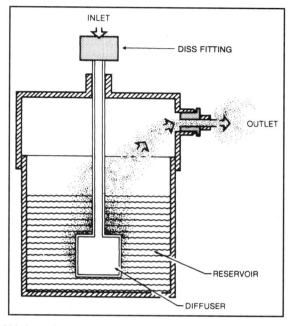

Figure 2-4 *A photograph and a functional diagram of a bubble humidifier.*

ting on the top of the unit. Gas flows down through a hollow tube to a diffusing element. The diffuser breaks the gas flow up into small bubbles. As the gas bubbles float to the surface, the water evaporates into them. The efficiency of these humidifiers is improved by the diffuser, which increases surface area and the time the gas is allowed to interface with the water.

A safety relief valve is incorporated into the upper housing of the humidifier to relieve pressure in the event the gas path becomes obstructed. Most of these relief valves operate at 2 psi. Many manufacturers incorporate an audible whistle alarm to alert practitioners when the relief is activated.

Ohmeda Ohio Jet Humidifier

The Ohmeda Ohio Jet Humidifier is a very efficient underwater jet bubble humidifier. This humidifier incorporates an aerosol generator with a bubble humidifier.

Gas flows into the humidifier through a DISS fitting on the top of the unit (Figure 2-5), then passes through a jet, below the surface of the water. The jet, using Bernoulli's principle, creates an aerosol. Bubbles containing aerosol generated from the jet form when the gas

passes through the diffuser. The bubbles float to the surface of the reservoir, absorbing more water. The presence of aerosol in the bubbles increases this device's efficiency. Gas flows from the reservoir through a nipple outlet where oxygen therapy equipment is attached.

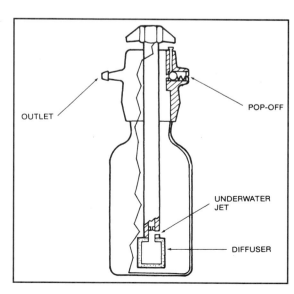

Figure 2-5 *A partial section of a bubble-jet humidifier.*

ASSEMBLY AND TROUBLESHOOTING

Assembly—Ohmeda Jet Humidifier

1. Separate the top and bottom portions of the humidifier by unscrewing the top.

2. Aseptically fill the reservoir to the indicated level using sterile distilled water.

3. Reconnect the top and bottom portions of the humidifier.

4. Attach the DISS fitting to a flowmeter.

5. Connect the oxygen tubing to the nipple outlet of the humidifier.

6. Turn on the flowmeter to the desired setting.

7. Check for bubbles and oxygen flow.

8. Check the safety relief valve by aseptically obstructing the outlet or pinching the oxygen connecting tube.

Troubleshooting

When troubleshooting this equipment, please follow the suggested troubleshooting algorithm (ALG 2-4).

If output is inadequate:

1. Check to ensure that the flowmeter is turned on.

2. Check to be sure the reservoir is filled.

3. Check the outlet for obstructions.

4. Check the oxygen connecting tube for obstructions or kinks.

5. If (1) through (4) are satisfactory, replace the humidifier. Remove the defective unit from service and take it to an authorized biomedical repair center.

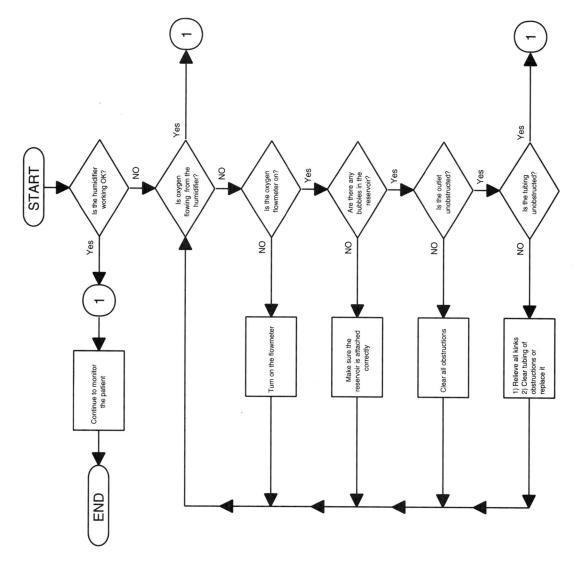

ALG 2-4 *An algorithm describing how to troubleshoot a bubble-jet humidifier.*

Misty Ox Laminar Diffuser Humidifier

Medical Molding Corporation of America (Misty Ox), has designed a new disposable humidifier which incorporates some unique features. The humidifier is unique in that aerosol produced by a high output nebulizer is evaporated into the gas flowing through the device, producing high humidity outputs, at high flow rates. When combined with the TurboHeater, the Laminar Diffuser Humidifier (LDH) is capable of producing heated molecular high humidity (HMHH) at flows of up to 80 L/min.

The design of the humidifier incorporates the Misty Ox Gas Injection Nebulizer (GIN) head (discussed later in this chapter) to produce a dense aerosol at high flow rates. The aerosol output from the nebulizer is directed downward into two perforated disks (Figure 2-6), which form an evaporation chamber. The perforated disks increase the turbulence of the gas/aerosol mixture flowing through them, while the large surface areas presented by the square-shaped perforations in the disks cause the suspended aerosol to deposit onto the disks, forming a thin film of water. Turbulent gas flowing through the disks, and the chamber created between them, evaporates the thin film of water, increasing the relative humidity of the gas. Gas flow is directed down through a converging duct into a conical-shaped mixing chamber. The shape of this chamber causes the gas to flow through it in a swirling pattern. Positioned along the outer wall of this mixing chamber are radially spaced baffles. The baffles further remove aerosol particles from the flowing gas by inertial impaction. The gas is then discharged through a short piece of tubing into the accumulator chamber where the gas comes into contact with the heater platen of

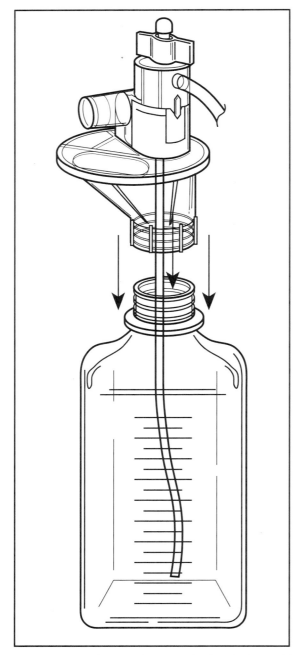

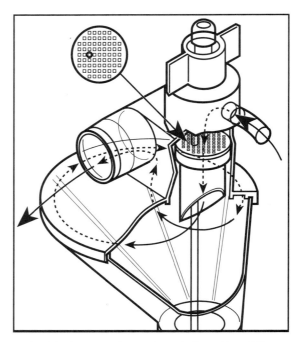

Figure 2-6 *A functional diagram (left) and a detailed diagram (right) of a Misty Ox Laminar Diffuser Humidifier*

ASSEMBLY AND TROUBLESHOOTING

Assembly—Misty Ox LDH Humidifier

1. Remove the cap from the sterile distilled water bottle you wish to use as a reservoir.

2. Aseptically remove the Laminar Diffuser Humidifier (LDH) from its package. Use caution not to contaminate the long capillary tube which will be immersed into the sterile reservoir.

3. Insert the capillary tube into the bottle and screw the nebulizer into place using the 38 mm threaded fitting. Make sure that the nebulizer is on tight and is not cross threaded.

4. Connect the primary gas source (DISS fitting on the top of the LDH) to a flowmeter (air or oxygen) or an oxygen blender. Be certain that you have screwed the DISS fittings together tightly, to preserve flow to the patient.

   a. If oxygen and air flowmeters are used for the primary and secondary gas sources, high range flowmeters (0-74 L/min) are recommended.

   b. In lieu of a high range flowmeter a standard 0–15 L/min flowmeter may be substituted for the primary gas source. When adjusting the flow, open the needle valve to its maximum open position (beyond flush). When opened this far, most standard flowmeters will deliver between 60–90 L/min. The nozzle in the GIN nebulizer head will limit flow through it to 40 L/min.

5. Attach large-bore (22 mm) aerosol tubing to the outlet of the LDH. Use of a drainage bag is recommended due to the high water vapor output of this humidifier.

6. Connect the desired delivery device to the aerosol tubing.

7. Adjust the flowmeters to the desired setting (Table 2-5 and Table 2-6, pp. 137, 141), or adjust the blender to the desired F_IO_2. Set the flow to maintain adequate flows to meet the patient's inspiratory demands.

8. Check the F_IO_2 level using a calibrated oxygen analyzer.

9. If using the TurboHeater, place an in-line thermometer near the patient to monitor the temperature of the delivered gas.

10. Replace the solution reservoir when the fluid level is 1/4 inch from the bottom of the container.

Troubleshooting

When troubleshooting this equipment, please follow the suggested troubleshooting algorithm (ALG 2-5).

No flow from the humidifier:

1. Check to ensure that there is an adequate oxygen supply when using cylinders.

2. Verify that the flowmeter is correctly connected to the 50 psi oxygen or air source.

3. Check the connection between the humidifier and the flowmeter.

   a. Make sure it is securely attached.

   b. Check for any obstruction where the nebulizer attaches to the flowmeter.

   c. Verify that the secondary gas inlet tube is free of obstruction or kinks.

   Little or no humidity output:

1. Check to ensure that the reservoir bottle contains fluid.

2. Check the capillary tube to ensure it is immersed into the solution in the reservoir bottle.

3. Check the capillary tube for obstructions.

4. Check the large bore aerosol delivery tubing for kinks or obstructions.

5. If using a standard flowmeter (0–15 L/min), verify that the needle valve has been opened to its maximum setting (beyond flush).

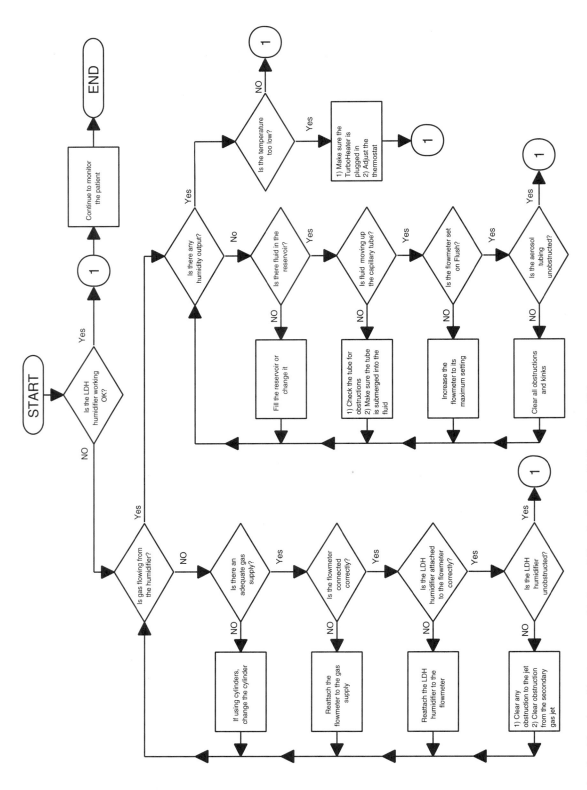

ALG 2-5 *An algorithm describing how to troubleshoot a Misty Ox Laminar Diffuser Humidifier.*

the TurboHeater. Increased pressure in the center of the humidifier and gravity cause the aerosol particles, which coalesce following removal from suspension, to flow down through the precipitate chamber (center of the humidifier) and to drain radially outward onto the heater platen. The hot platen causes the water to be vaporized, further increasing the relative humidity of the gas while also warming it. The heated, humidified gas flows radially through the accumulator chamber to the outlet where it then flows to the patient. It is important to note that the output from the humidifier is molecular water, or water vapor, which contains very few suspended aerosol particles.

The Gas Injection Nebulizer (GIN) head also provides greater flexibility in delivery of variable F_1O_2 levels and flow rates using a closed system. The nebulizer may be powered by oxygen or air (primary gas), while the injected gas (air or oxygen) provides additional flow. To determine the desired F_1O_2 and flow rates refer to Table 2-5 and Table 2-6 later in this chapter (pp. 137 and 141). The LDH humidifier, being a closed system, gives this humidifier further flexibility in that it may be used for positive pressure applications, such as CPAP, since oxygen dilution is not accomplished using jet mixing or air entrainment.

Cascade and Cascade II Humidifiers

The Puritan Bennett Cascade and Cascade II humidifiers are very efficient diffuser type humidifiers, capable of producing body humidity (BTPS) even with high flows of gas. This makes this humidifier suitable for adult mechanical ventilation or other high flow applications.

The efficiency of the Cascade humidifiers is accomplished by increasing surface area and incorporating a heating element. The Cascade II can deliver 100% relative humidity at body temperature at minute volumes up to 10 liters per minute. Gas entering the humidifier is directed down through the tower and passes through a one-way valve below the diffusion grid (Figure 2-7). The one-way valve prevents the gas from flowing back up the tower into the equipment attached to it. The bolus of gas entering below the diffusion grid causes the water to be displaced, increasing the water level and allowing some water to enter the diffusion grid. Water then enters a port above the grid, forming a thin sheet. The gas forms a

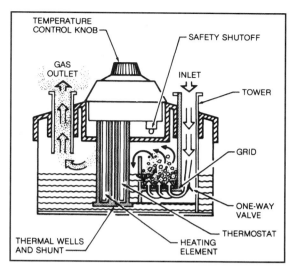

Figure 2-7 *A functional diagram of a Cascade humidifier.*

froth, which creates a large air-water surface area.

A small port located above the water level on the tower acts as a sensing port. Pressure changes created by the patient's inspiratory efforts can be conveyed to the equipment attached. Without the sensing port, the patient would need to generate a force equal to the depth of water in the reservoir.

A heating element increases the temperature of the reservoir, therefore increasing the rate of evaporation. The electrical heating element is not in direct contact with the water in the reservoir. Rather it is inserted into a well, which is a part of the reservoir assembly in contact with the water. A switch located on the heater assembly must close by contacting a raised part of the jar lid casting located in the depression. The switch closes when the jar assembly is attached to the heater. Failure to assemble the unit correctly will result in the heater not operating.

The Cascade II is similar to the Cascade humidifier except that it incorporates a servo controller that controls the temperature. The respiratory care practitioner adjusts the desired temperature level with the temperature control knob. A proximal sensor is placed near the patient's airway to measure the temperature there. Its signal is sent to the heater, which adjusts the output to maintain the temperature level established by the practitioner. This function is an example of servo feedback control.

ASSEMBLY AND TROUBLESHOOTING

Assembly—Cascade Humidifier

1. Be certain that the two red "O" rings are in place on the well where it attaches to the lid. Attach the heater well to the lid of the Cascade using the two small screws.

2. Attach the tower to the lid by inserting the top of the tower into the inlet on the lid. Secure it to the lid using the plastic stud. Verify that the one-way valve is installed correctly at this time.

3. Check to be sure the large "O" ring is in place on the lid where it attaches to the reservoir jar.

4. Aseptically fill the reservoir with sterile distilled water.

5. Screw the lid to the reservoir jar.

6. Attach the Cascade to its heater using the two twist tabs on the top surface of the lid.

7. Attach large-bore aerosol tubing to the inlet and outlet of the humidifier.

Troubleshooting

When troubleshooting this equipment, please follow the suggested troubleshooting algorithm (ALG 2-6).

If the Cascade fails to generate adequate foam or bubbles:

1. Check the water level in the reservoir.

2. Check to ensure that the tower is attached properly.

3. Check the tower for the one-way valve.

4. Check the inlet and outlet for obstruction to gas flow.

Leaks may be a problem when troubleshooting these humidifiers. Common sources include:

1. The large "O" ring in the lid.

2. The red "O" rings on the heater well. Presence of water in the lid's depression will alert you to a leak in this area.

3. Failure to tighten the lid sufficiently; cross threading the lid.

If the Cascade fails to heat properly:

1. Tighten the studs holding the locking tabs on top of the lid by gently tapping them further down into their seats. If these become loose, the lid may fail to activate a switch on the bottom of the heater assembly. Lift up on the reservoir and listen for the faint "click" of the switch closing.

2. If the switch is closed and the heater still fails to operate, replace the heater and take the other one to an authorized biomedical repair facility.

3. Check to see if a circuit breaker has tripped and reset it if required.

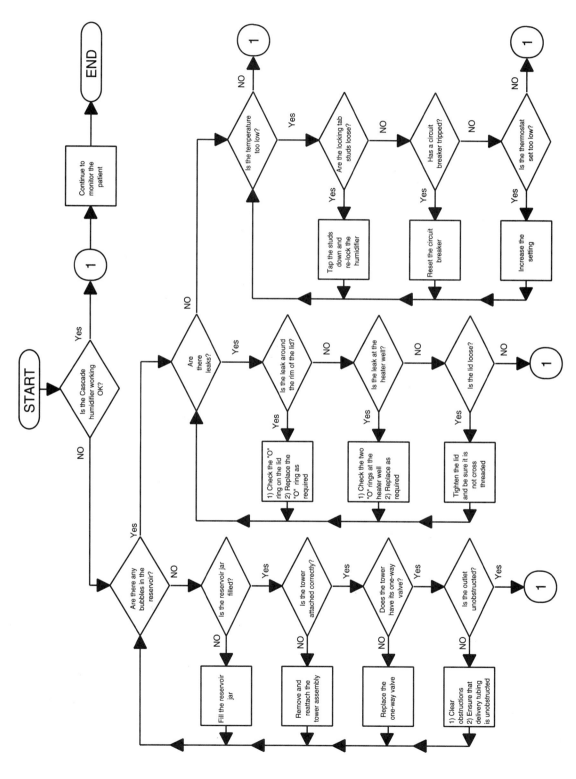

ALG 2-6 *An algorithm describing how to troubleshoot a Cascade humidifier.*

ASSEMBLY AND TROUBLESHOOTING

Assembly—Cascade II

Assembly of this humidifier is slightly different due to some design changes from the original Cascade humidifier (Figure 2-8).

1. Attach the "O" ring to the heating element.

2. Attach the heating element to the lid by mating the threaded portions.

3. Attach the large "O" ring to the outside of the reservoir jar.

4. Attach the plug to the jar by inserting the plug and mating the threaded portions together.

5. Attach the tower to the lid using the plastic stud. Ensure that the one-way valve is in place and moves freely.

6. Lock the lid to the reservoir jar and attach the assembly to the heating element.

Troubleshooting

Troubleshooting the Cascade II is similar to troubleshooting the Cascade humidifier. The exception is the servo controller. Occasionally, breaks will occur in the wire connecting the temperature probe to the heating element. Replacement of the probe and its wire will frequently cure problems with temperature sensing.

Other problems with the heating unit must be solved and repaired by a qualified biomedical repair technician.

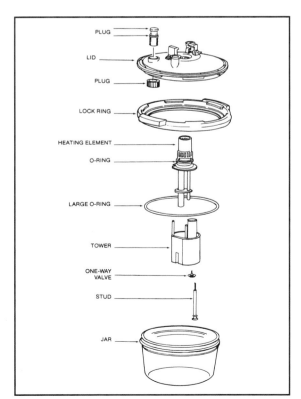

Figure 2-8 *An assembly drawing of the Cascade II humidifier.*

Bird Wick Humidifier

The Bird wick humidifier uses a cylinder of absorbent paper to draw water from the reservoir by capillary action. The water is drawn up the wick (paper cylinder), where it comes into contact with the gas moving through the humidifier. The wick provides a greater surface area for the gas and water to interface; therefore its efficiency is greater. A heating element surrounds the wick, increasing the rate of evaporation. The Bird wick humidifier is capable of delivering 100% relative humidity, at body temperature, at flow rates of up to 60 liters per minute.

Gas entering the wick humidifier is channeled down the hollow center column (Figure 2-9). The gas passes adjacent to the wick, absorbing water by evaporation. Gas then exits through a fitting for large-bore tubing.

The Bird wick humidifier incorporates an automatic feed system to replenish water lost through evaporation. Water flows down the inlet tube to the reservoir. As water enters the reservoir, the float rises. When the reservoir has filled to the correct level, the float obstructs the inlet tube, preventing more water from entering.

ASSEMBLY AND TROUBLESHOOTING

Assembly—Bird Wick Humidifier

1. Remove the cap that contains the water inlet tube and the gas inlet and outlet and install a wick.

2. Replace the cap, being careful to install the "O" ring properly.

3. Install the float into the bottom assembly, ensuring that the rubber seal is up.

4. Attach the bottom assembly to the humidifier, ensuring that the "O" ring is positioned properly.

5. Attach the assembly to the heating element by sliding the two components together.

6. Connect the heater to a 110 volt outlet.

7. Position the proximal temperature probe close to the patient's airway.

8. Adjust the temperature control to the desired temperature.

Troubleshooting

When troubleshooting this equipment, please follow the suggested troubleshooting algorithm (ALG 2-7).

Leaks can be a problem with these humidifiers. Sources include:

1. Top and bottom "O" rings.

2. Top or bottom assemblies are not attached tightly enough to the humidifier.

3. Large-bore aerosol tubing is not connected tightly enough to the inlet and outlet fittings.

If the humidifier fails to maintain the set temperature:

1. Check the temperature probe and wire for integrity and replace as required.

2. Verify that the 110 volt electrical outlet is good.

If the humidifier fails to produce adequate humidity:

1. Check the feed system for proper operation.

2. Check the temperature probe and wire for breaks and replace as required.

3. Ensure that the heater unit and the humidifier are mated properly.

A servo controller is also incorporated into the design of this humidifier. It has a proximal temperature probe much like that on the Bennett Cascade II, which operates in a similar fashion. The temperature probe measures the gas temperature at the proximal airway, and the heater automatically adjusts to maintain the desired temperature. This type of system is termed a "servo feedback control loop."

The humidifier also has three alarms—probe disconnect, temperature overheat alarm and a humidifier module disconnect alarm.

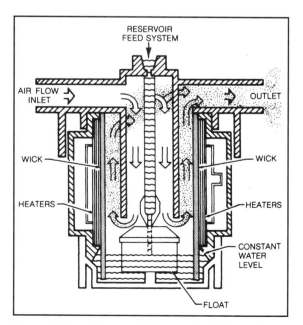

Figure 2-9 *A functional diagram of a Bird wick humidifier.*

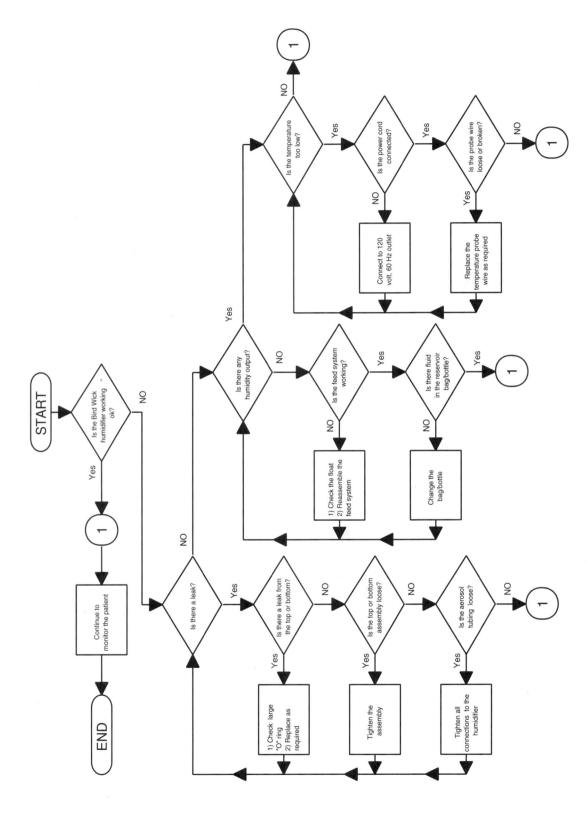

ALG 2-7 *An algorithm describing how to troubleshoot a Bird wick humidifier*

Hudson RCI ConchaTherm® IV Humidifier

The Hudson RCI ConchaTherm® IV humidifier is a microprocessor-controlled, wick-type humidifier that incorporates provisions for a heated wire circuit (Figure 2-10). The ConchaTherm® IV humidifier incorporates the same Concha-Column and feeds system employed on the earlier Conchapack and Conchatherm III designs, in which the wick assembly increases the surface area, thus improving output and performance. The wick assemblies are disposable and may be changed as frequently as required to maintain adequate asepsis.

The wick assembly consists of the wick, heating element, gas inlet and outlet, and water feed system fittings. Gas flowing into the unit flows down past the wick. The heating element surrounds the wick and increases the rate of evaporation.

The wick assembly mates to the ConchaTherm® IV heater control assembly. The heater/control assembly servo controls the airway temperature, servo controls the heated

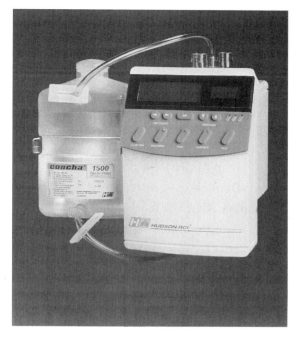

Figure 2-10 *The Conchatherm IV made by Hudson RCI, Inc.*

ASSEMBLY AND TROUBLESHOOTING

Assembly—Hudson RCI ConchaTherm® IV Humidifier

1. Mate a wick Concha-Column to the heater/control assembly by slipping it in from the top, ensuring that the plastic clamps on the feed tubes are closed.

2. Attach the disposable reservoir to the side of the heater assembly.

3. Connect the feed lines to the top and bottom positions on the reservoir by piercing them using a twisting motion. Open the clamps on the feed lines.

4. Attach the power cord to a suitable AC power source.

5. Connect the proximal airway probe to the patient circuit and, if you are using a heated wire circuit, connect the heated wire cables to the appropriate cables on the humidifier.

6. Select the correct mode (infant/adult), set the airway temperature and set the column-to-patient temperature gradient.

Troubleshooting

1. Feed system problems:
   a. Check the water level in the reservoir.
   b. Check for correct installation of the feed probes into the water reservoir.
   c. Check to be sure the clamps are in the open position.

2. Probe/Heated wire problems:
   a. Check connections at the humidifier and patient circuit.
   b. Check for breaks or faults in the cables and wires.

TABLE 2-3 Hudson RCI ConchaTherm® IV Alarms

Emergency Alarms (Red)

    High temperature

    Check probe

    Bad probe

    Adult

    Inspiratory wire and disconnect

    Service

Cautionary Alarms (Yellow)

    Adult/Infant

    Low temperature

    Expiratory wire and disconnect

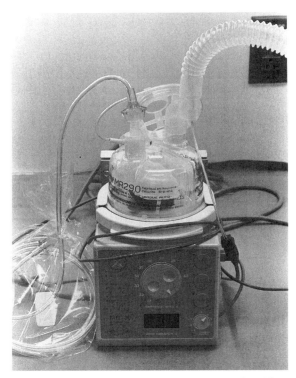

Figure 2-11 *The Fisher and Paykel MR 730 humidifier.*

wire circuit and provides alarm functions to alert the clinician of potentially dangerous events. The alarms incorporated into the ConchaTherm® IV humidifier are summarized in Table 2-3.

Fisher and Paykel Healthcare MR 730 Humidifier

The Fisher and Paykel MR 730 humidifier is a servo-controlled wick humidifier (Figure 2-11). This humidifier is capable of delivering heated humidified gas between 29° and 40° Celsius. These humidifiers may be used with heated wire circuits, which reduce condensate due to a more constant temperature distribution from the humidifier to the patient through the circuit.

Disposable and reusable chambers are available which slide into and lock into the computer controlled heater assembly. The chamber assemblies consist of the inlet, outlet, wick and heating platen.

ASSEMBLY AND TROUBLESHOOTING

Assembly—Fisher and Paykel

1. Slide the module onto the heater and lock into place with the locking tab.

2. Attach the water feed tubing from a disposable fill set to the center pole on the module.

3. Attach appropriate large-bore aerosol tubing to the inlet and outlet of the humidifier. Alternatively, a heated wire circuit may be used, in which case the appropriate electrical connections must be made at the servo controller, the chamber, and proximal to the patient's airway.

4. Place the proximal airway probe near the patient's airway.

5. Initiate gas flow through the unit, and adjust the temperature control to the desired temperature.

Troubleshooting

Troubleshooting primarily relates to breaks occurring in the cable from the temperature probe. Periodically these require replacement. Leaks are not a problem since it is a sealed unit.

Alarms include high and low chamber temperature, high and low airway temperature, probe disconnection and or heater wire disconnection, and microprocessor failure.

Bear VH-820 Humidifier

The Bear VH-820 humidifier is another example of a heated wick humidifier. This humidifier may be used for both infants and adults.

Gas entering the center of the humidifier passes by the heater rod (Figure 2-12). The gas is then channeled through a spiral-shaped chamber that contains the wick. The spiral shape ensures a large surface area and a longer time for gas to interface with water.

The humidifier is servo controlled with three temperature probe positions: proximal airway, heater rod and humidifier outlet. All three temperatures are monitored and the operation of the humidifier is regulated by a microprocessor.

The feed system is automatic and operates by a sensing system controlling a pinch valve. When the water level drops about 1 milliliter, the valve opens, admitting water to the humidity chamber. Gravity causes the water to flow from a reservoir bag (bottle) to the chamber. The volume within the chamber varies between 5 and 10 milliliters.

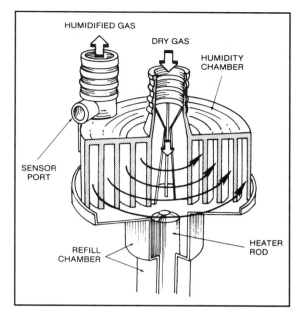

Figure 2-12 *A functional diagram of the Bear VH-820 humidifier.*

ASSEMBLY AND TROUBLESHOOTING

Refer to Figure 2-13 when following the assembly procedure.

Assembly—Bear VH-820

1. Attach the "O" ring to the chamber jar by seating it into the groove provided.

2. Mate the cover assembly and the jar together by twisting them. The outlet should be on the same side as the water feed port.

3. Insert the heater into the jar, ensuring that the heater is perpendicular to the feed tubing.

4. Insert the humidification chamber into the heater/control chamber.

5. Insert the water feed tubing into the pinch valve assembly.

6. Attach large-bore aerosol tubing to the inlet and outlet fittings.

7. Plug in the proximal airway probe and place it near the patient's airway.

Troubleshooting

Troubleshooting this humidifier relates primarily to alarm conditions and problems with the temperature probe cable.

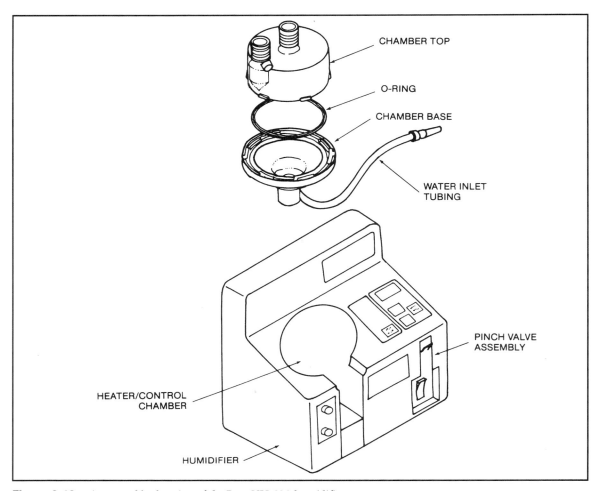

Figure 2-13 *An assembly drawing of the Bear VH-820 humidifier.*

Travenol HLC 37 S Humidifier

The Travenol humidifier is another example of a contemporary wick-type humidifier. Like the others, it is capable of producing body humidity with flows exceeding 60 liters per minute.

Gas entering the humidifier flows into the humidity chamber. The humidity chamber is a disposable unit that includes the wick, inlet and outlet fittings, and the feed system connection. The gas is heated and humidified by evaporation.

The heater assembly includes a microprocessor servo controlled heater, alarm system and feed system control. The microprocessor servo controller works in a similar way to that of the Bear VH-820. The feed system consists of a pinch valve that the feed tubing is inserted through and a controller that senses fluid level in the humidity chamber.

The alarm system on the Travenol humidifier is quite sophisticated and complex (Table 2-4).

ASSEMBLY AND TROUBLESHOOTING

Assembly—Travenol

1. Ensure that the humidifier is on a sturdy table or attached to a secure pole mount as it is quite heavy.

2. Attach the sterile reservoir bag to the pole so that gravity will feed the humidifier.

3. Ensure that the power switch is in the OFF position.

4. Connect the power cord to a 110 v, 60 Hz source.

5. Connect the temperature probe to the patient circuit, ensuring it is on the inspiratory side near the patient's airway or mouth. Connect the temperature probe plug to the receptacle on the humidifier.

6. Connect the gas supply to the inlet of the humidifier and connect the patient circuit to the humidifier canister outlet.

7. Attach the canister to the humidifier, matching the key way, and rotate it into the locked position.

8. Adjust the optic sensor arm so that the sensor contacts the light pipe on the canister lid.

9. Set the temperature control to the desired temperature.

10. Turn on gas flow through the humidifier.

11. Turn on the power switch.

12. Open the feed tube clamp and insert the feed tube. Connect the opposite end to the reservoir bag.

Troubleshooting

The alarm system facilitates rapid diagnosis and troubleshooting of problems. When troubleshooting this humidifier, refer to the key on the humidifier control panel or the instruction manual to diagnose alarm codes.

ARTIFICIAL NOSE (HEAT AND MOISTURE EXCHANGER)

The artificial nose is a simple device whose function can replace that of a humidifier. The heat and moisture exchanger consists of a honeycomblike-tubular structure made of aluminum or hygroscopic materials (Figure 2-14).

Moisture and heat from the patient's exhaled gas is absorbed into the tubular structure of the exchanger. The inspired gas is warmed and humidified by evaporation as it passes through the exchanger. The efficiency of these devices varies between manufacturers from 70% to 90% relative humidity between 30° and 31° Celsius.

The heat and moisture exchanger should be placed between the patient's artificial airway and the ventilator circuit or oxygen ther-

---

TABLE 2-4 Travenol HLC 37 S Alarms

P1	Checks integrity of the temperature probe. P1 will also alarm if the gas temperature at the probe is less than 15° Celsius or if excessive EMI/RFI interference is present.
P2	Alarms if the probe is shorted, if airway temperature is greater than 45° Celsius or if excessive EMI/RFI interference is present.
P3	Alarms if the probe has not detected a rise of at least 1° Celsius during a ten-minute period while the heater is on and the probe is more than 4° lower than the set point on the controller.
F1	The optic sensor arm is in the raised position or not lowered correctly.
F2	Feed tube is not in the feed clamp or is misaligned.
F3	Feed tube clamp has remained open for too long a time interval, potentially overfilling the humidifier.
F4	Feed tube clamp housing is not in the correct position.
HI	Probe temperature is equal to or greater than 40° Celsius.
LO	Probe temperature has dropped below 27° Celsius or the probe temperature has dropped more than 5° Celsius.
FF	Internal system malfunction.

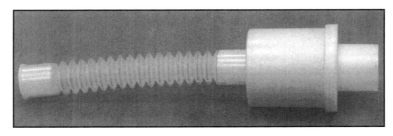

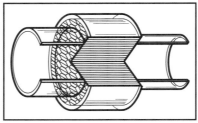

Figure 2-14 *A photograph and a functional diagram of a heat and moisture exchanger (HME).*

apy equipment. Minimizing resistance, dead space, and compliance are critical factors in a good design. Should these devices become obstructed with mucous, resistance can increase dramatically.

The placement and adjustment of external pressure disconnect alarms is also important for patient safety. The alarm should be set near the peak airway pressure and, if the sensor placement can be moved, it should be between the patient's airway and the moisture exchanger. This is due to the in-creased resistance that a moisture exchanger may develop, even if disconnected from the patient.

These devices are effective for short-term usage (less than 24 hours). For long-term use, a humidifier is recommended. Bronchial cast formation due to secretion retention from long-term use has been reported. This is caused by the comparatively low relative humidity and the fact that artificial airways bypass the upper airway.

ASSEMBLY AND TROUBLESHOOTING

Assembly—HME

1. Aseptically open the package containing the heat and moisture exchanger.

2. Using the adapters provided, match the 15 mm artificial airway connection on the patient side of the exchanger and the ventilator tubing or oxygen therapy equipment on the other.

3. Place the heat and moisture exchanger on the airway and attach the circuit to the other side.

4. If required, provide additional support to the artificial airway to prevent the weight of the heat and moisture exchanger from producing adverse traction on the airway.

5. Carefully monitor peak pressures (if mechanically ventilating the patient) before and after installation. If the patient is spontaneously ventilating, monitor respiratory effort and minute ventilation for adverse changes.

Troubleshooting

Troubleshooting primarily consists of monitoring the device for obstruction. Signs of obstruction would include increased peak airway pressures and increased work of breathing.

The heat and moisture exchanger should be replaced at the intervals recommended by the manufacturer. By replacing the device, problems with obstruction and bacterial contamination can be minimized.

AEROSOL THERAPY EQUIPMENT

MAINSTREAM AND SIDESTREAM NEBULIZERS

Mainstream and sidestream are two classifications of nebulizers based upon the nebulizer's placement in relation to the flow of carrier gas. The carrier gas is the main gas flow that carries the aerosol particles to the patient.

With a mainstream nebulizer, the nebulizer is placed directly in the path of the carrier gas (Figure 2-15). The aerosol produced by the nebulizer is conducted out of the device by the main flow of carrier gas. Particle sizes from this type of nebulizer tend to be larger since the aerosol flows in a relatively straight path.

Sidestream nebulizers have a nebulizer that is placed adjacent to the flow of carrier gas (Figure 2-16). The aerosol output must

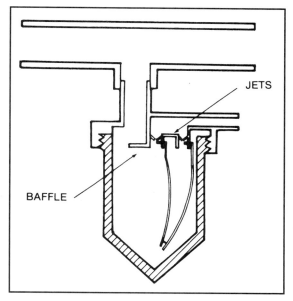

Figure 2-16 *A full section of the Puritan Bennett Twin-Jet nebulizer. This nebulizer is an example of a sidestream nebulizer.*

change direction before merging with the carrier gas. Due to this direction change, particle sizes are smaller in these nebulizers than in the mainstream type.

SMALL-VOLUME NEBULIZERS

Pneumatic nebulizers may be further classified by the volume of the reservoirs that they possess. A small-volume nebulizer is one with a volume of less than 30 milliliters and is primarily utilized for short-term medication delivery. These devices produce aerosol particles that range from 1.5 to 7 microns in diameter.

Bulb-Type Hand-Held Nebulizers

Bulb-type nebulizers are commonly used by outpatients receiving home therapy. These devices are small hand-held nebulizers that are powered by squeezing a rubber bulb (Figure 2-17).

Squeezing the bulb forces gas through the jet, creating a reduction in pressure and nebulization of the liquid in the reservoir (Bernoulli's principle). Each time the bulb is squeezed, a small amount of medication is delivered.

Patient instruction is critical with this type of nebulizer. Coordination of inspiration with the squeezing of the bulb sometimes becomes difficult. If the coordination is off, medication delivery is compromised.

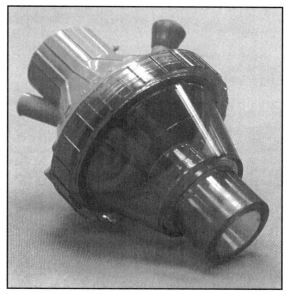

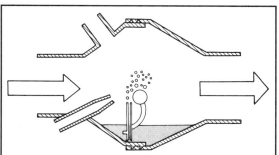

Figure 2-15 *A photograph and a functional diagram of a Bird Micronebulizer. This is an example of a mainstream nebulizer.*

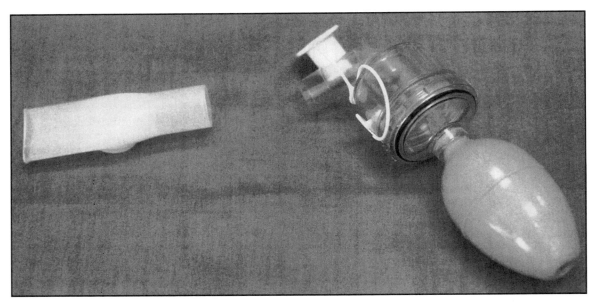

Figure 2-17 *A hand-powered bulb nebulizer for home use.*

ASSEMBLY AND TROUBLESHOOTING

Assembly—Bulb Nebulizer

1. Fill the reservoir with the ordered amount and dilution of medication.

2. Attach the bulb to the distal end of the nebulizer.

3. Insert the proximal end into the mouth.

4. Squeeze the bulb during a deep inspiration. Holding the breath at the end of inspiration for approximately 10 seconds helps to improve aerosol deposition.

Troubleshooting

Troubleshooting primarily consists of coordinating inspiration with squeezing the bulb. The nebulizer should be thoroughly cleaned after use to prevent the jet from becoming obstructed. Proper disinfection of home therapy equipment is also important to minimize infection.

Disposable Gas Powered Small-Volume Nebulizers

In the clinical setting, disposable gas powered small-volume nebulizers are very common. They are used to administer bronchodilators and other topical agents to the respiratory tract. The variety of styles and manufacturers are numerous. Most operate using similar principles.

Most small-volume nebulizers are updraft (draw medication up vertically) nebulizers that operate using choked flow, described earlier in this chapter. The liquid medication is atomized and entrained into the gas flow by a combination of shear forces and vorticity (Figure 2-18). The aerosolized medication is then directed into a baffle, stabilizing the particle size before the aerosol exits the nebulizer.

ASSEMBLY AND TROUBLESHOOTING

Refer to ALG 2-8 and Figure 2-19 when following the assembly and troubleshooting procedures.

Assembly—Small-Volume Nebulizer

1. Aseptically remove the component parts from the package.

2. Add the ordered volume and dilution of medication to the reservoir.

3. Attach the reservoir to the nebulizer top, screwing them together or pushing them together, depending upon the design.

4. Attach the aerosol T to the outlet of the nebulizer.

5. Attach the aerosol tubing reservoir to one end of the aerosol T and the mouthpiece to the other.

6. Attach the oxygen connecting tube to the nipple on the bottom of the nebulizer.

7. Attach the distal end of the oxygen connecting tube to a flowmeter. Adjust the flow between 5 and 7 liters per minute.

Troubleshooting

When troubleshooting this equipment, please follow the suggested troubleshooting algorithm (ALG 2-8).

If aerosol output is absent or low:

1. Check to be sure the oxygen connecting tube is attached to the flowmeter and nebulizer.

2. Check the flowmeter to ensure the flow is properly set.

3. Check the jet for obstruction.

4. If (1) through (3) are satisfactory, replace the unit with a new one.

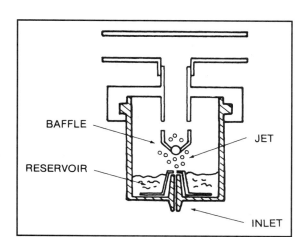

Figure 2-18 *A functional diagram of a small-volume nebulizer.*

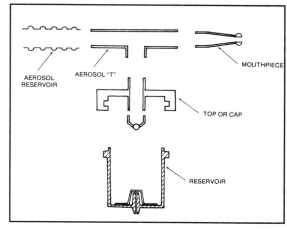

Figure 2-19 *An assembly drawing of a small-volume nebulizer.*

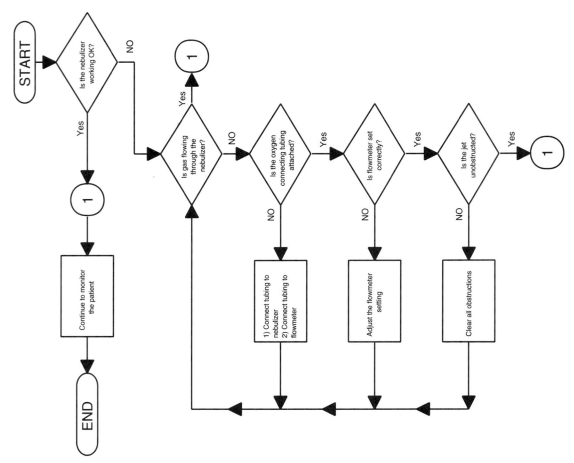

ALG 2-8 *An algorithm describing how to troubleshoot a small volume nebulizer.*

Respigard II Small-Volume Nebulizer

The Respigard II small-volume nebulizer (Figure 2-20) is a unique nebulizer which incorporates two one-way valves, a wye and an expiratory filter. These nebulizers are capable of producing particle sizes of less than 2 microns. The Respigard II is commonly used in the administration of Pentamidine, an antimicrobial drug used to treat Pneumocystis carinii pneumonia (PCP).

METERED DOSE INHALERS

Metered dose inhalers (MDIs) are small self-contained nebulizers designed for administration of medications (Part A of Figure 2-21). Many bronchodilators and steroids can be administered using MDIs. MDIs are advantageous in that they are very small and are easy to use.

How MDIs Operate

Contained in the MDI canister is the medication to be delivered (solution or powder) mixed with an inert liquified gas under pressure (Part B of Figure 2-21). The majority of MDIs use fluorocarbons as the propellant. When the patient depresses the mouthpiece toward the canister using a squeezing action, a valve opens, discharging a premeasured dose of medication along with the propellant. The propellant rapidly evaporates, leaving the medication in suspension as an aerosol. These devices operate in a way that is similar to an aerosol paint can.

There have been some reports of patient sensitivity to the propellant, causing bronchospasm and other unwanted side effects. More studies are currently being conducted regarding how safe and non-reactive these agents are in the population. These devices

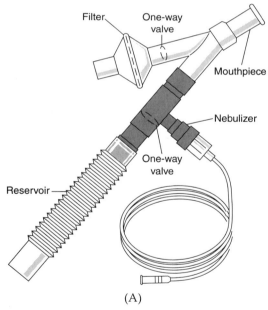

(A)

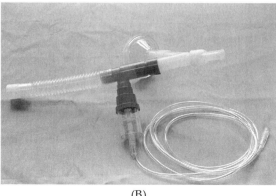

(B)

Figure 2-20 *(A) An assenbly drawing and (B) a photograph of the Bear VH-80 humidifier.*

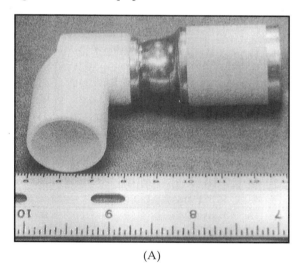

(A)

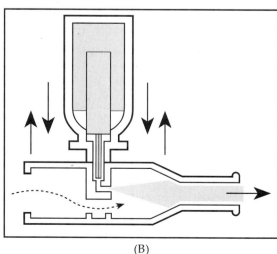

(B)

Figure 2-21 *(A) A photograph and (B) a functional diagram of a metered dose inhaler (MDI).*

are very popular and can be very cost-effective.

MDI Spacer Devices

The use of a spacer (Figure 2-22), enhances the effectiveness of aerosol deposition and improves delivery for patients who have problems coordinating the sequencing of squeezing the MDI and inspiration. The MDI is inserted into the spacer, at the opposite end from the mouthpiece (Figure 2-23). When the patient squeezes the MDI, the medication is discharged into the spacer, which acts as a reservoir and baffle device. The larger particles impact the walls of the spacer, removing them from suspension. The larger size of the chamber (reservoir) facilitates the further evaporation of the propellant. The net result is that smaller particles are inspired by the patient. If a patient has difficulty timing the release of medication with his/her ventilatory cycle, the spacer may improve medication delivery somewhat by acting as a holding chamber.

Patient Instructions for Use

The assembly and troubleshooting of the MDI device itself is relatively easy. The most difficult part of MDI use is educating the patient on how to correctly use it. The effectiveness of MDI administration is highly technique dependent. Therefore, it is important that you thoroughly instruct your patient on its proper use.

Use without a Spacer

Have the patient sitting or standing comfortably. It is important that the patient be upright to allow for good chest expansion to facilitate a deep breath. Make certain that the patient is not wearing restrictive clothing that may hamper his/her ability to take a deep breath.

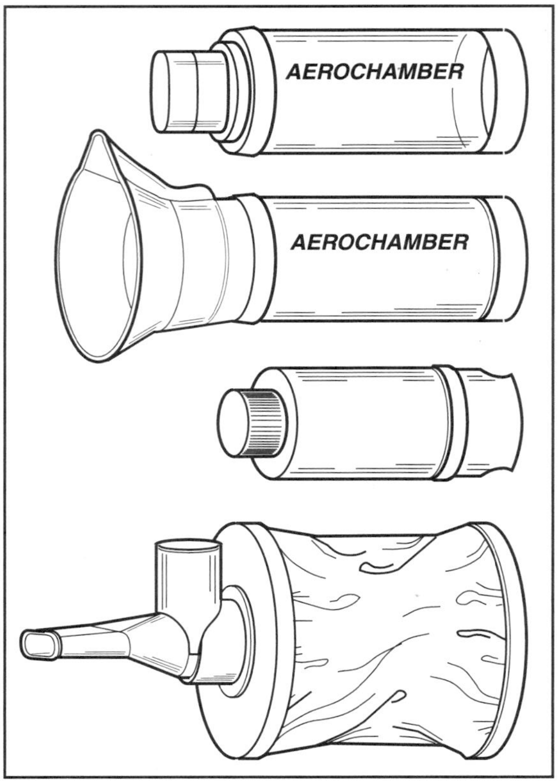

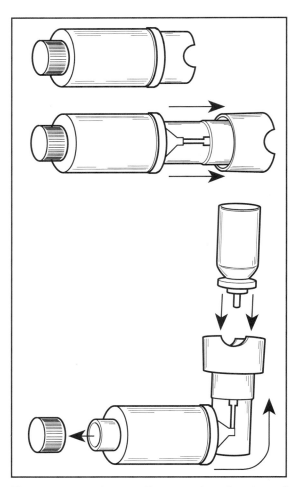

Figure 2-22 *A drawing showing several different types of spacers.*

Figure 2-23 *A drawing illustrating how the MDI and spacer are assembled together.*

Have the patient hold the MDI a few centimeters away from his/her open mouth. Have the patient exhale, then slowly inhale deeply a few times. Once the patient is cognizant of his/her breathing pattern, instruct the patient to squeeze the MDI just after beginning a breath, and to continue slowly inhaling deeply to a maximal inspiration. Have the patient hold his/her breath a few seconds (5 to 10 seconds) at the end of inspiration. Have the patient slowly exhale after MDI administration. Repeat the procedure as many times as ordered by the patient's physician, waiting between puffs.

Use with a Spacer

As discussed above, thorough patient instruction is important. Position the patient as described earlier. Connect the MDI to the spacer as shown in Figure 2-23.

Have the patient insert the mouthpiece into his/her mouth. Instruct the patient to exhale and to take a slow deep breath. Just after the patient begins a breath, have him/her squeeze the MDI delivering the medication. Have the patient continue his/her inhalation, performing a breath hold at the end of inspiration (5 to 10 seconds). Have the patient remove the spacer/MDI and slowly exhale following medication administration. Repeat the procedure as many times as ordered by the patient's physician, waiting between puffs.

ASSEMBLY AND TROUBLESHOOTING

Assembly—MDI

1. Remove the MDI from its box and assemble the mouthpiece by placing it on top of the canister.

2. Thoroughly shake the MDI vigorously for a few seconds.

3. If using a spacer, connect the MDI to the spacer as shown in Figure 2-23.

4. Instruct the patient on the use of MDIs.

Troubleshooting

When troubleshooting this equipment, please follow the suggested troubleshooting algorithm (ALG 2-9).

If the MDI fails to activate when the valve is depressed:

1. Check for correct assembly of the mouthpiece and how it mates to the propellant canister.

2. The MDI may be exhausted of propellant and medication. To check the contents of the MDI, float it in water in a small bowl or basin.
   a. If the MDI sinks to the bottom it is full.
   b. If the MDI floats upright it is partially full.
   c. If the MDI floats horizontally, it is empty.

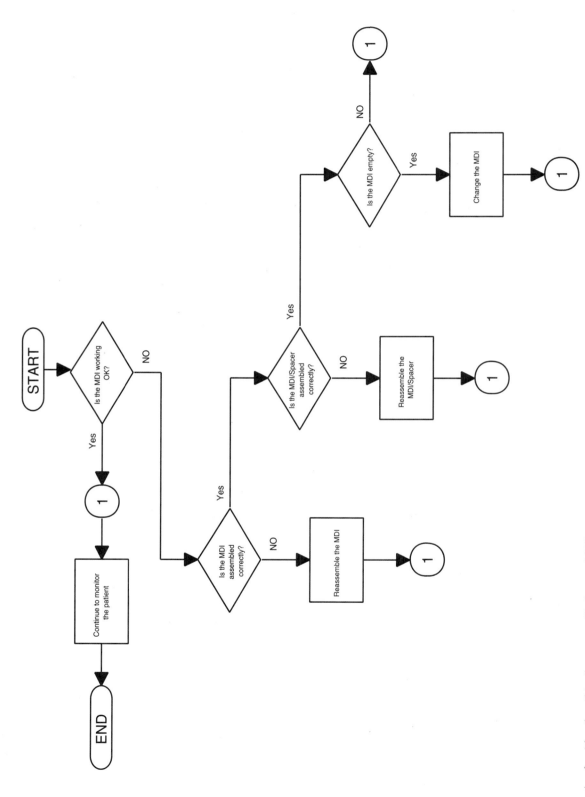

ALG 2-9 *An algorithm describing how to troubleshoot an MDI.*

Bird Micronebulizer

The Bird Micronebulizer is an example of a mainstream nebulizer. It is commonly used in conjunction with Intermittent Positive Pressure Breathing (IPPB, refer to Chapter 3) to deliver a medication. Its operation is similar to the disposable gas powered nebulizers using choked flow.

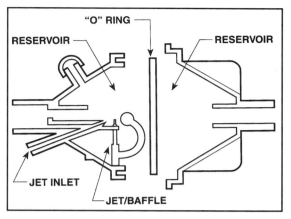

Figure 2-24 *An assembly drawing of the Bird Micronebulizer.*

ASSEMBLY AND TROUBLESHOOTING

Refer to Figure 2-24 when following the assembly procedure.

Assembly—Bird Micronebulizer

1. Attach the nebulizer jet/baffle assembly to the reservoir by pressing the two parts together.

2. Add the ordered dilution and amount of medication to the reservoir.

3. Join the two reservoir halves, ensuring that the "O" ring is in place and installed correctly.

4. Attach the main flow inlet and outlet tubing to the nebulizer.

5. Attach the nebulizer drive line to the fitting on the jet inlet.

Troubleshooting

Problems with this nebulizer are primarily related to incorrect assembly (leaving out the jet/baffle assembly) or obstructions of the jet. Both can be corrected quite easily.

Bennett Twin-Jet Nebulizer

The Bennett Twin-Jet nebulizer is an example of a sidestream small-volume nebulizer. It may be used as a hand-held nebulizer or attached to a ventilator circuit to provide medication delivery (Figure 2-25). The Bennett Twin-Jet nebulizer produces particles that range in size from 3.5 to 7 microns in diameter.

ASSEMBLY AND TROUBLESHOOTING

Refer to Figure 2-26 when following the assembly procedure.

Assembly—Bennett Twin-Jet

1. Attach the two capillary tubes to the jets on the cap of the nebulizer.

2. Add the ordered volume and dilution of medication to the reservoir.

3. Screw the reservoir to the cap of the nebulizer.

4. Attach oxygen supply tubing to the jet inlet.

5. Attach the main flow tubing to the inlet and outlet of the nebulizer.

Troubleshooting

Troubleshooting primarily consists of ensuring that capillary tubes are properly attached and checking the jets for obstructions.

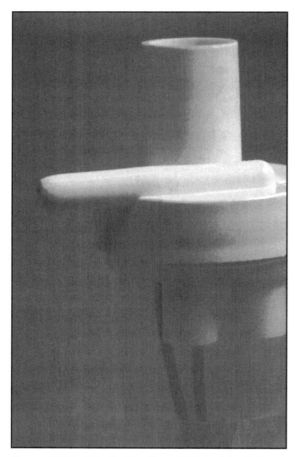

Figure 2-25 *The Puritan Bennett Twin-Jet nebulizer.*

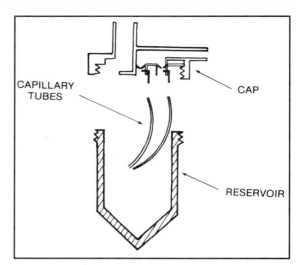

Figure 2-26 *An assembly drawing of the Puritan Bennett Twin-Jet nebulizer.*

LARGE-VOLUME NEBULIZERS

Large-volume nebulizers are used to provide continuous aerosol therapy. They are designed with large reservoirs that may require filling every four or eight hours, depending upon the flow through the nebulizer. All of these devices are designed to use large-bore aerosol tubing, to maximize gas and aerosol delivery.

Puritan Bennett All Purpose Nebulizer

The Puritan Bennett All Purpose nebulizer is designed to provide heated or cool continuous aerosol therapy (Figure 2-27 and 2-28). By adding an immersion heater, heated aerosol can be provided. The size of the reservoir is 375 milliliters. It requires refilling when it reaches 200 milliliters.

The Puritan Bennett All Purpose nebulizer operates using choked flow. Gas is forced through a jet causing the velocity of the source gas to increase to sonic velocities. Aerosol is

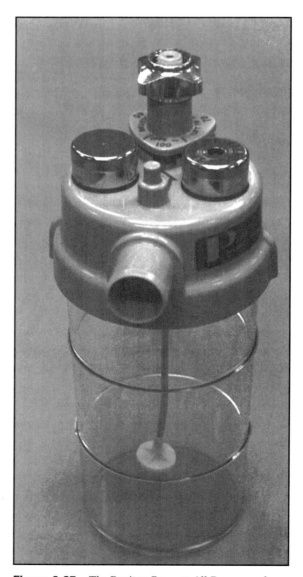

Figure 2-27 *The Puritan Bennett All Purpose nebulizer.*

ASSEMBLY AND TROUBLESHOOTING

Refer to Figure 2-28 when following the assembly procedure.

Assembly—Puritan Bennett All Purpose Nebulizer

1. Ensure that the jet assembly is installed. If it is not, install the assembly to the underside of the cap using the two small screws provided.

2. Attach the safety pop-off valve by screwing it into place on the fitting on top of the lid.

3. Attach the feed tube and filter assembly to the jet by mating the small diameter tube to the jet.

4. Aseptically fill the reservoir with sterile distilled water.

5. If heated aerosol is desired, insert the immersion heater into the other hole on the cap and connect the power cord to a suitable 110 v power source.

6. Attach the nebulizer to a flowmeter using the DISS fitting and adjust the flow to between 12 and 15 liters per minute.

Troubleshooting

When troubleshooting this equipment, please follow the suggested troubleshooting algorithm (ALG 2-10).

1. If aerosol output is absent or inadequate:

   a. Ensure that the flowmeter is set for the correct range and that the DISS fitting is tight.

   b. Clear the jet of any obstructions by depressing the jet cleaning button on the lid of the nebulizer.

   c. Ensure that the water level is adequate.

   d. Check the feed tube for kinks or obstructions.

   e. Check the outlet and aerosol tubing for obstructions to flow.

2. If the heater fails to function correctly:

   a. Ensure that the electrical outlet is functioning properly with a test lamp or other device.

   b. Check the cord for breaks or shorts.

   c. Replace the heater.

3. If the analyzed F_iO_2 varies from the entrainment setting:

   a. Verify the entrainment port setting (oxygen percent).

   b. If the F_iO_2 is higher than is set, check for tubing obstructions (water or kinks).

   c. If the F_iO_2 is lower than is set, check for correct assembly, such as loose fittings.

produced when the liquid is drawn into the high velocity gas stream. Furthermore, vorticity is used to entrain room air, allowing for variations in the F_iO_2.

Oxygen percentage adjustments include 40%, 70% and 100% oxygen. Understand, however, that as the oxygen percentage increases, total flow decreases. This is because less room air is entrained, decreasing total flow.

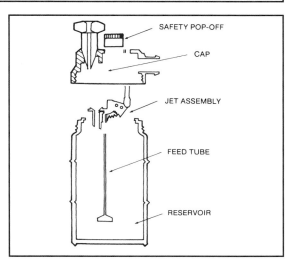

Figure 2-28 *An assembly drawing of the Puritan Bennett All Purpose nebulizer.*

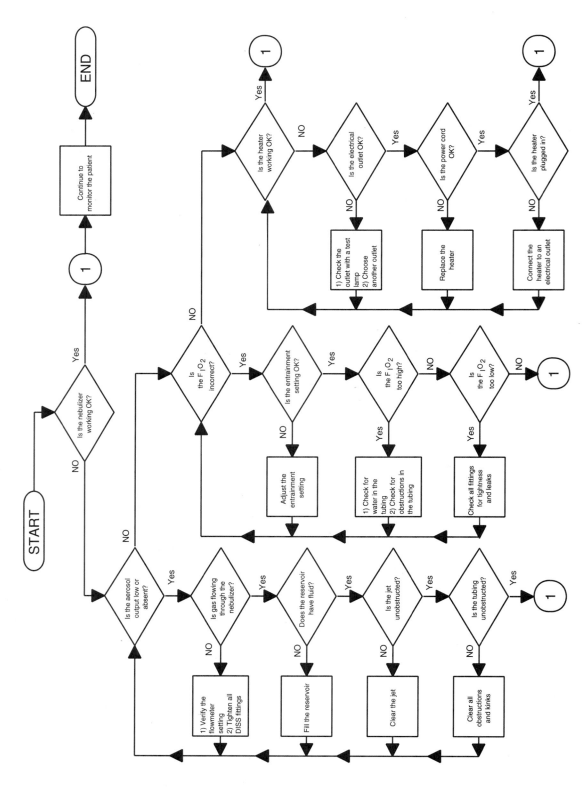

ALG 2-10 *An algorithm describing how to troubleshoot the Puritan Bennett All Purpose nebulizer.*

Ohmeda Ohio Deluxe Nebulizer

The Ohmeda Ohio Deluxe nebulizer is another large-volume nebulizer designed for continuous use. It uses choked flow in its operation in a way similar to the Puritan Bennett All Purpose nebulizer. Figures 2-29 and 2-30 show the Ohmeda Ohio Deluxe nebulizer. The reservoir on this nebulizer contains 800 milliliters. Oxygen percentages available include 40%, 60% and 100% settings. Heated aerosol is also available by clipping on a thermostatically controlled base heater.

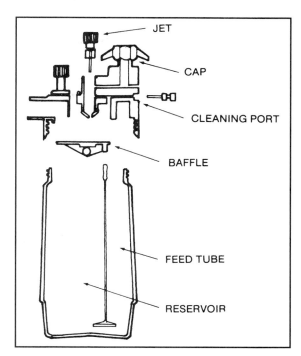

Figure 2-30 *An assembly drawing of the Ohmeda Ohio Deluxe nebulizer.*

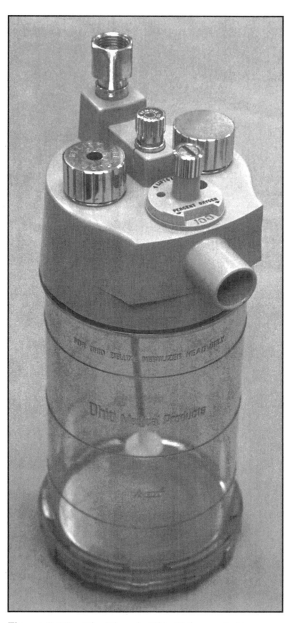

Figure 2-29 *The Ohmeda Ohio Deluxe nebulizer.*

ASSEMBLY AND TROUBLESHOOTING

Assembly—Ohmeda Ohio Deluxe Nebulizer

Follow Figure 2-30 in the assembly of this nebulizer.

1. Secure the jet to the nebulizer lid by screwing it into place.

2. Secure the cleaning port by screwing it into its seat.

3. Turn the lid over and place the baffle onto its seat. Secure it by screwing on the feed tube/filter assembly.

4. Ensure that the large "O" ring is in place around the inside of the lid.

5. Aseptically fill the reservoir with sterile distilled water.

6. Attach the lid to the reservoir by screwing the two pieces together.

7. Attach the nebulizer to a flowmeter using the DISS fitting and adjust the flow to between 12 and 15 liters per minute.

8. If heated aerosol is desired, connect the base heater to a suitable 110 v electrical outlet.

Troubleshooting

When troubleshooting this equipment, please follow the suggested troubleshooting algorithm (ALG 2-11).

1. If aerosol output is absent or inadequate:

   a. Ensure that the flowmeter is set for the correct range and that the DISS fitting is tight.

   b. Clear the jet of any obstructions by removing it and cleaning it.

   c. Ensure that the water level is adequate.

   d. Check the feed tube for kinks or obstructions.

   e. Check the outlet and aerosol tubing for obstructions to flow.

2. If the heater fails to function correctly:

   a. Ensure that the electrical outlet is functioning properly with a test lamp or other device.

   b. Check the cord for breaks or shorts.

   c. Replace the heater.

3. If the analyzed F_IO_2 varies from the entrainment setting:

   a. Verify the entrainment port setting (oxygen percentage).

   b. If the F_IO_2 is higher than was set, check for tubing obstructions (water or kinks).

   c. If the F_IO_2 is lower than was set, check for correct assembly such as loose fittings.

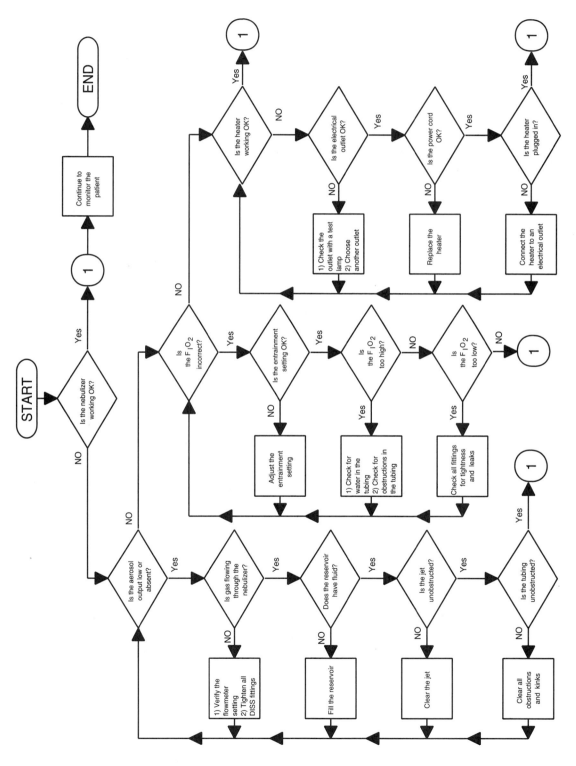

ALG 2-11 *An algorithm describing how to troubleshoot the Ohmeda Ohio Deluxe nebulizer.*

Misty Ox Hi-Fi Nebulizer

Medical Molding Corporation has designed a nebulizer that can provide F_iO_2 levels from .60 to .96 at flow rates between 42 and 77 liters per minute (Figure 2-31). The Hi-Fi nebulizer is similar in appearance to the MultiFit nebulizer, also marketed by the same company. The major difference is that the MultiFit has a maximum flow restriction through the nozzle of 14 L/min, while the Hi-Fi has a maximum flow restriction through the nozzle of 40 L/min. This design allows for sufficient total flows to meet or exceed the patient's inspiratory demand (43 L/min at F_iO_2 of .96, 77

L/min at F_iO_2 of .60). Without sufficient total flow to meet the patient's demand, you cannot achieve accurate oxygen concentration delivery to the patient.

The nebulizer operates using viscous shearing and jet mixing to nebulize water and entrain room air. Oxygen is conducted down through a small orifice jet, increasing the gas's velocity (Figure 2-32). Air is entrained at this point by viscous shearing, as described in Chapter 1. A capillary tube fitting, in close proximity to the jet, injects water into the high velocity gas stream by shear forces as described earlier in this chapter. The gas mixture and aerosol particles are directed through a converging duct downward and laterally form a swirling flow pattern in the mixing chamber. The swirling gas flow encounters baffles positioned radially along the edges of the mixing chamber which remove the larger aerosol particles from suspension. Careful design of the jet and mixing chamber allows the use of a 40 L/min jet (nozzle) to maintain higher total flow rates at higher F_iO_2 levels than other similar devices (Table 2-5). A TurboHeater is also available if heated aerosol is required.

The nebulizer is designed with a 38 mm threaded fitting to be used to attach the nebulizer to a reservoir bottle. The 38 mm fitting is a standard size fitting incorporated by many suppliers of sterile solutions. This is advantageous in that cost savings may be realized by using these solutions rather than purchasing prefilled nebulizers.

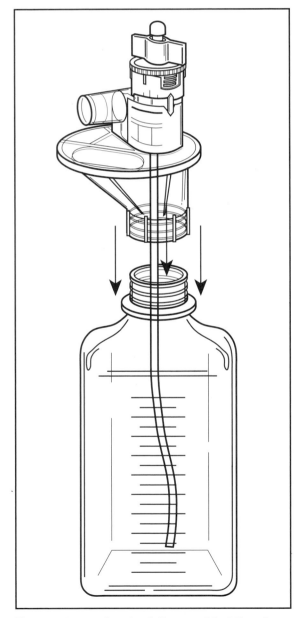

Figure 2-31 *A functional diagram of the Misty Ox Hi-Fi nebulizer.*

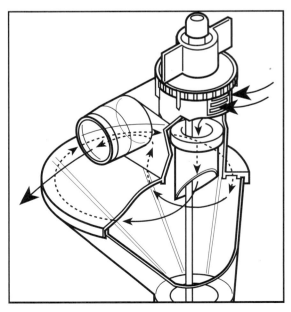

Figure 2-32 *A detailed diagram of the Misty Ox Hi-Fi nebulizer.*

ASSEMBLY AND TROUBLESHOOTING

Assembly—Misty Ox Hi-Fi Nebulizer

1. Remove the cap from the sterile distilled water bottle you wish to use as a reservoir.

2. Aseptically remove the nebulizer from its package. Use caution so that you do not contaminate the long capillary tube which will be immersed into the reservoir bottle.

3. Insert the capillary tube into the bottle and screw the nebulizer into place using the 38 mm threaded fitting. Make sure that the nebulizer is on tight and is not cross threaded.

4. Attach the nebulizer to a high range flowmeter (0–75 L/min). Connect the flowmeter to a 50 psi oxygen source.
   a. Alternatively, a standard flowmeter (0–15 L/min) may be substituted. Open the needle valve to its maximum position (beyond flush). Most standard flowmeters will deliver between 60-90 L/min at this setting. The nozzle design in the Hi-Fi nebulizer will limit flow through it to 40 L/min even if the flowmeter exceeds this setting.

5. Attach large-bore aerosol tubing to the nebulizer outlet. Secure a drainage bag to collect any condensate at the midpoint of the tubing.

6. Attach the delivery device to the aerosol tubing (aerosol mask, face tent, aerosol T, trach mask).

7. Set the entrainment control to the desired F_IO_2 (.60, .65, .75, .85, .96), and adjust the flowmeter to the desired setting. Reduction in the entrainment settings from .96 to .60 will increase total flow through the Hi-Fi nebulizer. Maximum achievable flow is 77 L/min.
   a. If you are using a standard flowmeter set on its maximum position, the nozzle in the Hi-Fi will limit flow to 40 L/min.
   b. Verify the oxygen concentration using a calibrated oxygen analyzer (refer to Chapter 1).

8. Replace the reservoir bottle when the solution level is 1/4 inch from the bottom of the container.

Troubleshooting

When troubleshooting this equipment, please follow the suggested troubleshooting algorithm (ALG 2-12).

No flow from the nebulizer:

1. Check to ensure that there is an adequate oxygen supply when using cylinders.

2. Verify that the flowmeter is correctly connected to the 50 psi oxygen source.

3. Check the connection between the nebulizer and the flowmeter.
   a. Make sure it is securely attached.
   b. Check for any obstruction where the nebulizer attaches to the flowmeter.

Little or no aerosol being generated:

1. Check to ensure that the reservoir bottle contains fluid.

2. Check the capillary tube to ensure it is immersed into the solution in the bottle.

3. Check the capillary tube for obstructions.

4. Check the large-bore aerosol delivery tubing for kinks or obstructions.

5. If using a standard 0-15 L/min flowmeter, make sure the flowmeter needle valve is opened to its maximum setting.

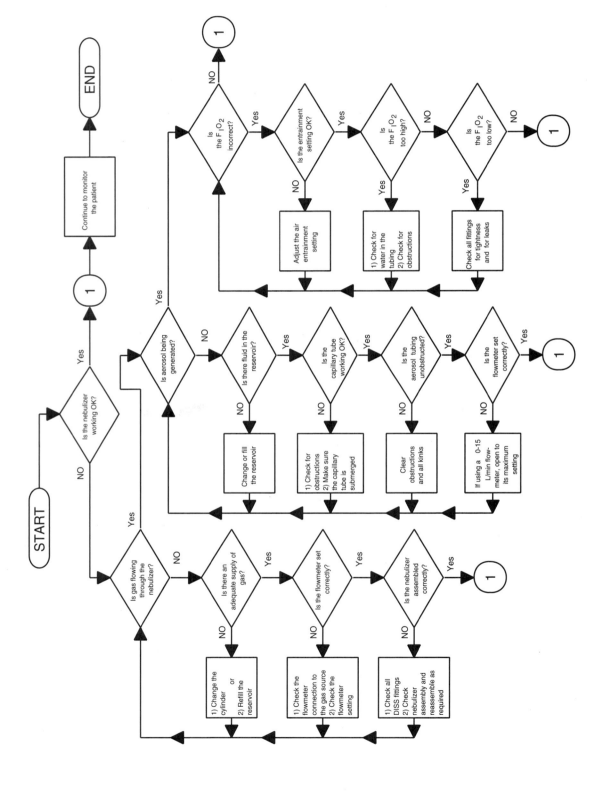

ALG 2-12 *An algorithm describing how to troubleshoot the Misty Ox Hi-Fi nebulizer.*

Table 2-5 Total Flow Rates Provided by Misty Ox Hi-Fi Nebulizer

ENTRAINMENT SETTING	OXYGEN FLOW (L/MIN)	TOTAL FLOW (L/MIN)
60%	20–30	40–61
65%	30–40	54–72
75%	30–40	44–58
85%	30–40	37–49
96%	40	42

Misty Ox Gas Injection Nebulizer (GIN)

Medical Molding Corporation has designed a nebulizer that can provide high F_IO_2 levels (.21–1.0) and at high flow rates (over 100 L/min). Unlike other nebulizers available, the Gas Injection Nebulizer (GIN) is not an entrainment device. It is a closed system device which requires two gas sources (oxygen and air). The second gas is injected via an attached titration tube to achieve any F_IO_2 at any total flow. Being a closed system, the nebulizer can provide a positive pressure (CPAP), as well as hydration and variable oxygen concentrations.

To achieve oxygen concentrations from .21 to .50, the device should be connected to an air flowmeter (driving primary jet) and titrate oxygen to blend specific concentrations. To achieve oxygen concentrations between .50 and 1.0, the device should be connected to an oxygen flowmeter (driving the primary jet) and titrate air to blend specific concentrations.

In either configuration, the titration tube is connected to a "nipple adapter" or "Christmas tree" adapter on a flowmeter to provide the secondary injected gas flow.

While the GIN part # 441G has a 40 L/min nozzle (same as the Hi-Fi) suited for adult applications, Medical Molding Corporation also produces another model (part # 441GB), the GIN Baby for pediatric and infant applications. The GIN Baby's nozzle restricts flow to a maximum of 14 L/min.

The nebulizer operates using viscous shearing and jet mixing to nebulize water and mix room air. Oxygen is conducted down through a small orifice jet, increasing the gas's velocity (Figure 2-33). Another gas is injected at perpendicular to the primary jet (through the titration tube). The injected gas is directed against a curved baffle, causing a swirling flow pattern in the mixing chamber. The two gases mix together by vorticity and turbulent flow.

A capillary tube fitting, in close proximity to the jet, injects water into the high velocity primary gas stream by shear forces as described earlier in this chapter. The gas mixture and aerosol particles are directed through a converging duct downward and laterally forming a swirling flow pattern in the mixing chamber. The swirling gas flow encounters baffles positioned radially along the edges of the mixing chamber which remove the larger aerosol particles from suspension.

The nebulizer is designed with a 38 mm threaded fitting to be used to attach the nebulizer to a reservoir bottle. The 38 mm fitting is a standard-size fitting incorporated by many suppliers of sterile solutions. This is advantageous in that cost savings may be realized by using these solutions rather than purchasing prefilled nebulizers.

The total flow from the nebulizer and the F_IO_2 level is dependent upon what gas (oxygen or air) is the primary source and its flow rate, and what gas (oxygen or air) is the secondary gas (injected) and its flow rate. The oxygen concentrations and total flow rates are outlined in Tables 2-6 and 2-7 on page 141.

One investigator was able to achieve an F_IO_2 of 1.0, with a total flow of 91.2 liters per minute, when running the GIN nebulizer using oxygen as a secondary source at a maximum flow setting, with the primary air source turned off.

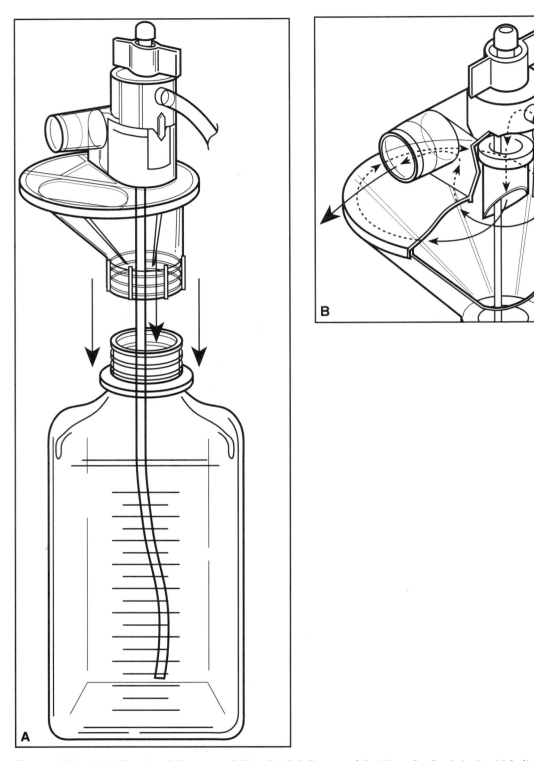

Figure 2-33 *(A) A functional diagram and (B) a detailed diagram of the Misty Ox Gas Injection Nebulizer (GIN).*

ASSEMBLY AND TROUBLESHOOTING

Assembly—Misty Ox GIN Nebulizer

1. Remove the cap from the sterile distilled water bottle you wish to use as a reservoir.

2. Aseptically remove the nebulizer from its package. Use caution so that you do not contaminate the long capillary tube which will be immersed into the reservoir bottle.

3. Insert the capillary tube into the bottle and screw the nebulizer into place using the 38 mm threaded fitting. Make sure that the nebulizer is on tight and is not cross threaded.

4. Attach the nebulizer to a high range flowmeter (0–75 L/min). Connect the flowmeter to a 50 psi oxygen or air source, depending upon the total flow and F_IO_2 desired.
   a. Alternatively, a standard flowmeter (0–15 L/min) may be substituted. Turn the needle valve to its maximum setting (beyond flush). Most flowmeters will produce a flow of between 60 and 90 L/min at this setting. The GIN nebulizer will limit flow through its nozzle to 40 L/min at this setting.

5. Attach the secondary gas inlet tube to a second flowmeter powered by the desired secondary gas (air or oxygen). Use of a high-range flowmeter is also recommended for the secondary gas source.

6. Attach large-bore aerosol tubing to the nebulizer outlet. Secure a drainage bag, to collect any condensate, at the midpoint of the tubing.

7. Attach the delivery device to the aerosol tubing (aerosol mask, face tent, aerosol T, trach mask).

8. Adjust the primary and secondary gas flows to achieve your desired F_IO_2 and total flow rate.
   a. Verify the oxygen concentration using a calibrated oxygen analyzer (refer to Chapter 1).

9. Replace the reservoir bottle when the solution level is 1/4 inch from the bottom of the container.

Troubleshooting

When troubleshooting this equipment, please follow the suggested troubleshooting algorithm (ALG 2-13).

No flow from the nebulizer:

1. Check to ensure that there is an adequate oxygen supply when using cylinders.

2. Verify that the flowmeter is correctly connected to the 50 psi oxygen or air source.

3. Check the connection between the nebulizer and the flowmeter.
   a. Make sure it is securely attached.
   b. Check for any obstruction where the nebulizer attaches to the flowmeter.
   c. Verify that the secondary gas inlet tube is free of obstruction or kinks.

Little or no aerosol being generated:

1. Check to ensure that the reservoir bottle contains fluid.

2. Check the capillary tube to ensure it is immersed into the solution in the bottle.

3. Check the capillary tube for obstructions.

4. Check the large-bore aerosol delivery tubing for kinks or obstructions.

5. If using a standard flowmeter (0-15 L/min), verify that the needle valve has been opened to its maximum setting (beyond flush).

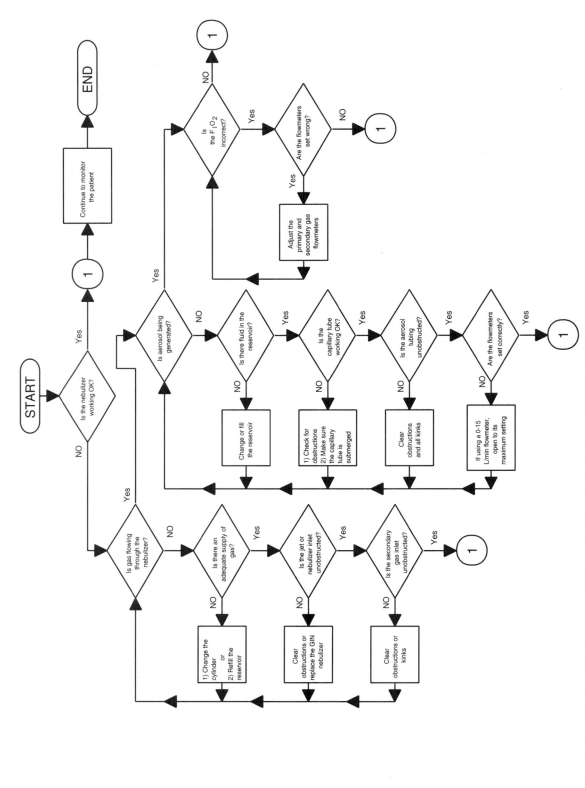

ALG 2-13 *An algorithm describing how to troubleshoot the Misty Ox Gas Injection Nebulizer (GIN).*

Table 2-6 Oxygen Concentration and Total Flow from the Misty Ox GIN Nebulizer

| OXYGEN (L/MIN) | | AIR (L/MIN) | |
PRIMARY GAS	SECONDARY GAS	TOTAL FLOW	CONCENTRATION
40	0	40	100%
40	10	50	84.2%
40	20	60	73.6%
40	30	70	66.1%
40	40	80	60.5%
40	50	90	56.1%
40	60	100	52.6%
40	70	110	49.7%

Table 2-7 Oxygen Concentration and Total Flow from the Misty Ox GIN Nebulizer

| AIR (L/MIN) | | OXYGEN (L/MIN) | |
PRIMARY GAS	SECONDARY GAS	TOTAL FLOW	CONCENTRATION
40	0	40	20.9%
40	10	50	36.8%
40	20	60	47.3%
40	30	70	54.9%
40	40	80	60.5%
40	50	90	64.9%
40	60	100	68.4%
40	70	110	71.3%

Bird 500-cc Inline Micronebulizer

The Bird 500-cc Inline Micronebulizer is primarily employed with the Bird infant ventilators. Both single and double jet models are available. The single jet model has one jet for aerosol production while the double jet has two. Figures 2-34 and 2-35 show the Bird nebulizer. This nebulizer uses a 500-cc reservoir and uses choked flow to produce an aerosol. It is designed to be interfaced with the Bird permanent ventilator circuits to provide aerosol during mechanical ventilation.

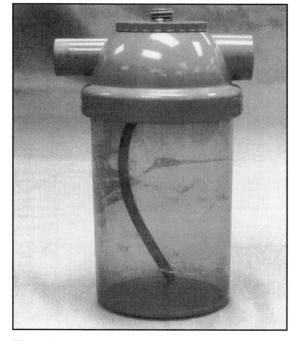

Figure 2-34 *The Bird 500 Micronebulizer.*

ASSEMBLY AND TROUBLESHOOTING

Assembly—Bird 500c Micronebulizer

Refer to Figure 2-35 when following the assembly procedure.

1. Connect the feed tube(s) to the fitting(s) on the crown (the part that fits onto the nebulizer top).
2. Attach the baffle(s) by pressing into place on the crown.
3. Insert the feed tubes through the opening in the nebulizer top and press the crown into place.
4. Fill the nebulizer with sterile distilled water.
5. Screw the reservoir to the nebulizer top.
6. Attach the inlet and outlet tubing.
7. Attach the lines that power the jets to the tallest fittings on the crown.
8. Plug the other crown fittings with the stoppers provided.
9. Attach the mantle by screwing it into place.

Troubleshooting

When troubleshooting this equipment, please follow the suggested troubleshooting algorithm (ALG 2-14).

1. If aerosol output is absent or inadequate:
   a. Ensure that the nebulizer drive lines are attached properly.
   b. Clear the jet of any obstructions.
   c. Ensure that the water level is adequate.
   d. Ensure that the jet/baffle spacing is not too close.
   e. Check the feed tube for kinks or obstructions.
   f. Check the outlet and aerosol tubing for obstructions to flow.
   g. Be certain that the baffle is in place.

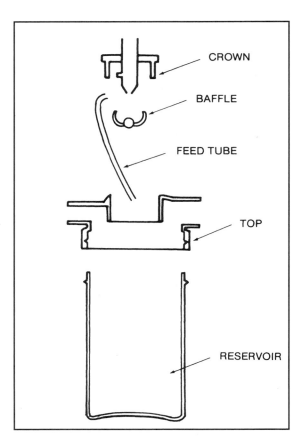

Figure 2-35 *An assembly drawing of the Bird 500 Micronebulizer.*

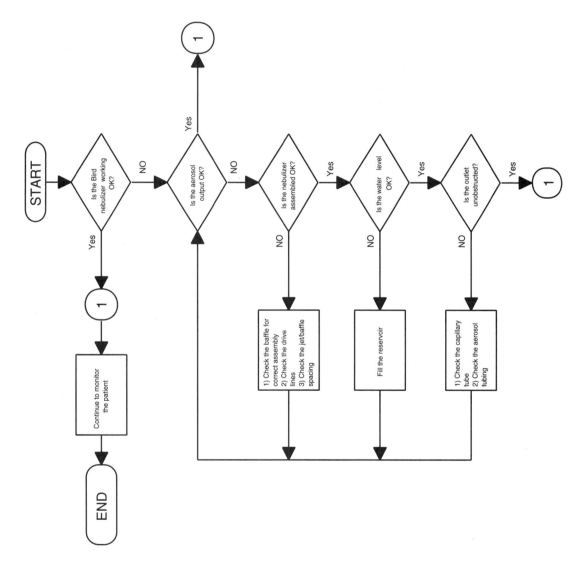

ALG 2-14 *An algorithm describing how to troubleshoot the Bird 500 Micronebulizer.*

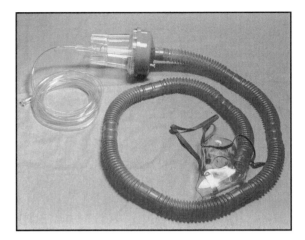

Figure 2-36 *A photograph of the HEART nebulizer.*

Vortan HEART Nebulizer

The Vortan HEART (High Output Extended Aerosol Respiratory Therapy) nebulizer is intended for continuous administration of aerosolized medication (Figure 2-36). In some patients, frequent administration of small-volume nebulizer treatments becomes ineffective, and continuous nebulization of bronchoactive agents is then warranted. The nebulizer has a 240 ml reservoir and obtains a particle size of between 3.5 and 2.2 microns in diameter.

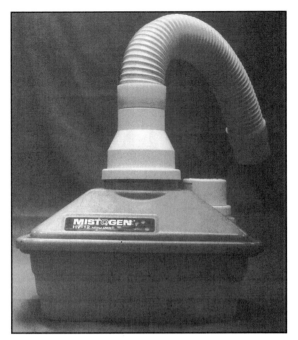

Figure 2-37 *The Mistogen HV-12 nebulizer.*

Mistogen HV-12

The Mistogen HV-12 is a high-volume nebulizer intended for use with the Mistogen CAM 3 tent. It can also be used for room humidity by placing it on a stand designed for this use (Figure 2-37). It is a pneumatic nebulizer that uses choked flow to create a dense aerosol.

ASSEMBLY AND TROUBLESHOOTING

Assembly—Mistogen HV-12

1. Push the inlet filter into the air dilution control fitting and secure the dilution control assembly to the lid of the nebulizer.

2. Attach the feed/filter assembly tube to the jet/baffle assembly by pressing the feed tube onto the jet.

3. Screw the jet/baffle assembly into place on the gas inlet elbow.

4. Fill the reservoir with sterile distilled water.

5. Mate the lid to the reservoir, using the two slide clips on the lid to attach them.

6. Connect the nebulizer to a 50 psi gas source set for between 12 and 15 liters per minute.

Troubleshooting

When troubleshooting this equipment, please follow the suggested troubleshooting algorithm (ALG 2-15)

If aerosol production is inadequate or absent:

1. Check the water level in the reservoir.

2. Ensure the feed tube is attached properly and not obstructed and that the jet/baffle assembly is attached securely.

3. Ensure that the gas source is adequate.

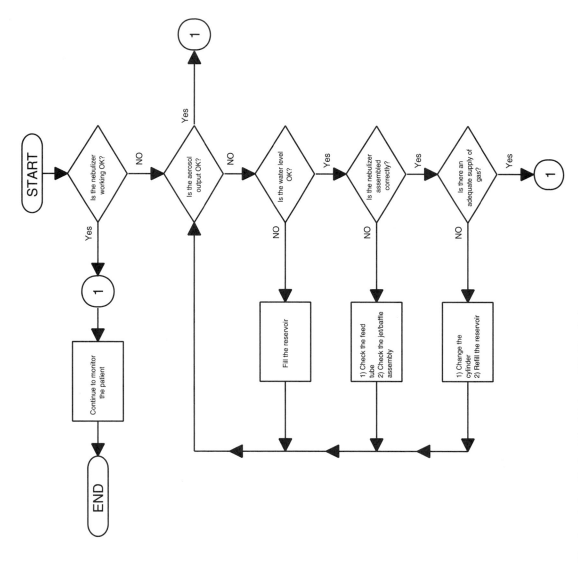

ALG 2-15 *An algorithm describing how to troubleshoot the Mistogen HV-12 nebulizer.*

BABBINGTON NEBULIZERS

Babbington nebulizers are pneumatically powered nebulizers that use the *Babbington principle* in their operation. The Babbington nebulizers have the brand names Solosphere, Hydrosphere and Maxicool. These are very efficient high output nebulizers that produce particle sizes ranging from 3 to 5 microns in diameter.

Gas entering the nebulizer is separated into two channels (Figure 2-38). One pressurizes a glass sphere and the other forms small bubbles that are pushed up a capillary tube to a reservoir above the glass sphere.

The bubbles carry small amounts of water up the tube to the reservoir, gradually filling it. The reservoir drains by gravity, and the water drips onto the glass sphere forming a very thin sheet.

Gas pressure exits the sphere through a very small hole, creating near supersonic velocities. The high velocity gas ruptures the thin sheet of water, producing a fine aerosol. A baffle placed in the path of the gas flow further reduces the particle size.

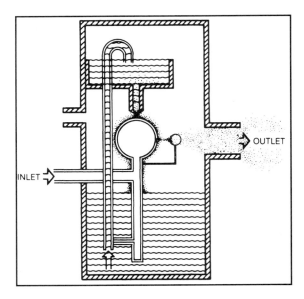

Figure 2-38 *A functional diagram of a Babbington nebulizer.*

Solosphere

The Solosphere nebulizer is intended for long-term aerosol therapy and may be used interchangeably with the other large-volume nebulizers discussed earlier. Figure 2-39 shows a photograph and an assembly drawing of the Solosphere nebulizer.

The Solosphere nebulizer also incorporates an adjustable air entrainment port. When the nebulizer is powered with oxygen, the air entrainment ports allow F_IO_2 adjustments of .40,

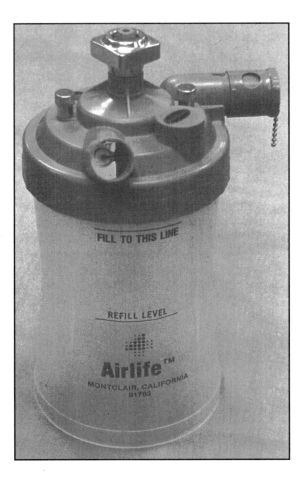

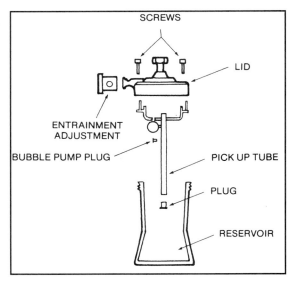

Figure 2-39 *A photograph and an assembly drawing of the Solosphere nebulizer.*

.50, .60, .80 and 1.00. Air is entrained into the nebulizer by jet mixing. As the air entrainment is decreased, total flow through the nebulizer also decreases.

As with any entrainment device, down-stream resistance in the tubing distal to the nebulizer will alter the room air entrainment characteristics of the device such that less air is entrained, increasing the delivered F_iO_2 and decreasing the total flow.

ASSEMBLY AND TROUBLESHOOTING

Assembly—Solosphere Nebulizer

1. Plug the bottom of the pick up tube (capillary tube) with the plug provided.

2. Push the bubble pump plug into place with the flat side facing the ball.

3. Be certain that the large "O" ring is in place on the lid assembly.

4. Insert the manifold assembly into the jar of the nebulizer and secure it in place using the two provided screws.

5. Fill the reservoir with sterile distilled water.

6. Screw the reservoir to the lid of the nebulizer.

7. Attach the nebulizer to a flowmeter and adjust to the ordered flow and F_iO_2.

Troubleshooting

When troubleshooting this equipment, please follow the suggested troubleshooting algorithm (ALG 2-16).

If aerosol production is inadequate:

1. Check the fluid level in the reservoir.

2. Check that the bottom and bubble pump plugs are in place.

3. Make certain the ball is in place and not damaged.

4. Check the DISS fitting for tightness.

5. Check the outlet and aerosol tubing for obstructions.

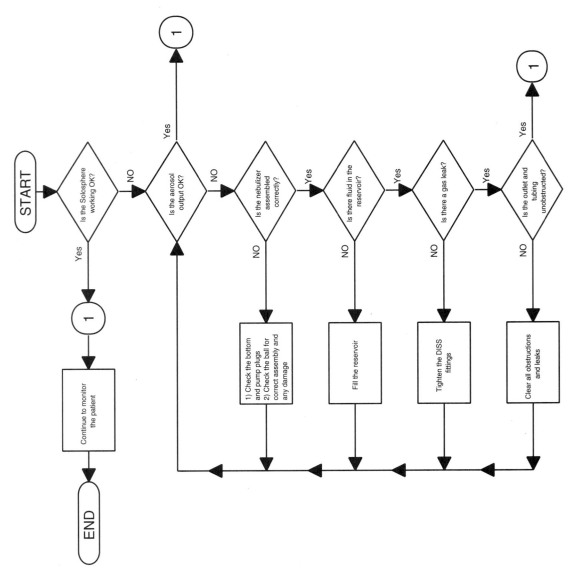

ALG 2-16 *An algorithm describing how to troubleshoot the Solosphere nebulizer.*

Maxi-Cool Nebulizer

The Maxi-Cool nebulizer is a dual ball Babbington nebulizer designed to be used with the Maxi-Cool aerosol tent. It operates using two Babbington nebulizers to produce a very fine dense aerosol. An air entrainment fitting is provided to adjust the F_IO_2 to between .28 and .98 when powered by oxygen.

Adjustment of the F_IO_2 control varies the air entrainment through the nebulizer. Total flows can vary from between 30 to 285 liters per minute, depending on the entrainment adjustment. If aerosol therapy without oxygen administration is the desired goal, the Maxi-Cool may be operated using compressed air.

ASSEMBLY AND TROUBLESHOOTING

Refer to ALG 2-17 and Figure 2-40 when following the assembly and troubleshooting procedures.

Assembly—Maxi-Cool Nebulizer

1. Install the pump plug onto the base of the manifold by pressing it into place.

2. Install the two ball/baffle assemblies, checking the integrity of the "O" rings on their seats. Lock the assemblies into place with the tabs on the manifold.

3. Ensure that the large "O" ring is in place on the top of the nebulizer lid.

4. Press the manifold and the lid together, mating the two pieces.

5. Fill the reservoir with sterile distilled water.

6. Attach the lid to the reservoir by twisting the two components together.

7. Place the reservoir/nebulizer assembly into the housing base and press the cover into position, locking the reservoir/nebulizer assembly.

8. Attach the air entrainment fitting to the inlet opening and attach the large bore delivery tubing to the other.

9. Connect the nebulizer to a 50 psi compressed gas source using a high pressure hose.

Troubleshooting

When troubleshooting this equipment, please follow the suggested troubleshooting algorithm (ALG 2-17).

If aerosol production is inadequate:

1. Check the fluid level in the reservoir.

2. Check that the bubble pump plug is in place.

3. Make certain the ball/baffle assemblies are in place and not damaged.

4. Check the DISS fitting for tightness.

5. Check the outlet and aerosol tubing for obstructions.

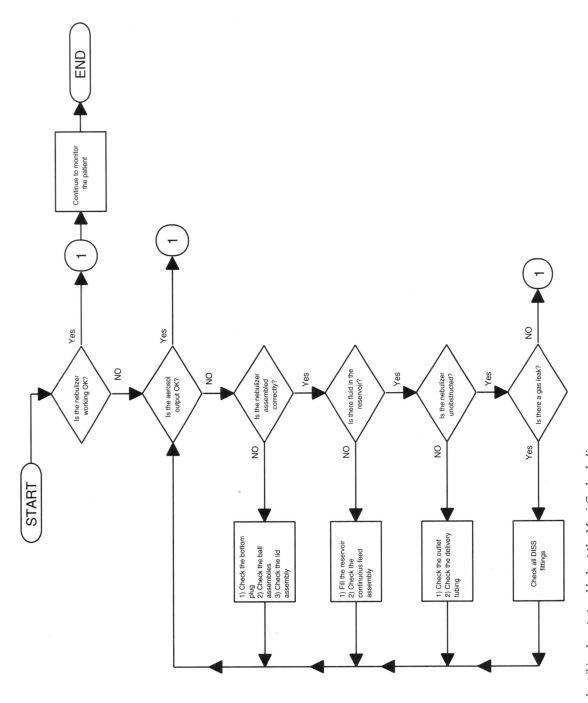

ALG 2-17 *An algorithm describing how to troubleshoot the Maxi-Cool nebulizer.*

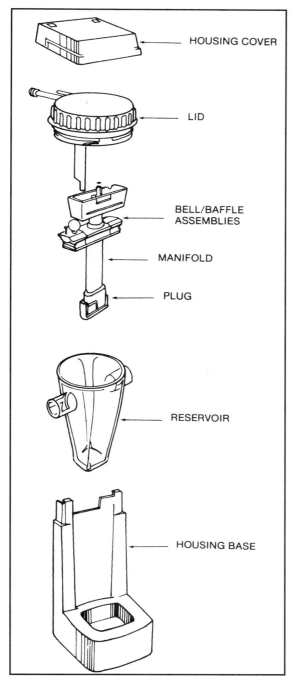

Figure 2-40 *An assembly drawing of the Maxi-Cool nebulizer.*

The labels in the figure from top to bottom read:
- HOUSING COVER
- LID
- BELL/BAFFLE ASSEMBLIES
- MANIFOLD
- PLUG
- RESERVOIR
- HOUSING BASE

SMALL-PARTICLE AEROSOL GENERATOR

ICN Pharmaceuticals, Inc., SPAG-2

The Small Particle Aerosol Generator-2 (SPAG-2) (Figure 2-41), manufactured by ICN Pharmaceuticals, Inc., is a pneumatically powered nebulizer designed specifically for the administration of ribaviran (Virazole®). Ribavirin is a medication that is specific for the treatment of respiratory syncytial virus (RSV), a common illness in infants and small children.

Ribaviran is a powder which is reconstituted by the addition of 300 ml of sterile water in the nebulizer flask or reservoir. Once the drug has been mixed, the nebulizer breaks the liquid into fine aerosol particles with a mean diameter of 1.3 microns.

The SPAG-2 is unique when compared to other nebulizers, in that it has its own regulated gas supply (26 psi) and a secondary gas supply for drying the aerosol particles. The secondary gas supply has a flow adjustment of 2 to 9 L/min. The secondary gas supply is directed through a drying chamber where the aerosol particles evaporate, further reducing the diameter of the particles.

Precautions

Since infants and young children are unable to cooperate using small-volume nebulizers, the SPAG-2 has been designed to administer ribaviran to a tent or hood. When administered in this way, aerosolized ribaviran may be released into the patient's room.

Ribaviran has caused toxicity effects in some care givers including conjunctivitis, rash and bronchospasm. Additionally, women who are pregnant or nursing should not be exposed to ribaviran. Because these effects have been reported, environmental and personal protective equipment precautions should be taken when administering this drug.

Environmental precautions should include a private room with negative-pressure ventilation of at least six air changes per hour. When the patient requires routine types of care, the aerosol therapy should be interrupted, and sufficient time allowed for the aerosol particles to clear. Personal protective equipment should include a HEPA mask, gloves, gown and goggles.

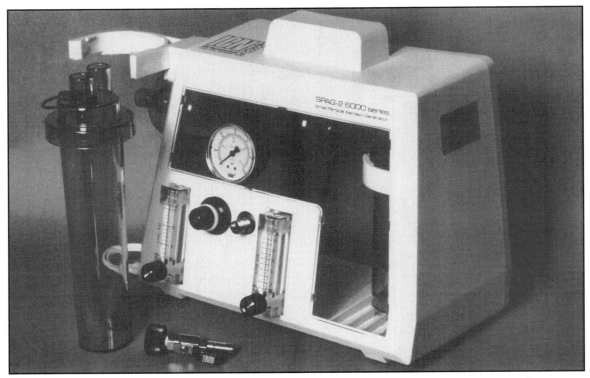

Figure 2-41 *A photograph of the ICN Pharmaceuticals, Inc., SPAG-2 nebulizer for the administration of ribaviran. (Courtesy of ICN Pharmaceuticals, Inc., Costa Mesa, CA)*

ASSEMBLY AND TROUBLESHOOTING

Assembly—SPAG-2 Nebulizer

1. Reconstitute the ribaviran in the reservoir flask by mixing one vial (6 grams) of lyophilized ribaviran into 300 mL of sterile water using aseptic technique.

2. Insert the nebulizer stem into the reservoir cap and place the cap onto the reservoir flask.

3. Insert the reservoir assembly into the nebulizer housing and snap it into place in the bracket.

4. Insert the drying chamber through the wall of the SPAG-2 housing, pressing it into the "O" ring of the cap assembly.

5. Connect the two gas supplies, one to the nebulizer air fitting and the other to the drying air fitting.

6. Connect the gas source (40–60 psi regulated range) to the regulator inlet and adjust the pressure to 26 psi.

7. Open the nebulizer flowmeter completely. The nebulizer flowmeter should indicate 6 1/2 to 8 1/2 L/min. Readjust the regulator to 26 psi, if required.

8. Turn on the drying air flowmeter and readjust the reducing valve to 26 psi, as required. Adjust the drying air flowmeter to 3 1/2 to 6 1/2 L/min. Total flow (nebulizer + drying air) should be 15 L/min. Verify that there are 3 spray spots with a pattern of approximately 2.5 cm diameter.

Troubleshooting

When troubleshooting this equipment, please follow the suggested troubleshooting algorithm (ALG 2-18).

Little or no aerosol output:

1. Check to be sure that there is reconstituted ribaviran in the reservoir assembly.

2. Check the nebulizer stem for correct assembly. Check for obstruction in the nebulizer orifices.

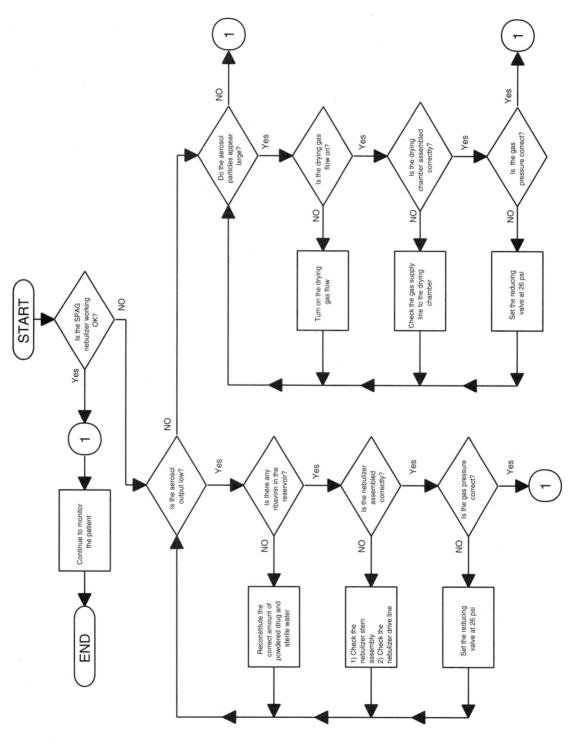

ALG 2-18 *An algorithm describing how to troubleshoot the SPAG-2 nebulizer.*

ULTRASONIC NEBULIZERS

Ultrasonic nebulizers operate by using high-frequency sound waves to produce a fine aerosol. The components of an ultrasonic nebulizer include a radio frequency generator, shielded cable, piezoelectric crystal or transducer, reservoir chamber and a fan.

Before discussing the operating principles of an ultrasonic nebulizer, it is important to understand the difference between frequency and amplitude of a wave form. *Frequency* refers to the number of wave forms per second, or hertz (Hz). The term *amplitude* refers to the height of the wave form from the crest to the trough. In an ultrasonic nebulizer, increasing the frequency causes a decrease in particle size because more waves impact the surface of the water. By increasing amplitude without altering frequency, aerosol output or quantity is increased. This is because each wave has more energy (amplitude). Figure 2-42 illustrates two waveforms with differing amplitudes and frequencies.

The radio frequency (RF) generator produces electromagnetic energy or waves at approximately 1.35 MHz (million cycles per second). The RF generator is an electrically powered electronically controlled RF oscillator (Figure 2-43). The frequency (1.35 MHz) is fixed, while the amplitude is usually variable.

The RF energy from the radio frequency generator is conducted to the *transducer* via a shielded cable. The term "shielded" means that the core of the cable conducting the RF energy is completely surrounded by a braided wire that is connected to an electrical ground. This prevents RF energy from being radiated and causing interference to other electrical equipment close by.

The transducer contains the *piezoelectric crystal.* The piezoelectric crystal has the ability to change shape as an electrical current is applied to it. Thus, electrical energy (RF energy) is converted to mechanical energy (sound waves). The piezoelectric crystal oscillates at the same frequency as the RF energy applied to it.

The sound waves are directed and focused against the surface of the water in the reservoir. The high-frequency sound waves break the water up into a fine aerosol with particle sizes ranging from 1 to 10 microns.

The fan evacuates the aerosol from the reservoir chamber. The aerosol is then conducted to the patient using large-bore aerosol tubing. Without the fan, the aerosol would be produced but would lack clinically significant flow.

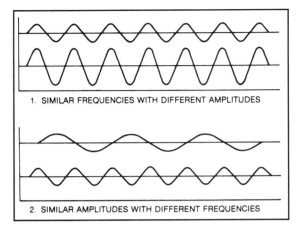

Figure 2-42 *A comparison between frequency and amplitude.*

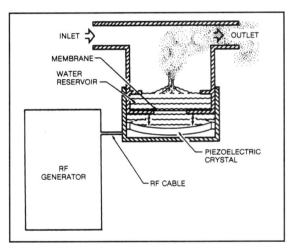

Figure 2-43 *A functional diagram of an ultrasonic nebulizer.*

Hazards of ultrasonic nebulizers include nosocomial infections and electrical shock hazards. Nosocomial infection transmission is a problem due to the large, stagnant reservoir. Furthermore, many nebulizers are taken from one room to another and used with different patients. Frequent reservoir changes and cleaning or the use of disposable reservoirs will reduce infection complications. Electrical shock may be prevented by ensuring that the surrounding floor is kept free of water spills and condensation from the nebulizer. A wet floor serves as an excellent ground pathway.

DeVilbiss Model 65

The DeVilbiss Model 65 is one example of an ultrasonic nebulizer (Figures 2-44 and 2-45). It is capable of producing 6 milliliters of aerosol output per minute. It may be pole-mounted on a small stand with castors to aid in its mobility.

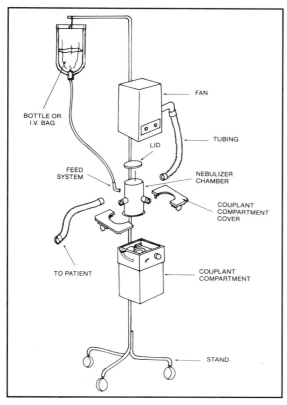

Figure 2-44 *An assembly drawing of the DeVilbiss Model 65 ultrasonic nebulizer.*

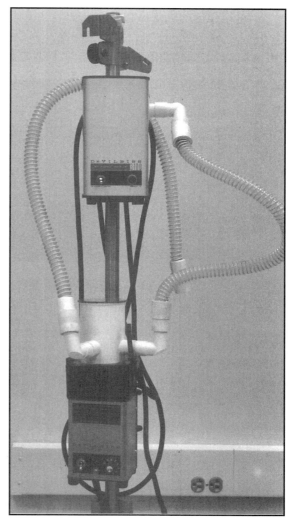

Figure 2-45 *A DeVilbiss Model 65 ultrasonic nebulizer.*

ASSEMBLY AND TROUBLESHOOTING

Assembly—DeVilbiss Model 65

Refer to Figure 2-44, an assembly drawing of this nebulizer.

1. Clip the drain tube onto its holder and fill the couplant chamber with sterile water until the float rises against its seat.

2. Assemble the two couplant chamber covers around the solution cup by clipping them together.

3. Place the solution cup assembly into the couplant chamber and snap it into place.

4. Fill the reservoir in the cup with the desired solution or attach a continuous feed system (reservoir and tubing) to the feed port on the side of the solution cup.

5. Attach large-bore tubing between the fan outlet and the solution cup, and

attach a longer length to the other side, which will go to the patient.

6. Connect the power cord to a suitable 110 volt power source and turn the nebulizer on.

Troubleshooting

When troubleshooting this equipment, please follow the suggested troubleshooting algorithm (ALG 2-19).

If aerosol output is low or absent:

1. Check the fan for proper operation and ensure that the aerosol tubing is connected between the fan and the solution cup.

2. Check the tubing to the patient for obstruction or accumulation of fluid.

3. Check the couplant chamber to verify that it is filled to the correct level.

4. Check the solution cup to ensure that it is filled properly.

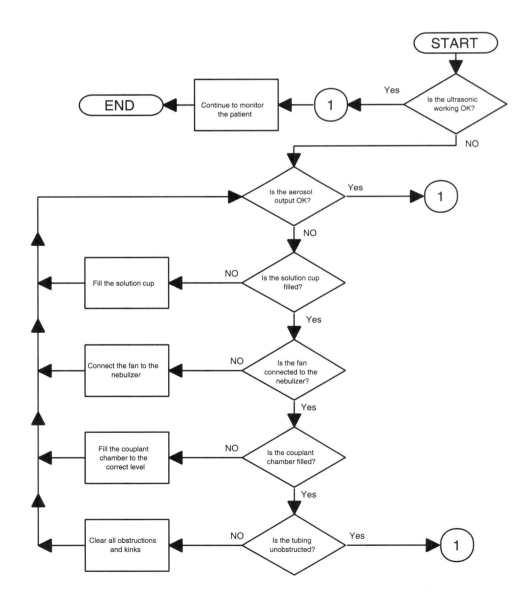

ALG 2-19 *An algorithm describing how to troubleshoot the DeVilbiss Model 65 ultrasonic nebulizer.*

DeVilbiss Ultra-Neb 99

The DeVilbiss Ultra-Neb 99 is an ultrasonic nebulizer capable of producing a minimum of 6 ml per minute of aerosol at the maximum setting (Figure 2-46). These nebulizers are commonly employed in the clinical setting both for direct aerosol application (aerosol mask or face tent) and at the bedside. A reservoir holds up to 200 ml of solution for nebulization.

ASSEMBLY AND TROUBLESHOOTING

Assembly—DeVilbiss Ultra-Neb 99

1. Connect the nebulizer to a 120 volt, 60 Hz power source.

2. Insert the nebulization chamber into the cylindrical receptacle at the front of the nebulizer. Align the nebulization chamber such that the slot matches the raised rib at the front of the receptacle.

3. Place the lid on the top of the nebulization chamber.

4. Attach the feed system to the reservoir bottle and clamp the feed tube. Invert the bottle and hang it from the bottle support arm.

5. Connect the feed system to the nebulization chamber by attaching the tubing to the nipple on the nebulizer lid. Unclamp the feed tubing, and the nebulizer will automatically fill.

6. Connect a short length of 22-mm diameter aerosol tubing between the nebulization chamber and the fan on the rear of the nebulizer. This will evacuate the aerosol from the nebulization chamber.

7. Connect a 60-inch length of 22-mm diameter aerosol tubing from the nebulization chamber to the patient.

8. If a disposable prefilled couplant chamber is to be used:
   a. Install the nebulization chamber as described in (2) above.
   b. Install the RF shield into the bottom of the nebulization chamber, aligning the notch on the circumference with the float assembly.
   c. Fill the chamber with sterile water to the fill line on the side of the chamber.
   d. Place the adapter ring onto the nebulizer chamber. Insert the disposable couplant into the nebulization chamber, seating it.
   e. Connect aerosol tubing to the prefilled chamber as described in (6) and (7).

Troubleshooting

When troubleshooting this equipment, please follow the suggested troubleshooting algorithm (ALG 2-20).

1. If the unit fails to operate and, when turned on, the "On/Off" switch does not illuminate:
   a. Ensure that the power cord is connected to a 110 v, 60 Hz outlet.
   b. Check the fuse at the rear of the nebulizer, and if necessary, replace it.

2. If aerosol output is diminished or absent:
   a. Check the "Check Chamber" indicator light. If the light is illuminated, the water level in the nebulization chamber is low.
   b. Check the delivery tubing for obstructions or accumulated condensate.
   c. Ensure that the tubing from the fan is attached to the chamber and that the fan is working.
   d. Check the float to ensure that it is free to travel up and down on its attachment rod.
   e. The chamber may have become contaminated. Wash the nebulizer chamber with alcohol or 2% acetic acid.

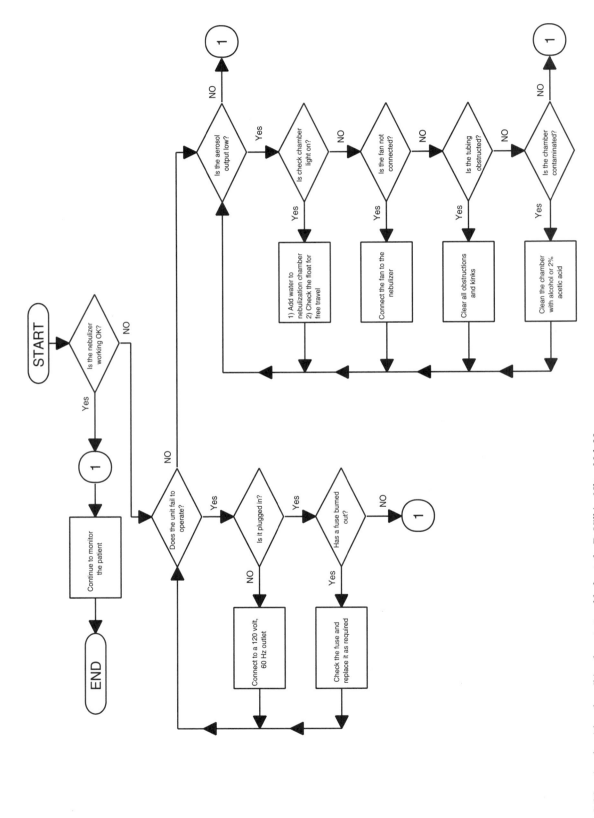

ALG 2-20 *An algorithm describing how to troubleshoot the DeVilbiss Ultra-Neb 99.*

Timeter Compu-Neb

The Timeter Compu-Neb is an ultrasonic nebulizer commonly used in the clinical environment (Figure 2-47). It operates using the principles discussed in this chapter.

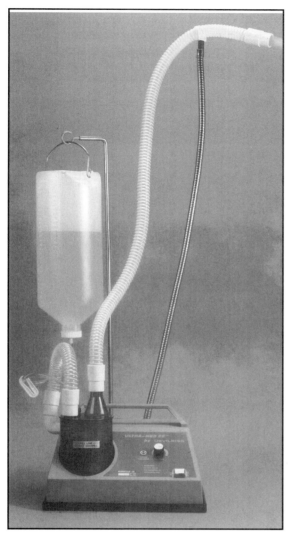

Figure 2-46 *The DeVilbiss Ultra-Neb 99. (Courtesy of DeVilbiss Health Care, Inc., Somerset, PA)*

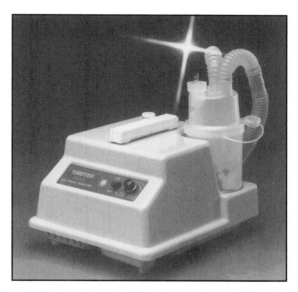

Figure 2-47 *The Timeter Model MP-500 Compu-Neb ultrasonic nebulizer. (Courtesy of Allied Healthcare Products, Inc.–Timeter Instrument Corporation. Timeter Instrument Corporation is a division of Allied Healthcare Products, Inc., St. Louis, MO.)*

ASSEMBLY AND TROUBLESHOOTING

Assembly—Timeter Compu-Neb

1. Place the transducer/couplant chamber into its well on the nebulizer housing.

2. Fill the chamber with the solution to be nebulized until the feed float rises. Alternately, a continuous feed system may be connected to the feed nipple on the transducer/couplant housing.

3. Attach the transducer/couplant cap to the housing by screwing it into place.

4. Attach a short piece of connecting tubing between the fan outlet and the transducer/couplant chamber.

5. Attach a long piece of aerosol tubing to the outlet of the couplant chamber for the patient.

6. Connect the power cord to a 110 volt source and turn the unit on.

Troubleshooting

When troubleshooting this equipment, please follow the suggested troubleshooting algorithm (ALG 2-21).

If aerosol output is low or inadequate:

1. Ensure that the power cord is connected to a 110 volt power source.

2. Verify that the transducer/couplant chamber is filled to the correct level.

3. Verify that the fan is connected to the transducer/couplant housing with aerosol tubing and that the fan is working.

4. Ensure that the aerosol delivery tubing is free of obstructions or condensate.

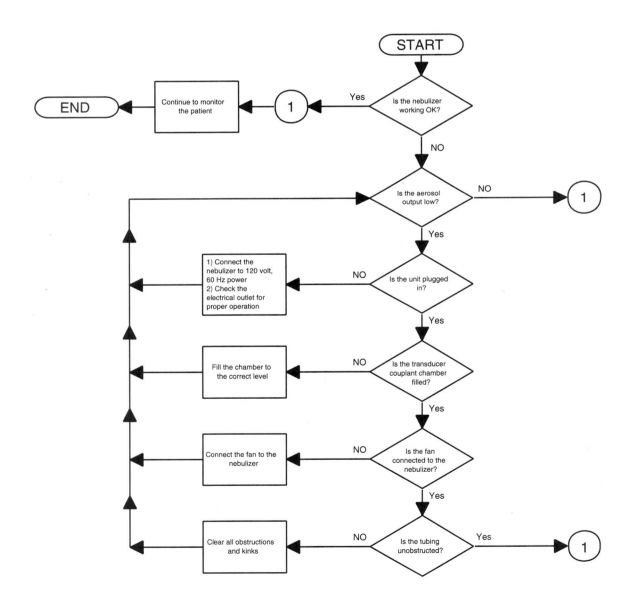

ALG 2-21 *An algorithm describing how to troubleshoot the Timeter Model MP-500 Compu-Neb ultrasonic nebulizer.*

SMALL-VOLUME ULTRASONIC NEBULIZERS FOR MEDICATION DELIVERY

Small-volume (less than 10 ml) nebulizers have been developed for medication delivery. These devices use ultrasonic transducers to break liquid medication into fine aerosol particles for inhalation. Since these are ultrasonic nebulizers, more aerosol particles fall into the small particle size ranges, which improves aerosol penetration. Unlike the larger, continuous ultrasonic nebulizers, these smaller versions are very light weight and portable. All of the units can be operated on internal battery packs, a 12 V DC power source or from a 120 volt, 60 Hz adapter. The portability of these nebulizers makes them very convenient for patient use in the home or other settings away from acute care facilities.

DeVilbiss Pulmosonic 5500 Nebulizer

The DeVilbiss Health Care, Inc. Pulmosonic 5500 ultrasonic nebulizer is a small, portable ultrasonic nebulizer designed for medication administration (Figure 2-48). Being truly portable (10.3 ounces, or 292 grams), it can operate from an internal battery pack, 12 V DC power or via a 120 v, 60 Hz power adapter.

Theory of Operation

When the patient depresses a switch plate on the front of the unit, ultrasonic energy is directed into the medication dome, breaking the

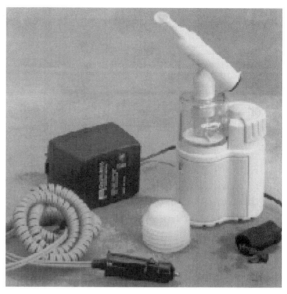

Figure 2-48 *A photograph of the DeVilbiss Pulmosonic 5500 ultrasonic nebulizer. (Courtesy of Sunrise Medical)*

liquid medication into a fine aerosol. Aerosol will only be produced as long as the switch plate is depressed. The patient is encouraged to release the switch plate during exhalation, conserving medication. A one-way valve on the mouthpiece assembly allows the patient to exhale through the mouthpiece without removing it from the mouth.

Flow through the unit may be adjusted by rotating the flow cap on the back of the nebulizer. Rotating the flow cap adjusts the amount of ambient air entering the dome. By increasing ambient air entrainment, flow is increased through the medication dome.

ASSEMBLY AND TROUBLESHOOTING

Assembly—DeVilbiss Pulmosonic 5500

1. Mix or dilute the medication ordered by the physician and place it into the medication reservoir.

2. Remove the dome by turning it counterclockwise until it separates from the control unit. Remove the medicine cup from the chamber assembly and fill the chamber with cold tap water to the top of the internal ribs (about 40 mL). Replace the medicine cup and baffle into the chamber assembly, making sure that water touches the base of the medicine cup. Attach the dome by rotating it a quarter-turn clockwise, locking it into place. Add medication to the medicine cup through the opening in the top of the chamber dome.

3. Insert the mouthpiece into the outlet of the chamber dome.

4. Plug the cord from the chamber assembly into the control unit, inserting it into the large receptacle on the front of the unit.

5. Determine which power source is to be used:
   a. To operate the unit on internal batteries, simply turn the control unit on.
   b. To operate the unit from an electrical outlet, attach the adapter to the power input receptacle on the front of the control unit. Then plug the adapter into a 120 volt, 60 Hz outlet.
   c. To operate the unit from a 12 volt power source, connect the supplied power adapter to the power input receptacle on the front of the unit. Connect the other end of the adapter to the auxiliary power supply (e.g., the cigarette lighter of an automobile.)

6. Turn the control unit on.

7. Instruct the patient as follows: Place the mouthpiece into your mouth and depress the switch plate on the chamber assembly. Slowly inhale, taking a deep breath. When you exhale, you may remove the mouthpiece or exhale through it and the one-way valve. Repeat this sequence until the medication has been delivered.

8. Once the medication has been delivered, turn the control unit off and disconnect the control unit from any external power source.

Cleaning

1. Disconnect the control unit from any power source.

2. Disassemble the chamber dome and mouthpiece from the chamber assembly.

   Note: Never use soap or detergent solution to clean this ultrasonic unit.

3. Soak the chamber dome and mouthpiece in a solution of one part white vinegar to one part water or in a cold disinfecting solution (Control III, Cidex, etc.).

4. Disconnect the chamber assembly from the control unit by unplugging the power cord.

5. Immerse the chamber dome assembly into the cleaning solution as described above. **DO NOT SUBMERGE THE CHAMBER ASSEMBLY ELECTRICAL CONNECTOR INTO ANY SOLUTION.** Gently clean the chamber assembly with a clean soft sponge.

6. Remove the chamber assembly and gently clean the transducer (gold disk at the bottom of the chamber assembly) using a cotton-tipped swab.

7. Rinse the parts under clean water and allow them to air dry.

8. Gently clean the control assembly with a damp sponge or cloth.

Troubleshooting

When troubleshooting this equipment, please follow the suggested troubleshooting algorithm (ALG 2-22).

The nebulizer will not turn on:

1. Check power source:
   a. Battery pack discharged. Twelve hours is required to fully charge the battery using the supplied adapter.
   b. The 12 V DC power source is exhausted.
   c. The 120 volt, 60 Hz adapter is not connected to an outlet. Ensure it is plugged in. If it still fails to operate, the adapter may be defective and need replacement.

2. The nebulizer has malfunctioned. Contact a DeVilbiss service center.

The nebulizer will not create a mist in the chamber dome:

1. The medication has been nebulized and none remains.

2. The 30-second shut off has been activated. Depress the button on the chamber assembly.

3. The thermal protection circuit has tripped, shutting the unit off. Wait 2 to 3 minutes and depress the button on the chamber assembly again.

4. The chamber assembly has become disconnected from the control unit. Ensure that the power cord is plugged into the control unit.

5. An air bubble has formed over the transducer. Gently tap and shake the chamber assembly.

6. The unit has malfunctioned. Contact a DeVilbiss service representative.

The nebulizer does not operate and the low battery light is illuminated:

1. The internal battery pack has lost its charge. Recharge the battery using the 120 volt, 60 Hz adapter for sixteen hours.

The battery will not hold a charge:

1. The battery has malfunctioned. Contact your DeVilbiss service representative for a replacement.

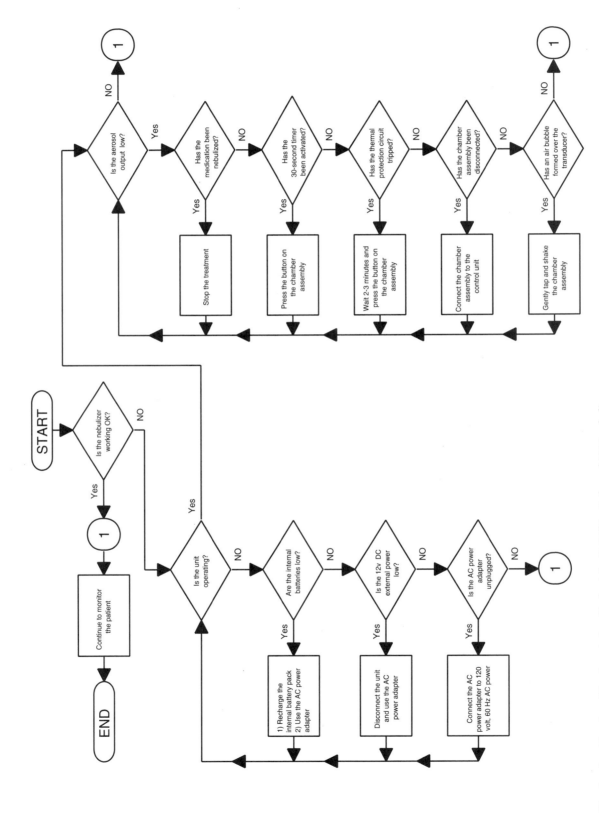

ALG 2-22 *An algorithm describing how to troubleshoot the DeVilbiss Pulmosol 5500 nebulizer.*

Microstat (CAIRE, Inc.)

The CAIRE, Inc., Microstat is a small, portable ultrasonic nebulizer designed for medication delivery (Figure 2-49). It weighs under 2 pounds, including the battery pack. The unit may also be powered by a 12 V DC power source or from a 115 v, 60 Hz electrical outlet, using the adapter provided by the manufacturer.

Theory of Operation

The Microstat uses ultrasonic energy to break the liquid medication into a fine aerosol. The aerosol particles range between 3 and 5 microns. As the aerosol rises toward the outlet of the medicine chamber, it passes through a spiral-shaped set of baffles, which removes larger particles from suspension. The larger particles fall to the base of the medicine chamber, where they will be nebulized again. The baffling system ensures delivery of a uniform, stable particle size.

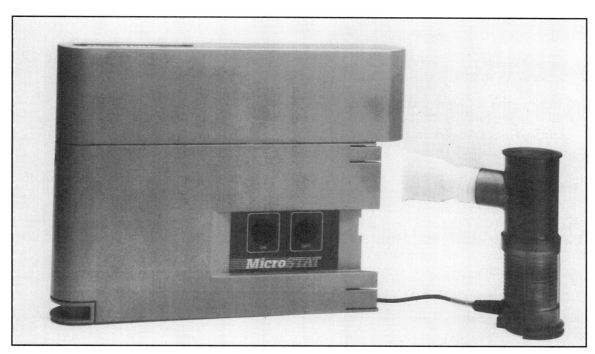

Figure 2-49 *A photograph of the Microstat ultrasonic nebulizer. (Courtesy of CAIRE, Inc., Littleton, CO)*

ASSEMBLY AND TROUBLESHOOTING

Assembly—Microstat

1. Detach the nebulizer head cover assembly from the nebulizer head (Figure 2-50).

2. Fill the medicine chamber using the medication and dilution prescribed by the physician.

3. Attach the nebulizer head cover assembly to the nebulizer head.

4. Attach a mouthpiece to the nebulizer head cover assembly.

5. Depress the "On" button on the front of the unit. Aerosolized medication will appear in the nebulizer head cover within 10 seconds.

6. Instruct the patient to take slow, deep breaths. A one-way valve allows medication delivery only during inspiration. To exhale, have the patient remove the mouthpiece from his/her mouth and exhale passively or exhale through his/her nose.

   a. During therapy keep the nebulizer upright (vertical). If it is tipped, medication may be lost.

Cleaning

After each use it is recommended that the unit be cleaned.

1. Disconnect the nebulizer head and nebulizer head cover from the nebulizer control unit by unplugging the end plug.

2. Remove the nebulizer head cover from the nebulizer head and disassemble it.

3. Gently wash the parts in a mild detergent and water. **Never immerse the End Plug in water or any solution.**

4. Rinse the parts in clean water and allow them to air dry.

5. Weekly, soak all parts (except the End Plug) in a solution of white vinegar and water or cold disinfecting agent (Control III, Cidex, etc.).

Troubleshooting

When troubleshooting this equipment, please follow the suggested troubleshooting algorithm (ALG 2-23).

The nebulizer is operating but a light is rapidly flashing:

1. The battery level is low. Recharge the battery for 24 hours using the supplied AC power adapter.

The nebulizer will not work and a light is slowly flashing:

1. There is insufficient power in the internal battery pack to power the nebulizer. Recharge the battery as described above.

The nebulizer will not operate. The "ON" light illuminates for a few seconds, then turns off.

1. The nebulizer is not connected properly to the control unit. Reattach the End Plug to the nebulizer control unit.

The nebulizer will not operate:

1. Check to ensure that the battery is properly installed.

2. Check to ensure the external power source and adapters are installed correctly.

3. The unit has malfunctioned. Contact your service representative.

4. The unit has overheated. Wait several minutes and restart the nebulizer.

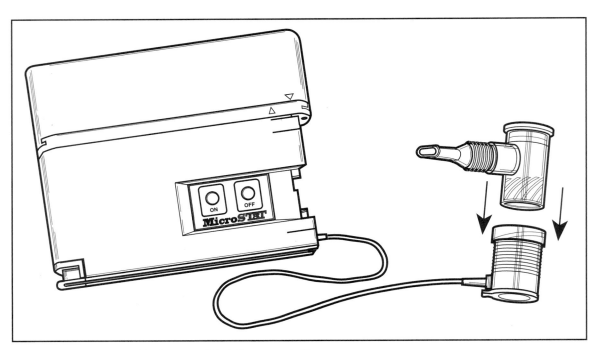

Figure 2-50 *An assembly drawing of the Microstat nebulizer.*

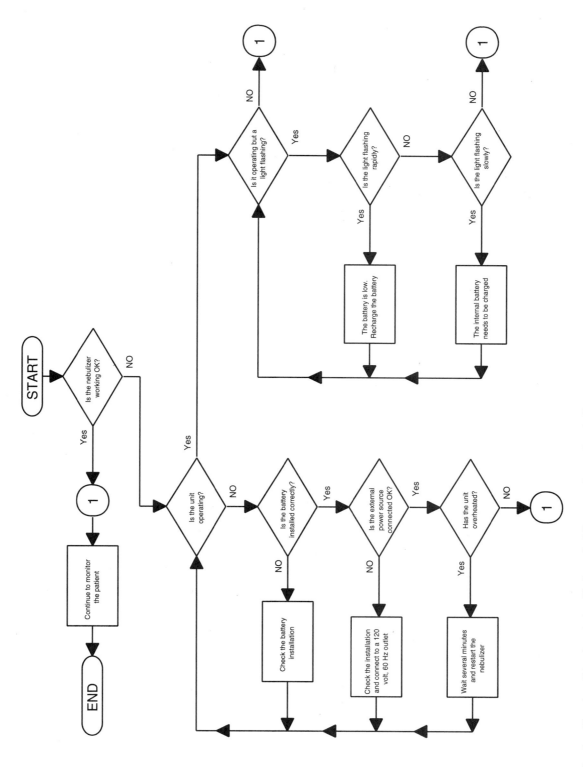

ALG 2-23 *An algorithm describing how to troubleshoot the Microstat ultrasonic nebulizer.*

AEROSOL ADMINISTRATION DEVICES

Aerosol produced by a nebulizer must be safely and effectively conducted to the patient. Various devices have been designed to improve aerosol delivery for a variety of clinical applications. These devices include the aerosol mask, trach mask, face tent, and Brigg's adapter or aerosol T.

The aerosol mask (Figure 2-51) is similar to the simple oxygen mask. The inlet, however, is designed for large-bore tubing. The two outlet ports are also large to facilitate evacuation of any exhaled aerosol.

The trach mask is designed to fit over a tracheostomy tube (Figure 2-52). It is secured by an elastic strap that surrounds the neck. A 22-mm large-bore inlet fitting accommodates the aerosol tubing and a single large outlet port evacuates exhaled aerosol.

The face tent is designed to be strapped under the chin, enclosing the lower part of a patient's face (Figure 2-53). This device is commonly used in the recovery room following general anesthesia or for patients with facial burns.

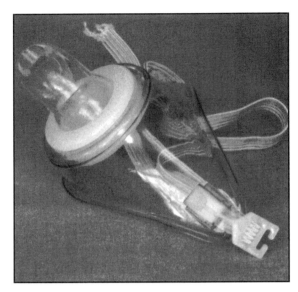

Figure 2-52 *A tracheostomy aerosol mask.*

The Brigg's adapter is designed to be used with an artificial airway. It is also commonly referred to as an aerosol T. The Brigg's adapter has two 22-mm ports opposite one another and a 15-mm port at right angles to them, forming a T (Figure 2-54).

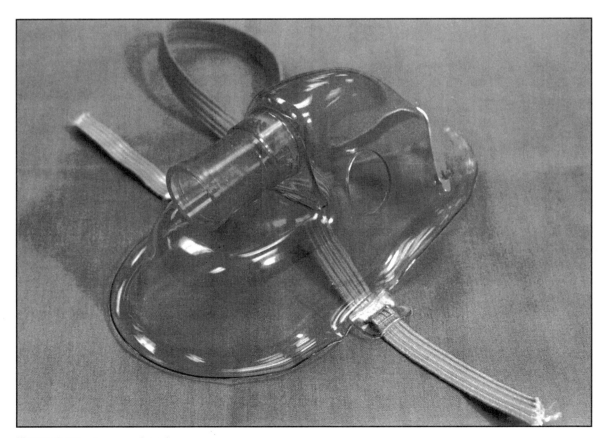

Figure 2-51 *An aerosol mask.*

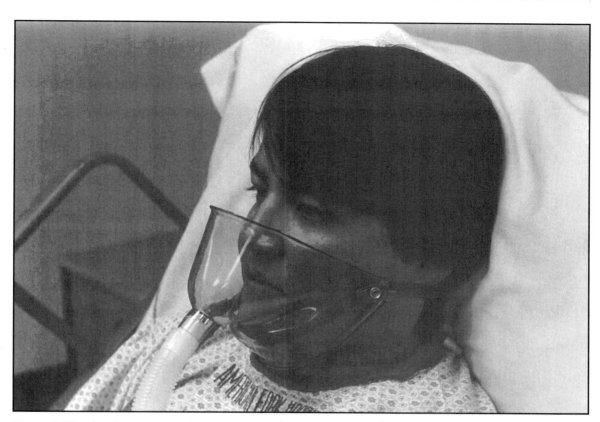

Figure 2-53 *A patient wearing a face tent.*

When using the Brigg's adapter with an artificial airway, it is important to install a short (approximately 6 inches) piece of aerosol tubing on the outlet of the adapter. This tubing serves as a reservoir, and prevents the patient from entraining room air during early inspiration. Adequate flow can be assured by observing the mist output through the reservoir. The flow of mist should never cease during the inspiratory phase; only then can you be sure that no air entrainment is occurring.

Although not technically an aerosol delivery device, drainage bags are an important part of an aerosol therapy circuit (Figure 2-55).

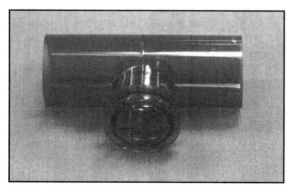

Figure 2-54 *An aerosol T. This is also known as a Brigg's adapter.*

The drainage bag is placed at a low point in the tubing between the aerosol generator and the patient. Its purpose is to collect water condensation, thus preventing contamination of the reservoir and the patient. With air entrainment devices, the drainage bag also prevents water accumulation, created by condensation, from causing an increase in F_IO_2 due to back pressure.

PEDIATRIC AEROSOL TENTS

Pediatric aerosol tents are environmental devices frequently used in the treatment of croup, epiglottitis and other pediatric upper airway disorders. They are designed to enclose the child in an atmosphere of cool aerosol. Oxygen may be administered, as well as aerosol, to correct hypoxemia, as required.

Croupette

The croupette is commonly used for pediatric aerosol therapy. The croupette was discussed in Chapter 1, in the section on enclosures. Refer to Chapter 1 for its assembly and troubleshooting.

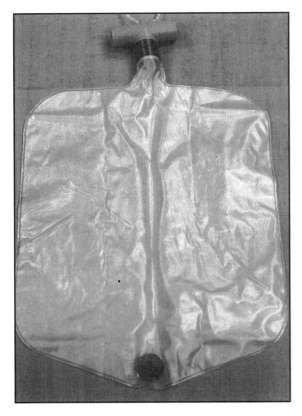

Figure 2-55 *A drainage bag. This bag is placed between the aerosol generator and the patient, to collect condensate.*

Ohmeda Pediatric Aerosol Tent

The Ohmeda Pediatric Aerosol tent is a self-contained refrigerated aerosol generator (Figure 2-56). The tent provides both aerosol generation and refrigeration to keep the atmosphere inside the tent cool.

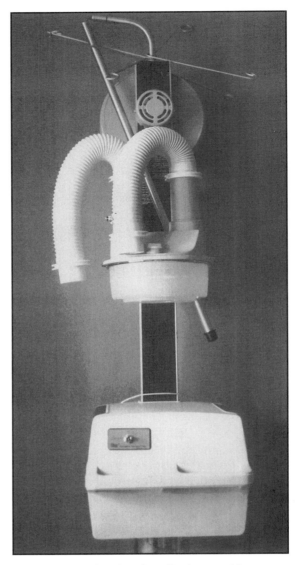

Figure 2-56 *The Ohmeda pediatric tent without a canopy attached.*

ASSEMBLY AND TROUBLESHOOTING

Assembly—Ohmeda Pediatric Aerosol Tent

1. Assemble the condensation bottle by screwing the cap on and attaching the condensate tube.

2. Place the condensation bottle into its bracket on the side of the main housing.

3. Assemble the cooling fan unit:
   a. Attach the radial finned plate to the evaporator bracket using the screws provided.

   b. Attach the blower wheel with the nut that secures it.
   c. Connect the condensation tube to the evaporator bracket.
   d. Attach the evaporator shroud by twisting it into place.

4. Attach the nebulizer to its bracket.

5. Erect the canopy support rod assembly over the bed or crib and secure it into place.

6. Attach the canopy to the frame, stretching the large opening over the rim of the evaporator shroud. Tuck the edges under the mattress for a tight seal.

7. Attach the large supply tubes to the two small holes in the canopy at the head of the bed.

8. Connect the nebulizer with high pressure hose to a flowmeter and set the flow between 12 and 15 liters per minute.

9. Fill the reservoir with sterile distilled water.

10. Connect the power cord to a 110 volt source.

11. Turn on the refrigeration unit.

Troubleshooting

When troubleshooting this equipment, please follow the suggested troubleshooting algorithm (ALG 2-24).

If aerosol output is low or absent:

1. Check to see if the reservoir is filled to the correct level.

2. Check the flowmeter setting and the high pressure hose connections.

3. Check the inlet tubing for obstructions.

4. Check the nebulizer jet for obstructions.

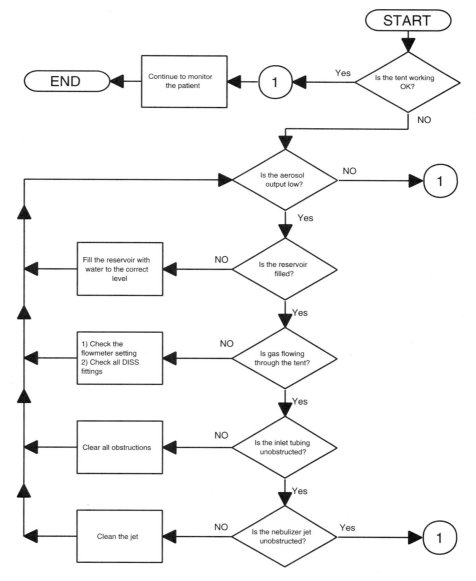

ALG 2-24 *An algorithm describing how to troubleshoot the Ohmeda pediatric tent.*

Mistogen Child Adult Mist (CAM) Tent

The Mistogen Child Adult Mist (CAM) tent (Figure 2-57) is designed to incorporate the Mistogen HV-12 nebulizer (discussed ear-lier) as its aerosol generator. In addition, the tent uses a refrigeration unit that chills and circulates water to cool the air inside the canopy.

ASSEMBLY AND TROUBLESHOOTING

Assembly—Mistogen CAM Tent

1. Assemble the tent frame and position it at the head of the bed with the lower assembly under the mattress.

2. Connect the cooling panel by latching it and connecting the lower portion to its support blocks.

3. Attach the canopy to the canopy frame.

4. Fill the cooler reservoir with distilled water to the indicated level.

5. Install the coolant tubing between the cooling panel and the control unit.

6. Connect the drain tubing to the condensation trap on the control unit.

7. Assemble the HV-12 nebulizer as discussed earlier in this chapter and place it onto the cover of the control unit.

8. Connect the nebulizer tubing to the opening in the tent.

9. Plug the power cord into a 110 volt source and turn on the power.

Troubleshooting

When troubleshooting this equipment, please follow the suggested troubleshooting algorithm (ALG 2-25).

If aerosol production is inadequate or absent:

1. Check the water level in the reservoir.

2. Ensure the feed tube is attached properly and not obstructed and that the jet/baffle assembly is attached securely.

3. Ensure that the nebulizer is connected to a high-pressure gas source and that the flowmeter is on.

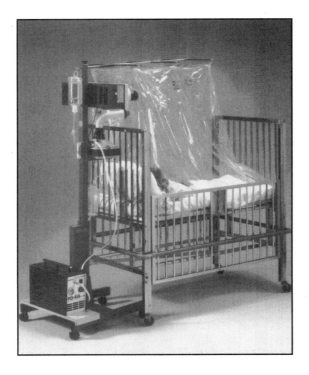

Figure 2-57 *The Mistogen CAM tent. (Courtesy of Allied Healthcare Products, Inc.–Timeter Instrument Corporation. Timeter Instrument Corporation is a division of Allied Healthcare Products, Inc., St. Louis, MO.)*

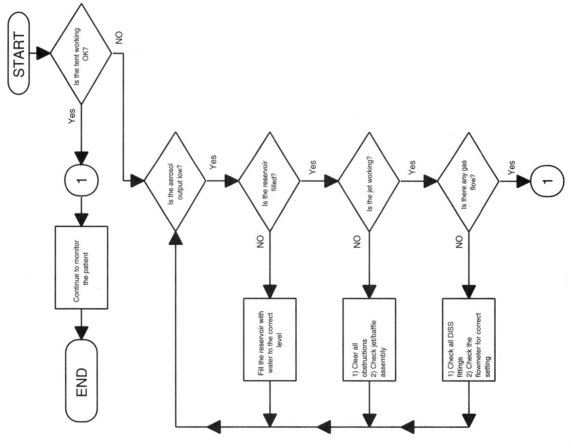

ALG 2-25 *An algorithm describing how to troubleshoot the Mistogen CAM tent.*

CLINICAL CORNER

Aerosol Therapy Equipment

1. You are taking care of a patient in an acute care setting and have just assembled a disposable, up-draft small-volume nebulizer. When you turn on the flowmeter, the liquid medication simply bubbles and does not aerosolize. Describe the steps you would take to correct the situation.

2. You are taking care of a patient in the intensive care unit (ICU) who is on a 65% heated aerosol, and the flowmeter is set for 12 L/min. The patient is desaturating. Describe how you would assess the situation in the case where the flow from the nebulizer is adequate for the patient's inspiratory needs.

3. In a role-play situation, teach your instructor how to take a Metered Dose Inhaler treatment using a spacer.

4. You are expecting a new admission from surgery. The new patient is postoperative, having just had a tracheostomy tube placed. What equipment should you gather and how would you set it up to deliver 35% oxygen?

5. You are called to the medical floor to evaluate a patient on low-flow oxygen. A care assistant has called to alert you that the patient seems short of breath. Upon your arrival, you note the patient to be tachypneic and dyspneic. When you glance at the oxygen flowmeter, you notice that the disposable bubble humidifier is bulging and no bubbles can be observed. Describe the steps you would take in troubleshooting this situation.

6. You are setting up an ultrasonic nebulizer in preparation for a 20-minute treatment. When you turn the nebulizer on, the fan runs and the water in the reservoir is agitated, but no aerosol is produced. Describe how you would troubleshoot the situation.

Self-Assessment Quiz

1. Humidity is measured by:
   I. Particle size.
   II. Partial pressure.
   III. Percentage.
   IV. Water content.
   a. I and II only
   b. II and III only
   c. I, II, and III only
   d. II, III, and IV only
   e. I, II, and IV only

2. An aerosol is defined as:
   a. Water contained in a gas as vapor.
   b. Particulate matter suspended in a gas.
   c. The maximum amount of water content a gas can contain at a given temperature.
   d. The actual water content of a gas at a given temperature.

3. The definition of capacity is:
   a. Water contained in a gas as vapor.
   b. Particulate matter suspended in a gas.
   c. The maximum amount of water content a gas can contain at a given temperature.
   d. The actual water content of a gas at a given temperature.

4. You must deliver a maximal amount of humidity to a patient's airway; how could this be accomplished using a diffusion grid humidifier?
   I. Increase the setting on the thermostat to a maximum of 37 degrees Celsius.
   II. Keep the water in the reservoir at the correct level.
   III. Ensure that the total flow through the humidifier exceeds the patient's requirements.

IV. Use water traps or a drainage bag in the circuit.
a. I
b. I and II
c. I, II and III
d. I, II, III and IV

5. You are administering oxygen to a patient via a bubble type humidifier. You know the humidity output is 14.5 mg/L (from a study published in Respiratory Care). What is the humidity deficit?
a. 14.5 mg/L.
b. 29.4 mg/L.
c. 43.9 mg/L.
d. 47.0 mg/L.

6. An advantage of the Misty Ox Laminar Diffuser Humidifier, when compared to a bubble jet humidifier, is:
a. High flow outputs at high humidity are possible.
b. It is designed for low flow oxygen delivery systems.
c. It only delivers cool aerosol.
d. None of the above.

7. The majority of humidifiers operate using the phenomenon of:
a. Bernoulli's principle.
b. Ultrasonic waves.
c. Evaporation.
d. Venturi's principle.
e. Pitot's principle.

8. Ways to improve a humidifier's efficiency include:
I. Increase the temperature.
II. Increase the jet's lateral pressure.
III. Increase the surface area.
IV. Increase the gas velocity through the device.
a. I and II only
b. I and III only
c. II and III only
d. II and IV only
e. III and IV only

9. The magnitude of the pressure exerted by water vapor is dependent upon:
I. Temperature.
II. Relative humidity.
III. Barometric pressure.
a. I
b. I and II
c. I and III
d. II and III

10. Factors that influence an aerosol's deposition in the lungs include:
I. Particle size.
II. Gravity.
III. Inertia.
a. I only
b. I and II only
c. II only
d. III only
e. I, II, and III only

11. The piezoelectric crystal in an ultrasonic nebulizer:
a. Converts electrical energy to mechanical energy.
b. Converts water to vapor.
c. Vibrates at a low frequency causing hydrolysis.

    d. When operated with the fan cools the aerosol.

    e. Operates using Bernoulli's principle.

12. Which of the following humidifiers would be suitable for use for a patient requiring a simple oxygen mask?

    I. Bubble humidifier.

    II. Wick humidifier.

    III. Bubble jet humidifier.

    IV. Misty Ox LDH humidifier.

    a. I and II

    b. I and III

    c. II and III

    d. II and IV

13. You must provide humidified gas for a patient who is intubated; which of the following devices would be the most appropriate?

    I. Bubble humidifier.

    II. Wick humidifier.

    III. Bubble jet humidifier.

    IV. Misty Ox LDH humidifier.

    a. I and II

    b. I and III

    c. II and III

    d. II and IV

14. When checking oxygen in a patient's room, you hear an audible chirping or whistling sound. The most likely cause is:

    a. The patient's inspiratory stridor.

    b. The nurse's call button.

    c. The humidifier pop-off.

    d. Flow through the patient's venturi mask.

    e. The ultrasonic nebulizer's circuit breaker.

15. Contemporary high output humidifiers employ which of the following in their operation?

    I. Bernoulli's principle.

    II. A wick.

    III. A piezoelectric crystal.

    IV. A heater.

    a. I and II only

    b. I and III only

    c. II and III only

    d. II and IV only

    e. I and IV only

16. The most common type of humidifier in clinical practice is:

    a. The bubble humidifier.

    b. The room humidifier.

    c. The Cascade Humidifier.

    d. The wick humidifier.

    e. The pass-over humidifier.

17. An indication that a heat and moisture exchanger is becoming obstructed would be:

    a. The temperature alarm is sounding.

    b. The patient's work of breathing is increased.

    c. The water reservoir rarely needs filling anymore.

    d. The resistance to gas flow decreases.

    e. Pressure decreases distal to the exchanger.

18. A heat and moisture exchanger should be:

    I. Placed between the ventilator circuit, or oxygen therapy equipment, and the patient's airway.

    II. Utilized for short term applications (less than 24 hours).

    III. Monitored for obstruction.

    a. I

b. I and II
c. II and III
d. I, II and III

19. Which of the following humidifiers would be suitable for use with a mechanical ventilator?
    I. Puritan Bennett Cascade humidifier.
    II. Ohmeda Ohio Bubble Jet humidifier.
    III. Respiratory Care Conchapack.
    IV. Room humidifier.
    a. I and II only
    b. I and III only
    c. III and IV only
    d. II and IV only
    e. I and IV only

20. Advantages of metered dose inhalers (MDIs) include:
    I. Small size.
    II. Ease of use.
    III. Inert nature of the propellants.
    a. I
    b. I and II
    c. II and III
    d. I, II and III

21. A spacer device may be helpful:
    I. To improve the patient's coordination and timing.
    II. To improve the particle size inhaled by the patient.
    III. In that it acts as a baffle and reservoir.
    a. I
    b. I and II
    c. II and III
    d. I, II and III

22. When using an MDI, the patient should be instructed to:
    I. Take a slow deep breath.
    II. Squeeze the MDI shortly after inspiration has begun .
    III. Hold his/her breath following inspiration.
    IV. Exhale passively.
    a. I
    b. I and II
    c. I, II and III
    d. I, II, III and IV

23. The most important aspect of using MDIs is:
    a. Equipment care and cleaning.
    b. Patient instruction.
    c. Use of a spacer.
    d. Infection control.

24. You are using a large-volume nebulizer to deliver aerosol and an F_IO_2 of 0.40 to a patient who is intubated. You measure the oxygen concentration and your analyzer reads 89%. The entrainment and flowmeter settings are correct. How might you troubleshoot this problem?
    I. Check for water in the tubing.
    II. Check for kinks or obstructions.
    III. Check for loose fittings.
    IV. Make sure the nebulizer is assembled correctly and is not leaking.
    a. I and II
    b. I and III
    c. II and III
    d. III and IV

25. An advantage of the Misty Ox Gas Injection Nebulizer (GIN) is:
    I. High flow rates are possible.

II. It may be heated.

III. It is permanent and may be reused.

IV. Only one gas source is required.

a. I and II

b. I and III

c. II and III

d. III and IV

26. Entrainment of a liquid into a near sonic stream of gas by shear forces and vorticity is an application of:

a. Evaporation.

b. Henry's law.

c. Choked flow.

d. Hemodynamics.

e. Thermodynamics.

27. A patient may have difficulty using a bulb nebulizer:

a. Because the volume is so large.

b. Because the particle size is too large.

c. Because it produces body humidity.

d. Because of the heating element.

e. Because of coordination.

28. Which of the following nebulizers employ choked flow in their operation?

I. Bear VH-12.

II. Solosphere.

III. Mistogen HV-12.

IV. DeVilbiss Model 65.

a. I only

b. I and II only

c. II only

d. III only

e. III and IV only

29. Increasing the amplitude of an ultrasonic nebulizer:

a. Increases the water temperature.

b. Increases the rate of evaporation.

c. Increases the amount of aerosol output.

d. Decreases the particle size.

e. Increases the flow of gas through the nebulizer.

30. Which of the following mist tents incorporate(s) refrigeration units into their design?

I. Croupette.

II. Ohio Pediatric Mist Tent.

III. Mistogen CAM tent.

a. I only

b. I and II only

c. II and III only

d. I and III only

e. III only

Selected Bibliography

Bagwell, Terry, *United States Patent Number, 4,767,576*, Medical Molding Corporation of America, Costa Mesa, CA, 1986.

Bagwell, Terry, *United States Patent Number, 4,629,590*, Medical Molding Corporation of America, Costa Mesa, CA, 1986.

Branson, Richard D., et al., "Laboratory Evaluation of Moisture Output of Seven Airway Heat and Moisture Exchangers," *Respiratory Care,* Vol. 32, No. 8, pp. 741–747.

CAIRE, Inc., *Microstat User's Guide,* Littleton, CO, 1990.

Darin, John, "An Evaluation of Water-Vapor Output from Four Brands of Unheated, Prefilled Bubble Humidifiers," *Respiratory Care,* Vol. 27, No. 1, pp. 41–50, 1982.

Des Jardins, Terry R., *Cardiopulmonary Anatomy and Physiology,* Delmar Publishers, Inc., 1988.

DeVilbiss Health Care, Inc., *DeVilbiss AeroSonic Ultrasonic Nebulizer Instruction Guide,* Somerset, PA, 1993.

Gagliardini, Fredric Jon, "Ultrasonic Nebulizers as Room Humidifiers" (abstract), *Respiratory Care,* Vol. 29, No. 10, p. 1025, 1984.

Greenway, Loren, et al., "Static Electricity Generated by Nebulizers" (abstract), *Respiratory Care,* Vol. 30, No. 10, p. 871, 1985.

ICN Pharmaceuticals, Inc., *Small Particle Aerosol Generator SPAG-2,* Costa Mesa, CA, 1986.

McPherson, Stephen P., *Respiratory Therapy Equipment,* 5th ed., Mosby-Yearbook, 1995.

Miller, Franklin, Jr., *College Physics,* Harcourt Brace Jovanovich, 1972.

Mortimer, Charles E., *Chemistry: A Conceptual Approach,* Van Nostrand Reinhold Company, 1971.

Op't Holt, Timothy, "Aerosol Generators and Humidifiers," in Barnes, Thomas A., et al. (eds.), *Respiratory Care Practice,* Year Book Medical Publishers, 1988.

Perch, Stanley A., Jr., et al., "Effectiveness of the Servo SH 150 Artificial Nose Humidifier: A Case Report," *Respiratory Care,* Vol. 29, No. 10, pp. 1009–1012, 1984.

Rau, Joseph L., *Respiratory Therapy Pharmacology,* Year Book Medical Publishers, 1978.

Waskin, Hetty, "Toxicology of Antimicrobial Aerosols: A Review of Aerosolized Ribaviran and Pentamidine," *Respiratory Care,* Vol. 36, No. 9, pp. 1026–1036, 1991.

CHAPTER 3

HYPERINFLATION THERAPY EQUIPMENT

INTRODUCTION

Incentive spirometry is a mode of therapy commonly used to promote deep breathing and coughing. Both disposable and permanent equipment are available for this therapeutic modality. In this chapter you will learn about the equipment, how to operate it, and how to correctly assemble and troubleshoot it.

Positive-Expiratory-Pressure (PEP) mask therapy uses the application of positive end expiratory pressure with the patient exhaling actively to FRC, ending the breath at ambient pressure level. This application of expiratory pressure splints the airways open, facilitating secretion clearance.

Flutter valve therapy is similar to PEP therapy except that the device excites pressure vibrations throughout the lung parenchyma. The flutter valve device incorporates a weighted ball valve that opens and closes at a high frequency, causing the vibrations in the lungs.

The use of Intermittent Positive Pressure Breathing (IPPB) has declined as a therapeutic procedure over the past several years. While most hospitals across the country still perform IPPB therapy, its frequency of use is low.

Some IPPB equipment may also be used for adult mechanical ventilation. The use of these machines for this purpose is uncommon due to the variability of the delivered tidal volume. The discussion in this chapter will focus primarily on their usage for hyperinflation therapy.

The two primary manufacturers of IPPB equipment, Bird Products Corporation and Puritan Bennett Corporation, still manufacture some IPPB machines. This chapter will be devoted to those machines still manufactured or supported with parts. In this chapter you will learn about IPPB equipment, its principles of operation, and how to assemble and troubleshoot it.

Intrapulmonary Percussive Ventilation (IPV®), although not considered IPPB therapy, has some elements which are similar to IPPB therapy, warranting its inclusion in this chapter. IPV® combines a high-frequency, pneumatically driven, time-cycled flow interrupter with a dense aerosol administration device. The combination of percussive, pulsed gas delivery with aerosolized medication delivery facilitates endobronchial secretion mobilization. As of this writing, one company has devices approved for sale and distribution (Percussionaire Corporation's IPV®-1, IPV®-2, and Spanker). Other companies have devices that are currently under clinical investigation for FDA approval.

In addition to volume enhancement, secretion mobilization is an important aspect of hyperinflation therapy. Various percussors are employed in the facilitation of secretion removal during chest physiotherapy and postural drainage. These devices, and their clinical application, are important for the practitioner to understand.

OBJECTIVES

After completing this chapter, the student will accomplish the following objectives:

PHYSICS OF HYPERINFLATION THERAPY EQUIPMENT

- Describe the two principles used by disposable incentive spirometers to measure inspired volumes.
- Describe how inspiratory flow and volume may be measured using a photoelectric sensor.
- Describe two ways gas pressure may be regulated.
- Describe how needle valves may be used to regulate gas flow.

INCENTIVE SPIROMETRY EQUIPMENT

- Describe the principles of operation, assembly and troubleshooting for the following incentive spirometers.
  - Sherwood Medical's
    - Voldyne
    - Triflo
  - Argyle Tru-vol
  - DHD Medical Volurex
  - Monaghan Spirocare

POSITIVE-EXPIRATORY-PRESSURE (PEP) AND FLUTTER VALVE THERAPY EQUIPMENT

- Describe how Positive-Expiratory-Pressure (PEP) and flutter valve therapy equipment work and how to use them.

INTERMITTENT POSITIVE PRESSURE BREATHING (IPPB) EQUIPMENT

Bird IPPB VENTILATORS

- For the Bird Mark 7, 7A and 8, identify the following components:
  - Ambient chamber
  - Pressure chamber
  - Center body
  - Venturi/venturi gate assembly
  - Ceramic switch/clutch plate assembly
  - Permanent magnets
- Describe the purpose and operation of the following controls on the Bird IPPB machines:
  - Sensitivity control
  - Flow rate control
  - Air mix control
  - Expiratory timer
  - Pressure control
  - Negative pressure control
  - Time/pressure cycle control
  - Apneustic time control
- Explain how adjustment of the controls affects F_IO_2, inspiratory time, expiratory time and tidal volume.
- Trace the gas flow through the Bird circuit.
- Describe the steps in assembly and troubleshooting of the Bird machines and their circuits.

Bennett IPPB Machines

- Describe the operation of the Bennett valve.
- Differentiate between the AP-5 and PR-2 and the clinical application of both.
- Describe the purpose and operation of the following controls on the Bennett AP-5 IPPB machine:
  - Pressure
  - Nebulization
- Describe the purpose and operation of the following controls on the Bennett PR-2 ventilator:
  - Pressure
  - Air dilution
  - Rate
  - Expiration time
  - Nebulizer
  - Negative pressure
  - Sensitivity
  - Terminal flow
  - Peak flow
- Describe the function of the two pressure manometers on the Bennett PR-2 ventilator.
- Explain how adjustment of the controls affects F_IO_2, inspiratory time, expiratory time and tidal volume.
- Trace the flow of gas through a Bennett circuit.
- Describe the steps in assembly and troubleshooting of the Bennett machines.

PERCUSSIONAIRE CORPORATION IPV® VENTILATORS

- Describe Intrapulmonary Percussive Ventilation (IPV®) and its clinical efficacy.
- Describe the Percussionator® and its function in IPV®.
- Describe the operation of the Phasitron® and the concept of fluid clutching.

- Differentiate between the Percussionaire IPV®-1, IPV®-2 and Spanker and their clinical applications and control features.
- Identify the components of the IPV® circuit and its correct assembly.
- Describe the steps in troubleshooting of the IPV® ventilators.

PHYSICS OF HYPER-INFLATION THERAPY EQUIPMENT

MEASUREMENT OF INSPIRED VOLUMES

Incentive spirometry is a therapeutic modality that relies on a patient's voluntary effort to perform a hyperinflation maneuver. Incentive spirometry equipment measures the inspired volumes and provides *biofeedback* to the patient using the device. When the patient can observe the inspired volume, he or she can be encouraged to work to inhale more. As the patient's effort increases, the transpulmonary pressures become greater, causing an increased inspired volume. This therapy is considered to be effective in the prevention and reversal of *atelectasis* and the promotion of coughing in postoperative patients.

Several methods of volume measurement are used in the operation of incentive spirometers, including flow dependent methods,

SECRETION MOBILIZATION DEVICES

- Describe the operation and clinical application of the following percussors:
  — Vibramatic
  — Flimm Fighter
  — MJ Percussor

volume displacement and photoelectric measurement. Accuracy varies, depending on the method employed.

Flow Dependent Methods

A flow of gas applied across the top of a tube will cause a subambient pressure to be developed in the tube (Figure 3-1A). If a float device is added to the tube, the subambient pressure will cause the float to rise (Figure 3-1B), overcoming gravity. The weight of the float and diameter of the tube determine how much flow is required to raise it.

If the flow measuring device is accurate, a known flow rate can be translated into a volume. For example:

An incentive spirometer requires a flow of 275 mL/second to raise a float. A patient inhales, raising the float, and sustains the flow (float is held up) for 3 seconds. How much volume did the patient inhale?

$$\text{Volume} = \text{Flow rate} \times \text{Time}$$
$$= 275 \text{ mL/sec.} \times 3 \text{ seconds}$$
$$= 825 \text{ mL}$$

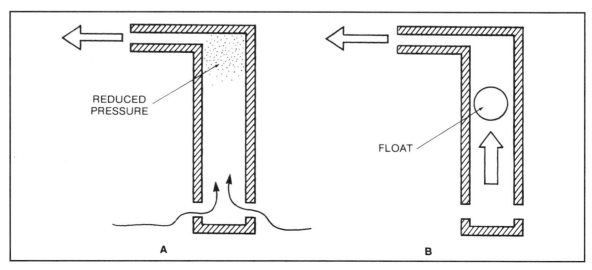

Figure 3-1 *(A) Flow vertically through a tube causing reduced pressure. (B) Float rising in the tube in response to a pressure differential.*

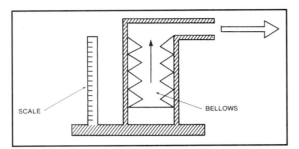

Figure 3-2 *A functional diagram of a bellows type incentive spirometer.*

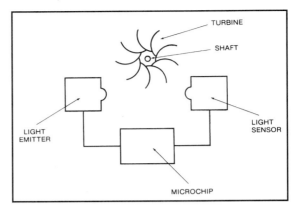

Figure 3-3 *A functional diagram of a photoelectric flow sensor.*

Volume Displacement

A patient who inhales air from a bellows causes the bellows to collapse as the gas is removed from it (Figure 3-2). Since one side is fixed and cannot move, bellows displacement is proportional to the inspired volume. This method of measurement can be quite accurate and is also used in some pulmonary function spirometers.

Photoelectric Measurement

A photoelectric flow sensor consists of a turbine or other flow measurement device, a light emitting and sensing device, and an electronic circuit card or microchip. The turbine, when placed in the path of a light beam, will interrupt the beam as it turns (Figure 3-3). As the flow through the turbine increases, the light beam is interrupted at a faster rate.

The circuit card or microchip counts the rate at which the light beam is interrupted and translates it to a flow rate. By calibrating the sensing device, "X" number of interruptions can equal "Y" amount of flow. Volume can be

measured by multiplying flow by the time the flow is sustained, as described above. This can all be accomplished electronically and virtually instantaneously.

GAS PRESSURE REGULATION

The reducing valves discussed in Chapter 1 are designed to reduce cylinder pressures to a working pressure of 50 psi. This pressure is too high to apply directly to a patient's lungs. *IPPB machines* reduce the pressure to between ambient pressure and 60 cmH$_2$O. Two different methods of reducing pressures are used by the manufacturers—a low pressure reducing valve (Puritan Bennett Corporation) and magnetic force opposing gas pressure (Bird Products Corporation).

Low Pressure Reducing Valve

Figure 3-4 shows a schematic of the Puritan Bennett reducing valve. Gas pressure entering

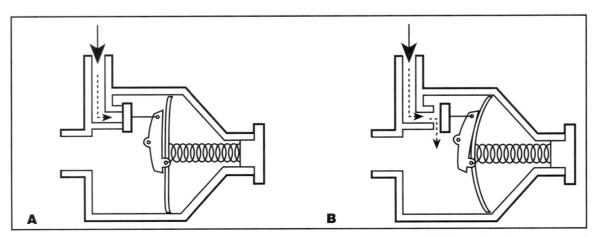

Figure 3-4 *The Puritan Bennett pressure control is a low pressure reducing valve. (A) Illustration showing the valve closed. (B) Illustration showing the valve open.*

the reducing valve displaces the diaphragm, opposing spring tension. When spring tension is overcome, the pivot closes the poppet valve. Gas escaping the pressure side reduces the pressure, causing spring tension to open the poppet valve again. This regulator functions in a way similar to those discussed in Chapter 1.

The spring tension may be varied by turning the knob on the face of the machine (pressure control). As spring tension is increased, the pressure from the regulator is also increased. Pressure is adjustable from zero to 45 cmH$_2$O.

Magnetic Attraction Opposing Gas Pressure

Figure 3-5 is a simplified schematic of the Bird IPPB machine's pressure chamber. Gas pressure within the chamber is conducted to a diaphragm through two holes in the center body. As gas pressure increases, the diaphragm moves to the left, causing a ceramic switch attached to it to close.

Magnetic attraction between a permanent magnet and a metal clutch plate opposes the movement of the diaphragm. Adjusting the pressure control causes the magnet to move closer to or further from the metal clutch plate, varying the degree of magnetic attraction. If the magnet is moved closer to the clutch plate,

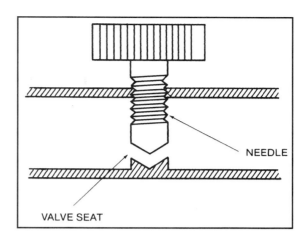

Figure 3-6 *A full section of a needle valve.*

it takes a greater pressure to move the diaphragm since magnetic attraction is greater.

GAS FLOW REGULATION

Needle valves are common devices used by manufacturers to regulate gas flow (Figure 3-6).

A needle valve designed to regulate gas flow operates much like a water faucet. Adjusting the valve by turning it moves the needle away from the valve seat (variable orifice), opening it and increasing gas flow. A larger

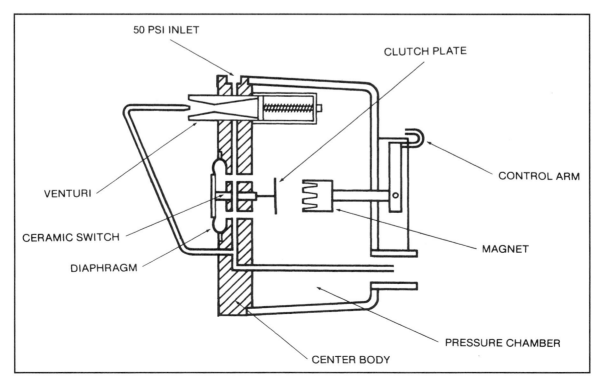

Figure 3-5 *A full section of the Bird pressure chamber. Note the proximity of the magnet to the metal clutch plate.*

opening allows more gas to pass through the valve seat in a given interval of time.

In addition to regulating flow, needle valves can be used to reduce pressure. Opening the valve causes a pressure drop across the valve seat. The pressure proximal to the valve seat becomes greater than the pressure distal to it. This pressure difference can be used to reduce a higher pressure to a lower pressure.

INCENTIVE SPIROMETRY EQUIPMENT

Several different types of incentive spirometers are employed in patient care. The majority are disposable, single-use devices. Others incorporate a permanent sensing/feedback device with disposable patient mouthpieces or flow sensors. All of the incentive spirometers in use today use one of the three principles of volume measurement discussed earlier in this chapter.

VOLDYNE

Sherwood Medical makes the Voldyne incentive spirometer (Figure 3-7), which is a disposable device that operates by the application of subambient pressure above a piston.

As the patient inhales, gas flows through a flow indication float, causing it to rise. The patient is encouraged to keep the yellow flow indicator centered in its chamber. The manufacturer maintains that keeping the float cen-

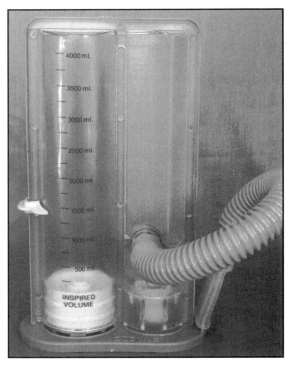

Figure 3-7 *The Sherwood Medical Voldyne incentive spirometer.*

tered promotes a more uniform distribution of air throughout the lungs.

Movement of gas through the Voldyne causes pressure to be reduced above the volume indication piston. As pressure is reduced, the piston rises in its tube. The top of the piston indicates the level of inspired vol-

ASSEMBLY AND TROUBLESHOOTING

Assembly—Sherwood Medical Voldyne

1. Aseptically remove the Voldyne, flexible tubing and mouthpiece from the package.

2. Attach the flexible tubing to the inlet of the spirometer.

3. Attach the mouthpiece to the free end of the flexible tubing.

4. Tip the spirometer to check for free movement of the flow indication float and the piston.

5. Instruct the patient on its use.

6. Adjust the volume pointer to the ordered or desired level.

Troubleshooting

Very little can go wrong with this relatively simple device. Check the tubing or mouthpiece for obstruction and ensure that the piston and flow indication float move freely. If the unit still fails to operate, replace it.

ume. The Voldyne's volume range is from 0 to 4000 milliliters.

A movable marker on the left side of the spirometer is adjusted to indicate to what volume the patient should inhale. The marker can be adjusted such that the patient is encouraged to work a little harder than normal, further expanding the lungs.

TRIFLO

The Triflo is a disposable incentive spirometer manufactured by Sherwood Medical (Figure 3-8). Like the Voldyne, it is a flow-dependent device.

The patient's inspiratory flow is drawn across the top of three chambers, creating a subambient pressure. If the patient's flow is less than 600 milliliters per second but greater than 300 milliliters per second, the float in the first chamber will rise. As the flow increases to 900 milliliters per second, the second float will rise. If the patient's flow exceeds 900 milliliters per second, all three floats will be suspended. The respiratory care practitioner should encourage the patient to sustain his inspiratory effort (flow), holding the float(s) up for at least 3 seconds. When the patient exhales, gravity pulls the floats back to the bottom of their chambers.

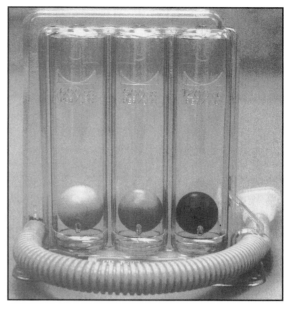

Figure 3-8 *The Sherwood Medical Triflo incentive spirometer.*

ASSEMBLY AND TROUBLESHOOTING

Assembly—Sherwood Medical Triflo

1. Aseptically remove the Triflo, flexible tubing and mouthpiece from the package.

2. Attach the flexible tubing to the inlet of the spirometer.

3. Attach the mouthpiece to the free end of the flexible tubing.

4. Tip the spirometer to check for free movement of the flow indication floats.

5. Instruct the patient on its use.

Troubleshooting

Very little can go wrong with this relatively simple device. Check the tubing or mouthpiece for obstruction and ensure that the floats move freely. If the unit still fails to operate, replace it.

VOLUREX

DHD Medical manufactures the Volurex incentive spirometer (Figure 3-9), which is another disposable incentive spirometer that operates using volume displacement with a range of 0 to 4000 milliliters.

The Volurex incorporates a flexible bellows. As the patient inhales, volume is removed and the bellows rises.

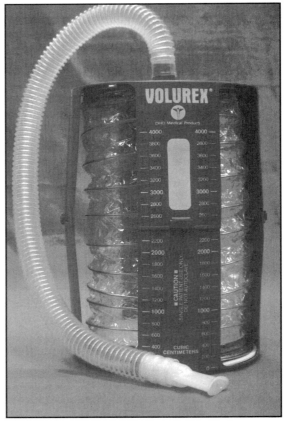

Figure 3-9 *The DHD Medical Products Volurex incentive spirometer.*

ASSEMBLY AND TROUBLESHOOTING

Assembly—DHD Medical Volurex

1. Aseptically remove the spirometer, flexible tubing and mouthpiece from its package.

2. Separate the top and bottom of the spirometer, expanding the bellows.

3. Align the volume scale on the top and bottom portions of the vertical support arms, and snap them together, locking them.

4. Attach the flexible tubing to the inlet and the mouthpiece to the free end.

5. Instruct the patient on its use.

Troubleshooting

The simplicity of these devices makes troubleshooting easier. Check the tubing and mouthpiece for obstructions. If the unit still fails to operate, replace it.

MONAGHAN SPIROCARE

Monaghan produces two models of the Spirocare spirometer (Figure 3-10). One model is small and is powered by batteries; the other is larger, operating from 110 volt electrical power.

Both Spirocares measure volume using the photoelectric principle discussed earlier in the chapter. The turbine is contained in a clear disposable mouthpiece, positioned longitudinally along its axis. The patient's inspiratory flow causes the turbine to spin. The photoelectric transducer and receiver are located in the handle of the spirometer. The electronic circuitry that interprets the signals from the photoelectric cells is located in the spirometer housing.

Adjustment of the desired inspiratory volume (inside the side door for the larger unit and under the spirometer housing for the smaller unit) causes colored lights to illuminate on the right indicator panel. As the patient inhales, the row of lights on the left panel illuminates, indicating inspired volume. The patient is encouraged to match the goal indicated on the right-hand row of lights. When the patient reaches the goal, a breath hold light or clown light (early larger models for pediatric patients) illuminates for 3 seconds to encourage breath holding.

A counter keeps track of the number of times the patient achieves the desired goal (volume). In this way a patient may be encouraged to use the spirometer a specified number of times between therapy sessions.

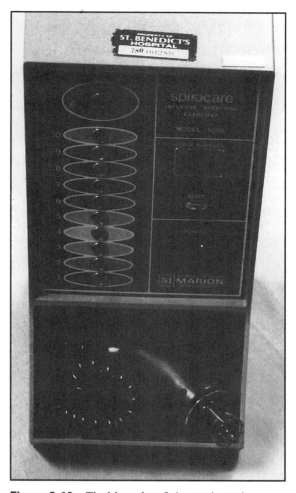

Figure 3-10 *The Monaghan Spirocare incentive spirometer.*

ASSEMBLY AND TROUBLESHOOTING

Assembly—Monaghan Spirocare

1. Ensure the spirometer has power (batteries in the smaller unit and 110 volts in the larger).

2. Attach the disposable mouthpiece to the handle by slipping it into place. Ensure that the tab on the mouthpiece matches the keyway on the handle. When assembled, the ring on the mouthpiece should be flush against the handle.

3. Turn the unit on.

4. Adjust to the desired goal using the adjustment provided on the spirometer. A scale is provided to convert the colored lights to volumes.

5. Instruct the patient on the spirometer's use.

Troubleshooting

If the lights fail to operate when the patient inhales:

1. Check for correct installation of the mouthpiece.

2. Ensure that the turbine spins freely without binding or excessive noise.

3. Ensure that light can be observed inside the handle. If light is not visible, take the spirometer to an authorized biomedical repair center.

POSITIVE-EXPIRATORY-PRESSURE AND FLUTTER VALVE THERAPY EQUIPMENT

Both Positive-Expiratory-Pressure (PEP) and flutter valve therapy apply positive expiratory pressure to mechanically splint the airways open, which facilitates the removal of secretions. Although they are both similar in the application of positive pressure during exhalation, they differ in that one provides continuous pressure while the other generates pressure pulses.

POSITIVE-EXPIRATORY-PRESSURE THERAPY EQUIPMENT

Positive-Expiratory-Pressure (PEP) therapy equipment consists of a mouthpiece, one-way valves, a T-assembly, a manometer, an adjustable resistance valve and an optional nebulizer and reservoir (Figure 3-11). The PEP level is adjusted by varying the diameter of the resistance valve's orifice, increasing or decreasing expiratory resistance (10 to 15 cmH$_2$O). The patient is instructed to take a deeper than normal breath and to exhale actively against the resistance, observing the manometer to maintain the desired expiratory pressure. Following 10 to 20 breaths, the patient is then instructed to remove the PEP device and forcefully cough.

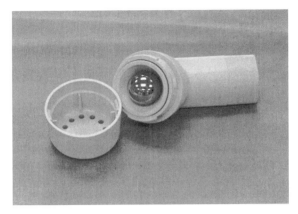

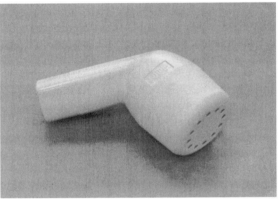

Figure 3-12 *Photographs of a flutter valve. Note the weighted ball (top) with the expiratory cap removed.*

FLUTTER VALVE THERAPY EQUIPMENT

The flutter valve consists of a single, weighted ball valve, which rapidly opens and closes during exhalation, creating positive pressure and a rapidly oscillating pressure wave within the patient's airways (Figure 3-12). Like PEP therapy, the patient takes a larger than normal tidal breath and then exhales against the flutter valve. This creates positive pressure in the airways in combination with an oscillating pressure wave caused by the valve's rapid opening and closing. Following 10 to 20 breaths, the patient is encouraged to vigorously cough.

INTERMITTENT POSITIVE PRESSURE BREATHING (IPPB) EQUIPMENT

Two common IPPB machines are made by two manufacturers, Puritan Bennett Corpora-

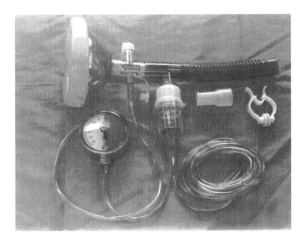

Figure 3-11 *A photograph of a PEP mask device. Note the attachment of an optional small-volume nebulizer for medication delivery.*

tion and the Bird Products Corporation. Currently only five models are being produced, the Bennett AP-5 and PR-2 and the Bird Mark 7, Mark 7A and Mark 8.

As indicated earlier in the chapter, the use of IPPB therapy has declined in the past several years. While it is still ordered and performed today, it is done so more selectively than it was in the past. It is still important to understand how the equipment functions and operates so that IPPB therapy can be administered safely and effectively.

BIRD IPPB VENTILATORS

The Bird Corporation developed an entire line of IPPB equipment based on the Mark 7. Figure 3-13 shows the present Bird line: the Mark 7, Mark 7A and Mark 8.

Ventilator classification systems enable a practitioner to categorize different ventilators based upon common characteristics. These common characteristics include power source, what variable is controlled during inspiration, how the ventilator is triggered, and how the ventilator is cycled. The ventilator power source may be electric, pneumatic or combined electric and pneumatic. The variable controlled during inspiration can be pressure, time, volume or flow. How a ventilator triggers a breath, or begins inspiration, can include pressure, flow, volume or time. How a ventilator is cycled, or ends inspiration, may include pressure, volume flow or time.

The Bird IPPB ventilators are classified as pneumatically powered pressure controllers. The ventilators are pressure or time triggered and are pressure cycled.

Various modifications were made to the Mark 7, to accomplish new and varied clinical goals. By understanding the operation of the Mark 7, the other models can be readily learned and understood.

Basic Components of the Bird Machines

The basic components common to all of the Bird machines are the ambient chamber, pressure chamber, center body, venturi/venturi gate assembly, the ceramic switch/clutch plate assembly and the permanent magnets. The ability to identify these components and to understand how they operate will enable you to apply these machines more effectively.

Ambient Chamber

As you face the front of the machine, the ambient chamber is the larger green transparent chamber on the left side of the machine. The ambient chamber is so named because it remains at ambient pressure. Room air is drawn through the chamber and into the venturi/venturi gate assembly if the machine is operating in air mix mode. The ambient chamber also contains the pressure manometer, which indicates the pressure contained in the pressure chamber.

Pressure Chamber

The pressure chamber is located on the right side of the machine. Gas pressure from source gas (or source gas and room air) builds in this chamber and pressurizes the patient circuit, resulting in gas delivery to the patient.

Center Body

The center body is a narrow casting made from aluminum alloy that separates the ambient and pressure chambers. It contains the venturi/venturi gate assembly, ceramic switch/clutch plate assembly, timing cartridge and other controls. The source gas supply attaches to the center body, where gas flow and its direction are controlled.

Venturi/Venturi Gate Assembly

The venturi/venturi gate assembly passes through the center body located at the top rear of the machine. When the machine is operating in air mix mode (Mark 7), source gas and room air mix in the venturi. The Mark 7A and Mark 8 operate using the venturi at all times.

The venturi gate is a spring-loaded gate that closes the distal end of the venturi with a spring tension equal to approximately $2 \text{ cmH}_2\text{O}$. This tension is necessary so that the patient's inspiratory effort will be sensed by the *sensitivity* system, and not be transmitted to the ambient chamber through the venturi. During ventilation when pressure in the pressure chamber reaches approximately $12 \text{ cmH}_2\text{O}$, the venturi gate closes. Once the gate closes, the only flow through the patient circuit is from the nebulizer.

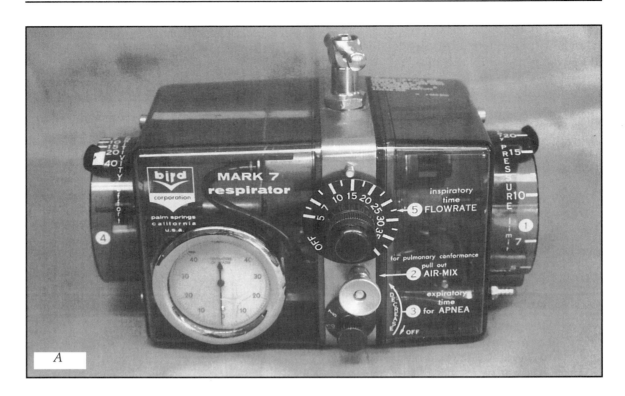

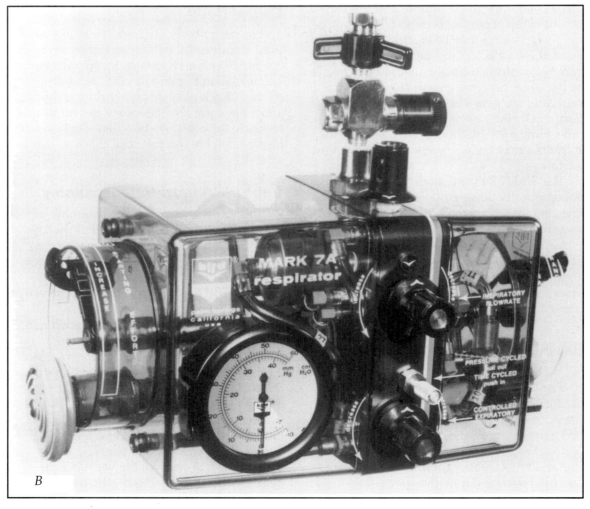

Figure 3-13 *(A) Bird Mark 7; (B) Bird Mark 7A; (continues)*

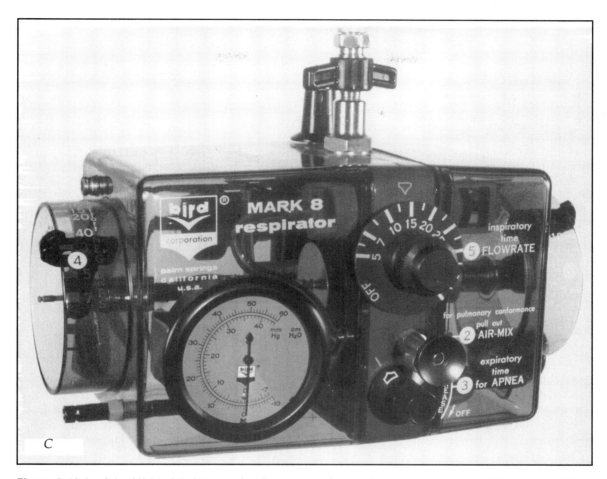

Figure 3-13 *(con't.)* *(C) Mark 8. (Reprinted with permission from Bird Products Corporation, Palm Springs, CA)*

Ceramic Switch/Clutch Plate Assembly

In the middle of the center body, passing through it, is the ceramic switch/clutch plate assembly (Figure 3-14). The assembly consists of the ceramic switch, diaphragm, two metal clutch plates and the hand timing rod.

The ceramic switch is an on-off switch made of a ceramic material. The switch is contained in a cylindrical housing. The ceramic material offers the advantages of ease of sealing and operation with little friction.

When the switch is positioned to the right (Figure 3-15A), gas flows through it and the center body. When the switch is in the left position, no gas flow occurs (Figure 3-15B).

The diaphragm is located on the ambient side of the center body. It is attached to the ceramic switch assembly and moves back and forth with it. Pressure in the pressure chamber is communicated to the diaphragm through two holes in the center body. The diaphragm plays an important role in the sensitivity system, which will be discussed later in this chapter.

Attached to each end of the ceramic switch/clutch plate assembly are two metal clutch plates. One is located in each chamber (ambient and pressure). The clutch plates operate in conjunction with permanent magnets to regulate pressure and sensitivity.

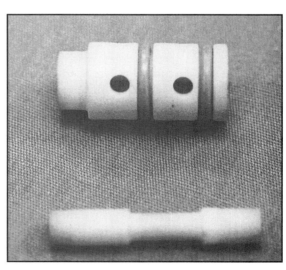

Figure 3-14 *The Bird ceramic switch.*

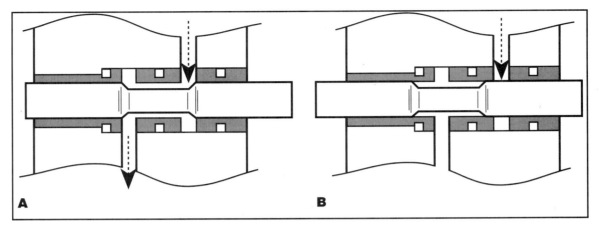

Figure 3-15 *A cross section of the Bird ceramic switch showing (A) the open (on) and (B) the closed (off) positions.*

The hand timing rod passes through the ambient chamber and protrudes through the center of the sensitivity control. Pushing the hand timing rod in moves the ceramic switch to the right and begins inspiration. Pulling the rod out moves the ceramic switch to the left and terminates inspiration. This rod provides a means for the operator to control the phase of ventilation (inspiration or expiration).

Control Operation

A complete understanding of how the controls operate and interact with one another is essential in the safe operation of these IPPB machines. In this section the controls will be individually discussed and their relation to other controls will be explained. The first four controls (sensitivity, flow rate, expiratory timer, and pressure control) are common to all of the Bird IPPB machines currently produced. The other controls in the discussion are unique to specific models.

Sensitivity Control

The sensitivity control is essentially a patient effort control. Adjustment of this control determines how much patient effort is required to initiate inspiration. The sensitivity ranges from 0 to 10 cmH₂O below ambient pressure.

The sensitivity control operates using the diaphragm, metal clutch plate (ambient side) and a permanent magnet. When the patient initiates a breath, the inspiratory effort (subambient pressure) is communicated through the circuit and the pressure chamber to the diaphragm. The diaphragm responds to the change in pressure by flattening out, which

moves the ceramic switch to the right, initiating inspiration (Figure 3-16).

Opposing the movement of the diaphragm is the magnetic attraction between the clutch plate and the permanent magnet. Adjustment of the sensitivity control moves the magnet closer or further from the clutch plate, varying the amount of magnetic attraction the patient must overcome. As the magnet gets closer to the clutch plate, it takes a lower pressure (subambient) to initiate inspiration.

When adjusting this control, the practitioner references the patient's inspiratory effort to the pressure manometer. The pressure manometer indicates the amount of negative pressure the patient must generate to initiate inspiration. Ideally, the control should be adjusted such that a pressure of 1 to 2 cmH₂O below ambient pressure will initiate inspiration.

Flow Rate Control

Gas entering the machine encounters the flow rate control first. It is located on the front of the center body (Figure 3-17) and is a needle valve. (The operation of needle valves was discussed in the Physics of Hyperinflation Therapy Equipment section earlier in this chapter.) Adjustment of the flow rate control regulates gas flow by opening and closing its valve seat. When the machine operates using the venturi, peak flows of up to 80 liters per minute are available.

Expiratory Timer

The expiratory timer is used to ventilate patients who are apneic. This control is not operated during IPPB therapy since it may

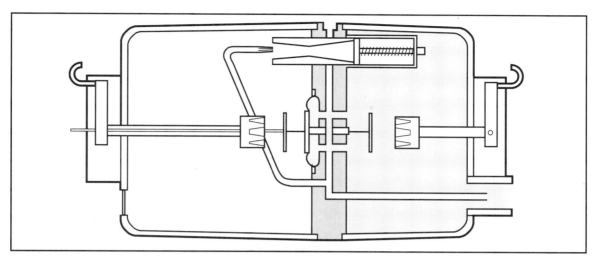

Figure 3-16 *A function diagram of the Bird sensitivity system.*

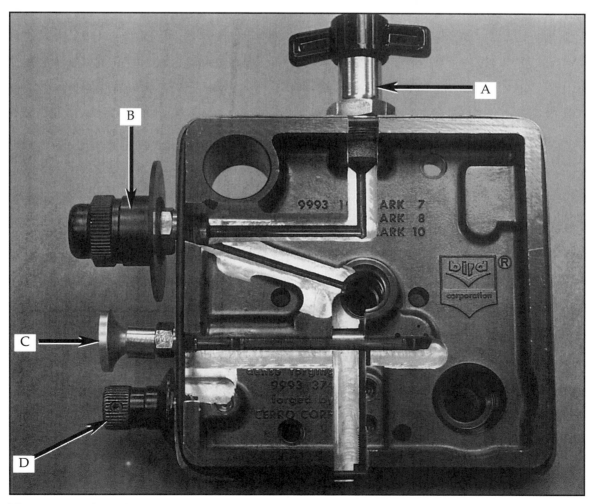

Figure 3-17 *The Bird center body with its controls labeled. (A) The gas inlet. (B) The pressure control. (C) The air mix switch. (D) Expiratory timer for apnea.*

cause *asynchronous ventilation*. An example of asynchronous ventilation is when a patient exhales while the machine delivers a breath.

The control operates using a timing cartridge, needle valve, and a timing arm.

During inspiration the cartridge is pressurized with source gas (Figure 3-18A). As the cartridge is pressurized, the diaphragm and spring opposite the inlet are compressed by the gas pressure. This increases the overall length of the cartridge slightly.

When the operator opens the needle valve (expiratory timer control), gas is allowed to leak from the timing cartridge into the pressure chamber. The needle valve regulates how fast the cartridge empties, and therefore regulates the expiratory time and, indirectly, the respiratory rate.

As the timing cartridge empties, the spring pushes the diaphragm to the right, decreasing the cartridge's overall length (Figure 3-18B). Attached to the diaphragm is a rod that is connected to the timing arm. As the spring compresses the diaphragm, the timing arm contacts the clutch plate (ambient side) and pushes it to the right. The timing rod pushes the clutch plate and slides the ceramic switch to the open position, beginning inspiration, and the cycle is repeated.

Pressure Control

The pressure control is located on the right side of the machine. The control operates using the ceramic switch/ clutch plate assembly and the permanent magnet in the pressure chamber.

Pressure building within the pressure chamber causes the diaphragm to distort and expand. As the diaphragm moves to the left, it also moves the ceramic switch. Once the switch moves far enough to the left, inspiration is terminated. Opposing the movement of the diaphragm is the magnetic attraction between the magnet and the clutch plate (pressure chamber).

Movement of the pressure control arm causes the magnet to be moved closer to or further from the clutch plate. The magnet's position varies the amount of magnetic attraction between it and the clutch plate (Figure 3-19). The closer the magnet is to the clutch plate, the greater the pressure needed to end inspiration, resulting in higher peak pressures.

Air Mix Control

The air mix control is unique to the Bird Mark 7. Essentially, it is an on-off switch that controls gas flow through the venturi/venturi gate assembly (Figure 3-17C).

In the out (on) position, source gas is conducted from the center body by plastic tubing to the venturi jet. If oxygen is the source gas, it is mixed with room air, diluting the oxygen. Oxygen percentage varies between 65 and 95% oxygen (depending on *tidal volumes* and peak pressures). Oxygen concentrations vary because, as pressure in the circuit increases, it causes less room air to be mixed with source gas (oxygen) through the venturi, increasing

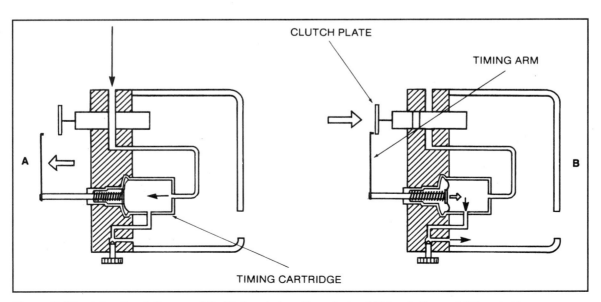

Figure 3-18 *A functional diagram of the Bird expiratory timer during (A) inspiration and (B) expiration.*

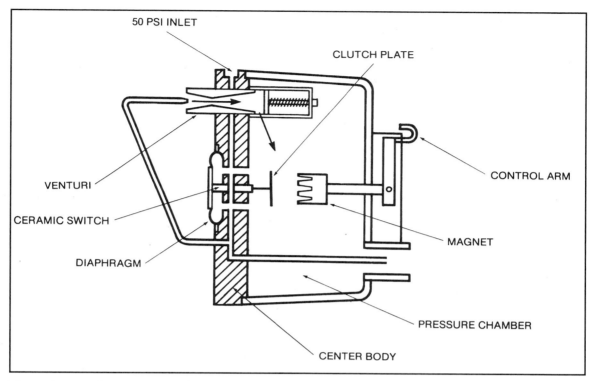

Figure 3-19 *A function diagram of the Bird pressure control operation.*

the oxygen concentration. Furthermore, when the spring-loaded venturi gate closes at approximately 12 cmH$_2$O, the only gas flow through the circuit is source gas through the nebulizer. When operated using the venturi, there is greater flow through the ventilator due to the additional air entrainment. The venturi causes a characteristic decelerating or tapered flow pattern (flow with respect to time). Flow throughout inspiration is not constant; it is greatest at the beginning of inspiration and decreases as inspiration proceeds.

When the control is pushed in, source gas alone powers the machine and the venturi/venturi gate system is bypassed. Furthermore, when operated in this mode, flow rates are significantly reduced. Reduction in flow rate occurs due to the loss of the additional flow provided by air entrainment when the control is pulled out. Although flow rates are decreased when operating the ventilator on source gas, the flow is constant. This produces a characteristic flow versus time curve that is square in shape. Thus, the air-mix control affects the flow pattern during inspiration; with the venturi activated, a decelerating flow pattern is produced. With the venturi disengaged (100% source gas), a square wave pattern (constant flow) is produced.

Expiratory Flow Control (Negative Pressure Control)

The expiratory flow control is unique to the Bird Mark 8. Its function is to control the flow of gas through an accessory nipple during expiration. This flow of gas can be used to drive negative end expiratory pressure (NEEP) or positive end expiratory pressure (PEEP) devices. It also may be used to provide expiratory nebulization. These applications were primarily restricted to the "Q" and "J" circles used for infant ventilation.

Activation of the control causes gas to be drawn from the expiratory flow cartridge, which is charged during inspiration. The control is a needle valve that adjusts the rate of flow.

Time/Pressure Trigger Control

This control was added to the Mark 7A and Mark 8 machines. It is a pneumatic switch that determines if the machine operates in a pressure triggered mode (IPPB therapy) or a time-triggered mode (apneustic ventilation).

If the control is in the pressure triggered mode, the machine will operate only when patient effort triggers it on. When the control is in the time triggered mode, the timing cartridge determines the machine's triggering.

Apneustic Time Control

The purpose of this control is to provide an inspiratory hold or pause to improve gas distribution within the lungs. It is unique to the Mark 7A and Mark 8.

During inspiration an apneustic flow cartridge is pressurized. If the control is activated, flow during expiration is directed from the cartridge to the nebulizer and auxiliary jets on the venturi. The additional flow from the nebulizer holds the exhalation valve shut while the venturi provides additional flow. The expiratory hold feature lasts between .3 and 3 seconds. Adjustment of the control moves a needle valve that regulates the flow rate from the apneustic cartridge.

How the Controls Affect Delivered F_IO_2

The Bird machines all employ the venturi/venturi gate assembly in their operation (provided the Mark 7 is operated with the air mix control pulled out). The way that back pressure distal to a venturi alters F_IO_2 was discussed in Chapter 1. As pressure distal to a venturi builds, air entrainment decreases, causing the F_IO_2 to increase.

When pressure in the pressure chamber reaches approximately 12 cmH$_2$O, the venturi gate closes and the only source of flow is from the nebulizer. Since the nebulizer is powered by source gas, this situation further increases the F_IO_2. These factors combine to cause a variation in the F_IO_2 delivered to the patient. This fluctuation in F_IO_2 is only true if the machine is powered by oxygen.

How the Controls Affect Inspiratory Time

Inspiratory time is affected by the pressure and flow rate controls. If these controls are improperly adjusted, it is possible to deliver *inverse (inspiratory-to-expiratory) (I:E) ratio* ventilation, which may have adverse effects on the patient. These effects may include cardiovascular compromise, increased intracranial pressure, and hypotension which is caused by a decrease in venous return. When the apneustic flow control is used on the Bird Mark 7A and Mark 8, it influences inspiratory time also.

If gas flows into a closed chamber at a constant rate, it will take longer to reach a high pressure than a low one. Therefore, if the pressure control is set to a higher pressure, a longer time period will pass before inspiration is terminated. The time from beginning to end of inspiration is termed the inspiratory time.

The flow rate control also affects inspiratory time. A closed chamber with a fixed size will fill faster at a higher flow rate than a low one. Increasing the setting of the flow rate control will shorten inspiratory time.

When the apneustic flow control is activated on the Mark 7A and Mark 8, an inspiratory pause occurs. The length of the inspiratory pause must be added to the inspiratory time to determine the total inspiratory time. One effect of this control is to lengthen inspiratory time, which may alter the I:E ratio.

How the Controls Affect Expiratory Time

Expiratory time is influenced when the expiratory timer is in operation. The expiratory timer control determines the length of expiratory time. Its operation was discussed earlier in the chapter.

How the Controls Affect Delivered Tidal Volume

Delivered tidal volume is the amount of gas delivered to the patient during a breath using the machine. One of the goals of IPPB therapy is hyperinflation, or the delivery of a breath larger than is possible spontaneously. Two controls on the machine can be adjusted to increase tidal volume.

The pressure control is the primary control influencing tidal volume. An increase in pressure causes more gas to be delivered before the machine pressure cycles into expiration (inspiration ceases). However, recall that an increase in pressure lengthens inspiratory time. To maintain the same inspiratory time at the higher pressure, the flow rate control must be increased.

The flow rate control may also influence delivered tidal volumes. If the flow rate is increased to the point where flow is turbulent, proximal pressure will build more rapidly. This may result in a lower volume delivery than is desired, since inspiration is terminated more quickly.

Gas Flow through the Bird Circuit

During inspiration, gas flows from the pressure compartment through the 22-mm large-bore tubing to the patient. This is some-

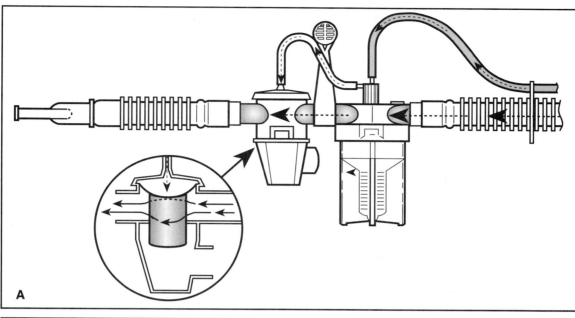

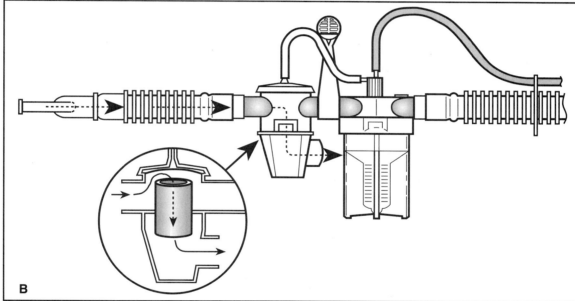

Figure 3-20 *Gas flow through a Bird circuit during (A) inspiration and (B) expiration.*

times referred to as "main flow" (Figure 3-20). It is this flow that is primarily responsible for the delivery of tidal volume to the patient. The gas flowing through the large-bore tubing also serves as the carrier gas for the medication nebulized in the nebulizer.

Source gas flows through small diameter tubing to the *exhalation valve* and to the nebulizer simultaneously with the main flow of gas.

The gas powering the exhalation valve ei-ther inflates a mushroom valve or pushes a diaphragm down, sealing the exhalation port. This prevents the gas from taking the path of least resistance away from the patient and out the exhalation port (Figure 3-21).

The gas also flows to the nebulizer jet. The nebulizer works just like the jet nebulizers discussed in Chapter 2, using choked flow. The nebulizer is a small-volume nebulizer that is either a main stream (Bird permanent circuit) or sidestream (disposable circuit) nebulizer.

ASSEMBLY AND TROUBLESHOOTING

Assembly—Bird IPPB Ventilator

Circuit Assembly:

1. Assemble the nebulizer drive line and exhalation valve drive line by attaching the adapter to the nebulizer nipple and the free end to the exhalation valve (Figure 3-22).
2. Attach the short flexible tubing to the outlet of the manifold (nebulizer/ exhalation valve assembly) and attach the mouthpiece to its free end. Figure 3-22 shows the circuit correctly assembled.
3. Connect the circuit to the machine by attaching the large-bore tubing to the machine outlet (disposable circuits may require an adapter) and the small diameter tubing to the accessory power line.

Ventilator Preparation:

1. Attach the machine to a 50 psi gas source with high pressure hose. If a cylinder is used, use a two stage regulator.
2. Adjust the controls to the following settings for the patient's first breath:
   a. Pressure between 10 and 20 cmH$_2$O.
   b. Flow at 15.
   c. Sensitivity at 10.
   d. Air mix control out (Mark 7).
   e. Expiratory time control off.
3. Instruct the patient on the machine's use.
4. Make further adjustments based on exhaled tidal volumes and the patient's tolerance to therapy.

Troubleshooting

A complete explanation of all events that can cause a malfunction is beyond the scope of this text. The more common ones are listed below and may serve as a useful guide. When troubleshooting please follow the suggested troubleshooting algorithm (ALG 3-1).

Machine cycles prematurely:

1. Check the flow rate control to determine if it is set too high. Adjust the control to a lower setting.
2. The patient may be obstructing the mouthpiece with the tongue. Explain the proper use of equipment again.
3. Pressure may be set too low to achieve the desired volumes. Increase the pressure as required.

Machine cycles on and off rapidly:

1. Adjust the sensitivity control to a lower setting (more difficult to initiate inspiration).
2. Coach the patient, explaining how the machine works when it senses a breath.

Inspiratory time is too long:

1. Increase the flow rate.
2. Check for leaks:
   a. In the patient circuit.
   b. Around the patient's mouthpiece.
   c. In some cases, nose clips, a mouth seal or a mask may be required.
3. Decrease the pressure. However, recall that this will decrease delivered tidal volumes.
4. Coach the patient to wait longer between breaths in order to lengthen expiratory time.

The pressure manometer indicates high negative pressures prior to inspiration:

1. Increase the sensitivity, reducing the patient's inspiratory effort.

The pressure manometer hesitates or rises erratically during inspiration:

1. Flow is inadequate. Increase the flow rate using the flow rate control.

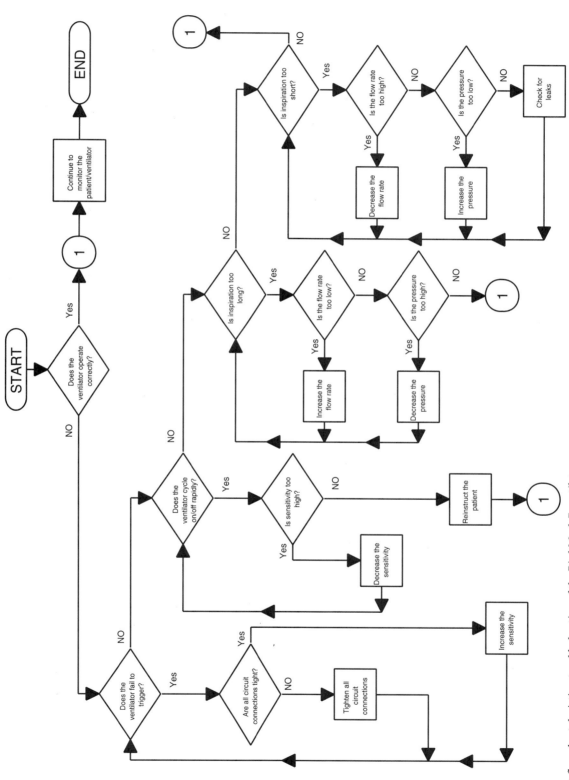

ALG 3-1 *A flow chart depicting troubleshooting of the Bird Mark 7 ventilator.*

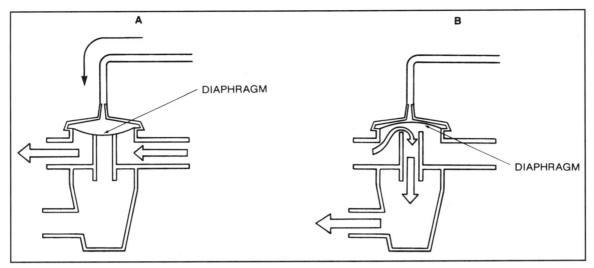

Figure 3-21 *A functional diagram of a typical exhalation valve during (A) inhalation and (B) exhalation.*

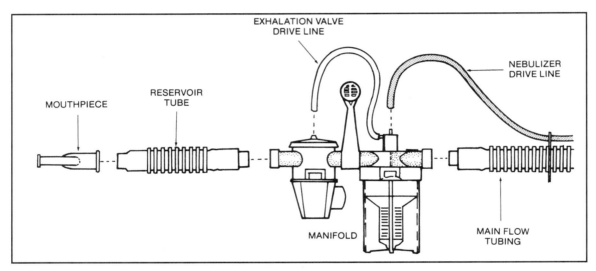

Figure 3-22 *An assembly drawing of the Bird circuit.*

BENNETT IPPB VENTILATORS

Puritan Bennett manufactures the AP-5 and the PR-2 models for sale and distribution.

The AP-5 shown in Figure 3-23 was designed for home use. It is an electrically powered ventilator with its own built-in compressor. The only other components required to operate the machine are a 120 volt power source and a patient circuit.

The Puritan Bennett PR-2 is a more complex machine designed for mechanical ventilation (Figure 3-24). It is a gas powered ventilator requiring a 50 psi source and is capable of ventilating an apneic patient.

The circuits are similar for both machines and will be discussed at the conclusion of this section.

The Bennett Valve

The Bennett valve functions as an on-off switch. The valve is flow sensitive and requires only .5 cmH$_2$O pressure to rotate it. Bennett literature describes the valve as "the valve that breathes with the patient."

The Bennett valve is composed of a drum, drum vane, counterweight and front and back plates.

The drum is a cylinder that is closed at the front and rear. Windows located at the top and bottom of the drum permit gas to flow through it. The valve rotates on jeweled bearings at the front and rear. The bearings have serial numbers that match and each is machined individually for a near perfect fit. The precision bearings allow the valve to rotate

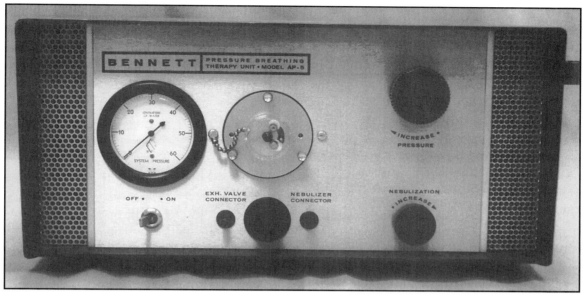

Figure 3-23 *The Puritan Bennett AP-5 ventilation.*

with little friction. Figure 3-25 shows the AP-5 and PR-2 Bennett valves; note that the PR-2 valve has two drum vanes.

As the patient begins inspiration, negative pressure is generated in the patient circuit and communicated to the Bennett valve. The reduced pressure rotates the valve (Figure 3-26). Once the windows are aligned with the inlet and outlet of the valve, gas flows through it.

As pressure builds within the patient circuit, flow diminishes. When the flow is reduced to between one and three liters per minute, gravity pulls down on the counterweight closing the valve (Figure 3-27).

Bennett AP-5 Machine

As indicated earlier the Bennett AP-5 is primarily designed for home use; it is, however, used in some hospitals. The AP-5 ventilator is an electrically powered ventilator. It is a pressure controller that is pressure triggered and flow cycled. The controls and their operation were designed simply, so that the average patient would be able to use the machine effectively. There are three controls on the Bennett AP-5: on-off switch, pressure control, and nebulizer control.

On-Off Switch

The on-off switch is located on the front of the machine below the pressure manometer. It is an electrical toggle switch that operates in a way similar to a light switch in your home.

Pressure Control

The pressure control on the AP-5 operates by using a spring-loaded disk that vents excess pressure to the atmosphere. Pressure output is limited to around 30 cmH2O.

Gas pressure is supplied to the pressure

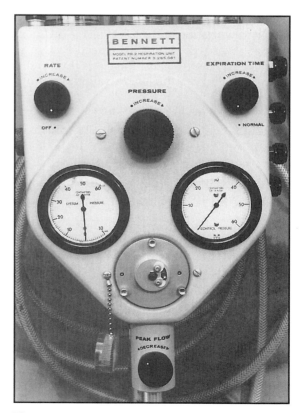

Figure 3-24 *The Puritan Bennett PR-2 ventilator.*

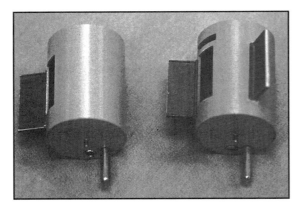

Figure 3-25 *Two Bennett valves. The AP-5 valve on the left has only one drum vane while the PR-2 valve on the right has two drum vanes.*

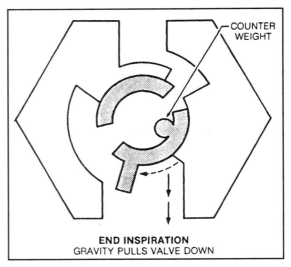

Figure 3-27 *A functional diagram illustrating how the Bennett valve closes at the end of inspiration.*

control by an internal electric compressor. Room air is drawn in through a 10-micron filter, compressed, then passed through a sub-micron filter. Flow is divided between the pressure control and the nebulizer.

Flow through the pressure control is augmented by a venturi. Ambient air enters the venturi through a 40-micron filter. The venturi boosts the flow out of the regulator providing total flow to the patient of between 75 and 90 liters per minute.

Nebulizer Control

The nebulizer on the AP-5 operates continuously (inspiration and expiration). Flow to the nebulizer is controlled by a needle valve. Opening the needle valve increases flow to the jet in the nebulizer, thus increasing the rate of nebulization.

The Bennett PR-2 Ventilator

The Bennett PR-2 has more controls than the AP-5 and is more complex in its operation. The PR-2 ventilator is one you will most likely encounter in the hospital environment. It is a pneumatically powered, pressure controller. The ventilator is pressure or time triggered and is flow cycled.

Pressure Control

The purpose of the pressure control is to reduce the 50 psi line pressure to a safe level. It is located in the center of the ventilator (Figure

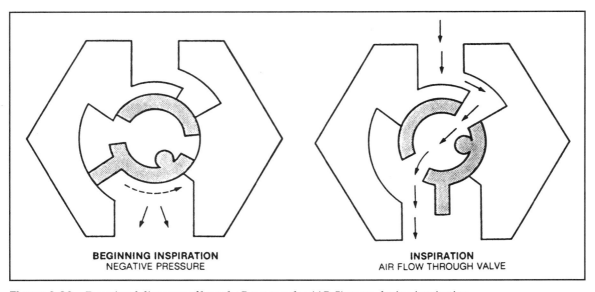

Figure 3-26 *Functional diagrams of how the Bennett valve (AP-5) opens during inspiration.*

ASSEMBLY AND TROUBLESHOOTING

Assembly—Puritan Bennett Corporation AP-5

1. Connect the machine to a 120 volt power source.

2. Assemble the circuit. (Refer to the section discussing the Bennett circuits.)

3. Attach the 22-mm diameter large-bore tubing to the large outlet on the machine.

4. Attach the small-diameter tube without the flared (large diameter) end to the exhalation valve nipple.

5. Attach the other small diameter tube (with the flared end) to the nebulizer nipple.

6. Turn the machine on and aseptically occlude the mouthpiece. Adjust the pressure to the ordered level by manually cycling the Bennett valve and adjusting the pressure until the desired pressure is registered on the manometer.

7. Turn on the nebulizer flow until aerosol is visible coming out of the mouthpiece.

Troubleshooting

When troubleshooting, please follow the suggested troubleshooting algorithm (ALG 3-2).

1. If the nebulizer fails to operate:

   a. Check the circuit for correct assembly and any obstructions or kinks in the nebulizer drive line.

   b. Check to ensure that the nebulizer drive line is attached to the nebulizer nipple on the machine and the nipple on the circuit.

   c. Ensure that medication has been added to the nebulizer cup.

   d. Check for flow coming out of the nebulizer nipple. If flow is absent, take the machine to a qualified biomedical repair facility.

2. If the machine fails to cycle properly:

   a. Check the circuit for correct assembly and tighten all connections.

   b. Clean the Bennett valve. This must be performed carefully since the valve is quite delicate. Gently remove the front cover and lay it on a flat surface where it will not be accidentally dropped. Carefully remove the drum by grasping the handle protruding from the front of the drum (Figure 3-28). Gently clean the valve with an alcohol prep pad and allow the alcohol to evaporate. Replace the valve, carefully aligning it and replace the front cover.

   c. If *a* and *b* are satisfactory and the machine still fails to operate correctly, take it to a qualified biomedical repair facility.

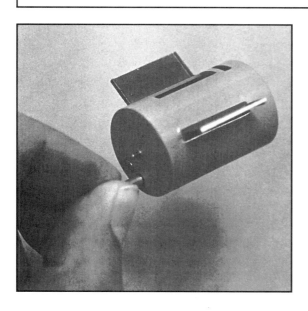

Figure 3-28 *This photograph illustrates the correct way to handle the Bennett valve.*

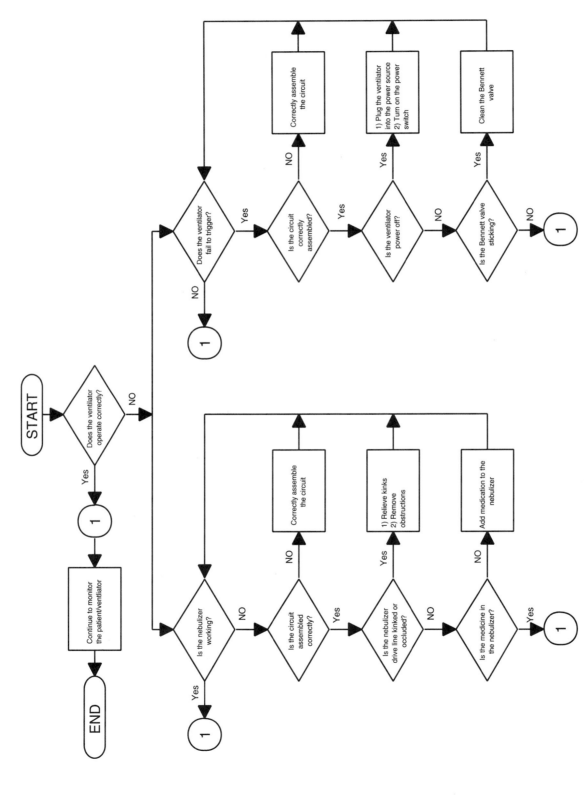

ALG 3-2 *A flow chart depicting troubleshooting of the Bennett AP-5 ventilator.*

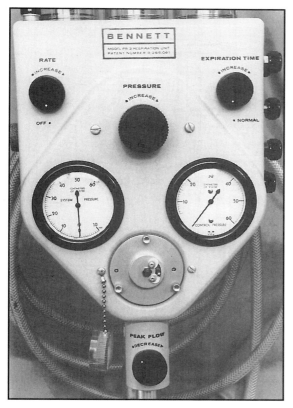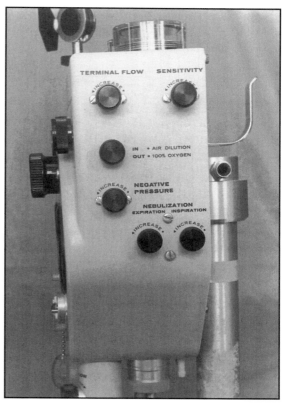

Figure 3-29 *The Bennett PR-2 ventilator. (A) Front panel controls; (B) side panel controls.*

3-29). Pressure reduction is accomplished by a single-stage, low pressure reducing valve. The operation of this valve was discussed earlier in this chapter. The pressure output from the reducing valve is between 0 and 45 cmH₂O.

Air Dilution Control

The purpose of the air dilution control is identical to the air mix control on the Bird Mark 7. Adjustment of the control determines whether 100% source gas or source gas diluted with ambient air is delivered to the patient. Pushing in the air dilution control activates a venturi, delivering source gas mixed with ambient air to the patient. Pulling the control out delivers 100% source gas to the patient. Since the venturi is an integral part of the reducing valve (pressure control), it does not affect gas flow as the venturi in the Bird machines does (Figure 3-30).

When the control is pushed in, gas is channeled through a venturi that supplies pressure to the reducing valve. In the out position, the venturi channel is closed, and pure source gas enters the reducing valve through the poppet valve.

Rate Control

The rate control is not used for IPPB therapy. It is utilized only when ventilating an apneic patient.

The purpose of the rate control is to establish a respiratory rate for an apneic patient. Activation of the control will time-cycle the ventilator. The operation of this control is quite complex. A complete discussion of gas pathways and control is not required for most practitioners. Enough of the operation will be discussed to understand its function without becoming too complex. (Refer to "Operating Instructions, Bennett PR-2 Respiration Unit," Bennett Respiration Products, Santa Monica, CA, 1979, for more specific discussion.)

Adjustment of the rate control opens or closes a needle valve. Gas flow from the needle valve is channeled to the left and right accumulators.

The accumulators are pneumatic timing switches that control the pathway of gas from many different lines. The PR-2 ventilator has three accumulators located on the top of the ventilator. Each accumulator has 6 ports (Figure 3-31). One port (number 6) supplies the

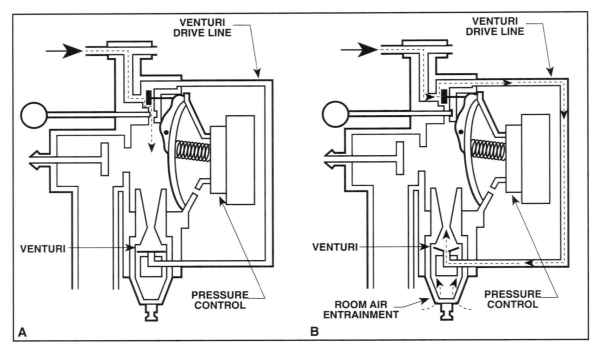

Figure 3-30 *A functional diagram of the Bennett PR-2 pressure control and venturi system. Air dilution control (A) pulled out and (B) pushed in.*

gas pressure that drives the accumulator. Depending on the accumulator's position (up or down) gas is routed through ports 2, 3, and 5 (up position) or ports 2 and 4 (down position).

Gas flows from the left and right accumulators pass through the center accumulator that phases inspiration and expiration. Gas supply for the center accumulator originates from a port directly below the Bennett valve. The center accumulator is only pressurized during inspiration. During inspiration, the balloon at the top of the accumulator is inflated, pushing the shaft downward, opening the even numbered ports (2 and 4), providing gas flow.

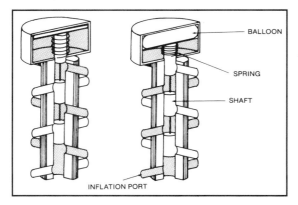

Figure 3-31 *This diagram of the PR-2 accumulators shows both the up and down positions.*

The number one accumulator (left most accumulator when facing the front of the ventilator), is phased to operate during expiration. The rate control is a needle valve which directs gas flow to port 6 of the number one and number three accumulators. Port 6 of the number one accumulator is connected to an even port on the center accumulator. When the even ports of the center accumulator are blocked during expiration, gas can only flow to the left accumulator (port 6) and up the accumulator shaft and inflate the balloon at the top of the port, driving the piston down. Once the left accumulator piston reaches the bottom of its travel, gas from the low pressure reducing valve is directed out port 4 of the left accumulator to a port above the upper drum vane, triggering the ventilator into inspiration by rotating the Bennett valve open (Figure 3-32).

Adjustment of the rate control determines the speed at which the left most accumulator travels downward, and therefore the length of the expiratory time.

The number three accumulator (right most accumulator when facing the front of the ventilator) is phased to operate during inspiration. Port 6 of the right accumulator is connected to an odd port (port 1) on the center accumulator. During inspiration, the center accumulator piston moves down, blocking the odd ports. Since

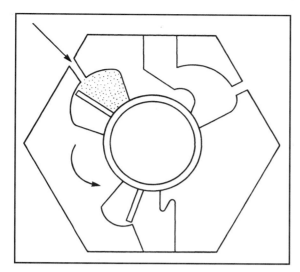

Figure 3-32 *The Bennett PR-2 valve opening in response to gas flow above the upper drum vane.*

the gas pathway for the number 6 port of the right accumulator is blocked, gas flows up the piston, inflating the balloon and driving the piston downward. Once the piston reaches the bottom of its travel, gas flow from the low pressure reducing valve flows through port 4 of the right accumulator to a mushroom valve located at the outlet of the dilutor regulator assembly. Gas pressure inflates the mushroom valve, blocking gas flow from the dilutor regulator to the Bennett valve, cycling the ventilator into expiration. Functionally, the speed of the right accumulator's inflation determines the inspiratory time. Since the right accumulator only inflates on inspiration, it lags slightly behind the center phasing accumulator.

Expiration Time

The expiration time control, like the rate control, is not used for IPPB therapy. The expiration time control modifies the function of the rate control to lengthen the expiratory time.

Functionally the expiration time operates by closing a needle valve. Closing the expiration time needle valve reduces flow to the left accumulator, increasing expiratory time.

Nebulizer Controls

The PR-2 ventilator has the ability to nebulize medication during both inspiration and expiration independently. The intent of the expiration nebulizer control is to fill the flexible

tubing, manifold, and mouthpiece with aerosol before inspiration begins. This is to ensure that the earliest part of inspiration (presumably the part that penetrates most deeply) contains aerosol.

The operation of these controls is regulated by an inflatable flapper valve, called a nebulizer pressure switch (Figure 3-33). During inspiration, the mushroom is inflated, directing gas to the needle valve. The needle valve controls the flow of gas to the nebulizer during inspiration.

During the expiration phase, gas no longer flows to inflate the mushroom valve in the nebulizer pressure switch. Hence, the valve is closed. Now gas flow may go to the expiration nebulizer needle valve only.

Negative Pressure Control

The negative pressure control is not used for IPPB therapy. Its use is primarily limited to the ventilation of neonates. The purpose of the control is to evacuate gas from the patient circuit. To operate, it requires an external attachment to the circuit.

The control operates by using the reduced lateral pressure from an internal venturi. The sub-ambient pressure (up to -6 cmH$_2$O) is applied to the patient circuit and also above the lower drum vane. The reduced pressure above the lower drum vane is to compensate for the application of reduced pressure below it (through the patient circuit) so the ventilator operates normally. Adjustment of the control varies the flow through the venturi and therefore the amount of reduced pressure generated.

Sensitivity

The sensitivity control on the PR-2 has the same function as the sensitivity control on the Bird ventilators. Both are patient effort controls.

The Bennett sensitivity control operates by using a needle valve. When the valve is opened, gas is directed to a port above the upper drum vane. This gas flow assists in rotating the valve open during inspiration. The center accumulator ensures that the valve is only rotated in the inspiratory phase.

Terminal Flow Control

Terminal flow is used to help cycle the ventilator off when leaks are present. Leaks can

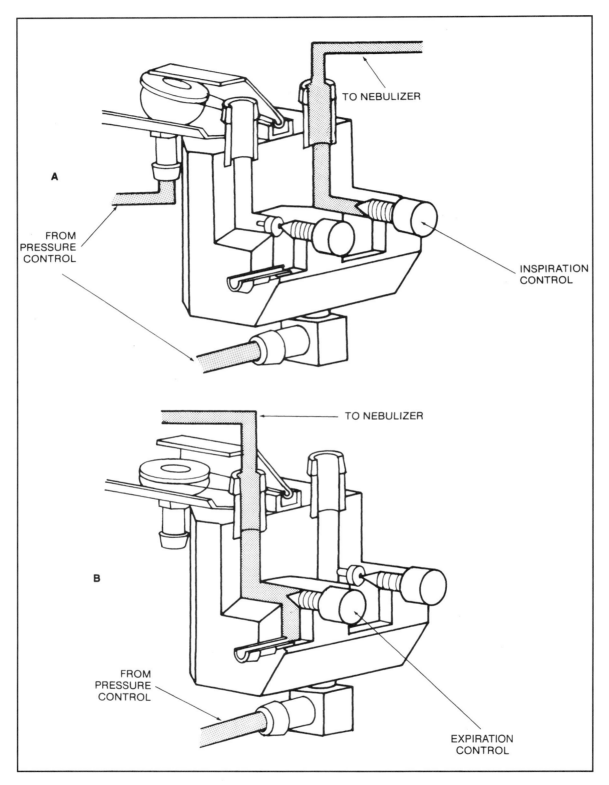

Figure 3-33 *A functional diagram of the PR-2 nebulizer control during (A) inspiration and (B) expiration. Note how the flapper valve determines which needle valve is operating.*

occur in the circuit or around the patient's mouth. The terminal flow control will compensate for a leak of up to fifteen liters per minute. If a leak is present, gas flow through the valve will not decrease sufficiently to close it.

Activation of the terminal flow control directs gas to a venturi below the Bennett valve. The additional flow provides assistance in closing the Bennett valve.

The use of terminal flow adds mixed gas (source gas mixed with ambient air) distal to the Bennett valve. Addition of terminal flow with the air dilution control out (source gas setting) will dilute the delivered F_IO_2.

Peak Flow

Distal to the Bennett valve is a variable orifice that is attached to the peak flow control. The purpose of the control is to slow the flow of gas delivered from the ventilator. It only limits maximum flow from the ventilator and does not operate in the same way as the Bird's peak flow controls. By turning the peak flow control clockwise, the orifice is restricted limiting peak flow from the ventilator. During IPPB therapy the control is normally turned fully counterclockwise.

Pressure Manometers

The PR-2 ventilator has two pressure manometers, control pressure (right) and system pressure (left). The control pressure tells the operator what the internal machine pressure is. The left one reflects the pressure in the patient circuit.

The control pressure manometer is connected between the Bennett valve and the low pressure reducing valve (pressure control). This manometer reflects the pressure output from the reducing valve.

The system pressure control is connected to a port below the terminal flow control. This manometer only reflects pressure in the patient circuit.

How the Controls Affect Ventilation

Adjustment of the ventilator controls affects inspiratory time, expiratory time, and F_IO_2 in a way similar to that in which the Bird ventilator controls are interrelated.

F_IO_2. As discussed earlier, F_IO_2 will be diminished when using the source gas setting (air dilution control pulled out) and by using terminal flow.

As with the Bird ventilator, when the PR-2 is operating using the venturi system, F_IO_2 will vary. This is because increased pressure in the circuit will cause a decrease in ambient air entrainment through the venturi. Actual F_IO_2 will vary between 40% and 60%.

Inspiratory Time. The inspiratory time of the PR-2 is primarily related to the pressure set on the pressure control. As with the Bird, when pressure is set at a higher level, a longer time is required to deliver that pressure.

The peak flow control will decrease the flow of gas at a given pressure. The effect of this control is to lengthen inspiratory time. Normally this is not desired during IPPB therapy.

Expiratory Time. During IPPB therapy, expiratory time is largely a function of patient coaching. Patients must usually be told to deliberately slow their respiratory rate when using an IPPB ventilator. Hyperventilation is a common adverse effect of this therapy.

When using the ventilator to ventilate an apneic patient, the expiratory time control will increase expiratory time by decreasing flow through the rate control system.

Tidal Volume. Tidal volume delivered from the PR-2 is altered by using the pressure control. Care must be used to ensure that pressures do not become excessive or that inspiratory time does not become too long when trying to deliver specific tidal volumes.

Gas Flow Through the Bennett Circuit

The Bennett circuit is composed of three lines: (1) a 22-mm, large-diameter main flow line; (2) a small-diameter line to power the nebulizer; and (3) a small-diameter line to power the exhalation valve (Figure 3-34).

The large, 22-mm tubing is connected to the outlet of the ventilator (underside for the PR-2). Gas from the Bennett valve flows through this line to the patient. The majority of volume delivery occurs through this line and it also serves as a carrier gas for the aerosol from the nebulizer.

The exhalation valve is simultaneously powered during inspiration. Gas inflates a mushroom (permanent circuit) or depresses a diaphragm (disposable circuit) to close the exhalation port during inspiration. During the

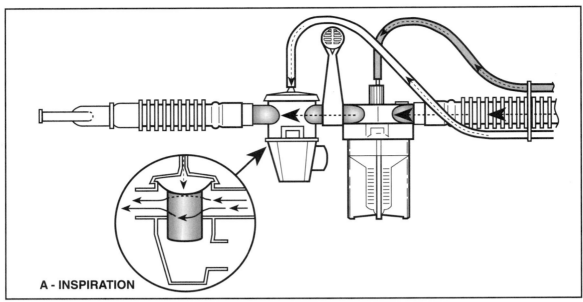

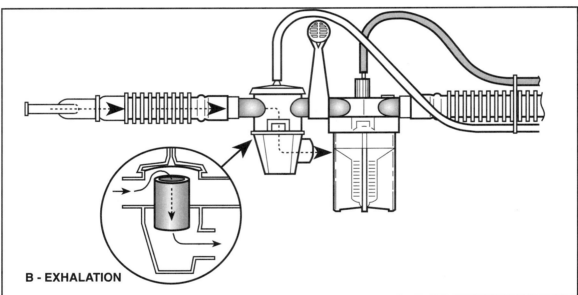

Figure 3-34 *This diagram illustrates flow through the Bennett circuit during (A) inspiration and (B) exhalation.*

expiratory phase, pressure is released and the patient's exhaled air is conducted through the exhalation port. The exhalation valve line is the smaller of the two small diameter lines in the circuit.

Flow to the nebulizer is delivered by the inspiration and expiration nebulizer controls. Output from the controls is conducted to the nebulizer by means of the small diameter tubing. The nebulizer drive line is the larger of the two small diameter lines in the Bennett circuit.

ASSEMBLY AND TROUBLESHOOTING

Assembly—Puritan Bennett Corporation PR-2 Ventilator

The following assembly procedure describes the use of the ventilator for IPPB therapy. For mechanical ventilation, a heated humidifier and monitoring equipment will need to be attached.

1. Assemble the circuit, as shown in Figure 3-35.

2. Connect the ventilator to a 50 psi gas source using high pressure hose.

3. Connect the circuit to the ventilator.

4. Adjust the following controls as indicated:
   a. Rate control fully counterclockwise (off).
   b. Expiration time fully counterclockwise (off).
   c. Peak flow fully counterclockwise (open).
   d. Terminal flow fully clockwise (off).
   e. Sensitivity fully counterclockwise (off).
   f. Negative pressure fully clockwise (off).
   g. Inspiration nebulizer counterclockwise about one-half turn (on).
   h. Air dilution control pushed in (on).

5. Add the ordered amount and dilution of medication to the nebulizer.

6. Adjust the pressure control to the ordered level or between 10 and 20 cmH$_2$O.

7. Adjust the expiration nebulizer until aerosol is just visible coming out of the mouthpiece.

8. Instruct the patient on the ventilator's use.

9. Make further adjustment in the controls based upon the ordered tidal volume and patient's tolerance.

Troubleshooting

A complete explanation of all events that can cause a malfunction is beyond the scope of this text. The more common ones are listed below and may serve as a useful guide. Proficient application of IPPB therapy requires practice and experience. When troubleshooting, please follow the suggested troubleshooting algorithm (ALG 3-3).

Ventilator cycles prematurely:

1. The patient may be obstructing the mouthpiece with the tongue. Explain the use of ventilator again.

2. Pressure may be set too low to achieve the desired volumes. Increase the pressure as required.

Ventilator cycles on and off rapidly:

1. Coach the patient, explaining how the ventilator works when it senses a breath.

2. Check for obstructions in the main tubing or a kinked tube.

3. Sensitivity may be set too high. Decrease the sensitivity.

4. The rate control may be on. Turn the rate control off.

Inspiratory time is too long:

1. Check to ensure the peak flow control is fully clockwise.

2. Check for leaks:
   a. Check the patient circuit.
   b. Ensure the patient has a tight seal around the mouthpiece.
   c. In some cases nose clips, a mouth seal or a mask may be required.

3. Decrease the pressure, recalling that delivered tidal volumes will decrease.

4. Coach the patient to wait longer between breaths in order to lengthen expiratory time.

Ventilator fails to cycle off:

1. Add terminal flow gradually to correct the problem.

2. Check for leaks in the patient circuit.

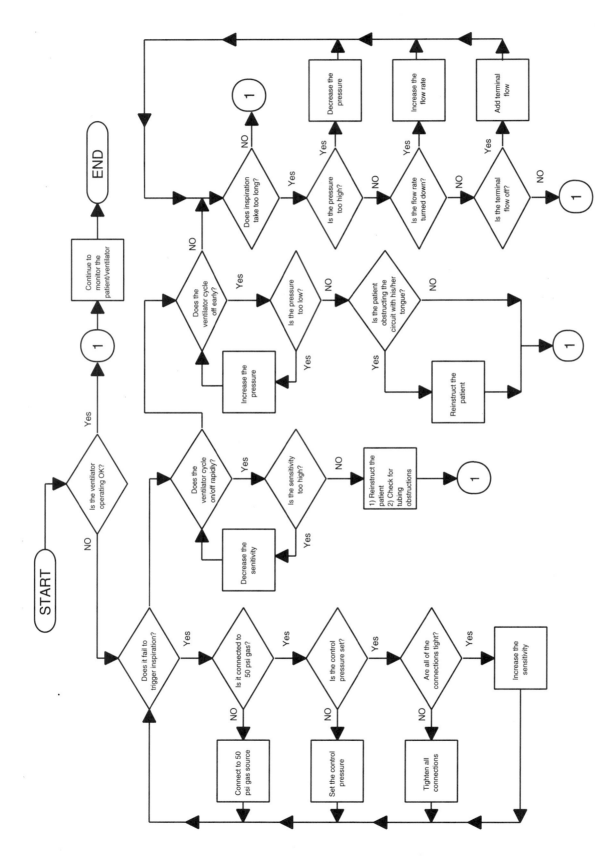

ALG 3-3 *A flow chart depicting troubleshooting of the Bennett PR-2 ventilator.*

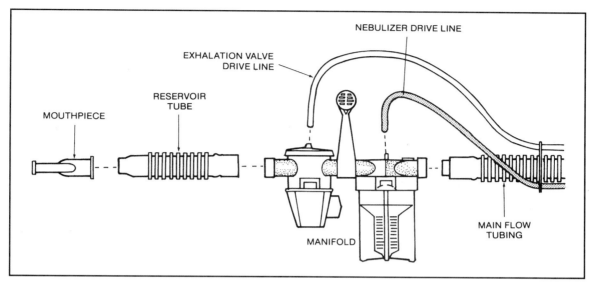

Figure 3-35 *An assembly drawing of a Bennett IPPB circuit.*

PERCUSSIONAIRE CORPORATION IPV® VENTILATORS

Intrapulmonary Percussive Ventilation (IPV®) is a combination of high frequency phased pulse gas delivery (100–250 cycles per minute) and the administration of a dense aerosol. The high frequency pulsed delivery of a sub-tidal volume of gas causes a pressure wedge to be developed in the pulmonary system (Figure 3-36). This controlled wedge of pressure is caused by gas trapping due to the high ventilatory rate and precisely regulated I:E ratio of gas delivery. This increase in pressure helps to augment the volume of inspired gas and to stabilize or enlarge the caliber of the airways. The percussive effect of gas delivery helps to ventilate past obstructions and to deliver air to the distal portions of the lungs.

Coughing following the percussive interval facilitates removal of retained secretions, further opening areas of the lung to ventilation.

The administration of a dense aerosol during IPV® allows the delivery of medications (vasoconstrictors, bronchodilators and mucokinetic agents) to promote bronchial hygiene, reduce edema, and decrease bronchoconstriction.

The clinical effect of IPV® is to combine an intrapulmonary percussion (similar in effect to external chest clapping) with the delivery of a dense aerosol. Advantages of IPV® over conventional aerosol administration and chest clapping is that practitioner technique and fatigue are no longer factors in determining the effectiveness of therapy.

PERCUSSIONATOR®

The Percussionator® is the mechanical device that delivers the pulsed gas to the Phasitron® in the patient circuit. A pneumatic

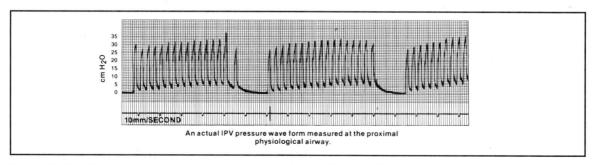

An actual IPV pressure wave form measured at the proximal physiological airway.

Figure 3-36 *Pressure versus time wave form of percussive ventilation while ventilating pulmonary structures (proximal airway pressure). (Courtesy Percussionaire Corporation, Sandpoint, ID)*

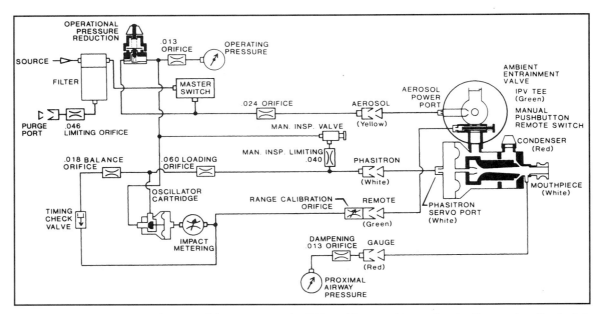

Figure 3-37 *A pneumatic diagram of the Percussionaire IPV®-1. (Courtesy Percussionaire Corporation, Sandpoint, ID)*

diagram of the IPV®-1 is shown in Figure 3-37. The Percussionator® is a pneumatically powered pressure controller which is time cycled. It is triggered by the patient when a thumb control is depressed.

Volume of pulsatile gas is controlled by adjusting the system pressure. Pressure is adjustable between 25 and 40 psi. As pressure is increased, volume delivery also is increased.

Frequency is controlled by the Impact control (IPV®-1), Frequency control (IPV®-2) or Percussion control (Spanker). The frequency is adjustable between 100 and 250 pulses per minute. I:E ratios will vary from 1:1.5 (higher frequencies) to 1:3 (lower frequencies).

PHASITRON®

The Phasitron® provides a mechanical and pneumatic interface between the percussionator and the patient's airway. During delivery of pulsed gas flow as shown in Figure 3-38, gas pressure is applied to an orificed diaphragm. As the diaphragm distorts from the applied pressure, the sliding body of the venturi is advanced forward, closing the exhalation port. Simultaneously, gas is ejected through a nozzle into the throat of the venturi. The venturi entrains room air through the entrainment port at a ratio of 1:5 (source gas to ambient air). Aerosolized medication is admitted through the entrainment port and delivered to the patient's airway through the Phasitron®.

As the pressure wedge develops in the pa-

tient's airways, entrainment through the venturi is decreased due to increased pressure distal to the entrainment port. This reduction in total flow through the Phasitron® protects the patient from barotrauma, acting as a pneumatic buffer to the Percussionator®.

When the thumb button is released, the percussive gas delivery from the Percussionator® ceases. The coil spring in the Phasitron® slides the venturi body back against the diaphragm, opening the exhalation port as shown in Figure 3-39. The patient may then passively exhale. While the exhalation port is open, the patient is free to breathe aerosol passively from the nebulizer without any percussive effect.

PERCUSSIONAIRE IPV®-2

The Percussionaire IPV®-2 is the most complex of the IPV® ventilators produced by the company. It is an advanced post-surgical model intended for acute care use. It has the most control features giving the practitioner great flexibility in the clinical application of the device.

Control Features
Master Switch

The master switch is an on/off valve that controls the operation of the IPV®-2 (Figure 3-40). In the on position, the IPV®-2 allows the practitioner to operate the ventilator deliver-

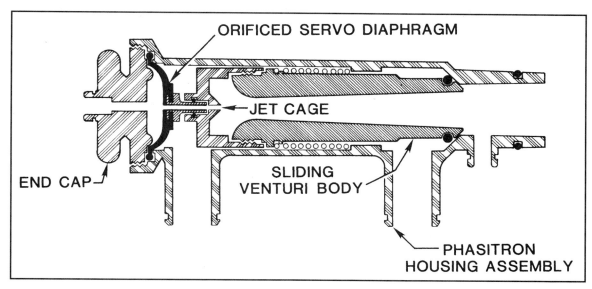

Figure 3-38 *A full section showing the Phasitron® during inspiration. (Courtesy Percussionaire Corporation, Sandpoint, ID)*

ing IPV® therapy, or IPV® therapy, with continuous positive airway pressure (CPAP). This is termed oscillatory demand CPAP (OD-CPAP). In the off position, the ventilator delivers aerosolized medication with traditional demand CPAP.

Inspiratory Flow

Inspiratory flow may be regulated during percussive ventilation by using the Inspiratory flow control. The control regulates the flow of gas going out of the oscillator cartridge (Figure 3-41). This control has the effect of reducing the percussive amplitude by modulating the output of the oscillator cartridge.

Inspiratory Time

The inspiratory time control gives the practitioner the ability to control the rate of inspiratory pressure rise during pulsed gas delivery. The control consists of a needle valve downstream from the oscillator (Figure 3-41).

Frequency Control

The frequency control allows the practitioner to control the frequency of pulsed gas

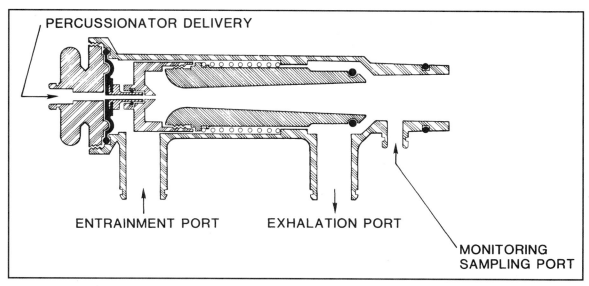

Figure 3-39 *A full section showing the Phasitron® during expiration. (Courtesy Percussionaire Corporation, Sandpoint, ID)*

Figure 3-40 *A photograph of the Percussionaire IPV®-2 ventilator. (Courtesy Percussionaire Corporation, Sandpoint, ID)*

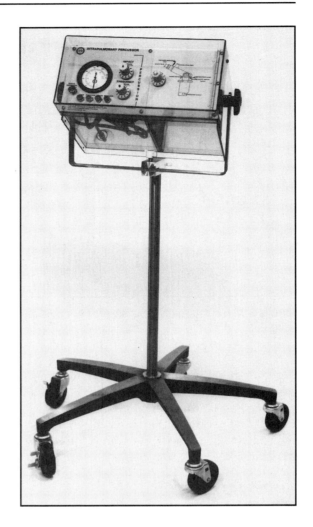

delivery to the Phasitron®. Frequencies from 100 to 250 cycles per minute are possible.

Source Pressure

The source pressure control is a pressure reducing valve that determines the impact velocity of the percussive pulses. Pressures are adjustable between 20 and 50 psi on the IPV®-2. It is recommended to begin therapy at pressures of 30 psi. The control is located on the side panel behind the hinged door on the front of the ventilator.

Nebulizer

The nebulizer control allows the practitioner to vary the output of the nebulizer in the patient circuit. A needle valve controls the flow of gas to the nebulizer.

Demand CPAP Control

The demand CPAP control is an adjustable regulator used to provide CPAP during oscillatory or demand ventilation. CPAP ranges are adjustable between 0 and 30 cmH$_2$O.

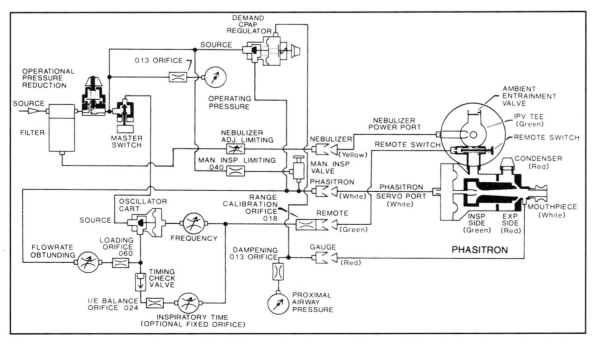

Figure 3-41 *A pneumatic diagram of the IPV®-2 pneumatic circuit. (Courtesy Percussionaire Corporation, Sandpoint, ID)*

Manual Inspiration

The manual inspiration switch is provided on the front panel to manually trigger the ventilator into the oscillatory mode. This is provided in the event the ventilator is used for cardiopulmonary resuscitation efforts.

PERCUSSIONAIRE IPV®-1

The Percussionaire IPV®-1 (Figure 3-42) is an acute care IPV® ventilator with fewer control features than the IPV®-2. It is suitable for the management of patients with cardiopulmonary disease in which secretion mobilization is desirable.

Control Features
Source Pressure

The source pressure control is a pressure reducing valve that determines the impact velocity of the percussive pulses. Pressures are adjustable between 20 and 50 psi on the IPV®-2. It is recommended to begin therapy at pressures of 30 psi. The control is located on the side panel behind the hinged door on the front of the ventilator.

Impact Control

The impact control controls the frequency of the pulsed gas delivery to the Phasitron®.

Frequencies are adjustable from 100 to 250 cycles per minute.

Manual Inspiration

The manual inspiration switch is provided on the front panel to manually trigger the ventilator into the oscillatory mode. This is provided in the event the ventilator is used for cardiopulmonary resuscitation efforts.

PERCUSSIONAIRE SPANKER

The Spanker IPV® therapy unit is a miniaturized version of the IPV®-1 and IPV®-2 (Figure 3-43). The ventilator is 6.5 inches long and 4 inches in diameter making it very portable. The Spanker does not have internal pressure regulation. Pressure is regulated by an external pressure regulator attached to the source gas supply.

Control Features
Percussion Control

The percussion control regulates the frequency of pulsed gas delivery. A frequency adjustment of 100 to 250 cycles per minute is possible.

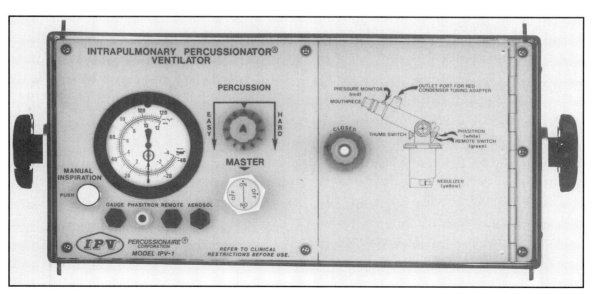

Figure 3-42 *A photograph of the Percussionaire IPV®-1 ventilator. (Courtesy Percussionaire Corporation, Sandpoint, ID)*

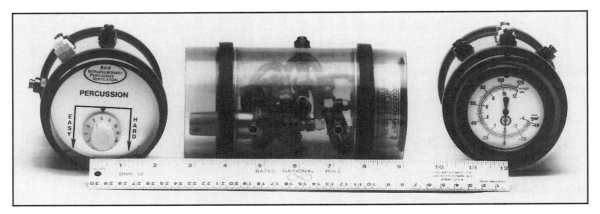

Figure 3-43 *A photograph of the Percussionaire Spanker ventilator. (Courtesy Percussionaire Corporation, Sandpoint, ID)*

ASSEMBLY AND TROUBLESHOOTING

Patient Manifold (Phasitron® and Nebulizer)—Percussionaire Corporation IPV®

As you complete the following sequence, refer to Figure 3-44 to identify the components of the circuit you are assembling.

Phasitron®

1. Attach the orificed diaphragm onto the stem of the venturi cage socket.

2. Check the distal end of the Phasitron® (opposite the diaphragm) for a black "O" ring, which seals against the exhalation port. If the Phasitron® is missing the "O" ring, install one.

3. Slip the coil spring over the venturi body and insert the venturi body into the Phasitron® housing.

4. Complete the Phasitron® assembly by installing the threaded white end cap by rotating clockwise until it is seated.

5. Install a mouthpiece onto the proximal end of the Phasitron®.

Nebulizer

1. Remove the reservoir assembly from the Nebulizer by rotating it counterclockwise.

2. Add the ordered medication to the nebulizer reservoir. The nebulizer can hold up to 20 ml of medication.

3. Reinstall the top of the Nebulizer which contains the thumb switch to the Nebulizer reservoir.

4. Mate the Phasitron® and the Nebulizer together using the port on the side of the Phasitron® at its distal end (near the diaphragm).

5. Set the completed assembly aside, being careful not to spill medication from the Nebulizer.

Drive Line Assembly

The drive lines for the IPV® circuit are color coded, facilitating their assembly to the Percussionator® and Phasitron®.

Percussionator® Connections

1. Mate the Red line to the red snap lock

fitting on the Percussionator® labeled Gauge.

2. Mate the White line to the white snap lock fitting on the Percussionator® labeled Phasitron®.

3. Mate the Green line to the green snap lock fitting on the Percussionator® labeled Remote.

4. Mate the Yellow line to the yellow snap lock fitting on the Percussionator® labeled Nebulizer.

Phasitron® Connections

1. Mate the Red line to the red snap lock fitting on the Phasitron®'s proximal airway port (at the proximal end).

2. Mate the White line to the white snap lock fitting on the Phasitron®'s white end cap.

3. Mate the Green line to the green snap lock fitting on the Phasitron®'s Nebulizer cap opposite the thumb button.

4. Mate the Yellow line to the yellow snap lock fitting on the Phasitron®'s Nebulizer at the base of the reservoir.

5. Finally connect red condenser tubing to the Phasitron®'s exhalation port to prevent aerosol from spraying yourself or the patient's clothing.

Operation of the IPV® ventilator

1. If you are using an IPV®-1 or IPV®-2, connect the 50 psi gas inlet to a suitable 50 psi medical gas supply (typically oxygen).

2. If you are using the Spanker, connect the drive lines to their appropriate snap lock fittings on the regulator supplied in the kit. Insure the regulator is attached to a medical gas cylinder with sufficient contents to deliver IPV® therapy.

3. When using the IPV®-1 or IPV®-2, adjust the operation pressure to 30 psi:
   a. Open the hinged door on the front of the ventilator.
   b. Depress the thumb button on the patient circuit, triggering pulsed gas delivery.

c. Release the red locking ring on the Source Pressure adjustment control by pulling it out away from the body of the Percussionator®.

d. Rotate the Source Pressure control clockwise to increase pressure or counterclockwise to decrease pressure. Monitor operational pressure adjustment by observing the pressure gauge on the top of the Percussionator® housing.

e. When the operational pressure is correctly set, lock the pressure adjustment by gently pushing the red locking ring, seating it against the Percussionator® housing.

4. IPV®-2 initial control settings:
   a. Rotate the Frequency control fully counterclockwise.
   b. Rotate the Insp. Time control fully clockwise.
   c. Rotate Insp. Flow control until the arrow is positioned at 12:00.
   d. Rotate the demand CPAP control clockwise to the "Off" position (inside the hinged door on the right of the Percussionator®).
   e. Rotate the Nebulizer control until the arrow points to the 12:00 position (inside the hinged door on the right of the Percussionator®).
   f. Rotate the Master Switch to the On position.
   g. Instruct the patient on IPV® therapy and carefully monitor the patient.

5. IPV®-1 initial control settings:
   a. Rotate the Impact control until the arrow is at the 12:00 o'clock position.
   b. Instruct the patient on IPV® therapy and carefully monitor the patient.

6. Spanker initial control settings:
   a. Rotate the Percussion control until the arrow is at the 12:00 position.
   b. Instruct the patient on IPV® therapy and carefully monitor the patient.

Troubleshooting

The IPV® unit fails to trigger delivering pulsed gas delivery. When troubleshooting, please follow the suggested troubleshooting algorithm (ALG 3-4).

1. Check to ensure that the IPV® unit is connected to a 50 psi medical gas power source.

2. Check for correct assembly of the drive circuit.
   a. Ensure that all color coded lines match to the appropriately color coded snap locks on both the Phasitron® and the Percussionator®.

3. Check for correct operational pressure adjustment. Initial operational pressure should be set at 30 psi.

The Nebulizer fails to generate any aerosol:

1. Check for correct assembly of the drive circuit.
   a. Ensure that all color coded lines match to the appropriately color coded snap locks on both the Phasitron® and the Percussionator®.

2. Check to ensure medication has been added to the nebulizer reservoir.

3. If using the IPV®-2, check to ensure that the Nebulizer control has been adjusted such that the nebulizer has sufficient output.

No pressure is indicated during percussive ventilation by the pressure manometer:

1. Check for correct assembly of the drive circuit.
   a. Ensure that all color coded lines match to the appropriately color coded snap locks on both the Phasitron® and the Percussionator®.

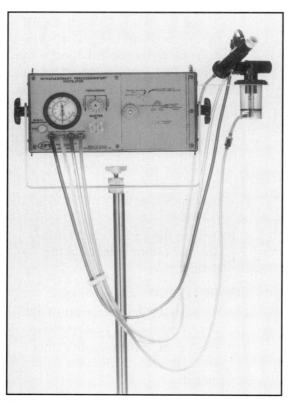

Figure 3-44 *A photograph of the Percussionaire IPV® circuit. (Courtesy Percussionaire Corporation, Sandpoint, ID)*

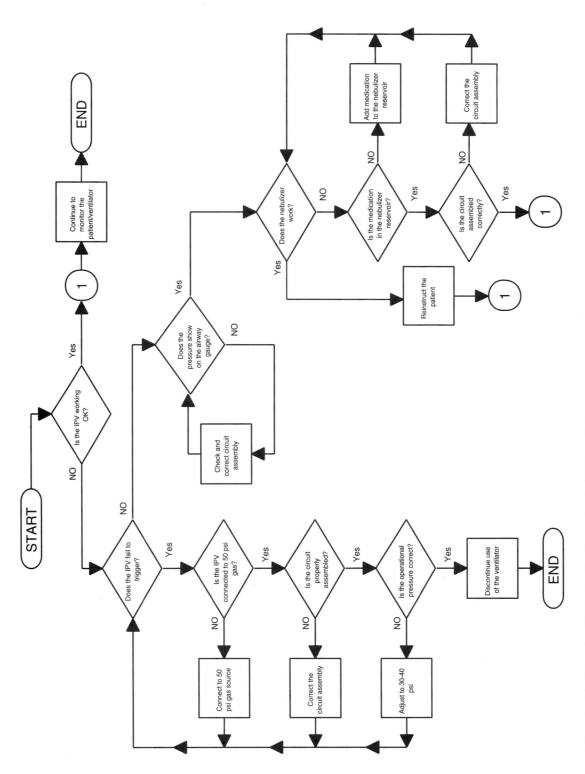

ALG 3-4 *A flow chart depicting troubleshooting the Percussionaire IPV® ventilator.*

PERCUSSORS USED FOR CHEST PHYSIOTHERAPY

Chest physiotherapy involves clapping on a patient's chest using cupped hands. By trapping a small pocket of air under the hands, vibrations are induced in the lung parenchyma that loosen pulmonary secretions. Manual percussion, although effective, can be tiring. Mechanical *percussors* have been developed to facilitate administration of chest physiotherapy and to ensure that all patients receive effective therapy.

Percussors are either electrically powered or gas powered. Both types will be discussed in this text.

VIBRAMATIC

The General Physiotherapy company manufactures both the Vibramatic and Flimm Fighter percussors. Both machines are electrically powered. An electric motor turns a flexible shaft that causes the head or applicator to vibrate.

The Vibramatic incorporates a timer and a frequency control (Figure 3-45). The timer may be set for a specific time interval of therapy. Once the time has elapsed, the percussor turns off. The frequency control may be adjusted to increase or decrease the frequency at which the applicator vibrates, allowing for variations in patient tolerance.

ASSEMBLY AND TROUBLESHOOTING

Assembly—Vibramatic Percussor

1. Connect the percussor to a 10 volt power source.

2. Adjust the frequency control to the desired setting.

3. Set the timer for the ordered length of therapy.

4. Apply the percussor head (applicator) to the patient's chest. (Do not push on the applicator. The weight of the head is sufficient for good therapy.)

Troubleshooting

Troubleshooting these devices in the clinical setting is primarily limited to checking for proper power connection. Any other malfunction should be referred to a qualified biomedical repair center.

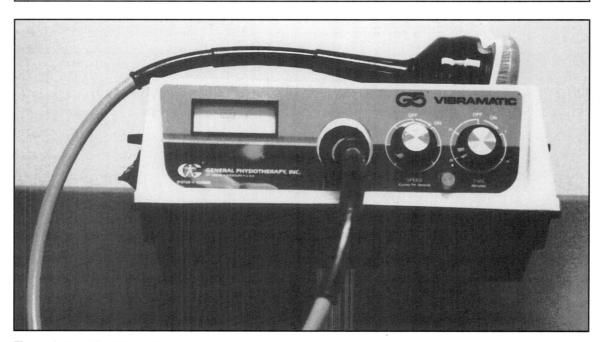

Figure 3-45 *The Vibramatic percussor.*

FLIMM FIGHTER

The Flimm Fighter is primarily intended for home use (Figure 3-46). It is a small portable percussor that allows self-therapy by the patient. A velcro pad and strap allow the patient to strap the applicator to his chest and then to assume the proper drainage position. Controls are limited to an "On/Off" switch.

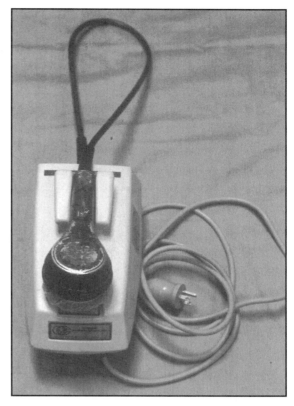

Figure 3-46 *The Flimm Fighter percussor.*

ASSEMBLY AND TROUBLESHOOTING

Assembly—Flimm Fighter

1. Connect the percussor to a 110 volt power source.

2. Apply the percussor head (applicator) to the chest. If self-therapy is desired, fasten the applicator in place using the belt. (Do not push on the applicator. The weight of the head is sufficient for good therapy.)

3. Turn on the percussor.

Troubleshooting

Troubleshooting these devices in the clinical setting is primarily limited to checking for proper power connection. Any other malfunction should be referred to a qualified biomedical repair center.

MJ PERCUSSOR

The MJ Percussor is a gas powered percussor. The components of this percussor include a high pressure supply hose, control head and applicator (Figure 3-47).

The high pressure hose is designed to use gas at 50 psi to power the unit. The gas may be oxygen or air. The use of air is recommended since one case of fire from an oxygen powered percussor has been reported.

The control head contains an electrically powered timing mechanism. The timing mechanism determines the frequency with which the gas powered piston is driven. The timer controls the operation of a solenoid valve that alternately applies gas pressure to the piston driving it. This electric control requires a 9 volt battery.

The applicator is a rubber suction cup. Disposable covers are available to promote aseptic usage of this device.

ASSEMBLY AND TROUBLESHOOTING

Assembly—MJ Percussor

1. Connect the applicator to the control head by screwing the two pieces together.

2. Install a 9 volt battery.

3. Connect the high pressure supply hose to a 50 psi source.

4. Install a protective cover over the applicator head.

5. Adjust the frequency to the desired level.

6. Apply the percussor to the patient's chest, using only the weight of the percussor.

Troubleshooting

Troubleshooting this percussor is limited to checking the battery and checking connections. Ensuring that all connections are tight will prevent many potential problems.

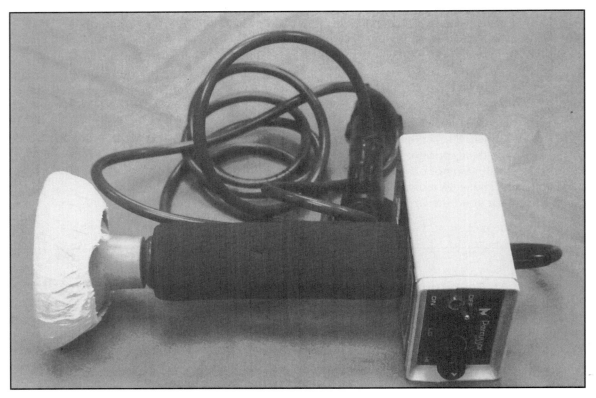

Figure 3-47 *The MJ Percussor.*

CLINICAL CORNER

Hyperinflation Equipment

1. You are asked to instruct a new adult postoperative patient on incentive spirometry. You learn in your review of her chart that she is blind. What incentive spirometer would you use and how you would instruct her?
2. Explain the advantages of flutter valve therapy as compared to chest physiotherapy for the ambulatory patient who is at home.
3. You are working with a 12-year-old cystic fibrosis patient, whom you are teaching to perform PEP therapy. During the session, he complains of being light-headed and adds that his fingers are numb. Explain what you should do and why.
4. You are asked to start an IPPB treatment on an elderly patient who wears a full set of dentures. The patient is not very cooperative and has a difficult time sealing his mouth around the mouthpiece. Decribe what device or devices could help to improve the outcome of the IPPB treatment and how they would be used.
5. You are giving an IPPB treatment to a patient with chronic lung disease in the emergency room. You are using a Bird Mark 7, set on air mix with the ventilator powered by oxygen. Ten minutes into the treatment you notice that the patient's respiratory rate has decreased markedly since you started. What do you suspect is occurring and what should you do about it?
6. A new physician in your area orders IPPB for a patient who is a new client of your homecare company. Explain which IPPB unit would be the best for home use and what you would need to properly instruct and set up the new patient.

Self-Assessment Quiz

1. The most accurate method of measuring inspired volumes is:
   a. Timing the duration of a flow of gas.
   b. Volume displacement.
   c. Photoelectric sensing.
   d. Ultrasonic measurement.
   e. Measuring chest expansion.

2. Three methods of volume measurement used in incentive spirometers include:
   I. Timing the duration of a flow of gas.
   II. Volume displacement.
   III. Photoelectric sensing.
   IV. Ultrasonic measurement.
   V. Measuring chest expansion.
   a. I, II and III
   b. II, III and IV
   c. I, III and IV
   d. III, IV and V
   e. II, IV and V

3. Gas pressure is regulated in the Bird ventilators by:
   I. A low-pressure reducing valve.
   II. Needle valve.
   III. Photoelectric sensing.
   IV. Magnetic attraction opposing gas pressure.
   V. A venturi.
   a. I and II
   b. I and III
   c. II and IV
   d. II and V

4. Gas pressure is regulated in the Bennett ventilators by:
   a. A low-pressure reducing valve.
   b. Needle valves.
   c. Magnetic attraction opposing gas pressure.
   d. Two opposing flows of gas.
   e. Using a venturi.

5. Needle valves are an effective way:
   a. To control gas temperature.
   b. To regulate gas pressure.
   c. To control gas flow.
   d. Of lengthening inspiratory time.
   e. Of increasing the F_IO_2.

6. Which of the following incentive spirometers operate by volume displacement?
   a. Voldyne.
   b. Spirocare.
   c. Volurex.
   d. Triflow.

7. Which of the following incentive spirometers operate using a photoelectric sensor?
   a. Voldyne.
   b. Spirocare.
   c. Volurex.
   d. Triflow.

8. A patient is using a flow-dependent incentive spirometer. The patient reaches a goal of 600 ml/second and holds that goal for 3 seconds. What inspired volume would you note in the patient's chart?
   a. 600 mL
   b. 1200 mL
   c. 1800 mL
   d. 2400 mL

9. An IPPB ventilator is failing to cycle off, and you suspect a leak. Possible places to check would include:
   I. The patient's ability to seal around the mouthpiece.
   II. All circuit connections.
   III. The exhalation valve.
   IV. The patient's nose.
   a. I
   b. I and II
   c. I, II and III
   d. I, II, III and IV

10. You are using a Bennett PR-2 ventilator to give an IPPB treatment. You want to increase the delivered tidal volume. You should:
    a. Increase the pressure.
    b. Increase the rate.
    c. Increase the terminal flow.
    d. Increase the peak flow.

11. When giving an IPPB treatment, the ventilator triggers on and cycles off rapidly. Which control should you adjust?
    a. Pressure.
    b. Peak flow.
    c. Sensitivity.
    d. Rate.

12. You are attempting to give an IPPB treatment with a Bird Mark 7 ventilator. The circuit has been assembled correctly and the ventilator is connected to a 50 psi gas source. However, the ventilator will not trigger into inspiration in spite of your patient's cooperative efforts. What

do you suspect is the problem?
a. The flow rate has been turned off.
b. The pressure is set too high.
c. The sensitivity is set too low.
d. The apnea control has been turned on.

13. The doctor wants an end inspiratory hold for his patient, who is receiving Albuterol via IPPB therapy. Which ventilator(s) can provide this?
I. Bird Mark 7.
II. Bird Mark 7A.
III. Bird Mark 8.
IV. Bennett PR-2.
a. I and II
b. I and III
c. II and III
d. II and IV
e. III and IV

14. Which of the following controls will dilute the F_iO_2 delivered from a Bennett PR-2 operating in the source gas setting?
a. Rate control.
b. Expiratory time control.
c. Peak flow control.
d. Pressure control.
e. Terminal flow control.

15. When giving IPPB therapy using a Bird Mark 7, changes in the delivered F_iO_2 can be attributed to:
I. The nebulizer.
II. The venturi gate.
III. The pressure.
IV. The flow setting.
a. I only
b. I and II
c. II and III
d. I, II and III
e. I, II, III, and IV

16. If an IPPB ventilator fails to cycle into exhalation (off), a common problem may be:
a. Too little pressure has been given.
b. Too much medication is in the nebulizer.
c. There is a leak.
d. Too much flow is going through the circuit.
e. The air dilution or air mix control should be turned off.

17. A control on the Bennett PR-2 that is designed to compensate for leaks is the:
a. Rate control.
b. Expiratory time control.
c. Peak flow control.
d. Pressure control.
e. Terminal flow control.

18. An IPPB ventilator designed primarily for home use is the:
a. Bennett AP-5.
b. Bennett PR-2.
c. Bird Mark 7.
d. Bird Mark 7A.
e. Bird Mark 8.

19. Ventilators that may be used to ventilate an apneic patient include the:
I. Bennett AP-5.

II. Bennett PR-2.
III. Bird Mark 7.
IV. Bird Mark 7A.
V. Bird Mark 8.
a. I only
b. II only
c. I and II
d. I, II and III
e. II, III, IV and V

20. When the patient attempts to trigger the IPPB ventilator on, a –8 cmH$_2$O is recorded on the pressure manometer. The respiratory care practitioner should:
a. Increase the flow.
b. Increase the pressure.
c. Increase the sensitivity.
d. Increase the terminal flow.
e. Increase the flow to the nebulizer.

21. Intrapulmonary percussive ventilation:
I. Is a form of internal percussion.
II. Delivers an aerosol.
III. Is a form of IPPB.
IV. Can only be used on apneic patients.
a. I and II
b. I and III
c. I and IV
d. II and IV

22. Which of the following delivers pulsed gas flow to the patient manifold on the Percussionaire IPV® ventilators?
a. The Phasitron®.
b. The Nebulizer.
c. The Percussionator®.
d. The Spanker.

23. Which of the following Percussionaire IPV® units is designed for portable use?
a. The Spanker.
b. The IPV®-1.
c. the IPV®-2.
d. The Mark 7.

24. Which of the following components of the Percussionaire IPV® units serves as a mechanical and pneumatic buffer to the high freqency generator?
a. The Phasitron®.
b. The Nebulizer.
c. The Percussionator®.
e. The Spanker.

25. Which of the following components in the Percussionaire IPV® circuit has an orificed diaphragm and a sliding venturi?
a. The Phasitron®.
b. The Nebulizer.
c. The Percussionator®.
e. The Spanker.

26. Which of the following controls governs the frequency of pulsed gas delivery when using the Percussionaire IPV®-1?
a. Percussion.
b. Inspiratory time.
c. Impact.
d. Inspiratory flow.

27. Which of the Percussionaire IPV® units has CPAP capability?
    a. IPV®-1.
    b. IPV®-2.
    c. Spanker.
    d. Mark 7.

28. Which of the Percussionaire IPV® units can control the nebulizer output?
    a. IPV®-1.
    b. IPV®-2.
    c. Spanker.
    d. Mark 7.

29. When troubleshooting the IPV®-1, it fails to initiate percussive ventilation when the thumb button is depressed. Likely sources of the problem are:
    I. No line pressure.
    II. The electric power cord is unplugged.
    III. The circuit is assembled wrong.
    IV. The nebulizer drive is disconnected.
    a. I and II
    b. I and III
    c. II and III
    d. II and IV

30. Which mechanical percussor facilitates self-therapy?
    a. Vibramatic.
    b. MJ Percussor.
    c. Flimm Fighter.
    d. Manual percussion.

Selected Bibliography

Bennett Respiration Products, "Operating Instructions, Bennett PR-2 Respiration Unit," Form 2131L, Santa Monica, CA, 1979.

Bird Corporation, "Instructions for Operating the Mark 7 and Mark 8 Respirators and Mark 10 and Mark 14 Ventilators," Form 1718, Palm Springs, CA.

Bird Corporation, "Understanding the Bird Mark 7 and Mark 8 Respirators with Apneustic Flow Time (A) and the Bird Ventilator," Form L929, Palm Springs, CA, 1977.

Bird, Forrest M., "Intrapulmonary Percussive Ventilation," *Flying Physician*, Vol. 30, No. 2, pp. 4–9, 1987.

Cheeseborough-Ponds, Valdyne Product Literature, St. Louis, MO, 1982.

Dupuis, Yvon, *Ventilators: Theory and Clinical Application*, C. V. Mosby Company, 1986.

Fluck, Robert R., Jr., "Intermittent Positive-Pressure Breathing Devices," in Barnes, Thomas A., et al. (eds.), *Respiratory Care Practice*, Year Book Medical Publishers, Inc., 1988.

Indihar, Frank F., et al., "A Prospective Comparison of Three Procedures Used in Attempts to Prevent Postoperative Pulmonary Complications," *Respiratory Care*, Vol. 27, No. 5, pp. 564–568, 1982.

Mahlmeister, Michael F., et al., "Positive-Expiratory-Pressure Mask Therapy: Theoretical and Practical Considerations and a Review of the Literature," *Respiratory Care*, Vol. 36, No. 11, 1991.

Mang, Harold, et al., "Imposed Work of Breathing During Sustained Maximal Inspiration: Comparison of Six Incentive Spirometers," *Respiratory Care*, Vol. 34, No. 12, pp. 1122–1128, 1989.

McPherson, Stephen P., *Respiratory Therapy Equipment*, C. V. Mosby Company, 1985.

Miller, Charles R., et al., "IPV Offers Cost-Effective Method for Self-Administered Therapy," *Advance*, Jan./Feb. 1993, pp. 2–34.

Natale, JoAnne E., et al., "Comparison of Intrapulmonary Percussive Ventilation and Chest Physiotherapy. A Pilot Study in Patients with Cystic Fibrosis," *Chest*, Vol. 105, No. 6, pp. 1789–1793, 1994.

Percussionaire Corporation, *Intrapulmonary Percussive Ventilation, a Twelve Year Learning Curve 1980–1993*, Sandpoint, ID, 1993.

Percussionaire Corporation, *Manual of Understanding, Operations and Clinical Restriction as They Relate to the Therapeutic Protocol for Bird Conceived Intrapulmonary Percussive Ventilation (IPV) and the Therapeutic Device the Bird Conceived IPV Percussionators® with the Therapeutic Breathing Head Assembly the Phasitron® and Percussive® Aerosol Generator Manufactured by the Percussionaire Corporation*, Percussionaire Corporation, Sandpoint, ID, 1985.

Reading, Paul M., et al., "Accuracy of Incentive Spirometer Indicators" (abstract), *Respiratory Care*, Vol. 29, No. 10, pp. 1025–1026, 1984.

White, Gary C., *Basic Clinical Lab Competencies for Respiratory Care*, 3ed Ed., Delmar Publishers, Inc., 1998.

CHAPTER 4

EMERGENCY RESUSCITATION EQUIPMENT

INTRODUCTION

This chapter will include discussions on artificial airways, manual resuscitators, vacuum regulation devices and secretion removal devices. Almost all of this equipment may be employed in the emergency setting.

In addition to the emergency management equipment, airways and other devices are discussed in this chapter, including tracheostomy weaning devices. A thorough understanding of the function and application of this equipment is important in the practice of respiratory care.

OBJECTIVES

After completing this chapter, the student will accomplish the following objectives:

PHYSICS OF THE PRINCIPLES

- Explain how the surface area of an endotracheal tube or tracheostomy tube affects the force exerted against the tracheal mucosa.
- Describe how a cuff pressure manometer measures the pressure inside an endotracheal or tracheostomy tube's cuff.
- Describe the common valve configurations employed in manual resuscitators and how gas flows in the desired direction.
- Explain how Poiseuille's law affects artificial airways and suction catheters.
- Explain how vacuum is regulated in secretion evacuation devices.

ARTIFICIAL AIRWAYS

- Distinguish between the following artificial airways, their placement, and how they open the airway:
  — Oropharyngeal airway
  — Nasopharyngeal airway
  — Esophageal Gastric Tube Airway (EGTA)
  — Pharyngeotracheal Lumen Airway (PTL Airway)
  — Laryngeal mask
  — Endotracheal tube
  — Esophageal obturator airway (EOA)
- Identify and explain the importance of the following components of an oral endotracheal tube:
  — Murphy eye
  — Cuff
  — Pilot tube
  — Markings on the tube
  — Pilot balloon
  — 15-mm connector
  — Radiopaque line
- Distinguish between the following tracheostomy tubes and their application:
  — Cuffed tracheostomy tube
  — Cuffed tracheostomy tube with a disposable inner cannula
  — Cuffed fenestrated tracheostomy tube
  — Hollinger or Jackson tracheostomy tube

CUFF PRESSURE MANOMETERS

- Differentiate between the following cuff pressure manometers and how each is used:
  — Manometer and a three-way stop cock

— Posey Cufflator
— DHD Cuff-Mate2
- Describe the differences between the following tracheostomy weaning devices and their application:
  — Pitt speaking tube/Communi-trach
  — Trach button
  — Kistner button
  — Passy-Muir Valve
  — Olympic Trach-Talk

MOUTH TO MASK VENTILATION DEVICES

- Describe purpose and correct use of mouth to mask ventilation devices.
- Describe the advantages and disadvantages of mouth to mask ventilation devices.

MANUAL RESUSCITATORS

- Differentiate between the following self-inflating manual resuscitators and their

valve configurations:
— Laerdal
— Hudson Lifesaver II
— Ambu Mark III
— Puritan Bennett PMR 2
- Differentiate between the following disposable manual resuscitators:
  — BagEasy
  — Pulmanex

SECRETION EVACUATION DEVICES

- Differentiate between the following suction regulators and their operation:
  — Puritan Bennett
  — Ohmeda Surgical/Free-Flow
- Differentiate between the following suction catheters:
  — Whistle tip
  — Argyle Aeroflow
  — Coudé tip
  — Trach Care

PHYSICS OF THE PRINCIPLES

FORCES EXERTED BY ARTIFICIAL AIRWAY CUFFS

As you may recall from physics, pressure is equal to a unit of force divided by the area over which the force is applied.

$$PRESSURE = \frac{FORCE}{AREA}$$

By rearranging the equation, force is a function of pressure multiplied by the area.

$$FORCE = PRESSURE \times AREA$$

As you can see in the second relationship, by increasing the surface area, a given force can be maintained at a lower pressure. This is the principle behind the design of the high-volume (increased surface area), low-pressure cuffs on endotracheal tube and tracheostomy tubes. By increasing the volume, and therefore the surface area, of the cuff, the pressure required to seal the tube against the tracheal wall is decreased. The

force that is applied is distributed over a larger area, reducing pressure trauma to the sensitive mucosa of the trachea.

CUFF PRESSURE MANOMETERS

Cuff pressure manometers are devices designed to measure the pressure contained in the inflated cuffs of endotracheal tubes or tracheostomy tubes. These manometers operate using simple diaphragms (mechanical manometer, see Chapter 1), or a diaphragm in conjunction with a strain gauge.

The mechanical manometer records changes in pressure which are directly proportional to the expansion and contraction of the diaphragm contained inside of the manometer (Figure 4-1). The needle is connected to the diaphragm by gear set, such that the linear motion of the diaphragm is converted to a rotary motion (needle indicator). These manometers are calibrated so that atmospheric pressure measures zero on the instruments scale.

The strain gauge type manometer also uses a diaphragm which changes shape with pressure changes (Figure 4-2). As the diaphragm moves, the strain gauge elongates or contracts proportionally with the diaphragm. As the

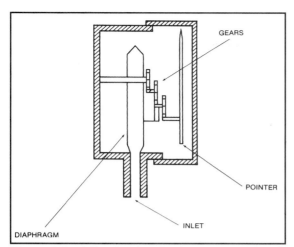

Figure 4-1 *A line drawing showing a cross section of a mechanical manometer. (Courtesy Delmar Publishers, Inc.,* Basic Clinical Lab Competencies for Respiratory Care *(3rd Ed.), 1998*

length of the strain gauge changes, electrical resistance increases or decreases. Therefore, a change in resistance is proportional to a change in pressure. Pressure is usually recorded digitally on a Liquid Crystal Display (LCD).

RESUSCITATOR VALVE TYPES

Diaphragm or Leaf Type

The simplest type of resuscitator valve is the diaphragm valve. It is made of a flexible rubber or plastic that will distort when pressure is applied. This type of valve will change shape in response to small pressure changes, which is advantageous in "sensing" a patient's spontaneous breathing efforts.

A diaphragm valve opens when pressure proximal to the valve seat distorts it (Figure 4-3A). The valve closes when pressure distal to the valve seat forces the valve against the seat closing it (Figure 4-3B).

Spring and Disk or Spring and Ball

This valve is composed of a rigid disk (diaphragm) or ball, spring, inlet and outlet (Figure 4-4). When pressure proximal to the disk or ball compresses the spring, the valve opens. When the pressure proximal to the disk decreases, spring tension overcomes gas pressure and the valve closes (Figure 4-4B).

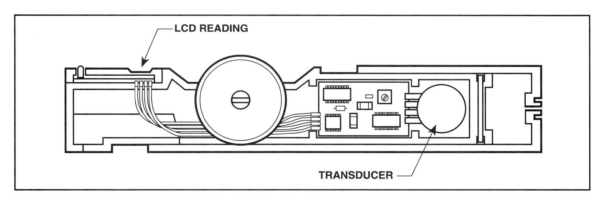

Figure 4-2 *A schematic diagram of a strain gauge cuff manometer.*

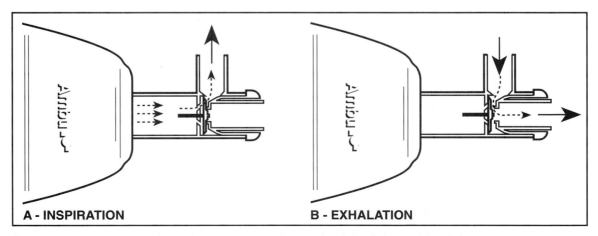

Figure 4-3 *The operation of a diaphragm-type resuscitator valve. (A) Inhalation. (B) Exhalation.*

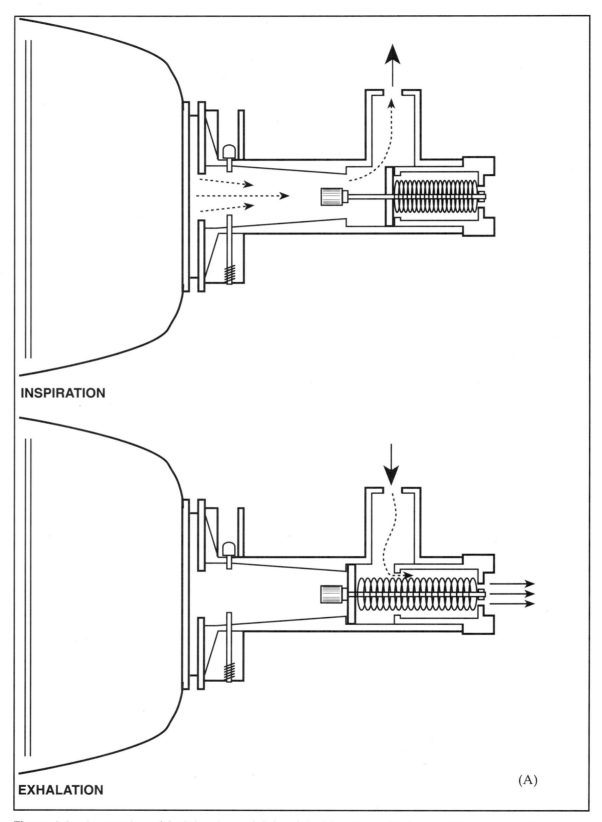

INSPIRATION

EXHALATION

(A)

Figure 4-4 *A comparison of the (A) spring-and-disk and the (B) spring-and-ball resuscitator valves (continues).*

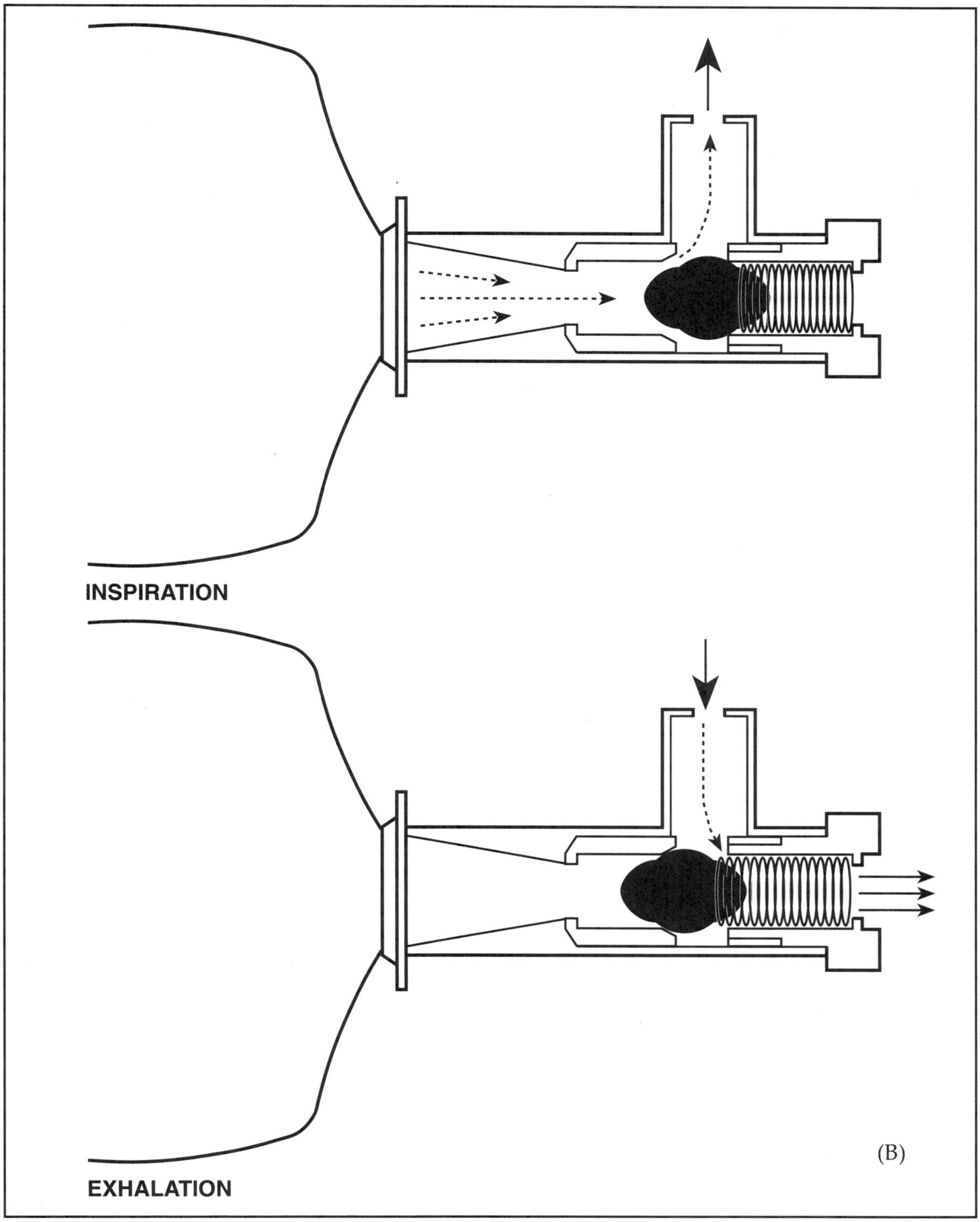

INSPIRATION

EXHALATION

(B)

Figure 4-4 *(continued)*

Duck Bill Valve

The duck bill valve is made from a flexible silastic or plastic (Figure 4-5). It, like the diaphragm valve, is very responsive to changes in pressure and is therefore sensitive to patient efforts.

The valve opens when pressure proximal to the valve seat distorts it (Figure 4-5A). The valve closes when pressure distal to the valve seat forces the valve against the seat, closing it (Figure 4-5B).

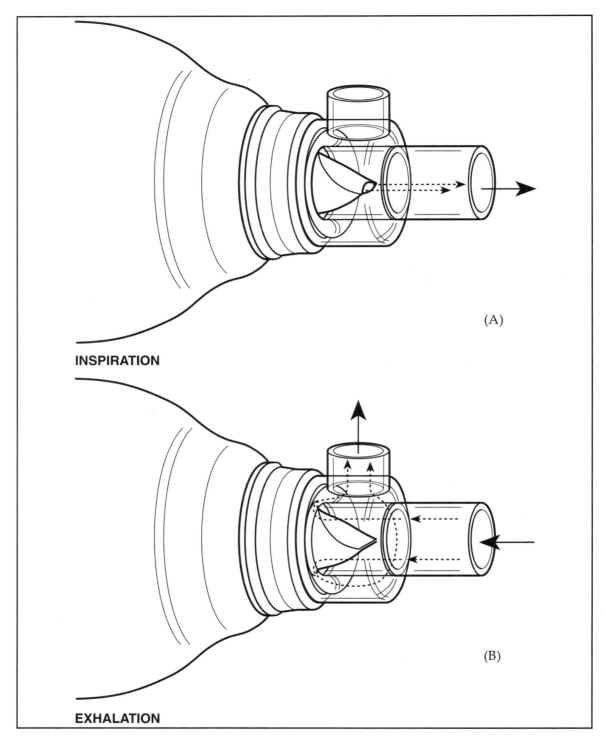

INSPIRATION

(A)

EXHALATION

(B)

Figure 4-5 *A duck bill–type resuscitation valve.*

THE IMPORTANCE OF POISEUILLE'S LAW

Poiseuille's law relates the diameter of a tube to the resistance imposed to gas flowing through it. This relationship is critical in both artificial airways and suction catheters.

A patient spontaneously breathing with a 6-mm internal diameter (ID) artificial airway will work harder than if using an 8.5-mm ID artificial airway. The imposed work of breathing from a narrow artificial airway can be significant. As the radius decreases by one-half, the resistance will increase 16 times. When a small artificial airway is placed, weaning from mechanical ventilation may be more difficult for that patient due to the increased work of breathing.

VACUUM REGULATION

The vacuum from the supply line in hospitals must be reduced to a safe physiological level for suctioning chest tubes and gastric tubes. Subambient pressure of between 400 and 600 mmHg from the supply lines must be reduced to 20 to 120 mmHg for clinical use.

Single-stage reducing valves are incorporated into the vacuum regulators to accomplish this. The operation of reducing valves is discussed in Chapter 1.

ARTIFICIAL AIRWAYS

Artificial airways are specialized medical devices that are designed to maintain a patent, or open, airway. Depending on the device, it may only displace the tongue or it may be inserted directly into the trachea. Artificial airways work by bypassing areas of obstruction or preventing vomitus or foreign material from obstructing the airway. Airways may be placed to prevent or to relieve airway obstruction.

OROPHARYNGEAL AIRWAY

The *oropharyngeal airway* is designed to relieve obstructions in the unconscious patient caused by the tongue or other soft tissue. Its curved shape separates the tongue from the posterior wall of the pharynx when properly placed (Figure 4-6).

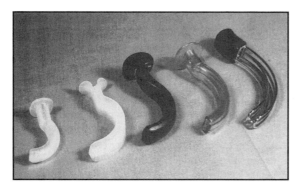

Figure 4-6 *A variety of oropharyngeal airways. Berman airways, a Guedel airway, and a Cath-Guide Guedel airway are shown.*

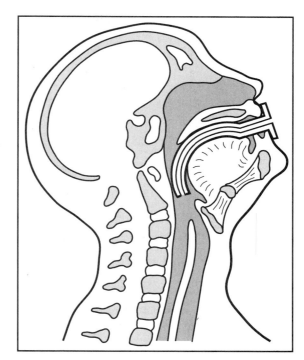

Figure 4-7 *The correct placement of an oropharyngeal airway. Note how the distal tip of the airway rests at the base of the tongue.*

By inserting the airway with the tip pointing toward the hard palate, then advancing it and rotating the airway 180°, the tongue will be separated from the posterior pharynx. The patient does not breathe through the airway itself, but through the opening created between it and the soft tissues.

The correct sizing of the oropharyngeal airway is important. If the airway is too small, the tongue may not be adequately separated from the soft palate, resulting in continued airway obstruction. If the airway is too large, it may actually push the epiglottis against the larynx, closing the airway. When correctly sized, the posterior tip of the airway should be positioned at the base of the tongue (Figure 4-7). These airways are rarely tolerated by the conscious patient. The gag reflex may be strongly stimulated, which could result in vomiting and aspiration.

NASOPHARYNGEAL AIRWAY

Like the oropharyngeal airway, the *nasopharyngeal airway* will relieve obstructions in the conscious or semiconscious patient caused by the tongue. The nasopharyngeal airway is a narrow hollow tube (Figure 4-8) made from a soft pliable rubber or plastic. It, like the oro-

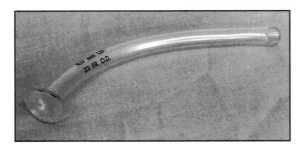

Figure 4-8 *A nasopharyngeal airway.*

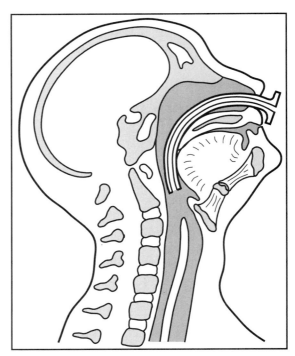

Figure 4-9 *The correct placement of a nasopharyngeal airway. Note how the tip of the airway separates the tongue from the soft palate.*

pharyngeal airway, separates the tongue from the soft palate.

The nasopharyngeal airway is inserted through the nose and nasal passage until the tip rests between the tongue and the soft palate. Airflow can pass through the airway as well as through the space created between it and the soft tissues.

Nasopharyngeal airways have many diameters and lengths. To size the airway, insert the largest diameter that can be easily passed with minimal force or trauma. The length may be sized by placing the distal end of the airway at the tragus of the ear and the proximal end near the nose. The airway should span from the tragus of the ear to the tip of the nose.

As described with oropharyngeal airways, if the size is not correct, airway obstruction may continue to be a problem. If the airway is too small, the tongue may not be separated from the posterior oropharynx. If the airway is too large, the epiglottis may be pushed inferiorly against the larynx, closing the airway. When properly sized, the distal tip of the airway should rest at the base of the tongue (Figure 4-9).

ENDOTRACHEAL TUBES

Endotracheal tubes are hollow pliable airways usually made from polyvinyl chloride (PVC) (Figure 4-10). The airway is inserted through the mouth or nose, through the larynx, and into the trachea. In proper position, the distal tip of the tube should be approximately 2 centimeters above the carina. Correct placement can be verified by examining the airway on a chest x-ray.

The endotracheal tube is hollow, allowing gas to flow through the airway. This type of airway may be used to bypass soft tissue obstructions. The component parts of an endotracheal tube include the cuff, pilot tube and pilot balloon, and murphy eye.

Cuff

The *cuff* is a large inflatable balloon near the distal tip of the endotracheal tube. When inflated, it is designed to seal against the tracheal wall (Figure 4-11). Positive pressure ventilation may be accomplished once the cuff is inflated and a patent airway is established. Since pressure is exerted on the tracheal wall, modern cuffs are designed to be low pressure, high volume cuffs. Low pressure, high volume cuffs exert less pressure against the tracheal wall because the pressure is distributed over a greater area. The greater surface area also helps to seal the cuff. Pressure exerted by these cuffs is typically less than 25 cmH$_2$O.

If cuff pressures are too high, damage to the tracheal mucosa may result. High cuff pressures may occlude blood flow to the mucosa by compression of the capillaries in the tracheal mucosa. This can lead to ischemic damage to the mucosal wall. Once ischemic damage occurs, it can progress resulting in tracheal stenosis, which causes a permanent narrowing of the tracheal lumen. These complications may be avoided by maintaining low cuff pressures and routinely monitoring the pressures within the cuff of the airway.

Another low-pressure cuff design is the foam cuff manufactured by Bivona. This cuff

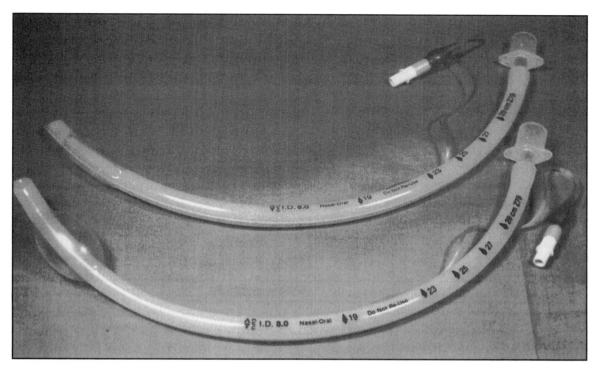

Figure 4-10 *Two adult endotracheal tubes (8.0 mm ID). Note that one cuff is inflated and the other is not. Also note the markings visible on the tubes.*

consists of a spongy foam covered with a thin silicone sheath (Figure 4-12). The cuff is exposed to ambient pressure (leaving the pilot tube uncapped), which allows the foam to expand to its normal size, sealing the tracheal wall. It is important not to inflate these cuffs with air like a conventional cuff. Addition of air will increase the pressure, defeating the purpose of the design. It is also important to size these tubes properly. If the tube is too

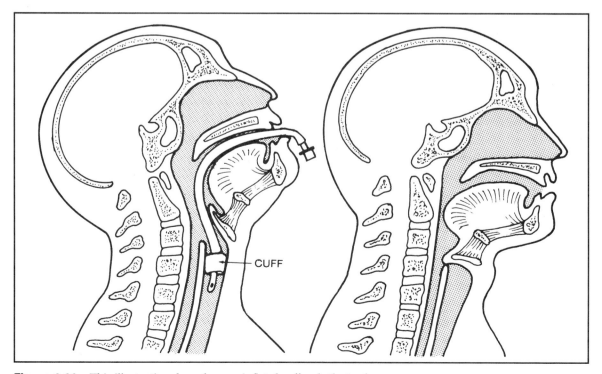

Figure 4-11 *This illustration shows how an inflated cuff seals the trachea.*

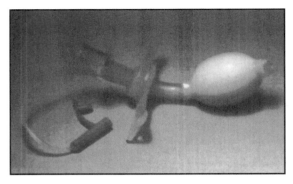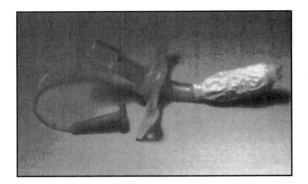

Figure 4-12 *A Bivona foam cuff on a tracheostomy tube.*

small, insufficient pressure may be exerted against the tracheal wall to seal it.

The Lanz tube is another design that minimizes endotracheal cuff pressures. This design incorporates a regulating valve and a control balloon made of latex within the large pilot balloon. The regulation valve and balloon limit cuff pressures to between 16 and 18 mmHg. As additional volume is injected into the cuff, the control balloon assimilates it without transmitting additional pressure to the cuff of the tube.

Pilot Balloon and Pilot Tube

Attached to the cuff is the pilot tube. The *pilot tube* is a small-diameter tube that conducts air to the cuff for inflation. On the proximal end of the pilot tube is the pilot balloon. When the cuff is inflated, the *pilot balloon* contains air to indicate that the cuff is inflated. The balloon therefore provides both a tactile and visual reference to whether the cuff is inflated. Close monitoring of cuff pressures is important to prevent adverse effects to the tracheal tissue.

Endotracheal Tube Markings

Endotracheal tubes have permanent markings to facilitate their usage. These markings include inside and outside diameters, length, and toxicity testing (Figure 4-10).

The endotracheal tube's inside and outside diameters are indicated in millimeters. Endotracheal tubes are manufactured in sizes varying from 2.5 to 9 mm internal diameters. When sizing artificial airways, the internal diameter is the diameter that is referenced.

The length from the distal tip is indicated in centimeters. This provides a rough guide as to how far the tube has been inserted into the airway. A chest x-ray should be obtained to confirm the exact tube placement. Once the correct placement of the endotracheal tube has been confirmed by x-ray, it is common practice to document the length of the endotracheal tube referenced to the patient's lips or incisors in the patient's medical record. This documentation provides a reference in the event that the endotracheal tube advances down the airway or is displaced outward.

A radiopaque strip runs along the length of the tube from the proximal tip to the end of the tube. This strip makes the tube more visible on a chest x-ray.

Toxicity testing is indicated by the markings *Z-79* or *IT*. One or both markings may be present. The Z-79 marking refers to the American National Standards Institute (ANSI) committee for anesthesia equipment. This committee requires specific cell culture testing to demonstrate a material's lack of human tissue toxicity. If the tube is marked *IT* (Implant Testing), a sample of the material was implanted into rabbit tissue to test for toxicity.

Murphy Eye

The murphy eye provides an alternate pathway for gas to flow in the event the proximal tip becomes obstructed (Figure 4-13). If the tip becomes obstructed, air will continue to flow but resistance will increase, due to the decreased airway diameter.

Fifteen-Millimeter Connection

A 15-mm connection at the proximal end of endotracheal tubes and tracheostomy tubes provides a connection to manual resuscitators and other ventilation equipment. The connection is tapered so that all connections may be made by simply pressing the two parts together. The 15-mm size has been adopted as a

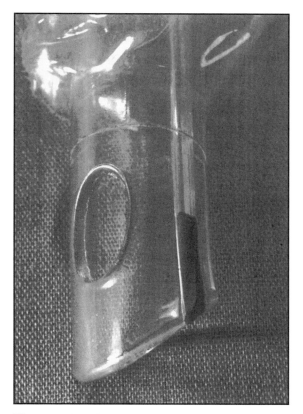

Figure 4-13 *The murphy eye is at the distal end of an adult endotracheal tube.*

standard for all resuscitation equipment so that all tubes will fit with all resuscitation equipment.

Radiopaque Line

A radiopaque line runs along the length of endotracheal and tracheostomy tubes. This thin line absorbs gamma rays emitted from an x-ray. The line facilitates the assessment of the artificial airway placement by appearing as a white (dense) line on a chest x-ray.

Mallinckrodt Hi-Lo® Evac Endotracheal Tube

The Mallinckrodt Hi-Lo® Evac endotracheal tube is a specialized endotracheal tube with an additional open lumen (suction lumen), which terminates proximal to the tube's cuff (Figure 4-14). The suction lumen has a separate suction line of its own and a fitting designed to interface with conventional suction lines. The purpose of the additional suction lumen is to evacuate secretions that pool above the endotracheal tube's cuff when inflated and therefore reduce the risk of their aspiration.

ESOPHAGEAL OBTURATOR AIRWAY

The *esophageal obturator airway* (EOA) is a combination of a mask and airway. Unlike the endotracheal tube, it is designed to intubate the esophagus and not the trachea. The advantage of this airway in the emergency setting is that the esophagus is more easily intubated blindly. The components of the EOA include the airway, mask, pilot balloon and line, and the cuff (Figure 4-15).

The airway itself is a hollow, flexible tube. The distal end is closed. Ventilation is achieved when gas flows through ports near the proximal end into the mouth and oropharynx. The mask seals against the face, facilitating positive pressure ventilation. If the mask is not tightly sealed, the patient will not be ventilated.

A large-volume, low-pressure cuff seals the esophagus, preventing aspiration. The pilot line and balloon serve the same function with the EOA as with the endotracheal tube.

ESOPHAGEAL GASTRIC TUBE AIRWAY

The Esophageal Gastric Tube Airway (EGTA) is similar in design and function to the EOA described earlier. The differences between the EOA and EGTA are that the EGTA does not have a blind blunt tip at its distal end (Figure 4-16). The long cuffed tube has an opening through which a gastric tube can be passed into the stomach to help relieve gastric

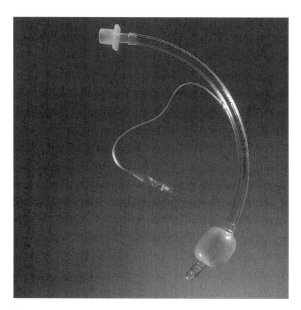

Figure 4-14 *Hi-Lo® Evac endotracheal tube. (courtesy of Mallinckrodt, Inc.)*

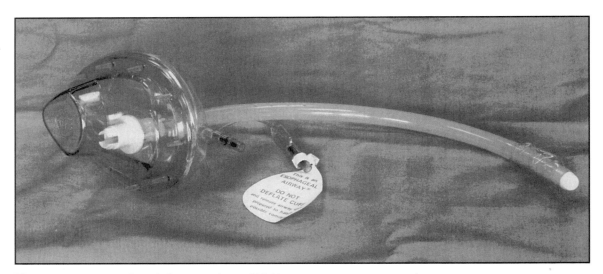

Figure 4-15 *An esophageal obturator airway (EOA).*

distension during ventilation of the lungs. Ventilation holes on the long cuffed tube are also absent. The mask of the EGTA has two ports, one to the long cuffed gastric tube and the other port for mask-to-mouth ventilation or for use in combination with a manual resuscitator. The EGTA is inserted in the same manner as the EOA. With the use of a gastric tube, the risk of aspiration is reduced over the use of an EOA. Care must be exercised when connecting a manual resuscitator to an EGTA to ensure that the manual resuscitator has been connected to the correct port on the mask.

Removal of an EOA or EGTA

Prior to the removal of either the EOA or

EGTA, it is recommended that the patient be intubated, orally or nasally, with an endotracheal tube and that the cuff of the endotracheal tube be inflated. Aspiration and vomiting following removal of the EOA or EGTA are common. It is important to protect the trachea from aspiration by intubating prior to removing either the EOA or EGTA. Suction equipment should also be available including a Yankaur suction catheter and a conventional suction catheter.

PHARYNGEALTRACHEAL LUMEN AIRWAY

The Pharyngealtracheal Lumen Airway (PTL airway) is a double lumen airway with

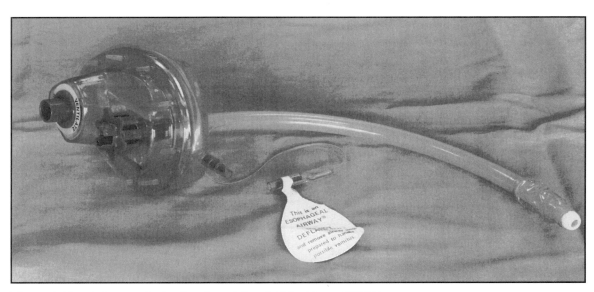

Figure 4-16 *A photograph of an Esophageal Gastric Tube Airway (EGTA).*

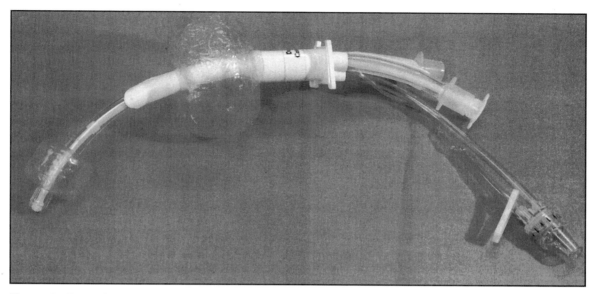

Figure 4-17 *A photograph of the Pharyngealtraheal Lumen Airway (PTL airway).*

the features of an Esophageal Tracheal Airway and an endotracheal tube (Figure 4-17). The tube is designed to be inserted blindly (without visualization, using a laryngoscope). Once inserted, the large cuff in the oropharynx is inflated, as is the second cuff at the distal end of the long tube. The rescuer attempts ventilation through the shorter tube and observes the patient's chest for adequate expansion and condensate in the tube from exhaled air. If adequate ventilation is not observed, then the rescuer ventilates through the longer lumen of the airway. The patient is again observed for adequate ventilation (Figure 4-18).

If the long tube is in the esophagus, ventilation is accomplished by ventilating through the shorter tube. Air is directed into the trachea since the esophagus is occluded by the cuff at the distal end of the long tube. When used in this way, the PTL functions in a similar way to the EGTA.

If the long tube has intubated the trachea, the airway performs in a similar way to an endotracheal tube. The cuff on the long tube

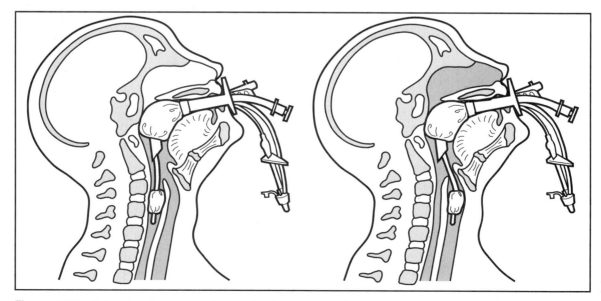

Figure 4-18 *A drawing showing the placement of the Pharyngealtracheal Lumen Airway (PTL airway) placed into the (A) esophagus and the (B) trachea.*

seals the tracheal wall, facilitating positive pressure ventilation.

LARYNGEAL MASK

The laryngeal mask is a small, triangular-shaped, inflatable mask secured to a tube, much like a cuff is secured to an endotracheal tube (Figure 4-19). The laryngeal mask is designed to be positioned such that when the mask is inflated, the tip rests against the upper esophageal sphincter and the sides face into the pyriform fossae and lie just under the base of the tongue (Figure 4-19). Like the EOA and EGTA, the laryngeal mask is designed to seal the esophagus, providing a more patent and easily maintained airway when compared with a conventional mask and oral airway combination.

Prior to insertion of the laryngeal mask, fully deflate the mask, using a syringe, and lubricate it well, using a water-soluble lubricant. Be certain to put on a pair of surgical gloves and wear appropriate personal protective equipment. Perform a manual head tilt maneuver and open the lower jaw widely, exposing the airway. With the aperture of the mask facing forward, guide it into the airway by holding it near where the mask joins the ventilation tube, just as one holds a pencil. Once the mask has advanced past the base of the tongue, use the ball of your finger to continue the mask's advance into position past the posterior portion of the pharynx, posterior to the tongue following the pharyngeal wall. Resistance will be felt when the mask rests against the isophageal sphincter. Inflate the mask and check for correct ventilation by observing chest rise and auscultation of the chest and by using exhaled carbon dioxide detection. Once ventilation is confirmed, secure the laryngeal mask in place using tape and protect it with a bite block. When positioned correctly, the black line on the ventilation tube should always face the patient's upper lip; do not rotate the laryngeal mask from the optimal position.

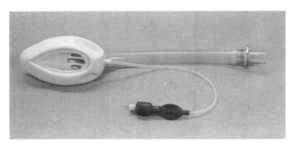

Figure 4-19 *A photograph of the Laryngeal Mask Airway.*

TRACHEOSTOMY TUBES

A *tracheostomy tube* bypasses the entire upper airway. When a tracheostomy tube is placed, an incision is made between the second and third tracheal rings and the tube is inserted directly into the trachea. Tracheostomy tubes are made in differing configurations including cuffed, cuffed with a disposable inner cannula, uncuffed fenestrated tubes, Hollinger tubes and Communi-trach tubes.

Cuffed, Disposable Tracheostomy Tube

The cuffed, disposable tracheostomy tube is one of the most common types of tracheostomy tubes (Figure 4-20). The design of the cuffed tracheostomy tube is somewhat similar to an endotracheal tube, in that a cuff, pilot tube and balloon are part of the design. This tracheostomy tube does not have a removable inner cannula; therefore it is recommended to change the cannula periodically, when needed. Like the endotracheal tube, it is typically made from PVC, providing a flexible, nontoxic appliance.

Cuffed Tracheostomy Tube with a Disposable Inner Cannula

A variation on the cuffed tracheostomy tube is one with a disposable inner cannula (Figure 4-21). Frequent changes of the inner cannula will ensure that the airway remains patent. This design change eliminates the need to change the tube unless the patency of the cuff is compromised.

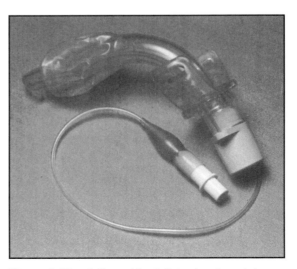

Figure 4-20 *A disposable adult tracheostomy tube.*

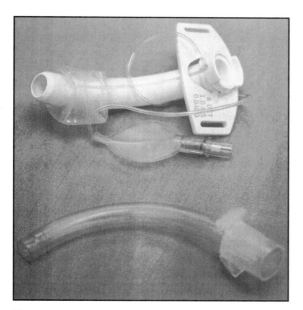

Figure 4-21 *An adult tracheostomy tube with a disposable inner cannula that may be replaced as required to maintain patency.*

Fenestrated Tracheostomy Tube

The *fenestrated tracheostomy tube* has a removable inner cannula like the one just described. The outer cannula, however, has a fenestration, or hole, in it (Figure 4-22). With the inner cannula removed and the cuff deflated, the patient may breathe through the upper airway, through the fenestration. This type of tracheostomy tube is frequently used for weaning purposes. In the event mechanical ventilation is required, the cuff can be inflated and the inner cannula replaced. In this configuration the tube performs like a regular cuffed tracheostomy tube.

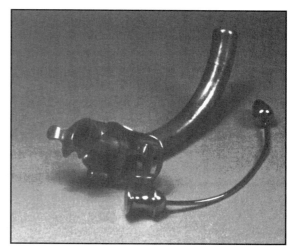

Figure 4-23 *A silver Jackson tracheostomy tube. This tube is permanent and is made from sterling silver.*

Silver Jackson Tracheostomy Tube

The silver *Jackson (or Hollinger) tracheostomy tube* is frequently used as a permanent tracheostomy tube. It is made from sterling silver and is cuffless (Figure 4-23). A silver tube is more durable and easier to clean than a PVC tube.

Communi-Trach

The *Communi-Trach* or *Pitt speaking tube* is a tracheostomy tube that facilitates speech when the cuff is inflated. A second line and tube are attached to the tracheostomy tube, which directs oxygen flow above the cuff through small holes (Figure 4-24). This flow of gas allows the patient to use the vocal cords to communicate even when the cuff is inflated. The

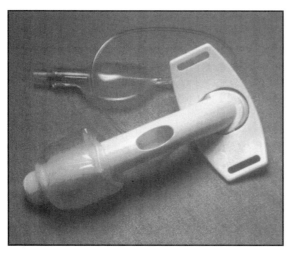

Figure 4-22 *A fenestrated tracheostomy tube.*

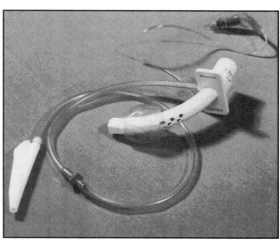

Figure 4-24 *A Communi-Trach. This is a variation of the Pitt Speaking tube.*

quality of the speech is different from normal communication, and the patient may have difficulty initially coordinating speech independent from diaphragmatic motion.

CUFF PRESSURE MEASUREMENT

As described earlier in this chapter, monitoring cuff pressure and maintenance of low cuff pressures are important to minimize some of the complications associated with endotracheal and tracheostomy tube cuffs. Two methods are frequently used to maintain the lowest cuff pressures while still allowing adequate positive pressure ventilation. These techniques are termed minimal occlusion volume and minimal leak techniques.

Minimal occlusion volume (MOV) is performed by slowly inflating or deflating the cuff during positive pressure ventilation. When cuff pressure is low, a leak can be heard at the patient's mouth. Once a leak is detected, enough air is added to the cuff to stop the leak. At this point, the cuff pressure is measured and recorded.

The minimal leak technique is performed by slowly removing air from the cuff until a very small leak is detected at the patient's mouth. At this point the cuff pressure is measured and recorded.

Cuff Pressure Manometers
Mechanical Manometer and Three-Way Stopcock

A mechanical manometer connected to a three-way stopcock and a syringe (Figure 4-25)

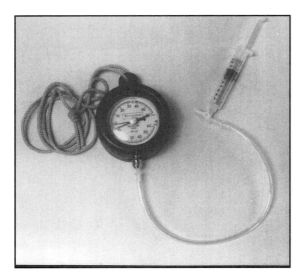

Figure 4-25 *A photograph of a mechanical manometer, a syringe and a three-way stopcock.*

is an effective way to measure and record cuff pressures. To effectively use this combination device, the practitioner must clearly understand which ports of the three-way stopcock are open as the valve is rotated (Figure 4-26). When the valve is rotated toward the distal port, the manometer and the syringe are open to one another. When the valve is rotated pointing to the syringe, the manometer and the distal tip are open to one another. When the valve is rotated toward the manometer, the syringe and the distal port are open. When the valve is rotated pointing opposite the syringe, all three ports are open. It is critical to know these positions from memory, since rotation to the wrong port, if the system is connected to an endotracheal or tracheostomy cuff, may cause loss of pressure to the cuff.

To use this device, fill the syringe with 5–10 ml of air and attach it to the three-way stopcock. Rotate the valve so it points to the distal tip of the three-way stopcock. Slowly add air to the system until the manometer reads 18 cmH$_2$O. Attach the distal tip of the three-way stopcock to the pilot tube of the airway. Rotate the valve to a position opposite the syringe, opening all three ports. Perform the MOV or minimal leak technique and record the cuff pressure.

Posey Cufflator

The Posey Cufflator combines the syringe, stop cock assembly and mechanical manometer into one easy-to-use device (Figure 4-27). A black rubber hand bulb replaces the syringe on this device. The silver port is connected to the pilot tube of the patient's airway. If there is insufficient air in the cuff, the bulb is gently squeezed adding air to the cuff. Changes in pressure are recorded on the mechanical manometer. If too much air is in the cuff, depressing the red toggle valve on the side of the Cufflator allows air to be vented to the atmosphere, reducing pressure in the patient's cuff. MOV or minimal leak techniques may be performed with the Cufflator and the pressure may then be recorded.

DHD Cuff-Mate2

The DHD Cuff-Mate2 combines a syringe (piston) and a diaphragm strain gauge combination (Figure 4-28). To use the Cuff-Mate2, withdraw the piston by grasping the device in the palm of your hand and rotating the thumbwheel toward the digital display until the calibrated indicator reads between 0.0

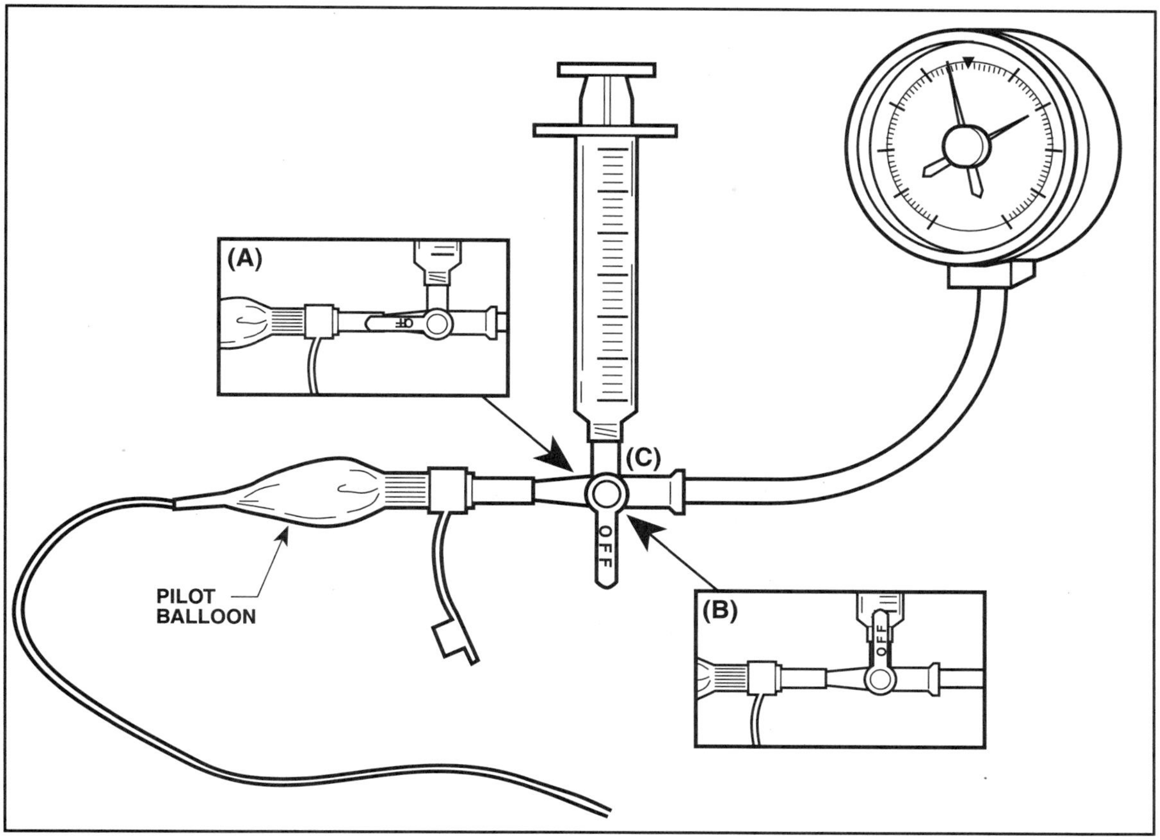

(A)

(C)

(B)

PILOT
BALLOON

Figure 4-26 *A line drawing showing three of the four stopcock positions. (A) Off to the pilot tube. (B) Off to the syringe. (C) All three ports open.*

and 5.0 cc. Connect the Cuff-Mate2 to the patient's pilot tube and depress the power switch (proximal to the digital display). Perform an MOV or minimal leak technique, by adding or subtracting air, using the thumbwheel to move the piston. When the desired condition is reached, record the pressure indicated on the digital display.

SPECIALIZED WEANING DEVICES

For many patients, it is desirable to remove the tracheostomy tube as their clinical course improves. Simply removing the tracheostomy

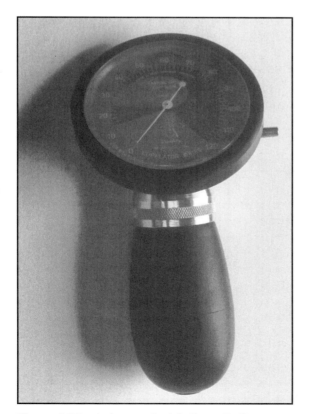

Figure 4-27 *A photograph of the Posey Cufflator.*

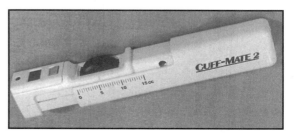

Figure 4-28 *The DHD Cuff-Mate2.*

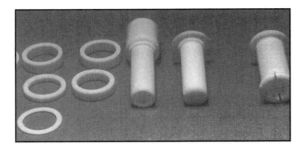

Figure 4-29 *A tracheostomy button. Note the spacers, plug and positive pressure adapter.*

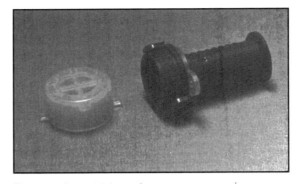

Figure 4-31 *A Kistner button.*

tube and covering the stoma can be a difficult transition. Temporary devices have been developed to ease this transition. In the event that the weaning trial fails, these devices maintain the patency of the stoma and, if it is required, mechanical ventilation can be accomplished with some of these appliances.

Trach Button

The *trach button* (Figure 4-29) is one type of weaning device. It is made from Teflon and consists of an inner cannula, plug, IPPB adapter and spacers. When the outer cannula is plugged, the stoma is closed and the patient is able to breathe through the upper airway (Figure 4-30). With the IPPB adapter in place, mechanical ventilation may be accomplished. However, since this device is cuffless, some volume leakage will occur through the upper airway. The spacers allow the appliance to be adapted to different neck thicknesses.

Kistner Button

The Kistner button is similar to the trach button, only it is made from a more pliable plastic. This device does not have any provisions for mechanical ventilation or a removable plug (Figure 4-31). The Kistner button maintains the stoma as does the trach button. A removable cap with a one-way valve forces the patient to

use his upper airway during exhalation. The cap assembly facilitates speech and also allows the patient to cough more effectively.

Olympic Trach-Talk

The Olympic Trach-Talk is an aerosol T with a spring-loaded, one-way valve. It is placed onto a tracheostomy tube (with the cuff deflated). A humidifier or aerosol generator provides oxygen and humidification to the airway. During inspiration, the valve opens, allowing the patient to inhale through the Trach-Talk and tracheostomy tube. During the expiratory phase, the valve closes and the patient exhales through the upper airway. This appliance should only be used when the patient is awake and able to manage the secretions effectively.

Passy-Muir Valve

Passy-Muir, Inc., manufactures the Passy-Muir tracheostomy valve (Figure 4-32). This

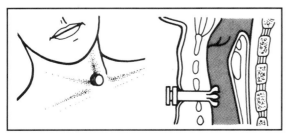

Figure 4-30 *This drawing shows the placement of a trach button.*

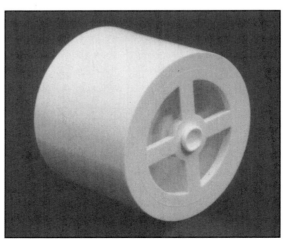

Figure 4-32 *A photograph of the Passy-Muir valve. (Courtesy of Passy-Muir, Inc., Irvine, CA)*

valve consists of a diaphragm valve which, during inspiration, allows the patient to inhale through the tracheostomy tube and, during exhalation, closes and forces air through the upper airway. When using this device it is important to deflate the cuff of the tracheostomy tube prior to placing the Passy-Muir valve onto the airway.

MOUTH-TO-MASK VENTILATION DEVICES

The Centers for Disease Control and the American Heart Association recommend the use of a barrier device when ventilating a patient prior to intubation or the use of a manual resuscitator during cardiopulmonary resuscitation. These barrier devices are designed to protect the practitioner from microorganism transmission from contact with the patient's saliva, or body fluids, during cardiopulmonary resuscitation efforts. These devices protect the practitioner by eliminating physical contact between the practitioner and the patient.

Mouth-to-mask devices incorporate a soft-seal mask for the patient and a one-way valve, or filter, to separate the patient from the practitioner (Figure 4-33). Additionally, some masks also incorporate an extension tube with a mouthpiece to further remove the practitioner physically from the patient. The masks are clear, to allow for observation of vomiting. Some devices also have a port on the mask, or near the one-way valve, for supplemental oxygen administration during manual ventilation efforts.

The use of a bacteria filter between the patient and the practitioner will further protect the practitioner from microorganism transmission.

To use these devices, the practitioner should be at the patient's head, facing the patient's feet. Each hand should grasp the ramus of the patient's jaw, thrusting the jaw anteriorly. The mask should be placed over the patient's mouth and nose, using the thumbs or thumb and forefinger of each hand (Figure 4-34). It is important to keep a tight seal, in that leaks hamper the performance of these devices.

Supplemental oxygen may be connected to the oxygen enrichment port on the mask or delivery tubing. Use of supplemental oxygen can increase oxygen delivery to approximately 70%. If the mouth-to-mask device lacks an oxygen enrichment port, the practitioner may wear a nasal cannula to provide additional supplemental oxygen.

MANUAL RESUSCITATORS

Manual resuscitators or bags are used in the emergency setting to manually ventilate apneic patients. They may also be used during intrahospital patient transport when a patient is moved from an acute care area to another area of the hospital. An example of the type of transport is taking a patient to have a Computerized Tomography (CT) scan, Magnetic Resonance Imaging (MRI) scan, Fluoroscopy

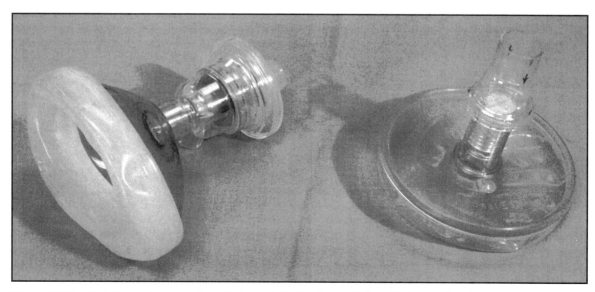

Figure 4-33 *A photograph of several mouth-to-mask devices for ventilation during cardiopulmonary resuscitation.*

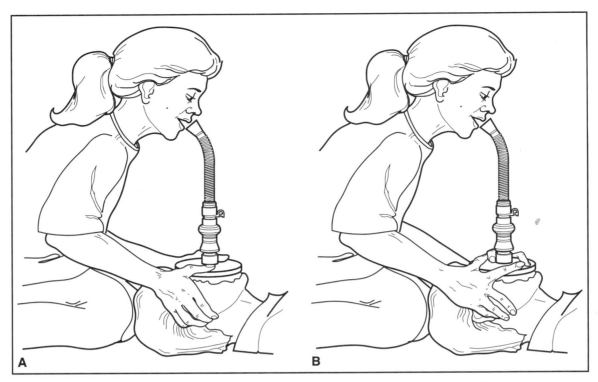

Figure 4-34 *An illustration showing the correct use of the mouth-to-mask barrier devices. (A) Use of the thumbs to seal the mask. (B) Use of the thumbs and index fingers to seal the mask.*

procedure, or to transport the patient from the Emergency Room (ER) to the Intensive Care Unit (ICU) or to the operating room (OR).

A manual resuscitator is classified based on inflation (flow-inflation or self-inflation) and whether it is disposable or permanent (reusable). The performance of these devices varies considerably and is well documented.

FLOW-INFLATING MANUAL RESUSCITATORS

As the name implies, *flow-inflating manual resuscitators* rely on gas flow to inflate them. Sometimes these devices are referred to as "anesthesia bags," due to their popularity in the operating theater. They are available as both permanent and disposable bags (Figure 4-35).

ASSEMBLY AND TROUBLESHOOTING

Assembly—Flow-Inflating Resuscitator

The following is a general guideline for assembling a permanent, flow-inflating manual resuscitator. Disposable resuscitators come preassembled, only requiring connection to an oxygen source.

1. Connect the reservoir bag to the anesthesia elbow.

2. Connect the oxygen connecting tube to the oxygen inlet on the elbow.

3. Connect the oxygen tubing to an oxygen flowmeter and adjust the flow to 8 to 12 liters per minute.

Troubleshooting

Troubleshooting these bags is relatively easy. The most common problems are connections that come apart. Therefore, it is important to ensure that all connections are tight prior to using the bag.

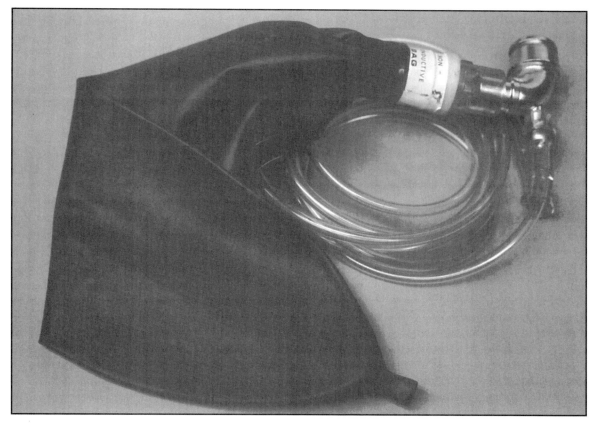

Figure 4-35 *A flow-inflating manual resuscitator. This may also be referred to as an anesthesia bag.*

Oxygen flowing into the reservoir inflates it when the tail of the bag is pinched closed. When the bag is manually compressed (while pinching the tail), a breath is delivered to the patient. When the bag is released, the exhaled gas flows out through the tail of the bag.

Due to the design of the oxygen inlet at the elbow, it is possible to deliver 100% oxygen with these manual resuscitators. Furthermore, since the bag offers little resistance when compressed, it is easy to assess the patient's compliance when using the bag.

PERMANENT, SELF-INFLATING MANUAL RESUSCITATORS

Permanent, *self-inflating manual resuscitators* are designed to be cleaned and reused between patients. They are quite expensive and must be treated carefully to prevent unnecessary damage when used in the emergency setting. Several types are available for clinical use including the Laerdal, Hudson Lifesaver II, and Ambu Mark III.

Laerdal Resuscitator

The Laerdal resuscitator (Figure 4-36) is a permanent resuscitator made from silicone. It has a 2,600 milliliter reservoir that improves the F_IO_2 delivery. This resuscitator uses the duck bill type of valve discussed earlier in this chapter. F_IO_2 delivery varies between .62 and 1.00 depending on oxygen flow, tidal volume and frequency.

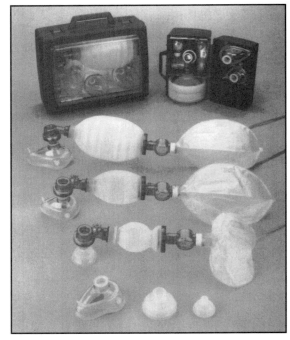

Figure 4-36 *Three permanent manual resuscitators manufactured by Laerdal™ Medical Corporation. The three sizes include infant, child, and adult resuscitators. (Courtesy of Laerdal™ Medical Corporation, Armonk, NY)*

ASSEMBLY AND TROUBLESHOOTING

Assembly—Laerdal Resuscitator

1. Place the duck bill valve into its seat facing the patient connection and screw the valve assembly together.

2. Snap the valve assembly to the bag.

3. Install the diaphragm into the tail-piece fitting and screw the assembly to the bag.

4. Attach an appropriately sized mask to the patient connection (if the patient is not intubated or trached).

5. Connect oxygen connecting tube between the bag and a flowmeter and set the oxygen flow to 10 to 12 liters per minute.

Troubleshooting

Troubleshooting this bag involves problems of improper assembly and loose connections. Careful inspection of the bag prior to use will eliminate many potential problems.

Hudson Lifesaver II

The Hudson Lifesaver II is another permanent, self-inflating manual resuscitator. It is made with transparent plastic and is capable of delivering up to 100% oxygen depending upon flow rate, tidal volume and frequency. This resuscitator uses the duck bill type of valve described earlier. A vinyl oxygen reservoir helps to increase the delivered F_IO_2.

ASSEMBLY AND TROUBLESHOOTING

Assembly—Hudson Lifesaver II

1. Install the duckbill valve on its seat and screw the two valve halves together.

2. Attach the pressure relief valve assembly to the valve by screwing it onto its fitting.

3. Push the completed valve assembly onto the bag ensuring that the fit is snug and that it is secure.

4. Attach the reservoir to the tailpiece of the bag.

5. Attach oxygen connecting tube to the oxygen inlet and attach the free end to an oxygen flowmeter.

6. Attach an appropriately sized mask to the outlet of the valve (if the patient is not intubated).

7. Adjust the oxygen flow to 8 to 12 liters per minute.

Troubleshooting

Troubleshooting this bag involves problems of improper assembly and loose connections. Careful inspection of the bag prior to use will eliminate many potential problems.

Ambu Mark III

Ambu Incorporated was one of the first companies to market a permanent manual resuscitator. In some areas the name *Ambu* is synonymous with a self-inflating manual resuscitator. The Ambu resuscitators are made from rubber that may be easily cold-sterilized or autoclaved (unlike the early versions, which contained foam rubber). The resuscitator is capable of delivering an F_IO_2 of between .4 and 1.00 depending on oxygen flow, rate and tidal volume. The Ambu Mark III uses a diaphragm type of valve for its operation. (Diaphragm valves were discussed earlier in this chapter.)

ASSEMBLY AND TROUBLESHOOTING

Assembly—Ambu Mark III

1. Screw the inlet valve to the valve housing with the patient outlet.

2. Push the valve assembly onto the bag, making sure it is tight.

3. Push the reservoir bag onto the inlet valve housing.

4. Attach oxygen connecting tube to the valve inlet and a flowmeter.

5. Attach an appropriately sized mask to the patient connection if the patient is not intubated.

6. Adjust the oxygen flow to 8 to 12 liters per minute.

Troubleshooting

Troubleshooting this bag involves problems of improper assembly and loose connections. Careful inspection of the bag prior to use will eliminate many potential problems.

PMR 2 Permanent Manual Resuscitator

Puritan Bennett Corporation manufactures and markets a permanent manual resuscitator, the PMR 2 (Figure 4-37). The resuscitator uses a diaphragm and leaf valve combination. When used without the oxygen reservoir, an F_iO_2 level of .35 can be maintained. When used with the reservoir, an F_iO_2 of .94 can be achieved.

ASSEMBLY AND TROUBLESHOOTING

Assembly—Puritan Bennett PMR 2

1. Patient valve assembly:
   a. Insert the diaphragm/leaf valve combination into the valve housing.
   b. Place the conical shaped spacer narrow end down against the diaphragm.
   c. Rotate the valve cap into its threaded seat.
2. Attach the silicone bag to the patient valve assembly.
3. Connect the bag fill valve to the distal end of the resuscitator bag.
4. Connect the oxygen supply tubing to the nipple on the fill valve.
5. Connect the accumulator to the bag by attaching it to the large threaded fitting on the fill valve body.

Troubleshooting

Problems with this bag usually involve incorrect assembly or loose connections. Always test the resuscitator prior to use to ensure that it functions properly. Missing valves or pieces may cause it to operate improperly.

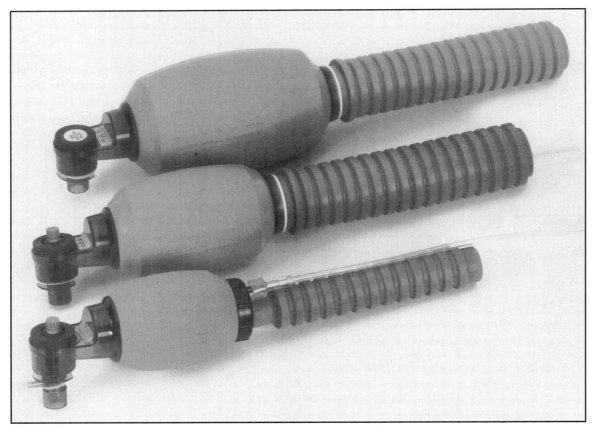

Figure 4-37 *A photograph of the PMR 2 manual resuscitator (Adult, Pediatric, Infant). (Courtesy Puritan Bennett Corporation, Lenexa, KS)*

POSITIVE END EXPIRATORY PRESSURE VALVES WITH MANUAL RESUSCITATORS

Positive End Expiratory Pressure (PEEP) may be needed to improve the oxygenation of critically ill patients. When these patients are ventilated manually, PEEP must be provided to maintain the patient's Functional Residual Capacity (FRC). To facilitate this, there are several PEEP valves that may be attached to the manual resuscitator's exhalation port.

These valves operate using spring tension and a diaphragm to adjust the PEEP level or by using a metal disk and a magnet. In both designs, resistance is created during exhalation creating positive pressure in the lungs. At a set pressure (adjustable by the operator), the valve closes, retaining that amount of pressure in the lungs. Figure 4-38 shows a PEEP valve attached to a manual resuscitator. Rotation of the valve will cause an increase or decrease in PEEP levels. PEEP pressures should be verified and monitored during use by using a manometer attached to the exhalation port.

DISPOSABLE, SELF-INFLATING MANUAL RESUSCITATORS

Disposable, self-inflating manual resuscitators have been available since 1985. Disposable resuscitators are effective, inexpensive, and reduce the threat of transmitting communicable diseases.

There are a variety of disposable self-inflating resuscitators available today. Their performance varies from one type to the next. Since function and assembly of most disposable resuscitators are nearly the same, only two will be discussed in this text.

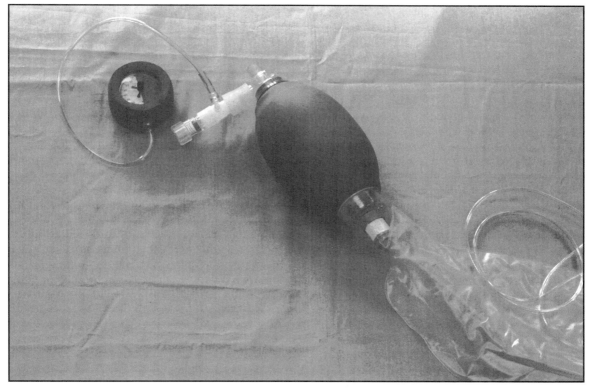

Figure 4-38 *A PEEP valve attached to the exhalation port of a manual resuscitator.*

BagEasy

The BagEasy resuscitator, manufactured by Respironics, Inc., is unique in that it is designed with a reservoir bag between the bag and the patient valve (Figure 4-39). This reservoir cannot be removed from the resuscitation bag. The bag delivers an F_IO_2 between .52 and .93 depending upon oxygen flow rate.

ASSEMBLY AND TROUBLESHOOTING

Assembly—Respironics, Inc., BagEasy

1. Attach the valve assembly to the bag.

2. Attach oxygen connecting tube to the oxygen inlet and an oxygen flowmeter.

3. Attach an appropriately sized mask to the patient outlet unless the patient is intubated.

4. Adjust oxygen flow to 8 to 15 liters per minute.

Troubleshooting

Troubleshooting this bag involves problems of improper assembly and loose connections. Careful inspection of the bag prior to use will eliminate many potential problems.

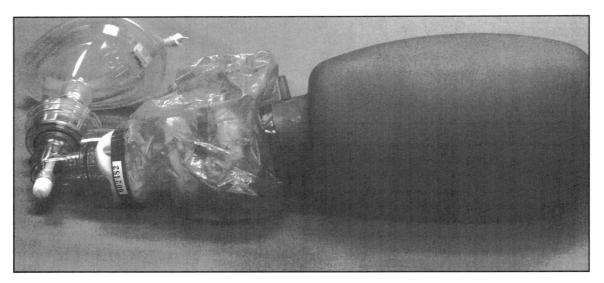

Figure 4-39 *A BagEasy disposable resuscitation bag.*

Pulmanex

The Pulmanex disposable resuscitator is manufactured by Life Design Systems (Figure 4-40). The bag is made from blue plastic and has a reservoir bag that attaches to the inlet of the bag. A duck bill valve is incorporated into the patient valve assembly. The F_IO_2 delivery varies between .38 and .86 depending upon oxygen liter flow and whether the reservoir is attached. Performance with the reservoir varies between .52 and .86.

ASSEMBLY AND TROUBLESHOOTING

Assembly—Pulmanex

1. Attach the reservoir to the inlet of the bag.

2. Ensure that the patient valve assembly is tight and that the duck bill valve functions properly.

3. Connect the oxygen connecting tube to the inlet and an oxygen flowmeter.

4. Attach a mask to the patient connector if the patient is not intubated.

5. Adjust the oxygen flow to 8 to 15 liters per minute.

Troubleshooting

Troubleshooting this bag involves problems of improper assembly and loose connections. Careful inspection of the bag prior to use will eliminate many potential problems.

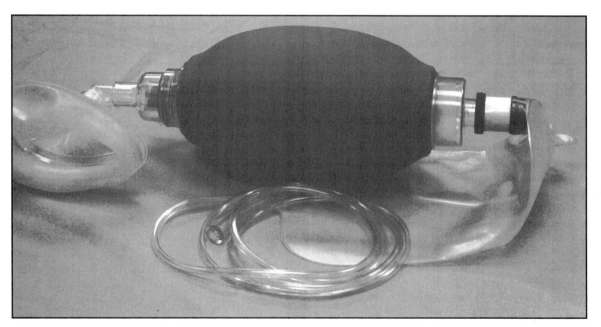

Figure 4-40 *A Pulmanex resuscitation bag.*

SECRETION EVACUATION DEVICES

SUCTION REGULATORS

As discussed earlier in the chapter, *suction regulators* provide a means of reducing the high negative pressures from the supply line to safe physiological levels. Suction regulators operate using a single stage regulator to control the pressure.

Puritan Bennett Suction Regulator

The Puritan Bennett suction regulator will control vacuum levels from 0 (off) to 200 mmHg (Figure 4-41). As discussed earlier, it controls vacuum using a single-stage reducing valve. Figure 4-42 shows a cross section of this regulator.

Note that the vacuum pressure opposes spring tension in much the same way that gas pressure in a cylinder opposes spring tension. Adjustment of the control increases or decreases spring tension, altering the vacuum

ASSEMBLY AND TROUBLESHOOTING

Assembly—Puritan Bennett Suction Regulator

1. Attach the vacuum regulator to a vacuum source using a DISS or quick-connect fitting.

2. Occlude the outlet and adjust the regulator to the desired pressure.

3. If using the regulator for suctioning, attach a drainage trap to the inlet of the regulator to protect the piping system from contamination.

Troubleshooting

Troubleshooting primarily consists of checking for leaks (connection to the vacuum line or suction trap). Ensure that all connections are tight. If the regulator fails to operate properly, have it serviced by a qualified biomedical repair center.

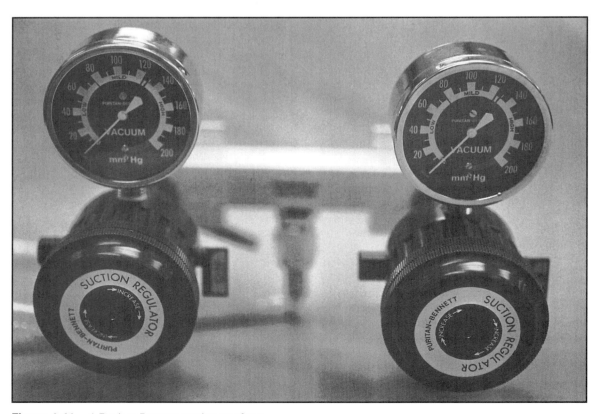

Figure 4-41 *A Puritan Bennett suction regulator.*

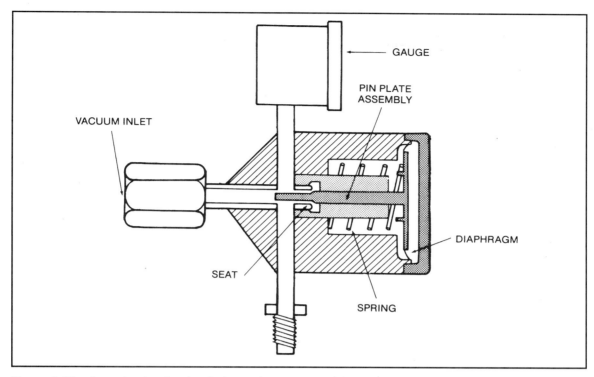

Figure 4-42 *A cross section showing the internal components of the Puritan Bennett suction regulator.*

level. Since the gauge is exposed to the same vacuum level at the outlet, the gauge measures the applied vacuum level.

In addition to the vacuum adjustment control, a safety lock on the side of the regulator prevents the accidental alteration of vacuum level when locked.

Ohmeda Surgical/Free-Flow

The Ohmeda Surgical/Free-Flow vacuum regulator is capable of regulating vacuum levels from 0 (off) to 200 mmHg (Figure 4-43). The regulator operates in a way similar to the Puritan Bennett regulator, using a single-stage reducing valve.

A mode selector offers the choice of "full vacuum," "vacuum off" and "regulated vacuum." In addition, this regulator incorporates a squamper bar, which regulates the vacuum flow rate as vacuum levels fluctuate. This allows the regulator to provide high flows even if the central vacuum pressure diminishes.

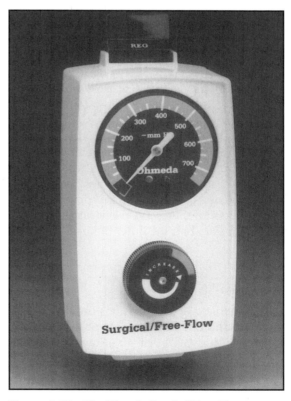

Figure 4-43 *The Ohmeda Surgical/Free-Flow vacuum regulator. (Courtesy of Ohmeda Critical Care, A Division of the BOC Group, Inc., Columbia, MD)*

ASSEMBLY AND TROUBLESHOOTING

Assembly—Ohmeda Surgical Free-Flow

1. Attach the vacuum regulator to a vacuum source using a DISS or quick-connect fitting.

2. Occlude the outlet and adjust the regulator to the desired pressure.

3. If using the regulator for suctioning, attach a drainage trap to the inlet of the regulator to protect the piping system from contamination.

Troubleshooting

Troubleshooting primarily consists of checking for leaks (connection to the vacuum line or suction trap). Ensure that all connections are tight. If the regulator fails to operate properly, have it serviced by a qualified biomedical repair center.

SUCTION CATHETERS

Suctioning a patient is necessary if the patient's cough is not effectively removing pulmonary secretions. Suctioning may be required in the emergency setting when a patient is intubated, in acute care facilities, in long-term care facilities, or at home.

Suction catheters are long, narrow catheters specifically designed to remove secretions from the airway. The designs vary slightly but the goal of efficient secretion removal with minimum trauma is common to all modern catheters. Suction catheters include the whistle tip, Argyle Aeroflow, Coudé tip and the Trach Care.

When using a suction catheter to aspirate an endotracheal tube, or tracheostomy tube, it is important to properly size the suction catheter. Never use a suction catheter that is greater than half the inside diameter of the airway. Use of a larger catheter may result in excessive negative pressures applied to the lungs, causing atelectasis and hypoxemia (Poiseuille's law). Always use a catheter that is smaller than half the inner diameter of the airway.

Whistle Tip

The whistle tip catheter has the tip cut at an angle and one or more side ports above the tip (Figure 4-44). An advantage of this design is that vacuum will be applied through the side ports even if the tip becomes occluded. Also, if the tip becomes lodged against the mucosal wall, the side ports will relieve vacuum levels and minimize tissue trauma.

Argyle Aeroflow

The Argyle Aeroflow catheter incorporates a ring at the tip with multiple side ports above it (Figure 4-45). The ring keeps the catheter separated from the mucosal wall when it is parallel to the airway. If the distal tip becomes occluded, the side ports relieve the vacuum applied at the tip. This type of catheter demonstrates less tissue trauma than other types.

Coudé Tip

The Coudé tip catheter incorporates a special bend at the distal end of the catheter. It is also known as a directional tip catheter (Figure 4-46).

The bend in the catheter allows the practitioner to selectively enter the right or left main stem bronchus by rotating and redirecting the catheter. Although it is not assured that the desired airway will be entered, chances are improved with this design.

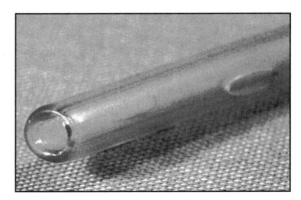

Figure 4-44 *A whistle tip suction catheter. Note the eyes a short distance proximal to the tip of the catheter.*

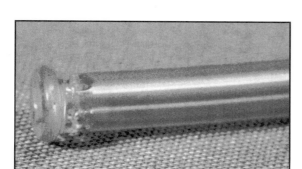

Figure 4-45 *The Argyle Aeroflow catheter. Note the doughnut shaped ring at the tip of the catheter and the multiple eyes for pressure relief.*

Closed Suction Systems

Closed suction systems consist of a control valve, suction catheter, sealed plastic sheath and a modified aerosol T (Figure 4-47). The closed system design allows the catheter to be used multiple times, reducing costs. One would assume that with reuse of the catheter, infection would be a concern. However, this type of catheter has shown no increased risk of infection when compared to other types of catheters.

The sealed plastic sheath allows the practitioner to use the catheter without having to glove up to maintain aseptic technique. However, as when performing all patient care, universal precautions should be taken, which assumes gloving using examination gloves for this procedure.

Additionally, the specialized aerosol T permits suctioning without having to disconnect

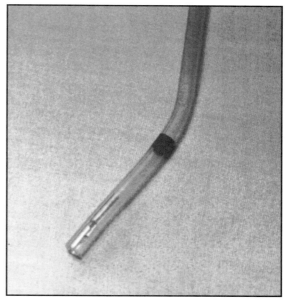

Figure 4-46 *A Coudé tip suction catheter. Note the angled catheter tip.*

the patient from oxygen to mechanical ventilation. This is advantageous because decrease of oxygen saturation can be minimized. Patients tend to desaturate less when suctioned without disconnection from mechanical ventilation or PEEP.

The control valve regulates the application of suction (on or off) and, additionally, incorporates a locking mechanism that is activated by lifting and turning the control valve.

ASSEMBLY AND TROUBLESHOOTING

Assembly—Closed Suction Systems

1. Aseptically open the package and prepare sterile solutions for irrigation as required.

2. Adjust the vacuum level to 80 to 120 mmHg.

3. Glove as required.

4. Connect the catheter to the suction tubing.

5. Suction as required.

Troubleshooting

Troubleshooting is limited to the operation of the suction regulators. Rarely will the catheter itself fail to function. Check all tubing connections to ensure that they are tight.

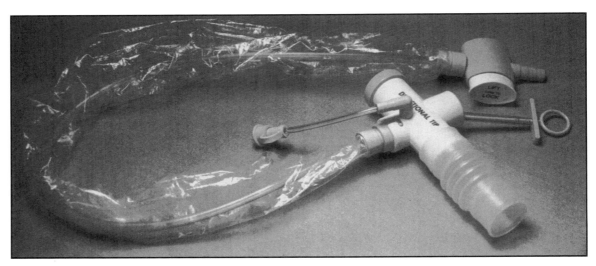

Figure 4-47 *An example of a closed suction system manufactured by Ballard Medical, Inc.*

CLINICAL CORNER

Emergency Resuscitation Equipment

1. You are a respiratory care practitioner in a small rural hospital. You are paged overhead to the emergency room. Upon your arrival, you learn that a patient who is en route via ambulance is in full cardiopulmonary arrest. Explain what equipment you would prepare and how you would organize it for the patient's arrival. Then answer questions (2) through (5) by referring to this patient.

2. The patient described in situation (1) has arrived. He is an elderly male who is being bag mask–ventilated by emergency medical technicians. The patient still has upper and lower dentures in place, and it is obvious that the mask is not sealing well. What should you do when you assume responsibility for the patient's ventilation?

3. You are successfully ventilating the patient, but the emergency room physician asks you to increase the respiratory rate to a rate twice as fast as what you are currently providing. Why does the physician want this increase?

4. You are asked to intubate the patient. Your facility uses Bivona endotracheal tubes. Describe how you would prepare a tube for insertion and how you would correctly secure it after placement.

5. After placing the endotracheal tube, you notice that it has become more difficult to bag the patient. The chest rise is not as great as before, and the patient appears to be doing less well. Explain how you would evaluate the situation and what you could do.

6. You are measuring the cuff pressure on a patient who is on mechanical ventilation and has a disposable tracheostomy tube. Using a mechanical manometer, you find the cuff pressure to be only 5 cmH_2O. You add air to the cuff, and then you note that the pressure gradually falls. What can you do to evaluate and correct the problem?

Self-Assessment Quiz

1. Which type(s) of manual resuscitation valves open in response to a patient's spontaneous effort(s)?
   I. Diaphragm.
   II. Duck bill.
   III. Spring-and-disk.
   IV. Spring-and-ball.
   a. I only

    b. II only

    c. III only

    d. I and II

    e. II and III

2. An increase in work of breathing caused by placement of an artificial airway that is too small is an application of:

    a. Charles' law.

    b. Poiseuille's law.

    c. Boyle's law.

    d. Henry's law.

    e. Bernoulli's principle.

3. Vacuum regulation is accomplished by:

    a. Single-stage regulators.

    b. Bleeding off excessive vacuum.

    c. Needle valves.

    d. Bernoulli's principle.

    e. Solenoid valves.

4. Simple, cuffless airways designed for use with a manual resuscitator or to facilitate suctioning include:

    I. Nasopharyngeal airway.

    II. Oropharyngeal airway.

    III. Endotracheal tube.

    IV. Esophageal Obturator Airway.

    a. I

    b. I and II

    c. II and III

    d. III and IV

5. Airway(s) that relieve laryngeal obstruction include:

    I. Nasopharyngeal airway.

    II. Oropharyngeal airway.

    III. Endotracheal tube.

    IV. Esophageal Obturator Airway.

    a. I only

    b. III only

    c. IV only

    d. I and II

    e. III and IV

6. Which of the following airways are inserted into the trachea?

    I. Nasopharyngeal airway.

    II. Oropharyngeal airway.

    III. Endotracheal tube.

    IV. Tracheostomy tube.

    a. I only

    b. III only

    c. IV only

    d. I and II

    e. III and IV

7. The marking *Z-79* on an endotracheal tube refers to:

    a. The fact that it was implanted into rabbit tissue to test for toxicity.

    b. The type of material it is made from.

    c. The serial number of the tube.

    d. The ANSI anesthesia subcommittee culture test.

    e. That it may be xenon gas sterilized for 79 minutes.

8. Examples of low-pressure endotracheal tube cuffs include:

    I. Low-pressure, high-volume.

II. Bivona Foam Cuff.

III. Lanz tubes.

a. I only

b. II only

c. III only

d. I and II

e. I, II, and III

9. Tracheal damage caused by endotracheal tube cuffs may be minimized by:

I. Correctly sizing the tube.

II. Maintaining cuff pressures less the 25 cmH$_2$O.

III. Adding only 3 ml more air after the cuff has sealed.

a. I only

b. II only

c. III only

d. I and II

e. I, II, and III

10. A type of tracheostomy tube that allows communication when the cuff is inflated is the:

a. Cuffed tracheostomy tube.

b. Cuffed tracheostomy tube with a disposable inner cannula.

c. Hollinger tube.

d. Communi-Trach.

e. Trach button.

11. A type of tracheostomy tube used for a permanent tracheostomy is the:

a. Cuffed tracheostomy tube.

b. Cuffed tracheostomy tube with a disposable inner cannula.

c. Hollinger tube.

d. Communi-Trach.

e. Fenestrated tube.

12. A device designed to preserve the patency of the stoma and allow weaning from a tracheostomy is the:

a. Cuffed tracheostomy tube.

b. Cuffed tracheostomy tube with a disposable inner cannula.

c. Hollinger tube.

d. Communi-Trach.

e. Trach button.

13. Advantages of disposable self-inflating resuscitation bags over permanent resuscitators include:

I. Cost savings.

II. Infection control.

III. Durability.

IV. Ease of cleaning.

a. I only

b. III only

c. I and II

d. II and III

e. I, II, III, and IV

14. Which of the following suction catheters allows the suctioning of a patient without disconnection from oxygen or ventilation?

a. Whistle tip.

b. Coudé tip.

c. Argyle Aeroflow.

d. Trach Care.

e. Fenestrated tube.

15. The primary purpose of mouth-to-mask resuscitation devices is:

a. Improve effectiveness of CPR efforts.

b. Infection control.

    c. Increase oxygen delivery.

    d. To open the airway.

16. Besides the use of the one-way valve or filter incorporated into the design of mouth-to-mask devices, it is recommended that the practitioner also use:

    a. An oropharyngeal airway.

    b. A bacteria filter.

    c. A nasopharyngeal airway.

    d. A PTL airway.

17. In order for the mouth-to-mask devices to be effective, it is important that the practitioner:

    I. Maintain a tight seal at the mask.

    II. Use good positional techniques to open the airway.

    III. Use both hands.

    IV. Utilize the supplemental oxygen fitting and supplemental oxygen if available.

    a. I

    b. I and II

    c. I, II and III

    d. I, II, III and IV

18. Use of supplemental oxygen through the oxygen enrichment port can increase oxygen delivery when using mouth-to-mask devices to:

    a. 40%.

    b. 50%.

    c. 60%.

    d. 70%.

19. An endotracheal tube cuff with a large surface area:

    I. Applies more pressure to the tracheal wall.

    II. Applies less pressure to the tracheal wall.

    III. Causes increased pressure trauma.

    IV. Causes decreased pressure trauma.

    a. I

    b. I and IV

    c. II

    d. II and IV

20. You are checking a cuff pressure on a patient's endotracheal tube. You deflate the cuff until a small audible leak is detected at the mouth. This technique is termed:

    a. Maximal pressure technique.

    b. Minimum seal technique.

    c. Minimal leak technique.

    d. Minimal occlusion volume.

21. When using a mechanical manometer and a three-way stopcock, the patient's cuff suddenly deflates. A probable cause is:

    a. The valve was turned the wrong way.

    b. There is a leak at the pilot line.

    c. There was too much pressure in the manometer.

    d. The patient coughed.

22. Which of the following combines a mechanical manometer with an inflation bulb?

    a. Mechanical manometer and a three-way stopcock.

    b. A Posey Cufflator.

    c. A DHD Cuff Mate2.

    d. The Puritan Bennett PMR 2.

23. Prior to removal of an Esophageal Gastric Tube Airway (EGTA), which of the following should be performed?

    I. Intubate the patient.

    II. Ensure that the gastric tube is functioning.

    III. Have suction supplies handy.

    IV. Ensure the endotracheal tube cuff is inflated.

a. I
b. I and II
c. I, II and III
d. I, II, III and IV

24. When using the Pharyngealtracheal Airway (PTL airway), you ventilate through the short tube and you don't see any chest rise. Which of the following should you perform?
    I. Ensure that both cuffs are inflated.
    II. Attempt to ventilate through the long tube.
    III. Remove the airway and intubate.
    IV. Continue to ventilate through the short tube.
    a. I
    b. I and II
    c. III
    d. II

25. Which of the following are differences between the Esophageal Obturator Airway (EOA) and the Esophageal Gastric Tube Airway (EGTA)?
    I. The EGTA does not have a blind end on the esophageal tube.
    II. The EOA has holes on the distal end of the esophageal tube.
    III. The EGTA has two ports on the mask.
    IV. The EGTA may be used with a gastric tube.
    a. I
    b. I and II
    c. I, II, and III
    d. I, II, III and IV

26. When using the Passy-Muir valve, the practitioner must:
    a. Inflate the cuff before use.
    b. Deflate the cuff before use.
    c. Connect supplemental oxygen to the valve.
    d. Verify that the cuff pressure is less than 25 cmH$_2$O.

27. When using the Olympic Trach-Talk, you neglect to deflate the patient's cuff. Which of the following will occur?
    a. The patient can inhale but not exhale.
    b. The patient cannot inhale.
    c. The patient will breathe normally.
    d. Coughing will be easier.

28. If an oral airway is too large or too small, which of the following may occur?
    I. The epiglottis may occlude the larynx.
    II. The airway obstruction may not be relieved.
    III. The esophagus may be intubated.
    IV. The cuff may not fit.
    a. I
    b. I and II
    c. I, II, and III
    d. I, II, III and IV

29. When sizing a suction catheter for use in an endotracheal tube, the diameter of the catheter should not exceed what portion of the inner diameter of the endotracheal tube?
    a. 1/3.
    b. 1/2.
    c. 3/4.
    d. 4/5.

30. From auscultating the patient's chest you know more secretions are on the left side than the right side. What suction catheter will improve your chances of aspirating the left side?
    a. Argyle Aeroflow.
    b. Whistle tip.
    c. Coudé tip.
    d. Trach Care.

Selected Bibliography

Barnes, Thomas A., "Oxygen Delivery Performance of Four Adult Resuscitation Bags," *Respiratory Care,* Vol. 27, No. 2, pp. 139–146, 1982.

Barnes, Thomas A., et al., "Oxygen Delivery Performance of Old and New Designs of the Laerdal, Vitalograph, and AMBU Adult Manual Resuscitators," *Respiratory Care,* Vol. 28, No. 9, pp. 1121–1128, 1983.

Barnes, Thomas A., et al., "Evaluation of Five Adult Disposable Operator-Powered Resuscitators," *Respiratory Care,* Vol. 34, No. 4, pp. 254–261, 1989.

Demers, Robert R., "Complications of Endotracheal Suctioning Procedures," *Respiratory Care,* Vol. 27, No. 4, pp. 453–457, 1982.

DHD Diemolding Healthcare Division, *Cuff-Mate2 Owner's Manual*, Canastota, NY.

Finucane, Brendan T., et al., *Principles of Airway Management*, F. A. Davis Company, 1988.

Fitzmaurice, Mary Watson, "Oxygen Delivery Performance of Three Adult Resuscitation Bags," *Respiratory Care,* Vol. 25, No. 9, pp. 928–936, 1980.

Gensia Pharmaceuticals, Inc., *The Intavent Laryngeal Mask Instruction Manual*, San Diego, CA, 1996.

Hess, Dean, "The Effects of Two-Hand versus One-Hand Ventilation of Volumes Delivered during Bag-Valve Ventilation at Various Resistances and Compliances," *Respiratory Care,* Vol. 32, No. 11, pp. 1025–1028, 1987.

Hess, Dean, et al., "Evaluation of Mouth-to-Mask Ventilation Devices," *Respiratory Care,* Vol. 34, No. 3, pp. 191–195, 1989.

Hess, Dean, et al., "Resistance to Flow through the Valves of Mouth-to-Mask Ventilation Devices," *Respiratory Care,* Vol. 38, No. 2, pp. 183–188, 1993.

Johannigman, Jay A., et al., "Oxygen Enrichment of Expired Gas for Mouth-to-Mask Resuscitation," *Respiratory Care,* Vol. 36, No. 2, pp. 99–103, 1991.

Jung, Ralph, et al., "Comparison of Tracheobronchial Suction Catheters in Humans," *Chest,* Vol. 69, No. 2, pp. 179–181.

Kester, Lucy, et al., "Fire in a Pneumatic Percussor" (letter), *Respiratory Care,* Vol. 31, No. 4, pp. 343–345, 1986.

LeBouef, L. Lynn, "Assessment of Eight Adult Manual Resuscitators," *Respiratory Care,* Vol. 25, No. 11, pp. 1136–1142, 1980.

Michael, T. A., et al., "The Esophageal Obturator Airway: A New Device in Emergency Cardiopulmonary Resuscitation," *British Medical Journal,* Vol. 281, pp. 1531–1534, 1980.

Naigow, Diane, et al., "The Effect of Different Endotracheal Suction Procedures on Arterial Blood Gases in a Controlled Experimental Model," *Heart and Lung,* Vol. 6, No. 5, pp. 808–815.

Neff, Thomas, et al., "A New Monitoring Tool—The Ratio of the Tracheostomy Tube Cuff Diameter to the Tracheal Air Column Diameter (C/T Ratio)," *Respiratory Care,* Vol. 28, No. 10, pp. 1287–1290, 1983.

Off, David, et al., "Efficacy of the Minimal Leak Technique, of Cuff Inflation in Maintaining Proper Intracuff Pressure for Patients with Cuffed Artificial Airways," *Respiratory Care,* Vol. 28, No. 9, pp. 1115–1120, 1983.

Puritan Bennett Corporation, *PMR 2 Owner's Manual*, Lenexa, KS.

Ritz, Ray, et al., "Contamination of a Multiple-Use Suction Catheter in a Closed-Circuit System Compared to Contamination of a Disposable, Single-Use Catheter," *Respiratory Care,* Vol. 31, No. 11, pp. 1086–1091, 1986.

Smith, J. P., et al., "The Esophageal Obturator: A Review," *Journal of the American Medical Association,* Vol. 250, pp. 1081–1084, 1983.

White, Gary C., *Basic Clinical Lab Competencies for Respiratory Care: An Integrated Approach*, 2nd Ed., Delmar Publishers, Inc., 1993.

CHAPTER 5

PHYSIOLOGICAL MEASUREMENT AND MONITORING DEVICES

INTRODUCTION

Physiological measurement and monitoring devices are very important in the medical field. Many of these monitors are employed at the bedside and provide instantaneous information about the patient's condition. These devices allow the measurement of physiological parameters to diagnose disease entities, alert practitioners to dangerous physiological changes, and analyze inspired, expired and dissolved gases.

The use of microprocessors has increased in recent years, providing this data nearly instantaneously. Therefore, more rapid and sophisticated monitoring systems have proliferated in the management of critically ill patients. This chapter will focus on measurement principles and how they apply to equipment used today.

OBJECTIVES

After completing this chapter, the student will accomplish the following objectives.

PULMONARY MEASUREMENT DEVICES

- Describe the methods used to measure inspired or expired gas volume and flows including:
  — Volume displacement
  — Body plethysmography
  — Flow measurement

OXYGEN ANALYZERS

- Describe the three physical principles of oxygen analysis and give an example of a specific oxygen analyzer using that principle:
  — Physical
  — Electrical
  — Electrochemical

BLOOD GAS ELECTRODES

- Explain the principle of operation for the following blood gas electrode systems:
  — pH
  — PCO_2 (Severinghaus electrode)
  — PO_2 (Clark electrode)
- Describe the operation of a transcutaneous O_2 and CO_2 electrode.
- Describe the four hemoglobin variants including those that can combine reversibly with oxygen.
- Describe how a pulse oximeter measures oxygen saturation.
- Describe how a CO-oximeter differs from a pulse oximeter.
- Describe the operation of an infrared end tidal CO_2 monitor.
- Describe the colormetric principle of carbon dioxide measurement.

PULMONARY MEASUREMENT DEVICES

Pulmonary measurement devices measure lung volumes and flow rates. Several different principles are used in this measurement. These include volume displacement, body plethysmography and flow measurement. Each will be discussed and examples of these devices will be given.

VOLUME DISPLACEMENT DEVICES

Volume displacement devices rely on the patient's exhaled volume or gas to expand a bellows and move a bell or a piston. The amount of movement (displacement) is proportional to the volume exhaled.

Water Seal Spirometers

Water seal spirometers have been the industry standard for over a decade. The patient's exhaled gas enters a counterweighted bell, displacing it upward. Figure 5-1 illustrates a Collins water seal spirometer. The counterweighted bell moves in proportion to the volume of gas entering the chamber below it. Linear movement of the counterweighted bell may be converted to a volume by multiplying the distance the bell moved by the bell factor (20.73 mL/mm or 41.27 mL/mm). Lined paper is available that is scaled correctly such that the volumes may be read directly from the paper.

The CO_2 absorber takes up the exhaled carbon dioxide, preventing it from being re-breathed during repeated maneuvers. Soda lime is a typical absorbing agent. An indicator turns a violet color when the soda lime needs to be changed.

A *kymograph* (moving pen recorder) turns at a specific speed (32 mm/min, 160 mm/min, and 1,920 mm/min) that allows the measurement of flows as well as volumes. If a patient exhales 3.0 liters in 32 mm while the kymograph is moving at 1,920 mm/min, the expired flow rate is 3 liters per second (there are 60 32-mm intervals in 1,920 mm; therefore, 32 mm = 1 second).

Another type of water seal spirometer is the Stead-Wells water seal spirometer (Figure 5-2). It differs from the Collins spirometer in that it uses a lightweight plastic bell that is not counterweighted. Since the mass of the plastic bell is less than the counterweighted metal bell, it is less susceptible to inertial affects. The Stead-Wells spirometer is more sensitive to subtle flow changes, when compared to the counterweighted spirometer, because of its lower mass and increased frequency response.

Dry Rolling Seal Spirometers

The best way to describe a *dry rolling seal spirometer* is to say that it operates like a frictionless piston (Figure 5-3). A volume of gas entering the spirometer causes the piston to be displaced. The piston moves on very low friction bearings, so that motion is not impeded. Lightweight plastic seals seal the walls of the cylinder with the piston, folding or unfolding as the piston moves. Oriented horizontally, mass is not a factor with the dry rolling seal spirometer. Therefore, counterweights are not required.

The recording pen can be directly attached to the piston rod, but more commonly a potentiometer is used instead. As the potentiometer rotates, electrical resistance changes. Therefore a change in resistance is proportional to a change in volume. The output from the potentiometer may be directly connected to an X-Y recorder for Flow-Volume loop recording or digitized by an analog to digital (A/D) conversion card in a microcomputer.

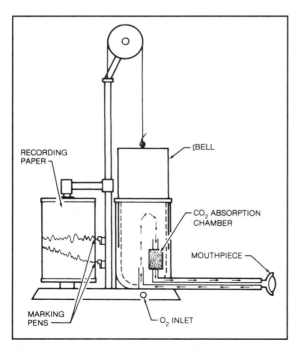

Figure 5-1 *A cross section of a Collins water seal spirometer.*

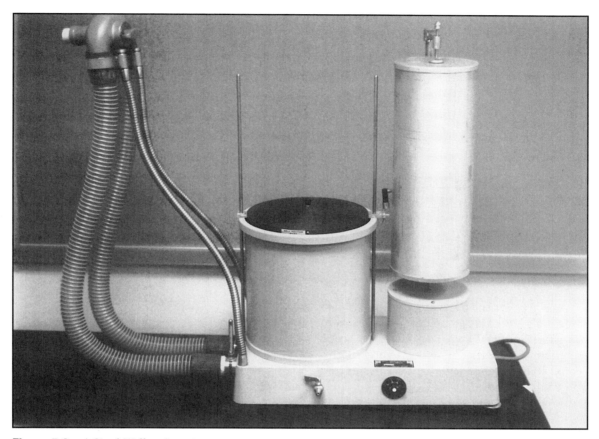

Figure 5-2 *A Stead-Wells spirometer.*

Bellows Spirometers

A bellows also may be used as a volume displacement device. Gas entering the bellows (Figure 5-4) causes it to expand. The bellows expansion is proportional to the change in volume. A pen attached to the bellows records its linear movement. The Vitalograph spirometer, which is an example of a wedge-type bellows spirometer, has the addition of a moving chart table. This allows the measurement of

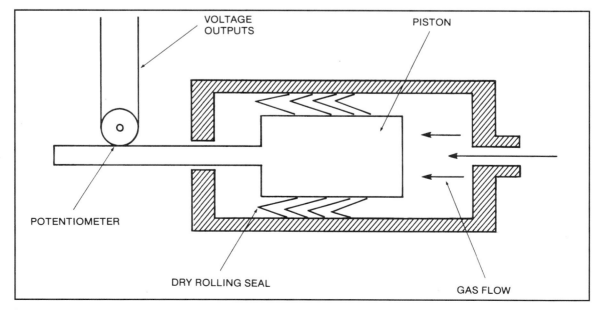

Figure 5-3 *A functional diagram of a dry rolling seal spirometer.*

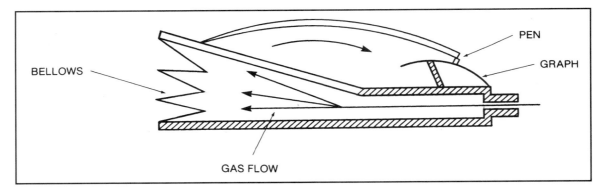

Figure 5-4 *A functional diagram of a bellows spirometer.*

flows as well as volumes. These devices are usually employed as bedside screening tools.

BODY PLETHYSMOGRAPHS

A *body plethysmograph* is a device that relies on Boyle's law to measure thoracic volume changes (Figure 5-5). A body plethysmograph completely encloses the patient in an airtight sealed chamber. As the patient's lungs expand and contract, the volume (V) that they occupy in the box increases and decreases ($P_1 \times V_1 = P_2 \times V_2$). The pressure (P) in the box will also change, providing that the temperature remains constant. By measuring the pressure change in the box, one can calculate the volume change of the thorax. This is accomplished by means of two pressure transducers. One transducer measures the pressure within the box and the other measures mouth pressures when a shutter is closed.

A *pneumotachometer* at the patient's mouth measures exhaled or inhaled gas flow. This pressure versus flow measurement ultimately yields the airway resistance (change in pressure divided by flow).

When the shutter is closed, the patient's airway is occluded. Pressure measurements in the box and at the patient's mouth are made directly, as he or she attempts to breathe. The box volume (pressure) versus mouth pressure measurement provides data that yield the functional residual capacity. The following relationships may be used to calculate the Functional Residual Capacity (FRC).

$$P \times V = P \times V$$
$$P \times V = (P + \Delta P) \times (V + \Delta V)$$
$$V = (P + \Delta P) \times \frac{\Delta V}{\Delta P}$$
$$V = P \times \left(\frac{\Delta V}{\Delta P}\right)$$

The final form of the equation assumes that the change in pressure (ΔP) produced by the patient's inspiratory efforts is small when compared to the atmospheric pressure. The change in volume divided by the change in pressure ($\Delta V/\Delta P$) is the slope observed on an oscilloscope or X-Y tracing. This method reflects the total gas volume within the thorax.

PNEUMOTACHOMETERS

Pneumotachometers are devices that measure gas flow. If volume is obtained, it is obtained indirectly by the following relationship.

$$\text{VOLUME} = \text{FLOW} \times \text{TIME}$$

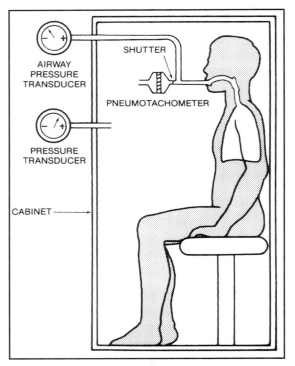

Figure 5-5 *A schematic diagram of a body plethysmograph.*

Time is measured by the computer (sample rate), and is further subdivided into inspiratory and expiratory times. Pneumotachometers operate using different principles. These devices may be employed in free-standing pulmonary function equipment, portable spirometers or incorporated into mechanical ventilators. It is important to understand the principles of operation of the various types of pneumotachometers and any limitations each design might have.

Thermal Anemometer

A thermal anemometer uses a heated element, elements, or a grid positioned in the gas flow (Figure 5-6). The heated element is maintained at a constant temperature by a sensitive thermostat. As gas flows past the element, it is cooled by convection. When the temperature of the element drops, additional current is called for by the thermostat circuit to maintain the constant temperature. Therefore, current flow is proportional to gas flow.

SensorMedics Corporation employs another type of thermal anemometer that uses two elements heated to different temperatures (Figure 5-7). By using two elements in series at different temperatures, gas composition and humidity cannot affect the accuracy of the measurements. Only the rate of gas flow influences the current flow through the device.

Fleisch Pneumotachometer

The Fleisch pneumotachometer relies on a pressure differential to measure flow (Figure 5-8). The heated capillary tubes cause a resistance to gas flowing through the pneumotachometer. The resistance grid is heated to prevent moisture from condensing on the grid, altering the resistance to gas flow. Gas flowing through the device will create a pressure dif-

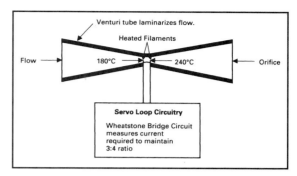

Figure 5-7 *A schematic diagram of the SensorMedics mass flow sensor. (Courtesy of SensorMedics Corporation, Yorba Linda, CA)*

ference before and after the resistance grid (the pressure differential is proportional to flow). A differential pressure transducer is employed to measure the pressure difference. (For a discussion of differential pressure transducers, refer to Chapter 6.) Microprocessors convert the differential pressure to a flow. If sample time is known, volume then is a function of time.

Fleisch pneumotachometers are frequently employed in laboratory type pulmonary function equipment. The output from the differential pressure transducer is easily interfaced with microprocessors to provide accurate data reduction.

Venturi Pneumotachometers

A venturi pneumotachometer incorporates a venturi tube and a differential pressure transducer (Figure 5-9). By placing pressure taps distal to the throat of a venturi and at the venturi throat, it is possible to measure flow. As gas flows through the venturi, the gas ve-

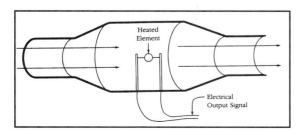

Figure 5-6 *A schematic diagram of a thermal anemometer. (Courtesy of Delmar Publishers, Inc., Madama,* Pulmonary Function Testing and Cardiopulmonary Stress Testing, *1993)*

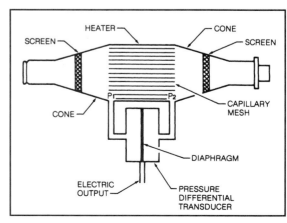

Figure 5-8 *A schematic diagram of a Fleisch pneumotachometer.*

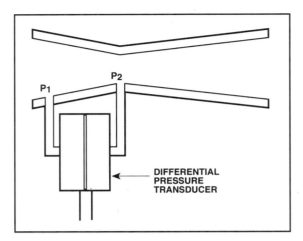

Figure 5-9 *A schematic diagram of a venturi pneumotachometer.*

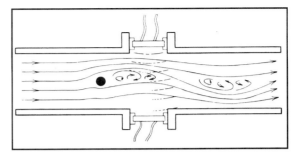

Figure 5-10 *A schematic diagram of a vortex sensor pneumotachometer employing the vortex shedding principle. (Courtesy of Bear Medical Systems, Inc., Riverside, CA)*

locity is a maximum where the cross sectional area is a minimum (refer to Chapter 1 to review a discussion of venturi tubes). At the point of maximum flow, pressure within the tube is at a minimum. Therefore, the difference in pressure between the proximal pressure port and the port at the venturi throat is proportional to the flow of gas through the tube.

The differential pressure transducer converts the pressure difference to an electrical signal. The voltage difference then becomes directly proportional to flow. The data can be displayed as an analog output (meter or digital display), or it can be converted to digital information by a computer's analog to digital conversion card (A/D card).

Vortex Sensor

A vortex sensor is a device that uses the vortex shedding principle to measure flow. The transmission of ultrasonic waves is impeded by turbulent gas flow. In a vortex sensor struts are strategically placed in a smooth walled tube to induce vortices distal to the struts (Figure 5-10). An ultrasonic transducer and receiver are placed into the vortex stream to measure their intensity. An increase in turbulence causes the strength of the ultrasonic energy to diminish. Therefore, the decrease in strength is proportional to the gas flow through the tube.

VANE-TYPE RESPIROMETERS

Wright Respirometer

The Wright respirometer is a portable respirometer that uses rotating vanes and a

gear mechanism to measure exhaled volumes (Figure 5-11 and 5-12). The rotating vane turns a gear mechanism, causing a dial to move and to indicate a change in volume. The gear mechanism resembles a watch. Directional vanes divert the gas flow in only one direction. This is advantageous, because the use of one-way valves is not required for tidal volume and minute volume measurements. These devices are most accurate between 10 and 20 liters per minute. Coaching is important to ensure that the patient will not blow hard into the respirometer, potentially damaging the unit. Flow rates in excess of 300 L/min can damage the delicate rotating vane.

A disadvantage of these respirometers is that inertia acting on the rotating vane may cause some inaccuracy in the measurement. Once an object is in motion, it tends to remain in motion unless acted upon (Newton's first law). This law applies to the rotating vane. Once it is in motion (caused by the gas flow),

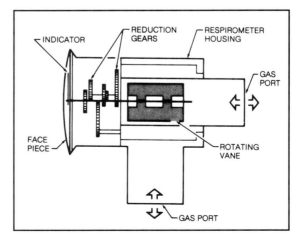

Figure 5-11 *A schematic diagram of a Wright respirometer.*

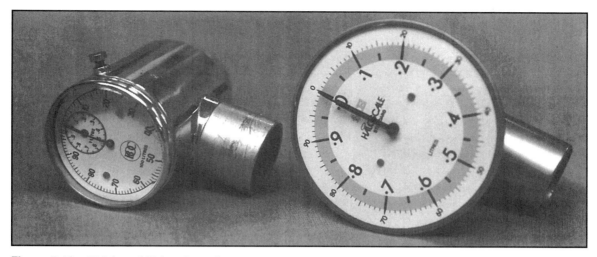

Figure 5-12 *Wright and Haloscale respirometers.*

ASSEMBLY AND TROUBLESHOOTING

Assembly—Wright Respirometer

1. It is recommended that a disposable bacteria filter be attached between the patient's mouthpiece and the respirometer. This will help to prevent contamination of the respirometer as the patient exhales into it.

2. Connect the mouthpiece/bacteria filter assembly to the respirometer inlet. Instruct the patient on how to perform the desired respiratory maneuver (tidal volume or vital capacity).

3. Place nose clips on the patient's nose to ensure that all exhaled gas is directed through the respirometer.

4. Have the patient hold the respirometer and place the mouthpiece into his or her mouth.

5. When measurement is desired, turn the ON/OFF switch on to record the exhaled volume.

Troubleshooting

1. Check all connections for leaks by hand tightening them.

2. If the spirometer fails to operate, verify that the ON/OFF switch is in the ON position.

3. If the spirometer still fails to function properly, send it to an authorized biomedical repair facility.

it tends to remain in motion, even if the flow stops. Therefore, at a high flow rate, actual volumes may be lower than those measured. Inertia also causes a slight lag, since at low flows (early inspiration) there is insufficient energy to rotate the vane.

PEAK FLOWMETERS

A *peak flowmeter* is a type of pneumotachometer that is used at the bedside to measure peak expiratory flow rates. Peak expiatory flows are useful in determining the effectiveness of a bronchodilator and the reversibility of airway obstruction.

A peak flowmeter is schematically represented in Figure 5-13. Exhaled flow displaces the diaphragm (spring loaded), opening a slot for the exhaled gas to escape. As the slot is progressively opened, more flow is required to move the diaphragm. Therefore, linear movement of the diaphragm is proportional to flow. The slot is calibrated and linear movement is read directly as a flow rate.

Other disposable devices are available that utilize a calibrated Thorpe tube to measure ex-

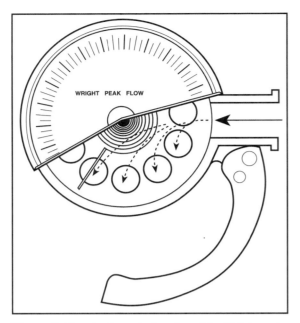

Figure 5-13 *A schematic drawing of the Wright peak flowmeter.*

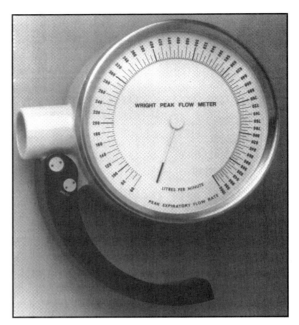

Figure 5-14 *The Wright peak flowmeter. (Courtesy of Delmar Publishers, Inc., Madama,* Pulmonary Function Testing and Cardiopulmonary Stress Testing, *1993)*

haled flows. As the patient exhales forcefully, a ball rises in the tube, which displaces an indicator marker. As the diameter of the Thorpe tube increases, greater flow is required to suspend the ball within the tube. These devices operate in a similar way to the Thorpe tube flowmeter described in Chapter 1.

Wright Peak Flowmeter

The Wright peak flowmeter is a permanent reusable peak flowmeter (Figure 5-14). It is commonly used at the bedside to assess the effectiveness of bronchodilator therapy. This device operates using a spring and a diaphragm. Linear motion of the diaphragm is proportional to the peak expiratory flow.

ASSEMBLY AND TROUBLESHOOTING

Assembly—Wright Peak Flowmeter

1. Attach a mouthpiece to the peak flowmeter inlet.

2. Instruct the patient on how to perform the desired expiratory maneuver.

3. Use nose clips to ensure that all exhaled gas flow is directed through the peak flowmeter.

4. Have the patient exhale forcefully (Forced Vital Capacity) into the peak flowmeter and record the results.

5. Reset the indicator, and if the patient has the pulmonary reserve, take the best of three attempts.

Troubleshooting

Very little can go wrong when using these devices. Problems can arise when the patient is not instructed thoroughly prior to performing the measurement. If the device fails to operate, send it to an authorized biomedical repair facility.

Mini-Wright Peak FlowMeter

The Mini-Wright peak flowmeter is a less expensive version of the Wright peak flowmeter. It is made from molded plastic components while the larger Wright Peak Flowmeter has cast metal parts. The Mini-Wright peak flowmeter operates using a principle similar to the larger peak flowmeter (Figure 5-15). The exhaled gas pushes against a spring loaded diaphragm. Linear motion of the diaphragm is proportional to peak expiratory flow. The Mini-Wright peak flowmeter, being made of molded plastic, is much lighter weight and easier for patients to use and handle.

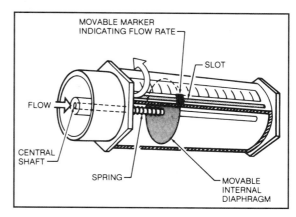

Figure 5-15 *A schematic diagram of the Mini-Wright peak flowmeter.*

ASSEMBLY AND TROUBLESHOOTING

Assembly—Mini-Wright Peak Flowmeter

1. Attach a mouthpiece to the peak flowmeter inlet.

2. Instruct the patient on how to perform the desired expiratory maneuver.

3. Have the patient hold the peak flowmeter, keeping the fingers clear of the indicator track. It is most effectively held by having the patient cradle it in the palm of the hand with the palm facing up.

4. Use nose clips to ensure that all exhaled gas flow is directed through the peak flowmeter.

5. Have the patient exhale forcefully (Forced Vital Capacity) into the peak flowmeter and record the results.

6. Reset the indicator, and if the patient has the pulmonary reserve, take the best of three attempts.

Troubleshooting

1. The most common problem that arises in the use of this device is the patient's fingers obstructing the indicator track. Ensure that the patient keeps his or her fingers clear of the indicator track.

2. Other problems that can occur relate to patient instruction. Be very through when you instruct the patient to perform the forced expiratory maneuver.

3. If the Mini-Wright fails to operate, little can be done at the bedside to repair it. Send it to an authorized biomedical repair facility.

Assess Peak Flowmeter

The Assess peak flowmeter is a disposable single patient use peak flowmeter manufactured by Healthscan Products, Inc. This peak flowmeter operates using a spring-loaded diaphragm, which is oriented vertically (Figure 5-16). Linear motion of the diaphragm is proportional to peak expiratory flow. A single patient use peak flowmeter eliminates the need for processing and cleaning the device between patients. Each patient requiring peak expiratory flow assessment may be given a peak flowmeter for individual use.

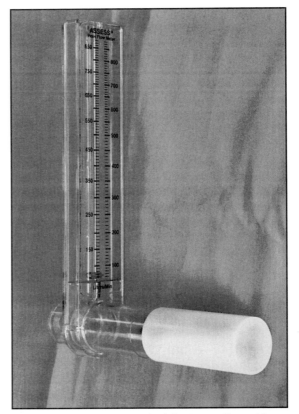

Figure 5-16 *A photograph of the Assess disposable peak flowmeter.*

ASSEMBLY AND TROUBLESHOOTING

Assembly—Assess Peak Flowmeter

1. Place a mouthpiece onto the inlet of the Assess peak flowmeter. (The longer tube should be at the base of the peak flowmeter.)

2. Move the red indicator to the base of the calibrated track.

3. Instruct the patient on the correct expiratory maneuver you wish him or her to perform.

4. Use nose clips so that all exhaled flow is conducted through the peak flowmeter.

5. Have the patient exhale forcefully (Forced Vital Capacity) into the peak flowmeter and record the results.

6. If the patient has sufficient pulmonary reserve, reset the indicator and take the best of three attempts.

Troubleshooting

The primary problems that occur with the use of this device is failure to communicate well during instruction of your patient. Be very thorough when giving instructions on how to use the device and what expiratory maneuver to perform.

If the peak flowmeter fails to operate, replace it with a new one.

OXYGEN ANALYZERS

Oxygen analyzers are used clinically to verify and adjust the F_iO_2. These analyzers employ three main principles of operation: (1) physical, (2) electrical, and (3) electrochemical. The electrochemical analyzers may be further subdivided into galvanic and polarographic types.

PHYSICAL OXYGEN ANALYZER

The physical oxygen analyzer uses the Pauling principle or the *principle of paramagnetism* to measure oxygen concentration. Gases are either paramagnetic (attracted to a magnetic field, aligning with flux lines) or diamagnetic (not aligned with magnetic flux lines). Oxygen is a paramagnetic gas. Therefore, if a magnetic field is present, oxygen will be attracted to it and its molecules will align themselves with the north–south magnetic flux lines.

The physical oxygen analyzer consists of two fixed permanent magnets with a hollow dumbbell filled with nitrogen between them (Figure 5-17). The dumbbell is suspended by a very fine quartz fiber. Attached to the quartz fiber is a mirror. Rotation of the dumbbell/fiber causes the mirror to rotate with the fiber. A light shines its beam onto the mirror, which is then reflected onto a scale on the front of the analyzer. Rotation of the mirror results in a deflection of the reading to a different part of the scale. The scale shows both partial pressure and fractional concentration, so it can be used at altitude, when properly calibrated.

When oxygen is drawn into the sensing cell, it is attracted to the magnetic field and the molecules align with the magnetic field, aligning with the poles. As the magnetic field is altered, the dumbbell rotates with changes in the field intensity. The degree of rotation is proportional to the oxygen concentration (partial pressure).

Disadvantages of this analyzer include: (1) it cannot continuously measure a flowing gas sample; (2) the gas sample must be anhydrous; and (3) it is very delicate and expensive to purchase and repair. Silica gel containing a cobalt chloride indicator is used as a desiccant to remove water vapor from the sample gas. The cobalt chloride indicator shows when the silica gel has been saturated with water vapor by changing color. If the silica gel is blue, the silica gel is still able to absorb water vapor. If it changes to a pink color, it must be replaced. An example of this type of oxygen analyzer is the Beckman D-2.

ELECTRICAL OXYGEN ANALYZER

Another type of oxygen analyzer is one that uses the principle of thermoconductivity to measure oxygen percentage. The principle of thermoconductivity states that a molecule of greater mass has a better ability to conduct heat. Oxygen has a greater mass, and therefore better thermoconductivity, than nitrogen, which is the primary gas in ambient air. Therefore, if more oxygen is present, there is a greater overall heat transfer.

An electrical oxygen analyzer uses four temperature sensitive resistors (thermistors)

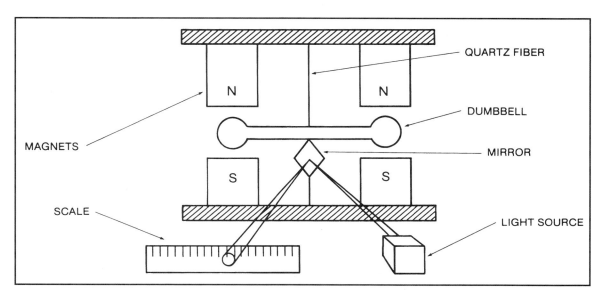

Figure 5-17 *A functional diagram of a physical oxygen analyzer.*

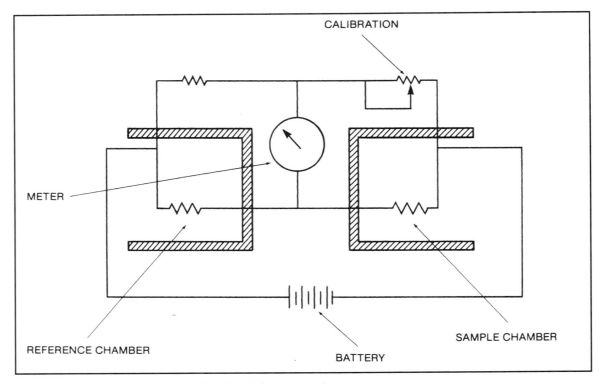

Figure 5-18 *A schematic diagram of an electrical oxygen analyzer.*

arranged into a circuit known as a *Wheatstone bridge* (Figure 5-18). The Wheatstone bridge is a special electrical circuit used to detect small changes of resistance. A small change in the resistance of one limb of the circuit will cause a change in current which may be easily measured.

The electrical oxygen analyzer in Figure 5-18 exposes one limb to ambient air, and the other to the sample gas (containing oxygen). The side exposed to the greater oxygen concentration cools, resulting in an unbalanced bridge state. Therefore, a current change is measured that is proportional to the oxygen concentration (percentage). A disadvantage of this analyzer is that it may only analyze static gas samples (moving samples would result in further cooling). Also, due to the heat and electrical components, these are not suitable for a flammable anesthetic agent environment. An example of this type of analyzer is the OEM.

ELECTROMECHANICAL OXYGEN ANALYZER

Electrochemical oxygen analyzers rely on a chemical reaction to produce a flow of electrons (current). The electrochemical analyzers may be further subdivided into galvanic and polarographic types.

GALVANIC OXYGEN ANALYZERS

The galvanic oxygen analyzer (Figure 5-19) relies on the chemical reaction that takes place when oxygen combines with water and electrons from the negative electrode (cathode) to form hydroxyl ions (OH^-). This is a reduction reaction. The hydroxyl ions migrate to the positive lead electrode (anode). At the lead anode, oxidation of the lead occurs to form PbO_2, free electrons and water.

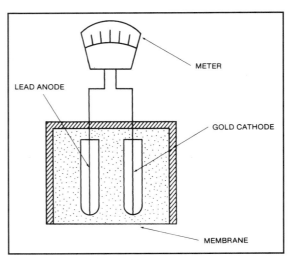

Figure 5-19 *A schematic diagram of a galvanic oxygen analyzer.*

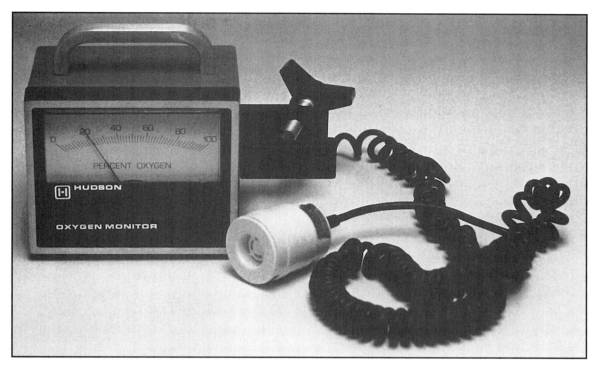

Figure 5-20 *The Hudson galvanic oxygen analyzer.*

$$O_2 + 2H_2O + 4e^- \rightleftharpoons 4OH^- + 2Pb \rightleftharpoons 2H_2O + 2PbO_2 + 4e^-$$

The free electrons flow through a sensitive meter (current meter), which measures the electrical current that is proportional to the partial pressure of oxygen. Although partial pressure is being measured, the analyzer's scale is calibrated in oxygen percentage. The semipermeable membrane ensures that only oxygen can pass through and other gases cannot. An example is the Hudson galvanic oxygen analyzer (Figure 5-20). An advantage of this type of analyzer is that moving gas samples may be analyzed. A disadvantage is that the chemicals in the fuel cell are continuously used, and the cell must be periodically replaced.

Polarographic Oxygen Analyzers

A polarographic analyzer is similar to a galvanic analyzer. The differences lie in the composition of the electrodes and the fact that a battery is used to polarize the system. The battery speeds the reduction reaction; therefore, the response time is faster.

The polarographic oxygen analyzer is shown in Figure 5-21. Oxygen passes through the semipermeable membrane while other gases do not. Electrons from the cathode combine with water and oxygen to form hydroxyl ions (OH⁻) and free electrons.

$$O_2 + 2H_2O + 4e^- \rightleftharpoons 4OH^- \rightleftharpoons 4OH^- + 2Ag \rightleftharpoons 2H_2O + 2AgO + 4e^-$$

The hydroxyl ions migrate to the positive anode, where the silver is reduced to AgO, water and free electrons. The free electrons result in a current flow measured by the current meter. The electrical current changes in proportion to the partial pressure of oxygen. This analyzer measures the partial pressure and displays its reading as an oxygen percentage.

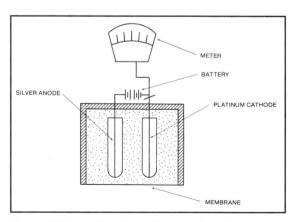

Figure 5-21 *A functional diagram of a polarographic oxygen analyzer.*

An example of this type of analyzer is the Teledyne Ted 60 (Figure 5-22). The advantages and disadvantages are similar to the galvanic analyzers, with the difference being response time (discussed earlier).

Teledyne Ted 60 Oxygen Analyzer

The Teledyne Ted 60 is an example of a polarographic oxygen analyzer (Figure 5-22). As described earlier, this analyzer uses a battery to polarize the electrodes, speeding the reduction reaction. This type of oxygen analyzer is used clinically to measure inspired oxygen concentrations for patient's receiving supplemental oxygen.

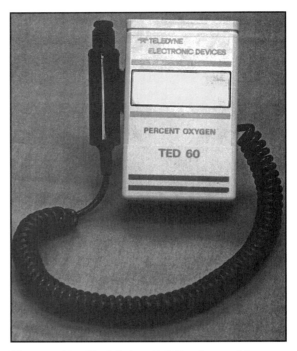

Figure 5-22 *The Teledyne Ted 60 polarographic oxygen analyzer.*

ASSEMBLY AND TROUBLESHOOTING

Assembly—Teledyne Ted 60

1. Open the battery compartment and install a 9-volt battery if the analyzer is not equipped with one. The Ted 60 uses a standard 9-volt transistor radio battery.

2. If you are installing a new polarographic sensor, turn the analyzer on/off switch to the "*" position. Wait for the reading to stabilize, and then place the on-off switch in the ON position.

3. Calibrate the analyzer at room air (21%) and 100% oxygen. The final calibration point should be close to the value you are attempting to verify. For example, if you are attempting to verify 30% oxygen, the last calibration point should be 21%. If you are attempting to verify 80% oxygen, the last calibration point should be 100%.

4. Place the analyzer probe in the desired position to analyze the patient's

inspired oxygen concentration and record the results.

Troubleshooting

When troubleshooting, please follow the suggested troubleshooting algorithm (ALG 5-1).

1. If the reading appears to be significantly different from what you expected, recalibrate the analyzer and measure the oxygen concentration once again.

2. If the analyzer fails to respond to calibration attempts, check the battery and replace it as required.

3. If the battery is good, the fuel cell may be bad. If the fuel cell is disposable, replace it. If the sensor is permanent, replace the electrolyte and re-membrane the sensor.

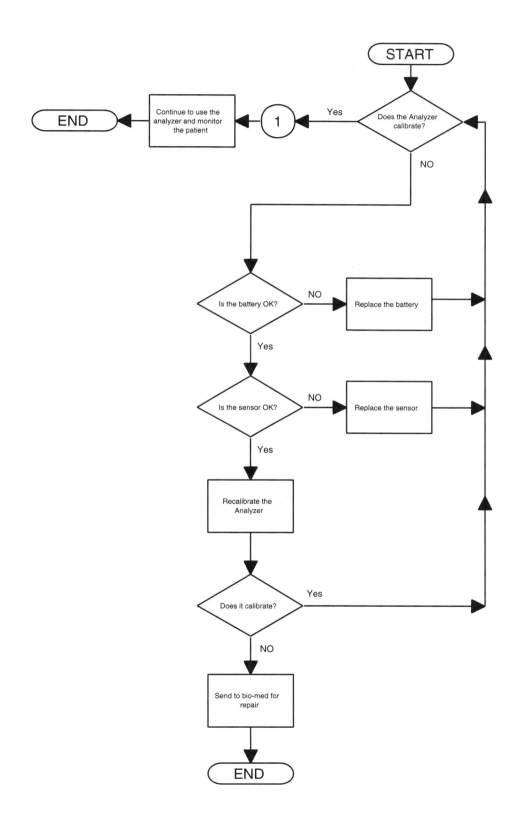

ALG 5-1 *A flowchart for troubleshooting oxygen analyzers.*

BLOOD GAS ELECTRODES

Blood gas analysis has become an essential component in the management of critically ill patients. Over the years blood gas analysis (measurement of oxygen and carbon dioxide tension and pH) has become rapid and reliable. The measurement of blood gases relies on three separate electrode systems, the pH, the PCO_2 and the PO_2.

THE pH SYSTEM

In this text the term "system" is used rather than "electrode" because, to an electrochemist, an electrode is the point at which electrical current enters or leaves the electrochemical cell. The pH system is in reality made up of two electrodes (half-cells) acting together to measure potential differences (voltage) that we term pH. Two electrodes or electrochemical cells make up the pH system: the reference cell and the measuring cell.

Reference Cell (Electrode)

The reference cell's purpose is to provide a constant potential or voltage. Several processes must occur so that the reference potential is constant: (1) the electrochemical reaction must be reversible; (2) the electrochemical reaction must be reproducible (it must be the same each time); and (3) the system must be stable. If all three requirements are met, a consistent voltage will be produced by a cell to serve as a reference. Common reference cells or systems include the calomel and the silver/silver chloride cells.

The calomel reference cell is composed of a metal and metallic paste electrode in contact with a salt solution. Figure 5-23 is an illustration of a calomel reference cell. The base of the electrode is a mercurous chloride paste (calomel) with a porous plug at the bottom. The calomel paste is blended into mercury metal. Finally, a wire conducts electrical current from the cell. The electrode itself is in a salt solution of saturated potassium chloride (KCl). The reaction that drives the cell is as follows:

$$KCL \leftrightarrows K^+ + Cl^-$$
$$Hg \leftrightarrows Hg^+ + e^-$$
$$2Hg^+ + 2Cl^- \leftrightarrows Hg_2Cl_2$$

As can be seen, the dissociation of mercury results in the formation of free electrons, and therefore a potential difference (voltage),

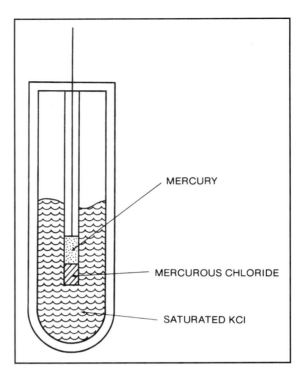

Figure 5-23 *A schematic diagram of a calomel reference electrode.*

which drives the cell. The electrons are conducted by the wire to a galvanometer (sensitive voltmeter), which measures the potential when compared with something else (serving as a reference). The calomel reference cell is the most common "reference electrode" used in clinical blood gas instruments.

The silver/silver chloride cell is depicted in Figure 5-24. It is simpler in design than the calomel reference cell. A silver wire has its end coated with silver chloride. The entire conductor is immersed in a solution of soluble chloride. The reaction that drives the cell is as follows:

$$Ag \leftrightarrows Ag^+ + e^-$$
$$AG^+ + Cl^- \leftrightarrows AgCl$$

The dissociation of silver produces electrons. As with the calomel reference cell, the silver/silver chloride cell produces free electrons creating a potential difference (voltage) that may be compared with something else.

pH Glass

One key component in the pH system is pH glass. The *pH glass* is said to be permeable to hydrogen ions (H^+). The exact method of ion or electrical transfer is not well understood. However, a potential difference (voltage) may be

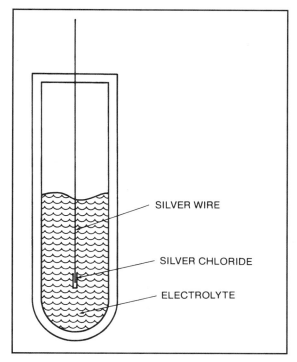

Figure 5-24 *A schematic of a silver/silver chloride reference electrode.*

produced by placing two solutions of differing pH on opposite sides of the glass. This potential difference may be used to determine the pH of an unknown solution.

pH System (or Cell)

One reference electrode and one sample electrode are placed on opposite sides of pH glass to measure the pH of a solution. This complete cell (two reference half-cells combined) is known as a pH cell or system (Figure 5-25).

The reference half-cell is immersed in its KCl bath and provides a constant reference voltage. The measuring half-cell has a known buffer solution on one side of the pH glass and an unknown pH solution (blood) on the other. The KCl bridge serves to complete the electrical contact between the reference half-cell and the measuring half-cell. The potential difference (voltage) between the buffer solution (known pH) and the unknown pH of the blood is proportional to the pH of the blood. The display is usually calibrated in pH units rather than voltage.

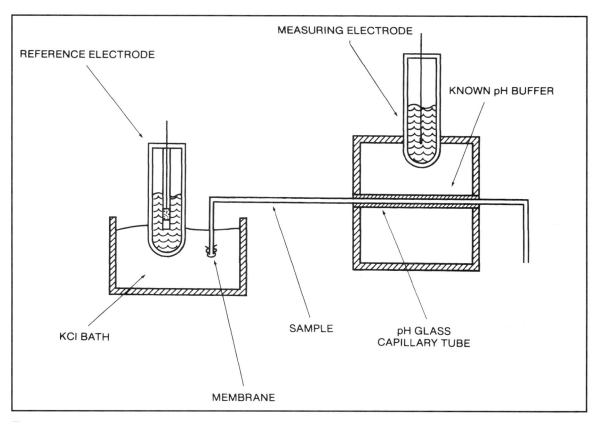

Figure 5-25 *A schematic diagram of the pH system in a blood gas analyzer.*

THE PCO₂ MEASURING SYSTEM

If the reader understands the pH measuring system, the CO_2 system will be easy to understand. This is because the PCO_2 system is a pH system modified to measure PCO_2. The modern PCO_2 system was developed by John Severinghaus in 1958. You may recall from your study of human physiology that the following reaction occurs in the blood.

$$CO_2 + H_2O \rightleftharpoons H_2CO_3 \rightleftharpoons H^+ + HCO_3^-$$

Carbon dioxide combines with water and forms carbonic acid, which dissociates to free hydrogen ions and bicarbonate ions. The PCO_2 cell is a system that takes advantage of this reaction to measure pH (which as you will see, is proportional to PCO_2).

The PCO_2 cell consists of two measuring half-cells (silver/silver chloride), as shown in Figure 5-26. The tip of the electrode has two special coverings. The inner one is a nylon mesh that allows only a thin film of sodium bicarbonate buffer to exist between the pH glass and the membrane. If the layer of buffer is thin, small changes in pH will produce a rapid change in hydrogen ions. The membrane is permeable only to carbon dioxide.

Carbon dioxide diffuses across the membrane from the blood and reacts with the sodium bicarbonate buffer and water to produce hydrogen ions. The hydrogen ions cause a measurable potential (voltage) to be produced between the buffer solution and the pH electrode. The voltage change (potential) is proportional to the partial pressure of dissolved carbon dioxide in the blood.

THE PO₂ MEASURING SYSTEM

The modern PO_2 system was developed by Leland Clark in 1958 (Figure 5-27). Frequently, the PO_2 electrode system is referred to as a *Clark electrode.*

The PO_2 cell is composed of a platinum cathode and silver/silver anode. The tip of the electrode is covered with a membrane that is permeable only to oxygen. Oxygen diffuses from the blood across the membrane and reacts with the potassium hydroxide buffer to drive the following reaction.

$$2O_2 + 2H_2O + 4e^- \rightleftharpoons 4OH^-$$

As you can see, four electrons will be consumed to form 4 hydroxide ions. The platinum cathode provides the electrons to drive the reaction and the hydroxide ions migrate to the silver/silver chloride reference cell (anode). The current flow from the anode to the cathode is measurable, and is proportional to the oxygen tension in the blood.

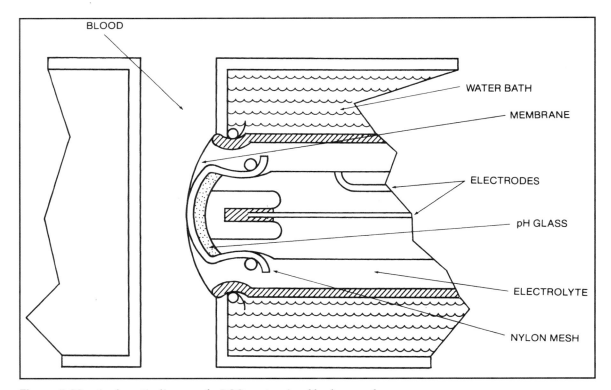

Figure 5-26 *A schematic diagram of a PCO₂ system in a blood gas analyzer.*

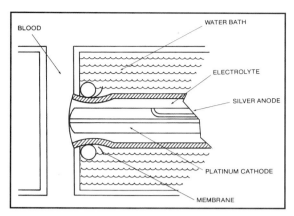

Figure 5-27 *A schematic diagram of a PO$_2$ system in a blood gas analyzer.*

CALIBRATION AND QUALITY CONTROL OF BLOOD GAS SYSTEMS

Life-and-death decisions in the management of critically ill patients are made from information provided by blood gas systems. To ensure clinical accuracy, calibration and quality control of the pH, PO$_2$ and PCO$_2$ systems are essential. *Calibration* is the process of comparing a measuring device (blood gas system) with a known physical standard. Periodic calibration of the blood gas instrument is one important part of ensuring clinical accuracy. *Quality control* is the application of statistical analysis with standardized control samples. Random testing is used to identify random errors that may affect clinical accuracy. A comprehensive calibration and quality control program will ensure that a blood gas instrument is accurate and that gross errors will not jeopardize patient safety.

Calibration

Blood gas instrument calibration involves the use of precision gases with concentrations known to within ±.05% and known buffer solutions. Gas mixtures (O$_2$, CO$_2$ and N$_2$) are used to calibrate the PO$_2$ and PCO$_2$ systems and buffer solutions are used to calibrate the pH system. To use the precision gases, the barometric pressure at the instrument must be known. Most laboratories have a mercury barometer to measure the barometric pressure. In some locations in the United States, barometric pressures can vary significantly with the passage of frontal weather systems. It is therefore important to check the barometric pressure frequently when weather changes are observed.

To determine the expected calibration readings for the PO$_2$ and PCO$_2$ systems, Dalton's law of partial pressures must be applied.

Example: Given the following gas mixture and barometric pressure, determine the calibration points for PO$_2$ and PCO$_2$.

Calibration Gas Mixture: 5% oxygen, 20% carbon dioxide, balance nitrogen

Barometric Pressure: 745 mmHg

Step 1: Since the blood gas instrument is at body temperature (37°C) and physiological solutions are being measured, water vapor pressure must be accounted for. The calibration gases are humidified with water creating a fourth gas (PH$_2$O), or water vapor. Subtract the water vapor pressure from the barometric pressure.

$$\begin{array}{r} 745 \text{ mmHg} \\ - \ 47 \text{ mmHg} \\ \hline 698 \text{ mmHg} \end{array}$$

Step 2: Apply Dalton's law using the corrected barometric pressure.

$$\begin{aligned} \text{O}_2 \ .05 \times 698 \text{ mmHg} &= \ 34.9 \text{ mmHg} \\ \text{CO}_2 \ .20 \times 698 \text{ mmHg} &= 139.6 \text{ mmHg} \\ \text{N}_2 \ .75 \times 698 \text{ mmHg} &= 523.5 \text{ mmHg} \end{aligned}$$

Since nitrogen is not measured, the value may be ignored. The values for PO$_2$ and PCO$_2$ are 34.9 mmHg and 139.6 mmHg, respectively.

Modern blood gas instruments will introduce a known buffer solution and the gases simultaneously to calibrate the instrument. Knowing the pH of the buffer and the calibration points for PO$_2$ and PCO$_2$, the instrument can be accurately calibrated to these known physical standards.

Both a high calibration and a low calibration are used to calibrate blood gas instruments. The difference between the two points is the gas concentrations and the buffer solutions used. Two common calibration points are listed below for one instrument manufacturer.

High Calibration		*Low Calibration*	
pH	6.840	pH	7.384
PCO$_2$	5%	PCO$_2$	12%
PO$_2$	0%	PO$_2$	10%

By calibrating at the high and low points of the physiological normals expected, the accuracy of the instrument between the two points is assured.

Quality Control

A quality control program involves random sampling of known solutions and statistical analysis to identify analytical variations that may impact the accuracy of a clinical instrument. The purpose of a quality control program is to differentiate between random analytical errors or variation and systematic, technical errors or variation. Quality controls are run following calibration and randomly with patient specimens according to the instrument manufacturer's approved quality control schedule.

Reference materials are manufactured by the blood gas instrument manufacturers and other companies for the purpose of quality control. The majority of these materials are aqueous solutions of a known pH with known partial pressures of dissolved gases (O_2 and CO_2). These materials are produced under very strict standards to ensure their accuracy and reproducibility in the clinical setting. Most companies manufacture aqueous solutions with different pH values and gas concentrations. Most manufacture three levels (different mixtures), ensuring that the instrument is tested over a wide physiological range of values. Some laboratories also employ tonometry of whole blood samples in their quality control programs.

Tonometry is the rapid equilibration of known gas samples with whole blood samples. An instrument known as a tonometer rapidly mixes a known gas mixture with whole blood until the gases are dissolved in the plasma. If the barometric pressure is known, and the gas mixture is also known, expected results may be calculated in a way similar to that described in the calibration section.

Statistical Analysis of the Results. As described earlier, statistical analysis plays an important role in a quality control program. When establishing a quality control program one must: (1) establish the allowable limits for variation, due to random analytical error; (2) evaluate all laboratory control data using those established limits; and (3) take corrective action in the event the limits are exceeded.

The limits for variation are established using the Gaussian distribution. The standard deviation is a measure of the distribution of values around the mean. The acceptable limits are established using plus and minus two standard deviations from the mean (± 2 SD). Variations due only to random analytical error will follow a Gaussian distribution; other

kinds of error will not. The ± 2SD confidence limits are the cutoff between random analytical errors versus mistakes in technique or systematic errors. If a control's value is less than ± 2SD from the established mean, then there is at least a 5% chance that a random error was the cause. If a control's value is greater than ± 2SD from the mean, there is less than a 5% chance of random analytical error being the cause. Therefore, there is a greater chance of technical or systematic error causing the deviation, and the result is out of control. The following example will illustrate how to calculate the mean and standard deviation given a set of data. The set of data represents 10 replicate assays of the same quality control sample. Normally at least 30 data points, collected over a period of time, are needed to establish the mean and standard deviation for a given lot number of quality control materials.

Number	Result (PCO_2)
1	20.4
2	21.6
3	19.8
4	20.8
5	20.2
6	20.4
7	21.0
8	20.8
9	20.5
10	20.6

$$\text{Mean} = \frac{\Sigma x}{n} = \frac{206.1}{10} = 20.61$$

The mean is the arithmetic average of the results. To find the mean, add all of the results and divide the sum (x) by the number of results (n). The standard deviation is found using the following formula.

$$SD = \sqrt{\frac{\Sigma(X_1 - X)^2}{n-1}}$$

To calculate the standard deviation (SD), one must first find the mean and then find the difference between each result and the mean. The sum of the differences is then squared and divided by the number of results (n) minus one. The square root of this number then becomes the standard deviation. To compute the standard deviation, it is convenient to work in columns as illustrated in the following example.

Number	Result	Mean	Difference	(Difference)²
1	20.4	20.61	-.21	.0441
2	21.6	20.61	.99	.9801
3	19.8	20.61	-.81	.6561
4	20.8	20.61	.19	.0361
5	20.2	20.61	-.41	.1681
6	20.4	20.61	-.21	.0441
7	21.0	20.61	.39	.1521
8	20.8	20.61	.19	.0361
9	20.5	20.61	-.11	.0121
10	20.6	20.61	-.01	.0001

The next step is to add all of the differences that were squared.

$$\Sigma \text{ (differences)}^2 = 2.129$$

To complete the calculation of the standard deviation, divide the sum of the differences squared by the number of results minus one and take the square root of this result.

$$SD = \sqrt{\frac{2.129}{9}} = .486$$

If ± 2 standard deviations is chosen as the acceptable limit, 95.5% of all values will be contained within these limits.

The standard deviation is used in conjunction with the mean to create a *Levey-Jennings chart* for graphing the quality control results. The sample data set analyzed earlier is shown plotted on a Levey-Jennings chart (Figure 5-28). All results are plotted, indicating their relationship to the mean and whether they fall within the limit of ±2 standard deviations. The Levey-Jennings chart is advantageous for quickly assessing whether a control value falls within the acceptable limits of variation but is used mainly for detecting shifts and trends. Levey-Jennings charts are available for the pH, PO_2 and PCO_2 results at each control level.

Not all quality control results will fall within the limit of limit of ± 2 standard deviations. Of those that do not, 5% may be due to random analytical error. The greatest probability is that they represent either technical or systematic error. These results are out of control. Not only will a single quality control result vary, but as a group, a set of results may display a predictable pattern (known as a *trend* or a *shift*) when compared to the mean.

A trend is six or more results that show an increasing or decreasing pattern (Figure 5-29). A trend may start on one side of the mean and cross over to the other side. Trends may be caused by worn electronic components, protein contamination on the electrodes or deterioration of reagents.

A shift is defined as six or more results falling on the same side of the mean (Figure 5-30). A shift is also an out-of-control result even though the results fall within the limit of ± 2 standard deviations. Shifts may be caused by use of a new standard (new lot number of control materials), electronic component deterioration, use of new reagents, or an incorrect calibration.

Once an out-of-control condition has been recognized, corrective action must be taken. Corrective action may include changing membranes, removing protein contamination, changing reagents, changing electrodes, and recalibration. Once the corrective action has been completed, repeat quality control results should be run to ensure accuracy and reproducibility.

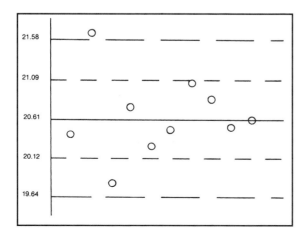

Figure 5-28 *The data points plotted on a Levey-Jennings chart showing the distribution about the mean.*

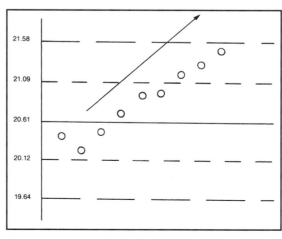

Figure 5-29 *A trend observed on a Levey-Jennings chart.*

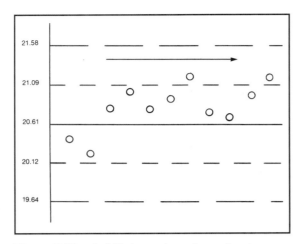

Figure 5-30 *A shift observed on a Levey-Jennings chart.*

TRANSCUTANEOUS ELECTRODES

The clinical measurement of dissolved gases in the arterial blood depends on the ability to draw an arterial blood sample for analysis. The operation of these systems were described in the previous section. In some cases, repeated sampling may be detrimental to the patient. Furthermore, real time monitoring, trending and immediate information regarding the patient's status are not available. Fortunately, a means to quantify dissolved oxygen and carbon dioxide transcutaneously (across the skin) is available. The *transcutaneous* carbon dioxide and oxygen *electrodes* are modifications of their blood gas counterparts. These systems provide immediate information as to the partial pressures of O_2 and CO_2 dissolved in the blood. They are used clinically at the bedside for monitoring and trending the patient's status, especially in the newborn intensive care setting.

TRANSCUTANEOUS PCO₂ ELECTRODE

The transcutaneous PCO_2 electrode is essentially the same as a *Severinghaus electrode* but modified slightly. The electrode incorporates pH glass formed into a flat surface that is perpendicular to the skin surface, separating the measuring and reference electrodes (Figure 5-31). A heater and a thermocouple maintain the electrode at 44°C to increase the circulation to the skin, "arterializing" the blood. The thermocouple near the skin adjusts the heater to maintain a constant skin temperature. The electrode must be moved frequently

to prevent skin burns. Like the Severinghaus blood gas electrode, a semipermeable membrane separates the electrode from the area of measurement (gases diffusing across the skin). An airtight seal around the electrode base prevents ambient air from entering the electrode, causing erroneous readings.

The reaction of carbon dioxide with water to ultimately form hydrogen ions and bicarbonate ions is the same. The H^+ concentration is proportional to the CO_2 concentration. Therefore a change in pH is proportional to the amount of carbon dioxide present.

Calibration

Calibration of transcutaneous PCO_2 monitors is performed in a way similar to that of blood gas electrode systems. Two gases of known CO_2 concentration (typically 5 and 10%) are used to calibrate the instrument. Knowing the barometric pressure, calibration values may be calculated. The known gas samples are introduced and the instrument is calibrated.

TRANSCUTANEOUS PO₂ MEASUREMENT

The transcutaneous PO_2 electrode also bears a strong resemblance to its blood gas counterpart (Figure 5-32). The electrode is a Clark electrode, modified with the addition of thermocouples and a heating element.

The heating element raises the skin temperature to 44°C and the thermocouple maintains it there. The thermocouple near the skin adjusts the heater to maintain a constant skin temperature. The electrode must be moved

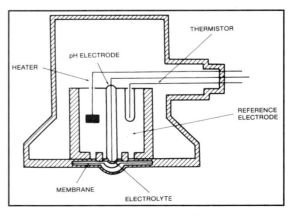

Figure 5-31 *A schematic diagram of a transcutaneous CO_2 electrode. (Courtesy of Novametrix Medical Systems, Wallingford, CT)*

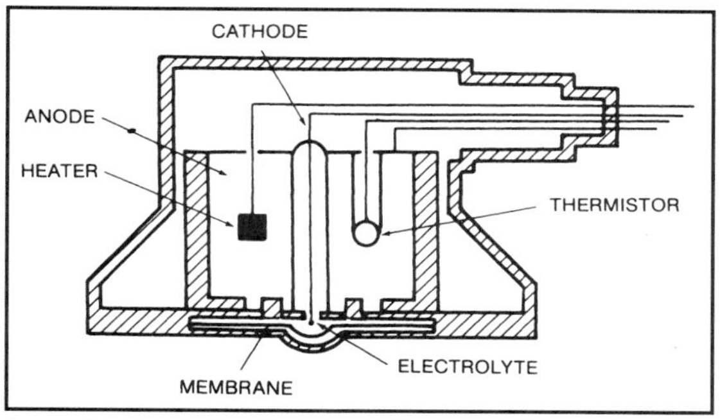

Figure 5-32 *A schematic diagram of a transcutaneous PO₂ electrode. (Courtesy of Novametrix Medical Systems, Wallingford, CT)*

frequently to prevent skin burns. Gases diffuse across the skin surface (circulation is improved with heating) and oxygen diffuses across the membrane. An airtight seal around the electrode base prevents ambient air from falsifying the reading. The oxygen tension is then measured in the same way it is measured in a blood gas analyzer.

The oxygen combines with water to form hydroxide ions, consuming electrons. The electron flow (current) is proportional to the oxygen tension.

Calibration

Like the transcutaneous PCO_2 electrode, the transcutaneous PO_2 electrode must also be calibrated at two points. A zero solution, which contains no oxygen (usually sodium sulfite), is used. A drop is placed on the electrode and the instrument is calibrated at the zero point. The instrument is then calibrated using room air (21% oxygen).

NOVAMETRIX MEDICAL SYSTEMS MODEL 840 PtcO₂/PtcCO₂ MONITOR

Novametrix Medical Systems, Inc. manufactures a transcutaneous $PtcO_2/PtcCO_2$ monitor (Figure 5-33), model 840 VFD (Vacuum Fluorescent Display). This instrument combines both the oxygen and carbon dioxide electrode into one electrode which is attached to the patient's skin. The single electrode monitors both transcutaneous oxygen and carbon dioxide noninvasively. The combined electrode is similar to the individual transcutaneous electrodes discussed earlier, but both have been combined into one electrode with a common heating element.

Controls

The Novametrix 840 VFD monitor uses a vacuum fluorescent display and four soft keys to control the many functions of the monitor. By depressing the appropriate soft key, alarm limits, calibration, temperature selection and other features may be adjusted or entered. The lower portion of the display is reserved for soft key labeling and for adjusting limits when working through the various menus.

Temperature Selection

To operate the monitor, the sensor temperature must be adjusted to the desired temperature. For monitoring $PtcO_2/PtcCO_2$ the recommended temperature setting for both adults and neonates is 44°C. To adjust the temperature, depress the Temp soft key in the main menu. The set temperature is displayed in the upper left portion of the display. The temperature may be adjusted up or down, by depressing the appropriate soft key (Up or Down Arrow). Once the desired set temperature is displayed, press the Main Menu key to exit the temperature menu.

Calibration

The 840 VFD monitor is calibrated by using the Model 989 Portable Gas Calibrator. To calibrate the monitor, connect the model 898 Portable Gas Calibrator to the AUTOCAL connector on the front panel of the monitor.

Once the sensor has reached the desired operating temperature, lift the black sensor port cover away from the calibrator to expose the calibration chamber. Place the sensor into the calibration chamber and release the cover.

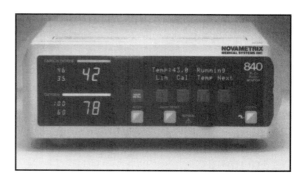

Figure 5-33 *The Novametrix Model 840 PtcO₂/PtcCO₂ Monitor. (Courtesy of Novametrix Medical Systems, Wallingford, CT)*

Make certain that the sensor fits tightly into the calibration chamber.

From the Main Menu, depress the Cal soft key. Depress the Start soft key from the calibration submenu. Verify the correct calibration values by referring to the precision gas calibration chart. During low calibration (approximately 2 minutes), an asterisk will flash on the display panel. Once calibration is complete, the monitor will display the calibration value, beep and automatically begin the high point calibration. A similar sequence will follow for the high point calibration. Once the sensor has calibrated, "Cal Done—Press Run" will be shown on the display. By depressing the RUN soft key, the monitor will return to the Main Menu. With each calibration, the site timer alarm will be reset to zero and will begin timing unless it is disabled.

Limits

The high and low alarm limits can be adjusted on the 840 VFD by depressing the LIM soft key from the main menu. Limits may not be adjusted any closer than 5 mmHg from one another. Once the LIM soft key is depressed, "O_2 Low Limit" will be displayed. The value may be adjusted by depressing the Up/Down Arrow soft key until the desired value is reached. Depressing the Next soft key advances the limit adjustment to the "High Limit" parameter.

Once the oxygen limits are set, depress the Next soft key to advance to the CO_2 Low and High limits. Adjust the CO_2 limits by using the Up/Down Arrow soft keys and the Next soft key to advance to the next limit.

Once all limits are adjusted, depress the Main Menu Key to capture the settings and return to the main menu. The new settings will be displayed to the left of the current $PtcO_2$ and $PtcCO_2$ displays. If the current value exceeds the set limits for more than 30 seconds, and audio and visual alert will sound.

Sensor Site Timer

The 840 VFD monitor has a built-in timer to alert the practitioner of the need to change the site of the transcutaneous electrode. Since the electrode is heated to enhance arterialization of the skin, prolonged exposure to one site may result in burns. The risk of a burn is dependent upon the temperature of the sensor and the length of time the sensor has been applied. Since the recommended temperature for monitoring $PtcO_2$ and $PtcCO_2$ is 44°C, it is recommended that the site be changed every 2 to 4 hours.

To set the site timer, while in the main menu press Next. Depress the Timer soft key. The current Set time may be increased, or decreased, in 0.5 hour increments by depressing the Up/Down Arrow soft keys until the desired time is reached. Depress the Prev soft key to capture the value and return to the main menu.

Two Minute Silence

The Two Minute Silence button will disable the audio alarm for two minutes after depressing this key. Once two minutes have passed, the alarm will be automatically reactivated.

Audio Off

This key disables the audible alarm. When this key is depressed, only the visual alerts will indicate if displayed values are outside of the set limits.

Audio Volume

The audio volume of the monitor may be adjusted by depressing the Next soft key from the Main Menu. Once in the Next submenu, depress the Vol soft key. The volume may be adjusted up or down by using the Up/Down Arrow soft keys. When the desired level is set, depress the Prev soft key to capture the value and return to the main menu.

Display Brightness

The brightness of the Vacuum Fluorescent Display can be adjusted from the Next submenu. Depress the Next soft key from the Main menu, then depress the Disp soft key. The brightness may be adjusted up or down by depressing the Up/Down Arrow soft keys. When the desired level is reached, depress the Prev soft key to capture the value and return to the main menu.

ASSEMBLY AND TROUBLESHOOTING

Assembly—Novametrix Model 840 (VFD)

1. Connect the O_2/CO_2 sensor to the monitor by pushing the cable connector into the Input connector on the rear of the Model 840 VFD monitor. Make sure the power is turned off.

2. Clean the O_2/CO_2 sensor:
   a. Using the black wrench supplied by the company, remove the old "Novadisk" assembly.
   b. Open a combination O_2/CO_2 sensor "Novadisk" membrane kit.
   c. Moisten a cleaning swab with distilled water or sterile water for irrigation.
   d. Rub the swab back and forth across the face of the sensor 24 times, rotating the swab 90 degrees every sixth time.
   e. Flush the cleaned sensor face with distilled water or sterile water thoroughly to remove any traces of abrasive from the cleaning swab.
   f. Dry the face of the sensor with tissue or gauze. Make certain that the sensor face is dry and free of any debris or abrasive from cleaning.

3. Apply a new membrane:
   a. Open an O_2/CO_2 Sensor Split Membrane kit.
   b. Remove the protective cap from the "Novadisk" assembly by rotating it counterclockwise. Leave the clear plastic cap and blue foam insert in place on the "Novadisk."
   c. Apply several drops of electrolyte onto the membrane inside of the "Novadisk."
   d. Turn the sensor upright and place a few drops of electrolyte onto the sensor face. Make sure that electrolyte completely fills the annulus of the sensor face.
   e. Invert the sensor into the "Novadisk" and tighten it securely by rotating it clockwise. Excess electrolyte will be expelled through a small vent hole.
   f. Wipe the exterior of the sensor with a tissue or gauze.
   g. Remove the protective cap and blue foam insert from the "Novadisk."
   h. Check the membrane for any trapped air. If more than 50% of the surface is covered by air, the sensor must be remembraned.
   i. Recap the sensor with the plastic cap and turn the monitor on. Set the temperature as described earlier and allow one hour for the sensor to stabilize.
   j. Once the sensor has stabilized, calibrate the sensor as described earlier.
   k. Once the monitor has been calibrated, it is now ready for patient use.

4. Apply the sensor to the patient.
   a. The selected site should be well perfused, flat and absent of any bony or fat deposits. Typical locations include the following:
      [1.] Upper chest
      [2.] Abdomen
      [3.] Inner thigh
      [4.] Inner aspect of the arm (adults and pediatrics)
   b. Attach an adhesive ring to the membrane and calibrated sensor, by pressing the self-adhesive ring onto the membrane assembly.
   c. Place a drop of transcutaneous contact gel onto the center of the sensor face. Distilled water may be substituted for the transcutaneous gel.
   d. Thoroughly clean the desired site with an alcohol prep pad. Allow the site to dry before applying the sensor.
   e. Pull the protective facing off of the adhesive ring, exposing the second self-adhesive side.
   f. Firmly press the sensor assembly onto the desired location on the patient's skin. Press around all of the edges of the adhesive disk to

form a complete seal.

g. To help stabilize the sensor, the sensor cable may be taped approximately one sensor assembly diameter away from the sensor head. Alternatively, a small roll of gauze may be used to stabilize the cable by placing it under the cable.

5. Adjust the alarm limits and audio level and adjust the sensor timer as required.

Troubleshooting

1. The sensor readings fluctuate or are significantly different from blood gas results.

   a. The sensor needs to be re-membraned.

   b. The site may need to be changed.

   c. Edema may be present at the sensor site.

   d. Medications may be affecting perfusion (vasopressors).

   e. An air leak is present around the self-adhesive ring.

2. Fault Condition Messages

   a. DELTA .05 TEMP ERROR RECYCLE SYSTEM POWER

      [1.] This error appears when there may be a fault in the sensor or monitor. The monitor will automatically shut down the heater power to the sensor head. To correct this, turn off the monitor and then turn it back on again. If the system operates appropriately, the condition has corrected itself. If the monitor/sensor fails to operate properly, contact authorized service personnel.

   b. HEATER DISABLED RECYCLE SYSTEM POWER

      [1.] This error appears when there may be a fault in the sensor or monitor. The monitor will automatically shut down the heater power to the sensor head. To correct this, turn off the monitor and then turn it back on again. If the system operates appropriately, the condition has corrected itself. If the monitor/sensor fails to operate properly, contact authorized service personnel.

   c. SITE TIMER EXPIRED RECYCLE SYSTEM POWER

      [1.] If the site timer has expired and has not been reset within 10 minutes, the monitor automatically shuts down power to the sensor heater. Change sensor sites and reset the timer.

      [2.] If it is inconvenient to change the site immediately (within 10 minutes), turn the monitor off and then on again. This will reset the monitor.

   d. TEMPERATURE FAILURE! RECYCLE SYSTEM POWER

      [1.] This error appears when there may be a fault in the sensor or monitor. The monitor will automatically shut down the heater power to the sensor head. To correct this, turn off the monitor and then turn it back on again. If the system operates appropriately, the condition has corrected itself. If the monitor/sensor fails to operate properly, contact authorized service personnel.

   e. UNRECOGNIZED PROBE RECYCLE SYSTEM POWER

      [1.] This message appears when a sensor that is not compatible with the model 840 VFD is connected to the monitor. Turn off the power, and replace the sensor with one that is compatible with the monitor.

OXYGEN SATURATION MEASUREMENT

HEMOGLOBIN

Hemoglobin is contained in the red blood cell and is capable of reversibly binding with oxygen. When hemoglobin binds with oxygen, it is termed oxyhemoglobin (HbO_2). When the hemoglobin molecule binds with oxygen forming oxyhemoglobin, it changes color to a bright red or scarlet.

When the hemoglobin molecule is not bound with oxygen, it is termed deoxyhemoglobin. Deoxyhemoglobin is also referred to as reduced hemoglobin (RHb). The term reduced hemoglobin does not imply that electrons have been added to the hemoglobin molecule, but rather that the molecule has not bound with or has released oxygen. Both oxyhemoglobin and deoxyhemoglobin exist in the Fe^{++} state. Deoxyhemoglobin has a darker bluish color when compared to the color of oxyhemoglobin. Since both oxyhemoglobin and deoxyhemoglobin can reversibly bind with oxygen, they are called functional hemoglobin.

Besides oxyhemoglobin and deoxyhemoglobin, there are two other common hemoglobin variants. These variants are carboxyhemoglobin and methemoglobin. These variants cannot combine reversibly with oxygen, and are therefore termed dysfunctional hemoglobin.

Carboxyhemoglobin (COHb) is hemoglobin that is bound to carbon monoxide. Hemoglobin has a strong affinity for carbon monoxide (CO). Its affinity for CO is 200–250 times greater than for oxygen. Once CO binds to and saturates a hemoglobin molecule, oxygen can not be carried on that molecule.

Methemoglobin (MetHb) is oxidized hemoglobin that has oxidized to the Fe^{+++} state. Like COHb, MetHb is not able to bind with oxygen. Oxidation of hemoglobin causes it to change color from red to brown.

Since the majority of oxygen carried in the blood is bound to hemoglobin, measurement of hemoglobin saturation provides useful clinical information. The saturation of hemoglobin is most often expressed as a percentage. Oxygen saturation can be determined two ways, fractional (HbO_2 in proportion to total Hb) or functional (HbO_2 in proportion to functional Hb).

$$Fractional\ SaO_2 = \frac{HbO_2}{RHB + Met\ Hb + COHb + HbO_2} \times 100$$

$$Functional\ SaO_2 = \frac{HbO_2}{RHb + HbO_2} \times 100$$

CO-OXIMETRY

A CO-oximeter is an instrument that is able to measure all hemoglobin variants and therefore determines oxygen saturation as a fraction of the total hemoglobin. A CO-oximeter measures hemoglobin saturation using spectrophotometry.

Each hemoglobin variant has a different absorption spectrum for red and infrared light (Figure 5-34). By using multiple wavelengths, the concentration of each hemoglobin variant may be determined.

At 548 nm, Hb, HbO_2, and HbCO all absorb the same degree of light. Since all three variants absorb the same degree of light at this wave length, it is termed an *isosebestic point*. Any wavelength where two or more variants have the same absorbance is termed an isosebestic point. At 568 nm, HbO_2 and RHb have the same absorbance while HbCO has a greater absorbance. At 581 nm, HbCO and RHb have the same absorbance while HbO_2 has a greater absorbance. By comparing the isosebestic points where two variants have the same absorbance with the third variant, its concentration can be determined. The 548 nm wavelength is used to determine

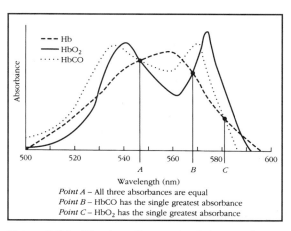

Figure 5-34 *The absorption spectrophotometry for hemoglobin. (Courtesy Delmar Publishers, Inc., Madama*, Pulmonary Function Testing and Cardiopulmonary Stress Testing, 2d Ed. *1998)*

changes in total hemoglobin. Since CO-oximetry measures the fractional saturation, the SaO_2 reported is the HbO_2 in proportion to the total hemoglobin.

A CO-oximeter requires a blood sample to measure the HbO_2 and all of the Hb variants. The red blood cells are hemolyzed (cell membranes are broken) by using chemicals or by bombarding them with ultrasonic waves. This releases the hemoglobin and provides a uniform distribution of hemoglobin in the sample for spectrophotometric analysis.

PULSE OXIMETRY

Pulse oximetry is a non-invasive method of measuring hemoglobin saturation. Being non-invasive, it does not require a blood sample to obtain a result. Furthermore, pulse oximetry may be performed continuously, providing real time information regarding oxygen saturation thus enhancing its usefulness at the bedside.

Like CO-oximetry, pulse oximetry uses spectrophotometry to measure hemoglobin saturation. The pulse oximeter uses two wavelengths of light, one red and one infrared. At 660 nm (red), deoxyhemoglobin (RHb) has an absorbance ten times greater than HbO_2 (Figure 5-35). At 940 nm (infrared), HbO_2 has an absorbance two to three times greater than RHb. Using only two wavelengths of light, only the functional hemoglobin variants may be determined (HbO_2 and RHb).

Pulse oximeters use two Light Emitting Diodes (LEDs) to transmit light through a capillary bed to a silicone photodiode detector. One diode emits light at 660 nm while the other emits light at 940 nm. The ratio of the two absorbencies forms the basis by which oxygen saturation is determined.

$$R = \frac{A_{660}nm}{A_{940}nm}$$

A calibration curve is determined by calculating various R values for different oxygen saturations from 0.00 to 100%. The calculated R values are compared to actual values and a calibration curve is then constructed.

Since the light passes through all tissue (venous, lymphatic, fat, skin, etc.), the pulse oximeter must be able to distinguish between light absorbed by hemoglobin and light absorbed by other tissues. In a capillary bed, the capillaries are subjected to two distinct states, venous (V) during diastole and arterialized

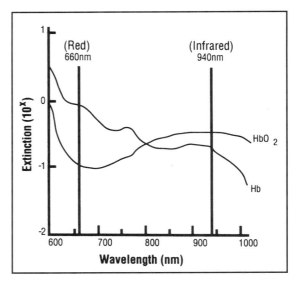

Figure 5-35 *Two-wavelength absorption spectrophotometry for hemoglobin. (Courtesy of Ohmeda Critical Care, a Division of the BOC Group, Inc., Columbia, MD)*

(A) during systole. The light absorbance between these two states varies.

During the venous state (V), the capillaries are the smallest in diameter and are not pulsating. During this state, light absorbance is constant, having a fixed value.

During the arterialized state (A), the vessels expand with blood, changing the absorbance of the tissue. The pulsating action of the capillary bed modulates light absorption (Figure 5-36).

The basis of oxygen saturation accounting for venous and arterialized states now becomes as follows.

$$R = \frac{A_{660}/V_{660}}{A_{940}/V_{940}}$$

This new ratio allows the oximeter to eliminate changes in absorbance by other tissues other than the arterialized blood.

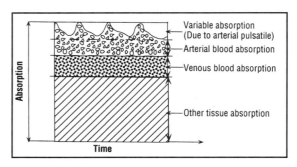

Figure 5-36 *A composite showing signal modulation with diastole and systole. (Courtesy of Ohmeda Critical Care, a Division of the BOC Group, Inc., Columbia, MD)*

Pulse oximetry is heavily dependent upon microprocessor technology. The microprocessor in the oximeter cycles the LEDs on and off at a rate of between 400 and 500 Hz. First the 660 nm LED is activated, then the 940 nm LED is activated and then both are turned off. This rapid cycling allows the instrument to measure the RHb and HbO₂ and compensate for changes in ambient light (when both LEDs are off). The microprocessor also permits the instrument to make rapid measurements so that real time monitoring is possible.

Comparison of Pulse Oximetry with CO-Oximetry

Pulse oximetry measures functional saturation while CO-oximetry measures fractional saturation (%HbO₂ compared to all hemoglobin variants). When comparing the results of pulse oximetry with the values obtained by CO-oximetry one must convert the fractional saturation (CO-oximetry value) to functional saturation in order to compare the results from the two different instruments.

$$\%SaO_2\ func = \left[\frac{\%SaO_2\ frac}{100 - (\%COHb + \%MetHb)}\right] \times 100$$

The percent COHb and Met Hb may be obtained from the CO-oximetry data and then applied in the above equation to convert the fractional saturation to the functional saturation. Once the factional saturation has been converted to functional saturation, the two instruments can be accurately compared with one another.

Pulse Oximetry Sensors

There are several different types of sensors employed in pulse oximetry. All sensors have some things in common. They all have two LEDs and one silicone photodiode. All sensors must transmit light through a capillary bed and receive that light on the opposite side of the capillary bed. Different sensors have been designed for adult, pediatric and neonatal patients (Figure 5-37).

When using a probe that is a wraparound type (usually self-adhesive), it is important to ensure that the LEDs and the silicone photodiode are opposite one another. Misalignment of the photodiode and LEDs can result in poor operation and signal strength or may result in not obtaining a signal at all.

Similarly, when using a finger probe, it is important not to force the finger or digit too far into the probe. This also may result in a misalignment of the LEDs and the photodiode (Figure 5-38).

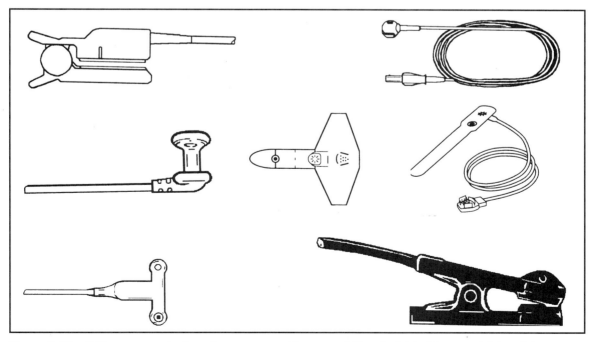

Figure 5-37 *Different types of pulse oximeter sensors. (Courtesy of Ohmeda Critical Care, a Division of the BOC Group, Inc., Columbia, MD)*

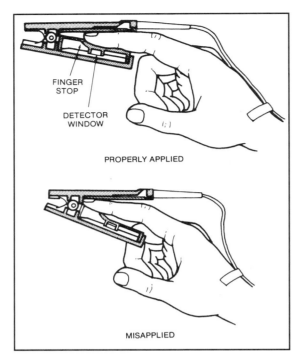

Figure 5-38 *A finger probe for a pulse oximeter misaligned by inserting the finger too far. (Courtesy of Ohmeda Critical Care, a Division of the BOC Group, Inc., Columbia, MD)*

When selecting a sensor site, convenience or access is only one consideration. The site should also be assessed for adequate circulation. Check the desired site for good skin color. Perfusion may be assessed by performing a capillary refill test. Depress the area firmly between your thumb and index finger for a few seconds. Once released, observe for rapid color return. If color does not rapidly return, this may be indicative of poor circulation and therefore the site may not be the best for monitoring.

Limitations of Pulse Oximetry
Sensor Position

As stated earlier, it is important to position the LEDs opposite the photodiode. If there is a significant misalignment, the result may be poor signal quality or the inability to measure saturation. If a sensor does not fit the patient or site well, select a different sensor to optimize LED/photodiode position.

Oxyhemoglobin Dissociation Curve

The oxyhemoglobin dissociation curve is not linear (Figure 5-39). There can be a signifi-

cant change in PaO_2 between a saturation of 85% and 95%. As the patient's PaO_2 falls on the portion of the curve where it plateaus, changes in SpO_2 may not be a good indicator of the patient's pending hypoxemia. Only when the PaO_2 falls far enough to cause significant changes in saturation will the SpO_2 be reflective of the hypoxemia. Therefore, measurements from pulse oximetry may not provide adequate warning of hypoxemia when the saturation and PaO_2 fall on the upper portion of the oxyhemoglobin dissociation curve.

Hemodynamics

The operation of the pulse oximeter depends upon adequate circulation to the site being monitored. Conditions such as shock, inadequate cardiac output, peripheral vasoconstriction and other conditions that affect peripheral perfusion and circulation may affect the accuracy of pulse oximeters. Many of these conditions will be encountered when caring for critically ill patients. Therefore, it is important to understand the patient's hemodynamics and how that may be influencing the accuracy of the pulse oximeter. When in doubt, obtain results from CO-oximetry which is less dependent upon peripheral hemodynamics.

Motion Artifact

With patient motion, the motion may amplify the difference the instrument perceives

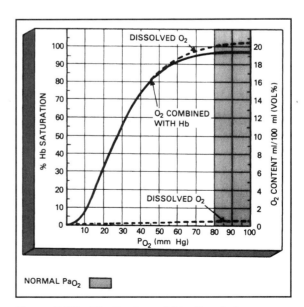

Figure 5-39 *The Oxyhemoglobin dissociation curve. (Courtesy of Delmar Publishers, Inc., Des Jardins, Cardiopulmonary Anatomy and Physiology, 3rd Ed., 1998)*

between the venous and arterialized states. This amplification may result in inaccuracies in both SpO_2 and heart rate measurements. Often motion artifact is more common in pediatric and neonatal patients. The use of sensors that have self-adhesive characteristics can help to reduce motion artifact.

Exogenous Dyes and Nail Polish

Since pulse oximetry relies on spectrophotometry to measure SpO_2 changes, the use of intravenous dyes can create an artifact. Dyes such as Methylene blue, indigo carmine and indocyanine green have similar absorption spectra as deoxyhemoglobin. Therefore, when these dyes are used diagnostically, the performance of the pulse oximeter will be affected. If you are in doubt, obtain arterial blood gases to accurately assess the patient's status.

Nail polish can also act as an additional filter to the light transmission through the capillary bed. If the pulse oximeter shows a poor signal strength or if the values obtained do not match the patient's clinical appearance, select another site or remove the nail polish. Often an ear or a toe may be used if the patient refuses to have the nail polish removed.

Ohmeda 3740 Pulse Oximeter

The Ohmeda 3740 pulse oximeter is one example of many pulse oximeters in clinical use (Figure 5-40). It uses the principle of spectrophotometry (described earlier in this section) to measure SpO_2. The oximeter may be used to monitor adult, pediatric and neonatal patients when employed with the correct sensor probe.

Controls

The Ohmeda 3740 pulse oximeter uses several soft keys (keys located to the right and left of the LCD display) and a large LCD display to operate the many functions of the pulse oximeter. By selecting the appropriate menu and soft key and using the Menu/Enter key, all features of the oximeter may be accessed and utilized. By using a large screen and soft key format, the number of controls have been reduced when compared to earlier models of this oximeter.

The display screen may be set in one of two formats. The "Large Waveform Display" utilizes the majority of the screen to display the plethysmographic wave form of the SpO_2. In this display mode, saturation and heart rate are displayed in smaller numbers when com-

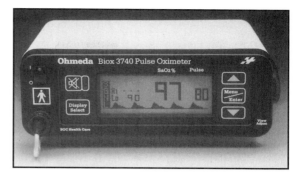

Figure 5-40 *The Ohmeda Model 3740 pulse oximeter. (Courtesy of Ohmeda Critical Care, a Division of the BOC Group, Inc., Columbia, MD)*

pared to the wave form. In the "Large Number Display," the saturation and heart rate are displayed in a large size while the plethysmographic wave form and high and low alarms are smaller in appearance. Both displays have a signal strength indicator to the left of the display. The higher the signal bar illuminates the stronger the signal is. The type of display may be selected by depressing the Display Select key located to the left of the display screen.

Screen Menus

All of the oximeters features and settings appear on three different menu screens. Figure 5-41 summarizes the three main screens.

By depressing the Menu/Enter key, you can scroll from one menu screen to the next. Once you have selected the desired menu screen, you can select items on the screen by depressing the Up/Down Arrow keys until the desired item is selected. Once selected, depressing the Menu/Enter key will enter an item from the menu or allow you to enter a new value.

Alarm Settings

One of the advantages of real time monitoring is that high and low alarms may be set for SpO_2 and for heart rate. The ability to utilize all of the features of this oximeter is dependent upon your ability to scroll through the three main screen menus to find the desired settings, alter them to match your patient's requirements, and then return to the display screen.

High and Low SpO₂ Alarms

The high and low SpO_2 alarms are found on screen 1 of the main menu. Select the menu

Screen 1	Screen 2	Screen 3
PULSE VOLUME	LOW PULSE ALARM	CALIBRATE RECORDER
ALARM VOLUME	HIGH PULSE ALARM	SET TIME hh:mm
LOW SpO$_2$ ALARM	RESPONSE TIME	SET DATE dd/mm/yy
HIGH SpO$_2$ ALARM	TREND OUTPUT	DIAGNOSTIC

Figure 5-41 *The screen display of the Ohmeda Model 3740 pulse oximeter. (Courtesy of Ohmeda Critical Care, a Division of the BOC Group, Inc., Columbia, MD)*

display by depressing the Menu/Enter key. Once screen 1 appears, use the Up/Down Arrow key to move the cursor to the desired alarm setting (high or low alarm). Depress the Menu/Enter key to select that item. By depressing the Up/Down Arrow key, you can adjust the alarm setting to the value that you wish. Once the value is displayed, depress the Menu/Enter key to capture that value. Press the Display key to return the display screen.

High and Low Pulse Alarm

The high and low pulse alarms are found on screen 2 of the main menu. Select the menu display by depressing the Menu/Enter key. Once screen 2 appears, use the Up/Down Arrow key to move the cursor to the desired alarm setting (high or low alarm). Depress the Menu/Enter key to select that item. By de-

pressing the Up/Down Arrow key, you can adjust the alarm setting to the value that you wish. Once the value is displayed, depress the Menu/Enter key to capture that value. Press the Display key to return the display screen.

Pulse and Alarm Volume

The pulse and alarm volumes can be adjusted from screen 1 of the main menu screens. Using the Menu/Enter key, depress it until screen 1 appears. Using the Up/Down Arrow keys, move the cursor to the desired volume (pulse or alarm). Press the Menu/Enter key to select that item from the menu. Using the Up/Down Arrow key, adjust the volume to the desired setting. Press the Menu/Enter key to capture the new value and depress the display screen to return to the display screen.

ASSEMBLY AND TROUBLESHOOTING

Assembly—Ohmeda 3740 Pulse Oximeter

1. Connect the power cord to a 110 volt, 60 Hz electrical outlet.

2. Connect the oximeter probe to the monitor by plugging it into the connection on the rear of the monitor.

3. Turn on the power by depressing power switch to the left of the display screen. Verify that CALIBRATION PASSED SYSTEM OPERATIONAL appears on the display screen. This message will appear after the oximeter passes a self-diagnostic test.

4. Wipe the probe clean with an alcohol

prep pad prior to applying it to the patient.

5. Apply the probe to the patient.

6. Observe for an adequate signal indicated by a good wave form and adequate signal strength. Compare the heart rate to an ECG monitor or count the radial pulse.

7. Set the alarms to the desired values.

Troubleshooting

ALG 5-2 will serve as a useful guide when troubleshooting the various alarm conditions on the model 3740 pulse oximeter.

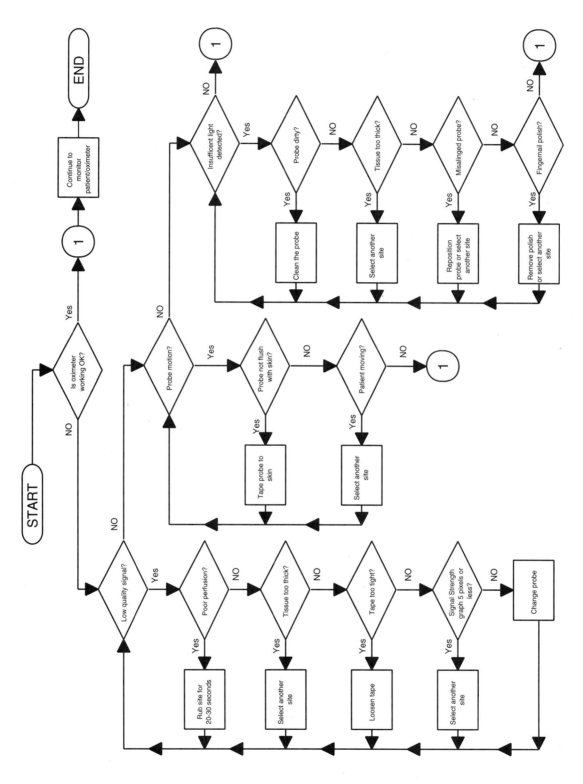

ALG 5-2 *A flowchart to assist in troubleshooting the Ohmeda Model 3740 pulse oximeter.*

Nellcor N-180 Pulse Oximeter

The Nellcor N-180 pulse oximeter is another free-standing pulse oximeter that uses spectrophotometry to determine oxygen saturation (SpO_2). The Nellcor N-180 is a microprocessor controlled monitor that allows real time monitoring of oxygen saturation and heart rate (Figure 5-42). The monitor uses two Light Emitting Diode (LED) displays for heart rate and SpO_2 and LED bar graph for signal strength. The monitor also has built in alarms for high and low SpO_2 and heart rate.

Controls
On/Off Switch

The main power switch is located on the back panel of the monitor. Toggling the switch to the on position delivers power to the monitor. Prior to turning on the power, connect a sensor probe to the sensor connector on the front panel of the monitor.

On/Stdby Switch

The On/Stdby switch turns the monitor on or will place the monitor in standby mode. When turned on, the monitor has full capability. In the standby mode, all displays are inactive and power consumption is minimized (extends battery life when not in use). When the switch is toggled to the on position, the monitor automatically performs a self-diagnostic test. When the test is completed, the monitor displays measurements and the pulse amplitude bar graph indicator rises and falls with each heartbeat.

Control Knob

To the right of the front panel is a large round control knob. Its function is that it changes instrument functions and allows you to adjust alarms setting desired values.

High and Low Sat Buttons

By depressing the appropriate button (High or Low Sat), the alarm setting is displayed in the oxygen saturation LED display. The alarm settings may be changed by depressing the appropriate button (High or Low Sat) and simultaneously rotating the control knob clockwise or counterclockwise to adjust the display to the desired setting. Once the button is released, the new alarm parameter will have been set.

High and Low Rate Buttons

By depressing the appropriate button (High or Low Rate), the alarm setting is displayed in the pulse rate LED display. The alarm settings may be changed by depressing the appropriate button (High or Low Rate) and simultaneously rotating the control knob clockwise or counterclockwise to adjust the display to the desired setting. Once the button is released, the new alarm parameter will have been set.

Alarm Volume

To adjust the audio alarm volume, press the High Sat and Low Sat buttons simultaneously and hold them down. Rotate the control knob clockwise to increase the volume and

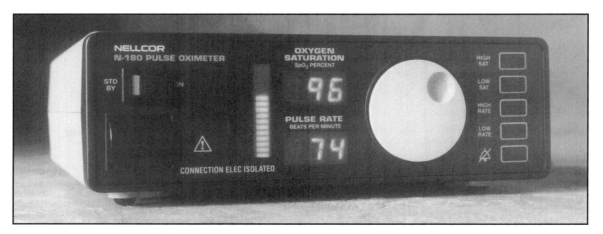

Figure 5-42 *The Nellcor N-180 pulse oximeter. (Photos courtesy Courtesy of Nellcor, Incorporated, Pleasanton, CA)*

counterclockwise to decrease the volume. Once the volume has been adjusted, release the High and Low Sat buttons.

Alarm Silence and Alarm Off

The audio alarm may be temporarily silenced by depressing the Audio Alarm Off button. When depressed the audio alarm will remain off for 60 seconds before it is reactivated. The duration of the alarm silence may be adjusted by holding the Audio Alarm Off button down and rotating the control knob until the desired time interval is displayed in the Oxygen Saturation Display. The time interval may be adjusted between 30 and 120 seconds.

The audio alarm may be disabled by holding down the Audio Alarm Off button and rotating the control knob clockwise until "OFF" appears in the Oxygen Saturation Display.

ASSEMBLY AND TROUBLESHOOTING

Assembly—Nellcor N-180 Pulse Oximeter

1. Connect the power cord to a 115 volt, 60 Hz electrical outlet.

2. Turn the main power switch (back panel of the oximeter) to the "ON" position.

3. Select an appropriate sensor probe and connect it to the oximeter by plugging it into the sensor connector and front panel of the monitor. Close the plastic cover over the sensor plug to lock it into place.

4. Turn the oximeter on by pushing the Stdby/On rocker switch to the "ON" position.

   a. Once turned on, the monitor will perform a self-diagnostic test.

5. Connect the probe to the patient and observe for the signal strength bar to rise and fall with each heartbeat. The pulse tone will also sound with the strength of the heartbeat. The pulse tone volume may be adjusted by rotating the Control Knob clockwise or counterclockwise until the volume is at the desired level.

6. Set the High and Low Sat and High and Low Rate alarms to the desired settings as described earlier.

Troubleshooting

ALG 5-3 will serve as a useful guide when troubleshooting the Nellcor Model N-180 Pulse Oximeter.

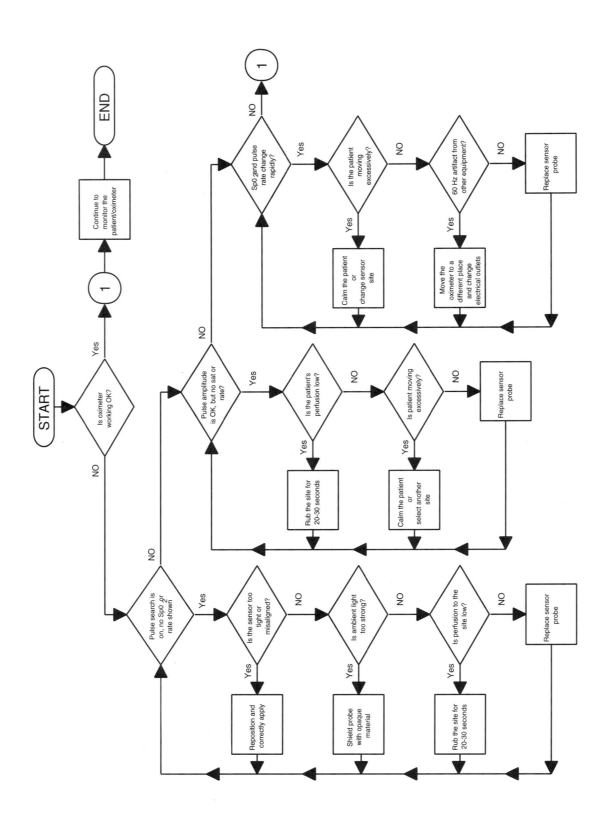

ALG 5-3   *A flowchart for troubleshooting the Nellcor N-180 pulse oximeter.*

Novametrix Oxypleth Pulse Oximeter Model 520A

Novametrix Medical Systems manufactures a pulse oximeter, the Oxypleth Model 520A, that utilizes the principle of spectrophotometry to measure oxygen saturation and heart rate. It is a microprocessor controlled monitor with many features including alarms and the ability to monitor saturation and heart rate continuously (Figure 5-43).

Controls

The Novametrix Oxypleth uses a large Liquid Crystal Display (LCD) and several soft keys to control the many features of the oximeter. The display screen is divided into a main menu (Alert, Trend and Menu) and several submenus. By depressing the soft key directly under the desired selection, the appropriate submenu will appear.

System Menu

By depressing the "Menu" soft key from the main menu, the "System Menu" will be displayed on the main LCD display screen. From the "System Menu," you may adjust audio volumes and display screen brightness and SpO$_2$ averaging times by depressing the appropriate soft keys.

To adjust the Alert Volume, press the "Menu" soft key from the main menu display. Select the "Audio" soft key from the "System Menu" screen display. Press the "Alert" soft key from the "Audio Features" menu. Adjust the volume by pressing the Up/Down Arrow to reach the desired setting. Press "Run" to return to the main menu.

To adjust the "Beep" volume, press the "Menu" soft key from the main menu display. Select the "Audio" soft key from the "System Menu" screen display. Press the "Set Pulse Volume" soft key from the "Audio Features" menu. Adjust the volume by pressing the Up/Down Arrow soft keys until the desired setting is reached. Press the "RUN" soft key to return to the main menu.

To adjust the screen brightness, press the "Menu" soft key from the main menu display. Select the "Lite" soft key from the "System

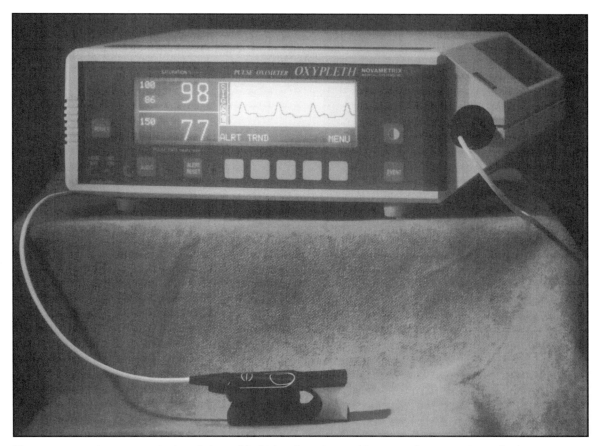

Figure 5-43 *The Novametrix Oxypleth Model 520A pulse oximeter. (Courtesy of Novametrix Medical Systems, Inc., Wallingford, CT)*

Menu" screen display. The "Lite" soft key will switch the background between bright and dim settings. To return to the main menu, press the "RUN" soft key.

Alert Menu

The alert menu allows the operator to adjust the limits for SpO_2 and Pulse rate. Each of these alerts can be adjusted by the user to match the patient's condition and needs.

To set the SpO_2 High or Low limit, press the "Alert" soft key from the main menu. Use the SEL soft key to move the cursor to the desired limit (SpO_2 High or Low limit). Use the Up/Down Arrow soft key to adjust the limit to the desired value. Note that limits may not be set closer than 5 digits of one another. To adjust the High or Low Pulse rate limit, follow the same procedure as described, only use the "SEL" soft key to select the desired Pulse rate

limit. When the limits have been adjusted, press the "Run" soft key to return to the main menu.

Alert Reset and Audio Keys

The "Alert Reset" key located below the numeric displays is used to reset alert conditions that may have corrected themselves. If the probe becomes disconnected from the patient, pressing the "Alert Reset" key will silence the alarms until the probe can be reconnected and the monitor is able to detect appropriate signals from the sensor.

The "Audio" key is used to silence the audio portion of a limit or alarm. To silence the audio portion for two minutes press and release the "Audio" key. To disable the audio alarms, press and hold the "Audio" key until the audio off indicator illuminates.

ASSEMBLY AND TROUBLESHOOTING

Assembly—Novametrix Model 520A

1. Connect the power cord on the rear of the monitor to a 115 volt, 60 Hz electrical outlet.

2. Select an appropriate sensor probe and connect the probe to the SpO_2 Sensor Input connector on the right front of the monitor.

3. Depress the Power key to turn on the monitor. The monitor will perform self-diagnostic checks when the power is turned on.

4. Apply the sensor probe to an appropriate site on the patient and observe the monitor for SpO_2, Pulse Rate and Signal Strength.

5. Adjust the alert limits and audio volumes as described earlier.

Troubleshooting

ALG 5-4 will assist you in troubleshooting the Novametrix Oxypleth Pulse Oximeter.

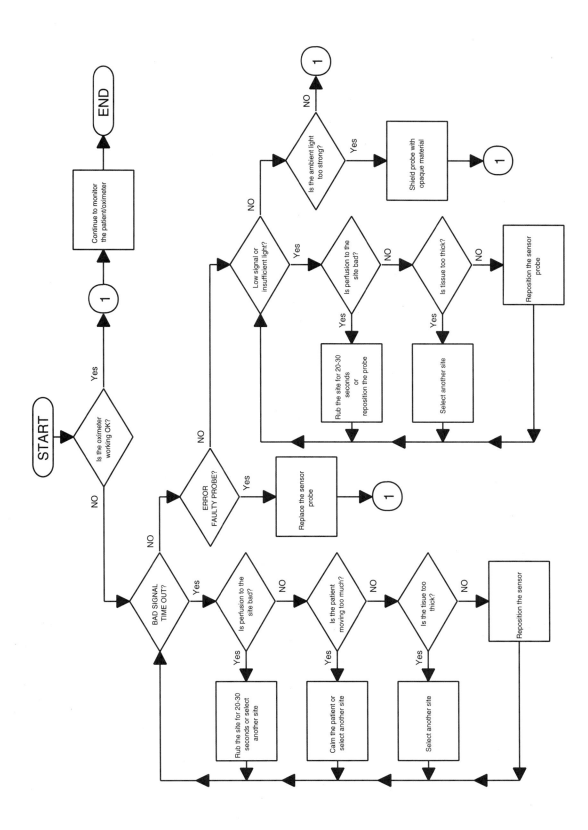

ALG 5-4 *A flowchart for troubleshooting the Novametrix Model 520A pulse oximeter.*

BCI International 3301 Oximeter

BCI International manufacturers a hand-held battery operated portable oximeter (Figure 5-44). Weighing less than one pound, including batteries, it can be easily carried or inserted into a lab jacket pocket making it ideal for "spot checks" or patient transport settings. The oximeter uses the principle of spectrophotometry to measure oxygen saturation and pulse rate. The oximeter may be used with a permanent finger probe or disposable self-adhesive probes for adults, pediatric and infant patients.

Controls and Displays
On/Off keys

The On/Off keys are the only user-activated keys on the oximeter. Depressing the appropriate key turns the oximeter on or off.

Displays

The SpO_2 and Pulse are displayed on an Light Emitting Diode (LED) display. Both are real-time displays.

A pulse strength bar graph indicator is located below the digital displays. The bar graph indicates the signal strength of the site selected for monitoring. To the left of the signal strength bar graph is a Low Battery Indicator. The Low Battery Indicator will illuminate when approximately two hours of battery life is left.

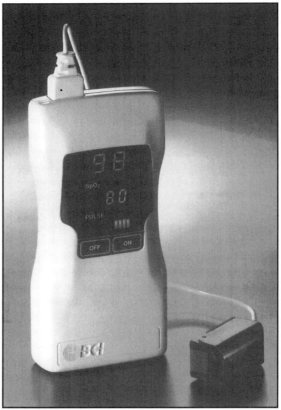

Figure 5-44 *The BCI Model 3301 hand held pulse oximeter. (Courtesy of BCI International, Waukesha, WI)*

ASSEMBLY AND TROUBLESHOOTING

Assembly—BCI Model 3301

1. Open the battery compartment on the rear of the oximeter, and install three "C" size alkaline batteries, following the polarity indicated in the battery compartment. Once the batteries are installed, replace the battery compartment cover.

2. Select an appropriate sensor probe and connect it to the sensor probe connector on the top of the oximeter.

3. Connect the probe to the patient at the selected monitoring site and turn on the oximeter.

4. Observe the bar graph signal display and the SpO_2 and Pulse Rate displays.

Troubleshooting

ALG 5-5 will provide a useful guide when troubleshooting the BCI 3301 Oximeter.

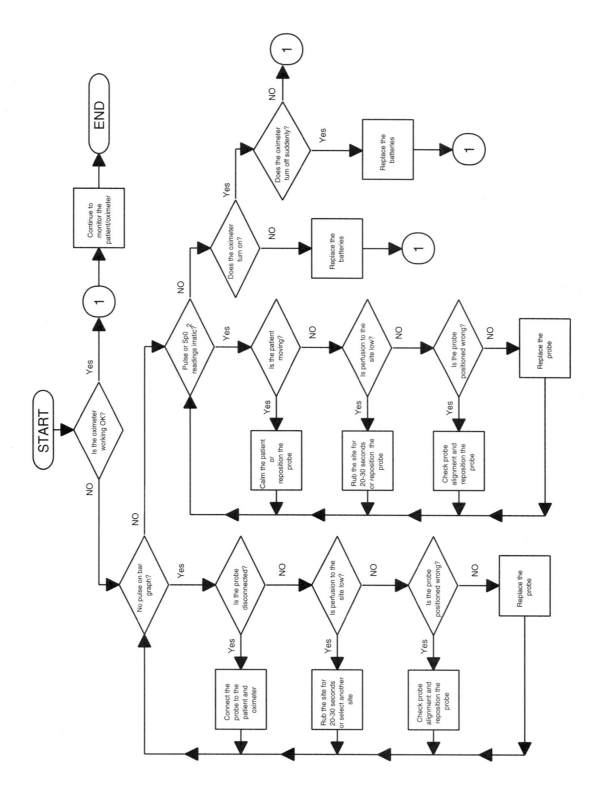

ALG 5-5 *A flowchart for troubleshooting the BCI Model 3301 hand-held pulse oximeter.*

Nonin Model 8500M Pulse Oximeter

Nonin Medical manufacturers a hand-held, battery operated, portable oximeter (Figure 5-45). Weighing only 10 ounces, including batteries, it can be easily carried or inserted into a lab jacket pocket making it ideal for "spot checks" or patient transport settings. The oximeter uses the principle of spectrophotometry to measure oxygen saturation and pulse rate. The oximeter may be used with a permanent finger probe or disposable self-adhesive probes for adults, pediatric and infant patients.

Controls and Displays
On/Off keys

The On/Off keys on the oximeter are marked *1* and *0*. Depressing the appropriate key turns the oximeter on or off.

Display Intensity

By depressing the display intensity button, the intensity of the digital LED displays may be adjusted. The brightness of the display may be altered by using this feature. The display intensity will cycle through the entire intensity range as long as the button is depressed. Once the desired brightness is obtained, release the button.

Perfusion LED Indicator

The perfusion LED indicator will blink with each heartbeat. The indicator has three colors: green, yellow and red. Each color signifies to the operator the condition of the signal strength at the selected monitoring site.

If the indicator is green, the signal strength is good and the SpO_2 and pulse rate are accurate. If the indicator is yellow, the signal is of marginal quality and the operator should consider selecting an alternate site. The data obtained may be acceptable, however, even if the indicator is blinking yellow. If the indicator is red, there is insufficient signal strength for a reliable reading.

SpO_2 and Heart Rate Displays

The SpO_2 and pulse are displayed on Light Emitting Diode (LED) displays. Both are real-time displays.

Battery Low Display

If the numerical displays blink off and on, this is an indicator that the battery power is low and the batteries should be changed.

ASSEMBLY AND TROUBLESHOOTING

Assembly—Nonin Model 8500M

1. Open the battery compartment on the rear of the oximeter, and install six "AA" size alkaline batteries, following the polarity indicated in the battery compartment. Once the batteries are installed, replace the battery compartment cover.

2. Select an appropriate sensor probe and connect it to the sensor probe connector on the top of the oximeter.

3. Connect the probe to the patient at the selected monitoring site and turn on the oximeter.

4. Observe the Perfusion Indicator and the SpO_2 and Pulse Rate displays.

Troubleshooting

ALG 5-6 will provide a useful guide when troubleshooting the Nonin 8500 Oximeter.

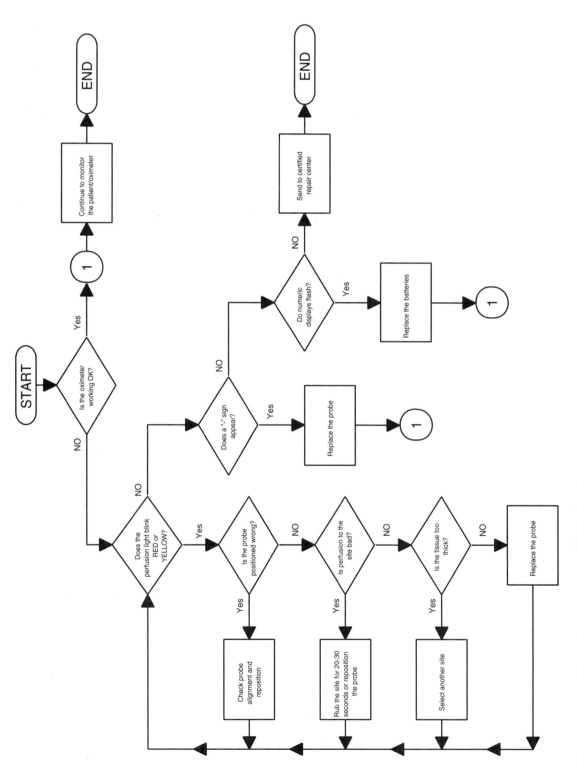

ALG 5-6 *A flowchart to troubleshoot the Nonin Model 8500M pulse oximeter.*

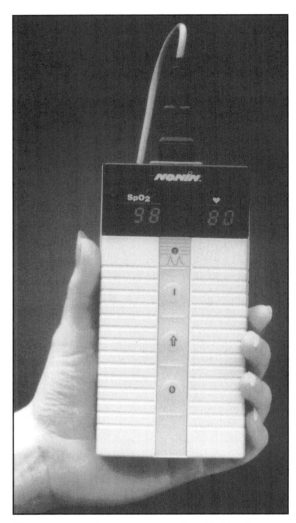

Figure 5-45 *The Nonin 8500M hand-held pulse oximeter. (Courtesy of Nonin Medical, Inc., Plymouth, MN)*

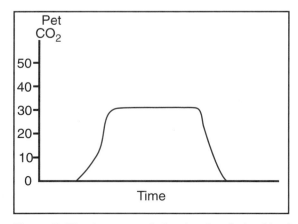

Figure 5-46 *A capnograph showing the relationship of exhaled carbon dioxide tension and time.*

END TIDAL CO₂ MONITORING

End tidal carbon dioxide monitoring allows continuous and instantaneous measurement of the exhaled carbon dioxide. Furthermore, contemporary equipment allows a concentration versus time curve to be plotted graphically on Liquid Crystal Diode (LCD) displays. The morphology (shape of the waveform) has been shown to be more significant clinically in patient management than the actual end tidal carbon dioxide value.

CAPNOGRAPHY

Terms Used during End Tidal CO₂ Monitoring

Capnography is the graphic display of CO_2 concentration versus time (Figure 5-46). As described earlier, the shape of the waveform is more important clinically than the actual concentration displayed numerically. The capnograph (wave form) can be displayed at both fast and slow speeds. The fast speed is useful for trending data, while the low speed is useful in the evaluation of the wave form's morphology or shape.

Capnometry is the measurement of end tidal CO_2 concentration. This data is a numeric display that changes with time and the ventilatory cycle. A capnometer is the instrument that provides this numeric information.

Most often, capnometry and capnography are combined together in the same instrument. This has the advantage of providing both types of data simultaneously. When combined, the validity of the numeric display can be verified by comparing it to the graphic display.

Principle of Operation

End tidal CO_2 monitors rely on nondispersive infrared technology to detect the concentration of CO_2 in a gas sample. When infrared light at a specific wave length is passed through a sample containing carbon dioxide, the gas absorbs some of the infrared light. If a detector is placed opposite the light source, infrared light transmission is proportional to CO_2 concentration in the sample.

At a wavelength of 4.26 μm (infrared light), CO_2 absorption of light is at maximum.

Two other gases (CO and N_2O) have absorption spectra very close to CO_2. These two gases may be differentiated from CO_2 by using a very narrow band pass filter, which only passes the 4.26 μm wavelength, allowing the instrument only to detect changes in transmission that are proportional to the CO_2 concentration.

WAVEFORM MORPHOLOGY

The normal capnograph has a distinct shape (Figure 5-47). The capnograph can be divided into four distinct phases. Phase I contains no exhaled CO_2. The first part of the capnograph shows an absence of CO_2 because it originates from the conducting zone of the lungs, which is primarily dead space gas, and therefore does not participate in ventilation (gas exchange). Phase II has a steep slope as the exhaled CO_2 concentration increases. This gas is mixed dead space gas and alveolar gas. Since some of the gas in this phase has participated in ventilation, the CO_2 concentration rises. Phase III represents alveolar gas. The concentration of CO_2 plateaus as the alveoli empty their contents during this part of the expiratory phase. The maximum concentration at the end of the alveolar plateau (phase III), is the end tidal CO_2 concentration. The CO_2 concentration rapidly falls to zero once inspiration begins. Phase IV represents the inspiratory portion of the capnograph.

Abnormal Capnograph Morphology

As described earlier, the morphology of the capnograph can be important in interpreting

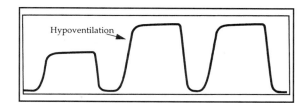

Figure 5-48 *Hypoventilation. Note how the carbon dioxide tension is greater than normal. (Courtesy of Novametrix Medical Systems, Inc., Wallingford, CT)*

changes in the patient's status. Changes in ventilation and distribution can be detected by observing the capnograph morphology.

Hypoventilation

Hypoventilation may be caused by a decrease in respiratory rate, tidal volume or both. Increases in metabolic rate, or a rapid rise in body temperature, will also cause a patient to produce higher than normal CO_2 concentrations. The morphology of hypoventilation is illustrated in Figure 5-48. Notice how the concentration (height) of the capnograph has increased.

Hyperventilation

Hyperventilation may be caused by an increase in respiratory rate, tidal volume or both. Decreases in metabolic rate or a decrease in body temperature will also cause the CO_2 concentration to fall. The morphology of hyperventilation is illustrated in Figure 5-49. Notice the decrease in the height (concentration) of the capnograph.

Rebreathing

If a patient is rebreathing part of his or her exhaled gas, CO_2 concentrations in the exhaled gas will rise. This may be performed intentionally (addition of dead space) or not intentionally. Inadvertent causes of rebreathing can

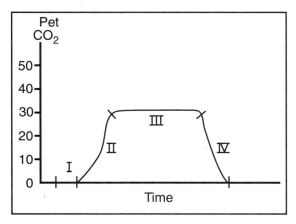

Figure 5-47 *The four phases of a capnograph. (I) anatomical dead space. (II) Mixed dead space and alveolar gas. (III) Alveolar gas. (IV) Inspiration.*

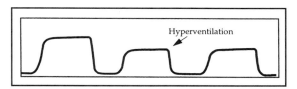

Figure 5-49 *Hyperventilation. Note how the carbon dioxide tension is less than normal. (Courtesy of Novametrix Medical Systems, Inc., Wallingford, CT)*

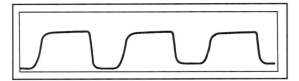

Figure 5-50 *Rebreathing. Note how the baseline of the capnograph has become elevated. (Courtesy of Novametrix Medical Systems, Inc., Wallingford, CT)*

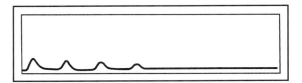

Figure 5-52 *A capnograph illustrating esophageal intubation. (Courtesy of Novametrix Medical Systems, Inc., Wallingford, CT)*

include insufficient expiratory time (inverse I:E ratios), faulty exhalation valves of ventilator circuits, or inadequate inspiratory flow. Note how the baseline of Phase I increases from zero with rebreathing (Figure 5-50).

Obstruction

Obstruction is characterized on a capnograph by a decrease in the slope of phase II (Figure 5-51). Obstruction may be caused by pulmonary pathophysiology (emphysema, asthma, bronchitis, etc.), a foreign body in the airway, partial obstruction of ventilator tubing, kinking of the endotracheal tube or bronchospasm.

Esophageal Intubation

Esophageal intubation is characterized by a sudden decrease in CO_2 concentrations (Figure 5-52). Since the stomach has little or no CO_2, the capnograph quickly plateaus to zero in a few breaths. When the endotracheal tube is repositioned properly, a normal capnograph will result.

SENSOR POSITION

The sensor for a capnometer may be positioned in one of three ways (Figure 5-53), mainstream, sidestream and proximal diverting. Each sensor position has advantages and disadvantages.

The mainstream sensor is positioned directly at the patient's airway in line with the inspired and expired gases. The sensor must be very lightweight to prevent torsion or traction on the endotracheal tube or tracheostomy tube. This sensor position results in the most instantaneous and well-defined capnographs.

The sidestream sensor position is where the sensor/monitor is removed from the patient and exhaled gas is diverted to the sensor through small-diameter tubing. This sensor

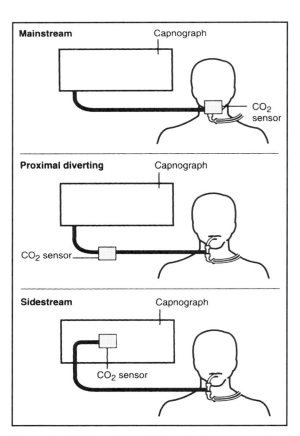

Figure 5-53 *The three positions for the capnograph sensor. (1) Mainstream. (2) Proximal diverting. (3) Sidestream. (Copyrights Nellcor, Incorporated, Pleasanton, CA)*

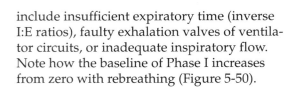

Figure 5-51 *Obstruction. Note how the slope of phase II has become decreased. Obstruction can be at the level of the circuit or airway or can be related to bronchospasm. (Courtesy of Novametrix Medical Systems, Inc., Wallingford, CT)*

position has an advantage in that a heavy sensor is not applying force or torque on the airway. However, the small-diameter line may become occluded with mucous or secretions, disrupting flow. Also an adequate flow rate must be maintained to the sensor to prevent artifact from showing on the capnograph.

The proximal diverting position places the sensor adjacent to the airway, where some of the exhaled gas is diverted to the sensor. This combines some of the best features of the mainstream and sidestream positions while attempting to minimize the disadvantages.

END TIDAL CO₂ MONITORING EQUIPMENT

Novametrix Capnogard 1265

Novametrix Medical Systems manufactures an end tidal CO_2 monitor that operates using nondispersive infrared technology (Figure 5-54). The monitor provides capnometry, capnography and alarms for ETCO₂ and respiratory rate.

Principle of Operation

The Capnogard Model 1265 uses a lightweight solid state sensor (Capnostat) that can

be used in the mainstream or sidestream sampling position. The Capnostat (Figure 5-55) uses a pulsed infrared light source that cycles at a frequency of 86 Hz. The pulsed infrared light passes through the airway adapter to a beam splitter. The beam splitter splits the infrared light beam into two beams. Each infrared light beam passes through an optical filter. One filter only passes light at 4.2 μm and the other only passes light at 3.7 μm. A detector then converts the transmitted light into an electrical signal.

The two signals from each sensor are compared electronically. During the time that the infrared light source is off, the signals are forced to be zero. During the time the infrared light source is on, the ratio between the 3.7 and 4.2 μm sensors are compared. The 4.2 μm wavelength is absorbed in proportion to any CO_2 present in the sample. The 3.7 μm wave length is unaffected by any respiratory gases (including CO and N₂O). The ratio of the two signals is therefore proportional to the CO_2 concentration in the gas sample.

Controls

The Novametrix Medical Systems Capnogard Model 1265 uses a Cold Cathode

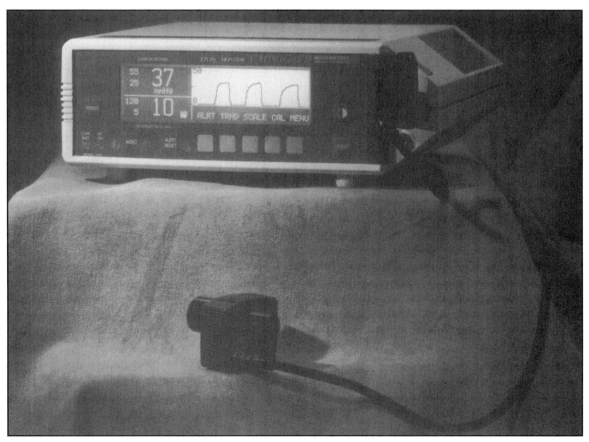

Figure 5-54 *The Novametrix Capnogard 1265. (Courtesy of Novametrix Medical Systems, Inc., Wallingford, CT)*

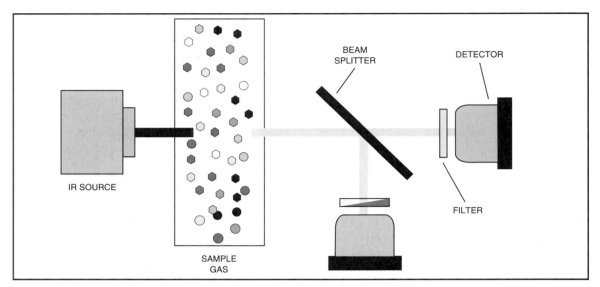

Figure 5-55 *A schematic drawing of the Novametrix Capnostat sensor. (Courtesy of Novametrix Medical Systems, Inc., Wallingford, CT)*

Display (CCD) to present numeric data (capnometry and respiratory rate) and graphic data (capnography). The monitor is controlled by soft keys and is menu driven.

Main Menu

The main menu consists of the following selections: Alert, Trend, Scale, Calibration, and Menu. By depressing the appropriate soft key, the desired submenu can be accessed.

ASSEMBLY AND TROUBLESHOOTING

Assembly—Novametrix Model 1265

1. Connect the Capnogard monitor to a 115 volt, 60 Hz electrical outlet. Ensure that the monitor is off.

2. Select an airway adapter to use with the Capnostat sensor.

3. Verify that the windows on the Capnostat are clean and dry. If necessary, carefully clean the windows on the Capnostat.

4. Snap the Capnostat onto the airway adapter.

5. Calibrate the monitor as described earlier.

6. Place the capnostat in the mainstream position, or if using in the sidestream position, the airway adapter at the patient's airway and route the monitoring tubing to the sensor located away from the patient.

7. Press the "Power" soft key to turn the monitor on.

8. Adjust the Alert limits, scale and screen brightness to the desired levels as described earlier.

Troubleshooting

ALG 5-7 will assist you in troubleshooting the Novametrix Medical Systems Capnogard Model 1265.

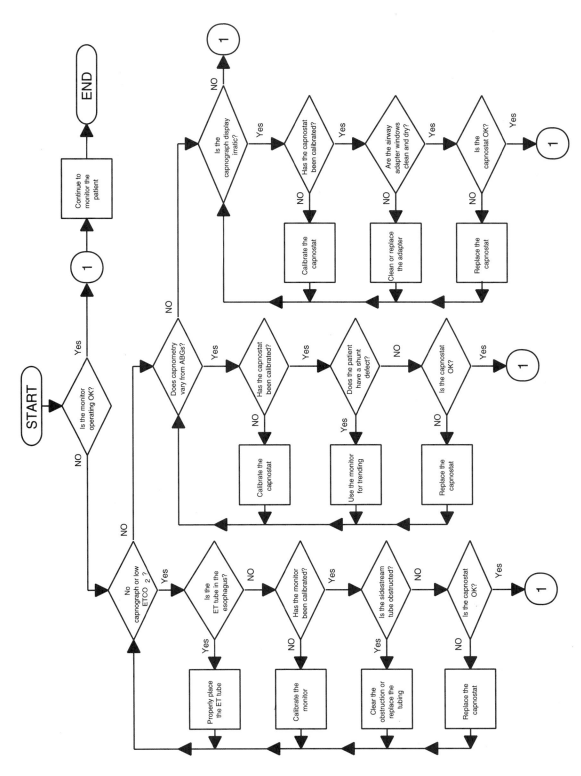

ALG 5-7 *A flowchart for troubleshooting the Novametrix Capnogard Model 1265.*

Alert Settings

The alert settings are adjusted by depressing the Alert soft key from the main menu. Once accessed, "Set Alert Limits" appears on the display. By using the "Select" soft key, the cursor can be moved to the desired limit (High, Low, Respiration Rate) and then that limit may be adjusted using the Up/Down Arrow soft keys. Once the desired value is obtained, press the RUN soft key to capture that value and return to the main menu.

The alert volume may be adjusted by depressing the "Menu" soft key from the main menu display. Once pressed, "CO₂ Options" appears in the display. Press the "Next" soft key and the next submenu "System Options" will appear. Select the "Audio" soft key and adjust the volume using the Up/Down Arrow soft key to the desired level. Press the "Run" soft key to capture the value and return to the main menu.

Display Brightness

The brightness of the CCD display may be user adjusted between bright and dim. From the main menu select the "Menu" soft key. Once pressed, "CO₂ Options" appears in the display. Press the "Next" soft key and the next submenu, "System Options," will appear. Press the "Lite" soft key. Pressing the key will toggle the display from bright to the dim settings. Once the desired brightness has been selected, press the "Run" soft key to return to the main menu.

Scale

The vertical scale of the capnogram can be adjusted from 0 to 50 mmHg or 0 to 75 mmHg.

To set the scale, press the "Scale" soft key from the main menu. Once the desired scale has been set, press the "Run" soft key to return to the main menu.

Calibration

To calibrate the Capnogard, place the Capnostat sensor into the Zero cell. Press the "Cal" soft key from the main menu. Once pressed, a "Time Remaining" counter is displayed. After the counter has timed out, place the Capnostat on the Reference cell (furthest from the monitor face). The prompt "Checking Calibration" should be displayed. "Calibration Verified" will appear on the display when calibration is complete.

Nellcor Ultra Cap™ N-6000

Nellcor, Inc. manufacturers the Ultra Cap™ N-6000 pulse oximeter and capnograph monitor (Figure 5-56). This monitor combines pulse oximetry with end tidal CO₂ monitoring into one monitor. The monitor can display the plethysmographic waveform of end tidal CO₂ or SpO₂ and numeric data for pulse rate, respiratory rate and end tidal CO₂. All information is displayed on a large vacuum fluorescent display. Alarm systems are incorporated for both the pulse oximetry and end tidal carbon dioxide monitors.

Principle of Operation

The pulse oximeter uses the principle of spectrophotometry to measure the hemoglobin saturation. The N-6000 monitor may be interfaced with any compatible Nellcor oximeter probe.

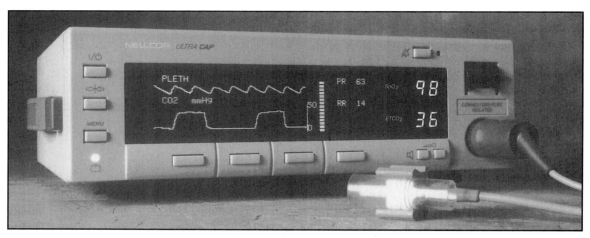

Figure 5-56 *The Nellcor Ultra Cap™ N-6000 monitor. (Photo courtesy of Nellcor Incorporated, Pleasanton, CA)*

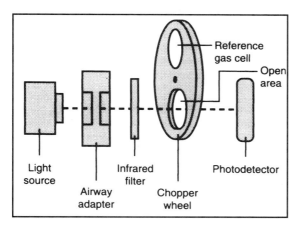

Figure 5-57 *A schematic drawing of the Nellcor Ultra Cap N-6000 CO_2 sensor. (Copyrights Nellcor Incorporated, Pleasanton, CA)*

The capnograph uses nondispersive infrared technology to measure the end tidal CO_2 concentration. The sensor consists of a light source, airway adapter, filter, chopper wheel, and a photodiode detector (Figure 5-57). The infrared light passes from the light source, through the airway adapter and filter, to the chopper wheel, and then to the photodetector. The optical filter assures transmission of the specific wavelength for carbon dioxide, while filtering other infrared wavelengths.

The chopper wheel is motor driven and rotates. The photodiode alternately senses no light transmission (solid areas between the reference and open areas), light transmitted through the sample gas (airway), and light transmitted through the reference-plus-sample. The concentration of $ETCO_2$ becomes a ratio between reference-plus-sample and sample measurements (reference + sample / sample).

Controls

The Nellcor Ultra Cap™ N-6000 uses a large vacuum fluorescent display and several function keys or soft keys to control the many features of the monitor. The main monitoring display screen is shown in Figure 5-58. From this display screen, the operator may select from several submenus using the Menu key or the soft keys along the lower part of the monitoring screen. Figure 5-58 illustrates the four primary menus or screens and their respective submenus using a branching directory tree.

System Screen

The system screen allows the operator to perform the following: select what parameters will be monitored, set the monitor to compen-

sate for nitrous oxide or high F_iO_2 levels, disable the graphics display to conserve power when running on batteries, or adjust system variables.

To select what parameter you wish to monitor, press the Menu key and from the menu screen, press the System key. The operator may turn off the SpO_2 display, $ETCO_2$ display or monitor both parameters simultaneously from the system screen, by pressing the Monitored Parameters key until the desired option is selected. Once the desired option has been selected, press the Menu key to return to the monitoring screen.

To compensate for the presence of nitrous oxide or high F_iO_2 levels, press the Menu key and press the System key from the display. Select the COMP. key and press the key until the desired parameter is displayed. Press the Menu key to return to the monitoring screen. It is recommended that compensation be used for F_iO_2 levels greater than 0.60.

Alarm Screen

By depressing the Menu key and then the Alarms key, the alarm screen can be selected. From the alarm screen you may set limits, configure the alarms (silence, volume, time periods), or disable alarms.

To set the alarm limits, press the Menu key and then the Alarms key. Once the alarms screen is displayed, press the Set Limits soft key. You may scroll through the various alarm parameters by pressing the Select soft key. Continue pressing the Select soft key until the desired alarm limit is highlighted. Press the increase or decrease soft key to adjust the alarm to the desired level. Press the Menu key to return to the monitoring screen.

To configure the alarms, press the Menu key and then the Alarms key. Select Configure by pressing the appropriate soft key. From the configure alarms screen, the length of alarm silence, alarm volume and apnea periods may be adjusted. Press the Menu key to return to the monitoring screen.

The Disable key from the Alarms screen allows the operator to disable the audible portion of an alarm for any of the monitored parameters. To disable an alarm, press the Disable soft key from the Alarms screen display. Use the Select soft key to move through the screen until the desired parameter is highlighted. Press the Change soft key to change the alarm status. Press the Menu key to return to the monitoring screen.

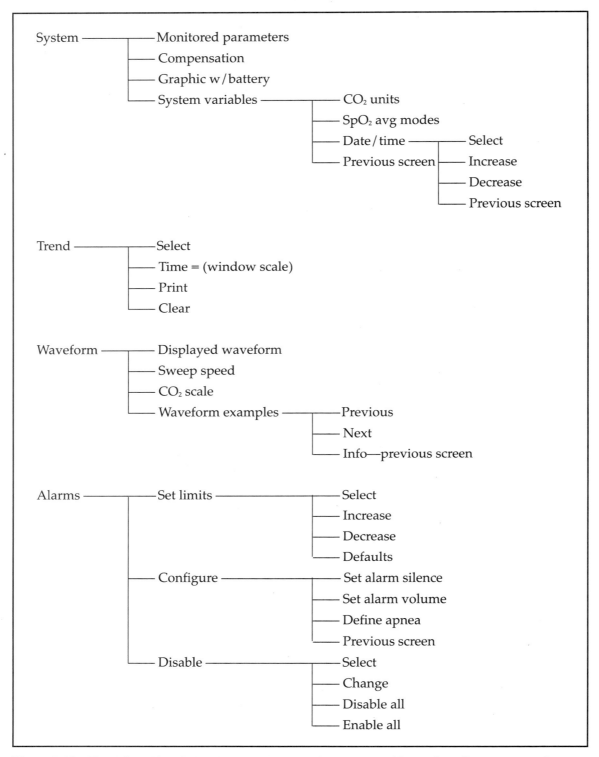

Figure 5-58 *The Nellcor Ultra Cap™ N-6000 main monitoring menu tree. (Copyright Nellcor Incorporated, Pleasanton, CA)*

Waveform Screen

The waveform screen allows the operator to adjust what waveform is displayed, sweep speed and CO_2 scales. To enter the Waveform screen, press the Menu key and then the Waveform soft key.

To select the waveform display, press the Displayed Waveform soft key and continue depressing the soft key until the desired waveform is highlighted. Press the Menu key to capture your selection and return to the monitoring screen.

Sweep speed is adjustable from 6.25 to 50 mm/sec. To adjust the sweep speed, press the Sweep SPD soft key from the Waveform screen until the desired speed is selected. Press the Menu key to capture the parameter and return to the monitoring screen.

The CO_2 scale may be adjusted from 0.00 to 50 mmHg to a maximum of 0.00 to 99.00 mmHg. To adjust the scale of the screen, press the CO_2 Scale soft key from the Waveform screen display. Continue to press the soft key until the desired scale is highlighted. Press the Menu soft key to return to the monitoring screen.

Trend

The Trend function may be used to record trends for SpO_2, $ETCO_2$, pulse rate and respiratory rate. The trends may be displayed individually or in any combination. Use the Select key to display the desired trend(s). Press the Menu key to return to the monitoring screen.

To select the time scale for monitoring the trend, press the Time soft key from the Trend screen. Continue pressing the soft key until the desired time interval is highlighted (2, 4, 8, 12, and 24 hours). To return to the monitoring screen, press the Menu key.

ASSEMBLY AND TROUBLESHOOTING

Assembly—Nellcor Model N-6000

1. Connect an appropriate pulse oximeter sensor to the monitor by plugging it into the SpO_2 connector on the front of the monitor and sliding the latch of the sensor lock over the plug to hold it securely.

2. Connect the mainstream sensor to the patient's airway and connect the sensor cable to the monitor by plugging it into the connector labeled CO_2 on the front of the monitor.

3. Connect the power cord to a 115, 60 Hz power outlet and verify that the power cord is connected to the monitor by checking the rear panel of the monitor.

4. Turn the monitor on by pressing the On/Standby button.
   a. The monitor will warm up for about 45 seconds. During warm up the monitor will display "CO_2 sensor warming up."
   b. The first screen display will be the Nellcor Copyright screen, which will be active for 3 seconds.
   c. The Copyright screen will be replaced with the alarm limit screen. You may adjust alarm limits at this time using the procedure described earlier, or accept the default limits.

5. Press the Menu key to return to the Monitoring screen.

6. System parameters, trends, waveforms and alarms may be adjusted as described earlier in this section.

Troubleshooting

Oximeter

To troubleshoot the oximeter, refer to ALG 5-3 (earlier in this chapter).

End Tidal CO_2 Monitor

ALG 5-8 will assist you in troubleshooting the $ETCO_2$ monitor.

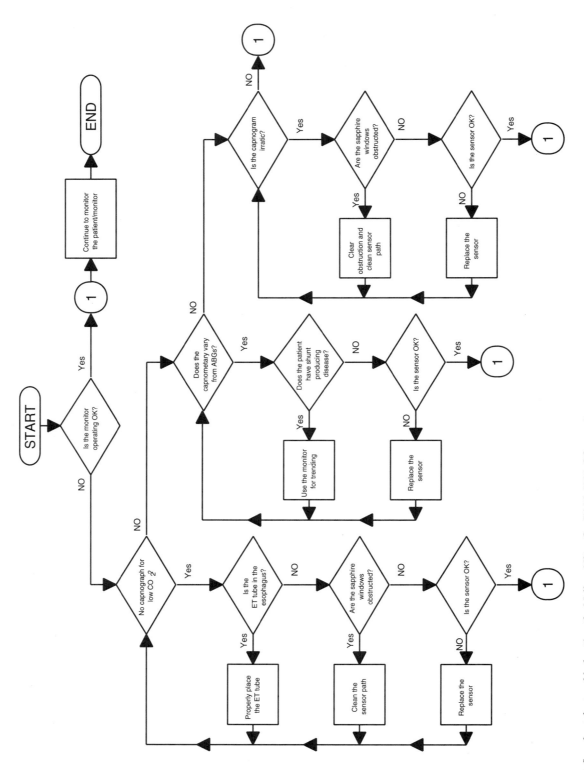

ALG 5-8 *A flowchart for troubleshooting the Nellcor Ultra Cap™ N-6000 CO₂ monitor.*

Colormetric End Tidal CO₂ Determination

Besides nondispersive infrared spectroscopy to detect CO_2, a chemical method may be used to detect end tidal CO_2. When a chemical with a color indicator is exposed to CO_2, and the color changes are due to the chemical used for detection, the reaction is reversible, allowing breath-to-breath determination. Nellcor markets a colormetric detector called "Easy Cap™."

Easy Cap™ (Figure 5-59) is a disposable single patient–use, nonelectronic monitor that measures ETCO₂ using a chemical reaction and color change (colormetric). It is designed to be used following intubation to detect esophageal intubation (no exhaled CO_2). To use the Easy Cap™, place it on the airway following intubation and observe for a color change from purple to yellow in the center of the monitor. If the color changes from inspiration (purple) to yellow (expiration), the endotracheal tube is in the trachea and CO_2 has been detected. If the color in the center remains purple, esophageal intubation has occurred.

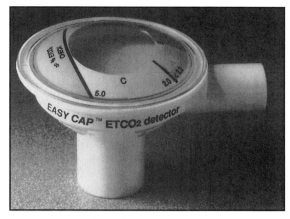

Figure 5-59 *The Nellcor Easy Cap™ colormetric CO₂ monitor. (Photo courtesy Nellcor Incorporated, Pleasanton, CA)*

CLINICAL CORNER

Pulmonary Measurement Equipment

1. You are using a standard range peak flowmeter to assess an asthmatic patient in your emergency room. The peak flowmeter is calibrated from 60 to 800 L/min. The patient is unable to achieve even 60 L/min. What should you report for peak flow, and what other device could you use?

Oxygen Analyzing Equipment

1. You are checking the F₁O₂ on a Nellcor Puritan Bennett 7200ae ventilator using a polarographic oxygen analyzer. The oxygen percent control is set at 60%, and your oxygen analyzer reads 67%. Describe the steps you should take to verify the oxygen concentration.
2. You are using a polarographic oxygen analyzer to measure the F₁O₂ on a heated nebulizer. While attempting to use the analyzer, it fails to calibrate. You suspect the battery is low, so you change it, but the analyzer still fails to calibrate. Describe the steps you should take to troubleshoot the analyzer.

Blood Gas–Analyzing Equipment

1. You are performing quality control on your blood gas instrument. The control results for the oxygen electrode fail to come in within plus-or-minus two standard deviations. Upon review of the Levey-Jennings chart, you note a trend. What could you do to bring the electrode back into plus-or-minus two standard deviations?

Transcutaneous Monitoring Equipment

1. You are tending a PtcCO₂ monitor with a patient's blood gases. The mon-

itor values are drifting away from the blood gas results. What could you do bring the monitor more closely in line with the current blood gas results?

Pulse Oximetry Equipment

1. The pulse oximeter you just connected to a patient's finger is indicating that the signal strength is poor. What can you do to improve the ability of the oximeter to give you the desired results, and what other means can you use to verify the signal strength?

End Tidal CO₂ Equipment

1. You are resuscitating a patient in the emergency room, and the emergency room physician asks you to intubate. How can you verify placement of the endotracheal tubes before the chest x-ray returns? Discuss at least three ways.

Self-Assessment Quiz

1. Which of the following pulmonary function measuring devices are volume displacement devices?
   I. Collins spirometer.
   II. Vortex shedding pneumotachometer.
   III. Stead-Wells spirometer.
   IV. Fleisch pneumotachometer.
   a. I and II
   b. I and III
   c. II and III
   d. I and IV
   e. III and IV

2. A body plethysmograph measures thoracic volume by:
   I. Changes in pressure.
   II. Flow measurements.
   III. Temperature changes.
   IV. Rotating vanes.
   a. I only
   b. II only
   c. III only
   d. I and II
   e. III and IV

3. A type of pneumotachometer that depends upon a resistive element that causes a pressure drop is:
   a. The Fleisch pneumotachometer.
   b. The vortex shedding pneumotachometer.
   c. The venturi pneumotachometer.
   d. The Wright respirometer.
   e. The Wright peak flowmeter.

4. A pneumotachometer that is susceptible to damage from high flow rates is:
   a. The Fleisch pneumotachometer.
   b. The vortex shedding pneumotachometer.
   c. The venturi pneumotachometer.
   d. The Wright respirometer.
   e. The Wright peak flowmeter.

5. Which gas law is used in the body plethysmograph to measure lung volumes?
   a. Charles' law.
   b. Gay-Lussac's law.
   c. Henry's law.
   d. Boyle's law.

6. A type of pneumotachometer that is dependent upon a temperature change to measure flow is:
   a. A vortex sensor.
   b. A thermal anemometer.
   c. A vane respirometer.
   d. A Fleisch pneumotachometer.

7. A venturi pneumotachometer works by measuring:
   a. A difference in ultrasonic energy.
   b. A difference in voltage.
   c. A difference in current.
   d. A difference in pressure.
   e. The height of a ball in a Thorpe tube.

8. A physical oxygen analyzer measures oxygen using:
   a. The chemical reaction of oxygen-forming hydroxyl ions.
   b. The paramagnetic property of oxygen.
   c. A Wheatstone bridge.
   d. The chemical reaction of oxygen-forming hydrogen ions.
   e. The principle of thermoconductivity.

9. An electrical oxygen analyzer measures oxygen using:
   a. The chemical reaction of oxygen-forming hydroxyl ions.
   b. The paramagnetic property of oxygen.
   c. Infrared absorption.
   d. The chemical reaction of oxygen-forming hydrogen ions.
   e. The principle of thermoconductivity.

10. A galvanic oxygen analyzer measures oxygen using:
    a. The chemical reaction of oxygen-forming hydroxyl ions.
    b. The paramagnetic property of oxygen.
    c. Infrared absorption.
    d. The chemical reaction of oxygen-forming hydrogen ions.
    e. The principle of thermoconductivity.

11. A polarographic oxygen analyzer is similar to a galvanic analyzer with the exception of:
    a. The addition of a battery.
    b. The deletion of an anode.
    c. A separate reference and sample chamber.
    d. The addition of a quartz fiber.
    e. The addition of a heating element and thermocouple.

12. The most common reference half-cell for the pH system is:
    a. The silver/silver chloride cell.
    b. The calomel cell.
    c. The polarographic cell.
    d. The galvanic cell.
    e. A platinum cathode.

13. The PCO₂ blood gas electrode directly measures:
    a. PCO_2.
    b. Hydrogen ion concentration.
    c. Carbon dioxide percentage.
    d. Hydroxyl ions.
    e. Free electrons.

14. The PO₂ blood gas electrode measures oxygen by:
    a. Changes in electrical current.
    b. Changes in mass.
    c. Using a photospectrometer.
    d. Using an infrared analyzer.
    e. Using a Wheatstone bridge.

15. A blood gas PO₂ electrode measures oxygen:
    a. Percentage.
    b. Mass.
    c. Tension.
    d. Reactivity.
    e. Weight.

16. A transcutaneous carbon dioxide electrode is a modified:
    a. Clark electrode.
    b. Galvanic electrode.
    c. Severinghaus electrode.
    d. Polarographic electrode.
    e. Paramagnetic electrode.

17. A transcutaneous carbon dioxide electrode directly measures:
    a. PCO_2.
    b. Hydrogen ion concentration.
    c. Carbon dioxide percentage.
    d. Hydroxyl ions.
    e. Free electrons.

18. Both an end tidal carbon dioxide monitor and a pulse oximeter work using:
    a. Changes in electrical current.
    b. Changes in mass.
    c. A photospectrometer.
    d. An infrared analyzer.
    e. A Wheatstone bridge.

19. The occurrence of six or more blood gas quality control results that show an increasing pattern is termed a:
    a. Shift.
    b. Trend.
    c. Standard deviation.
    d. Drift.

20. The presence of six or more blood gas quality control results on the same side of the mean is termed a:
    a. Shift
    b. Trend
    c. Standard deviation
    d. Drift

21. Which of the following hemoglobin variants are unable to combine reversibly with oxygen?
    I. Oxyhemoblobin.
    II. Reduced hemoglobin.
    III. Methemoglobin.
    IV. Carboxyhemoglobin.

a. I and II
b. I and III
c. I and IV
d. II and III
e. III and IV

22. Which of the following hemoglobin variants exists in the Fe^{+++} state?
    a. Oxyhemoblobin.
    b. Reduced hemoglobin.
    c. Methemoglobin.
    d. Carboxyhemoglobin.

23. The term functional hemoglobin refers to which of the following variants?
    I. Oxyhemoblobin.
    II. Reduced hemoglobin.
    III. Methemoglobin.
    IV. Carboxyhemoglobin.
    a. I and II
    b. I and III
    c. I and IV
    d. II and III
    e. III and IV

24. Which of the following factors may influence the accuracy of a pulse oximeter?
    I. Ambient light.
    II. Nail polish.
    III. The patient's hemodynamics.
    IV. Patient motion.
    a. I
    b. I and II
    c. I, II and III
    d. I, II, III and IV

25. The term isosebestic point refers to:
    a. Hemoglobin's freezing temperature.
    b. The wavelength where two or more variants have similar absorptions.
    c. The wavelength where all variants have differing absorptions.
    d. The wavelength of light that is not affected by hemoglobin.

26. Pulse oximeters measure hemoglobin saturation:
    I. Continuously.
    II. During systole.
    III. During diastole.
    a. I
    b. I and II
    c. I and III
    d. III

27. Which of the following pulse oximeters are hand-held instruments?
    a. Nellcor N-180.
    b. Ohmeda 3740.
    c. Novametrix Oxypleth.
    d. Nonin 8500M.

28. Which of the following end tidal CO_2 monitors positions the sensor on the patient's airway?
    I. Mainstream.
    II. Sidestream.
    III. Proximal diverting.
    a. I
    b. II
    c. III
    d. II and III

29. Which of the following removes some exhaled gas and measures the CO_2 concentration away from the patient's airway?
    I. Mainstream.
    II. Sidestream.
    III. Proximal diverting.
    a. I
    b. II
    c. III
    d. II and III

30. When is the use of a colormetric CO_2 monitor most useful?
    a. For continuous monitoring.
    b. For trending data over time.
    c. To detect esophageal intubation.
    d. None of the above.

Selected Bibliography

Adams, A. P., and C. E. W. Hahn, *Principles and Practice of Blood-Gas Analysis*, Franklin Scientific Projects, 1979.

Aloan, Claire A., *Respiratory Care of the Newborn*, J. B. Lippincott Company, 1987.

Barnes, Thomas, et al., *Respiratory Care Practice*, 2nd Ed., Mosby-Yearbook, 1994.

BCI International, *BCI 3301 Oximeter Operation/Service Manual*, Waukesha, WI, 1992.

Beer, Ferdinand, and Russell Johnston, *Vector Mechanics for Engineers*, 5th Ed., McGraw-Hill Book Company, 1988.

Burton, George, Hodgkin, John, et al., *Respiration Care: A Guide to Clinical Practice*, 3rd Ed., J. B. Lippincott Company, 1984.

Datex Division Instrumentarium Corporation, *First Steps in CO_2 Monitoring*, Helsinki, Finland, 1992.

East, Thomas D., "What Makes Noninvasive Monitoring Tick? A Review of Basic Engineering Principles," *Respiratory Care*, Vol. 35, No. 6, 1990.

Hess, Dean, "Capnometry and Capnography: Technical Aspects, Physiologic Aspects and Clinical Applications," *Respiratory Care*, Vol. 35, No. 6, 1990.

Instrumentation Laboratory, Inc., *Blood Gas Quality Control*, Lexington, MA, 1973.

Kacmarek, Robert, et al., *The Essentials of Respiratory Therapy*, 2nd Ed., Mosby-Yearbook, 1985.

Kinasewitz, Gary T., "Use of End-Tidal Capnography during Mechanical Ventilation," *Respiratory Care*, Vol. 82, No. 27, 1982.

McPherson, Steven P., et al., *Respiratory Therapy Equipment*, 5th Ed., Mosby-Yearbook, 1995.

Nellcor, Incorporated, *Measurement of Functional and Fractional Oxygen Saturation*, Hayward, CA, 1987.

Nellcor, Incorporated, *Operator's Manual Nellcor N-180 Pulse Oximeter*, Hayward, CA, 1991.

Nellcor, Incorporated, *Ultra Cap™ N-6000 Pulse Oximeter and Capnograph Operator's Manual*, Hayward, CA, 1993.

Nonin Medical, *Instruction and Service Manual Model 8500 and Model 8500M Hand Held Pulse Oximeter*, Plymouth, MN, 1992.

Novametrix Medical Systems, Inc., *Capnogard ETCO2 Monitor User's Manual*, Wallingford, CT, 1992.

Novametrix Medical Systems, Inc., *Oxypleth Pulse Oximeter User's Manual*, Wallingford, CT, 1992.

Novametrix Medical Systems, Inc., *PtcO₂/ PtcCO₂ Monitor Model 840 User's Manual,* Wallingford, CT, 1992.

Ohmeda, a BOC Health Care Company, *Ohmeda 3740 Pulse Oximeter Operation and Maintenance Manual,* Louisville, KY, 1988.

Portnoy, Alan L., *A Review of the Principles of Quality Control: A Programmed Text,* Fisher Diagnostics, n.d.

Pulwer, Ed, and David Plaut, *Quality Control,* Miami, FL, American Dade, 1979.

Ruppel, Gregg, *Manual of Pulmonary Function Testing,* 6th Ed., Mosby-Yearbook, 1994.

Severinghaus, John W., "Transcutaneous Blood Gas Analysis,"*Respiratory Care,* Vol. 27, No. 82, 1992.

Welch, James P., and Richard DeCesare, "Pulse Oximetry: Instrumentation and Clinical Applications," *Respiratory Care,* Vol. 35, No. 6, 1990.

White, Gary C., *Basic Clinical Lab Competencies for Respiratory Care,* 2nd Ed., Delmar Publishers, Inc., 1993.

CHAPTER 6

MECHANICAL VENTILATOR THEORY AND CLASSIFICATION

INTRODUCTION

Mechanical ventilators play a very important role in the management of critically ill patients. A wide variety of both newborn and adult ventilators are used in multiple patient care settings.

Despite the variety in ventilators, certain features are common to all. The first section will focus on the common elements of ventilation. A classification system will be developed to help you group ventilators having similar function or operation. You will also learn how gas laws, gas control systems, and flow and pressure measuring devices are applied to a ventilator's design. Once this knowledge is attained, you will understand the advantages and disadvantages of the ventilator control systems in use today.

The next section of the chapter will discuss special ventilatory procedures. These include how to modify or add PEEP, CPAP, or intermittent mandatory ventilation (IMV) to a ventilator not having these mode capabilities. Although the majority of the contemporary adult ventilators incorporate these features, a careful study of an external circuit will facilitate your understanding of a contemporary ventilator's operation.

OBJECTIVES

After completing this chapter, the student will accomplish the following objectives:
- Explain how Poiseuille's and Boyle's law can be applied when mechanically ventilating a patient.
- Explain how the following detect, or measure, gas flow or pressure:
  — Strain gauge
  — Vortex sensor
  — Heated wire grid
  — Strain gauge pressure transducer
  — Variable reluctance pressure transducer
  — Differential pressure transducer
- Explain the operation of the following valves:
  — Solenoid valve
  — Proportional solenoid valve
  — Servo-controlled scissor valve
  — Demand valve
- Define work in physical science terms,

and apply that definition to pulmonary work.
- Define ventilator support in relation to pulmonary work.
- Explain the ventilator control circuit including:
  — Input power
  — Power conversion or transmission
  — Identify the types of control circuits including:
    a. Mechanical
    b. Pneumatic
    c. Fluidic
    d. Electric
    e. Electronic
- Define the term *control variable* and what conditions must be met for a ventilator to be classified as one of the following:
  — Pressure controller
  — Volume controller

— Flow controller
— Time controller
- Define the term *phase variable* and state how that variable may be used during the four phases of ventilation:
  — limit variable
  — cycle variable
  — baseline variable
  — conditional variable
- Describe the different output wave forms and their characteristics.
- Describe the characteristics of the ventilator/patient circuit including:
  — Single versus double
  — Compliance
  — Resistance
  — Washout time
- Explain the operation of the following PEEP/CPAP devices:
  — Boeringer valve
  — Downs' valve

— Magnetic valve
— Emerson water column
— Water seal
- Explain how PEEP, IMV, and IMV with CPAP may be added externally to a ventilator.
- Explain the purpose of ventilator alarm systems and the types of alarms that are used.
- Describe different types of ventilator alarms:
  — Input power
  — Control circuit
  — Output alarms
- Describe the modes of ventilation and classify them according to Chatburn's ventilator classification system.

PHYSICS OF MECHANICAL VENTILATORS

GAS LAWS THAT APPLY TO MECHANICAL VENTILATION

Knowing how Boyle's and Poiseuille's laws apply to mechanical ventilation is important to the understanding of mechanical ventilator operation and airway management (see Chapter 1).

Boyle's law is applied in the determination of *tubing compliance and compressible volume.* Compliance, by definition, is a change in volume per unit of pressure.

To calculate these values, the ventilator is adjusted to deliver 200 mL of volume, the patient wye is occluded and a spirometer is placed at the expiratory limb to measure expiratory volumes. The ventilator is allowed to cycle for 10 to 12 breaths, permitting an accurate determination of expired volume. The peak pressure on the pressure manometer is also recorded. To calculate tubing compliance and compressible volume, complete the following steps.

Measured volume: 200 mL

Measured pressure: 70 cmH$_2$O

Compliance = Volume / Pressure
= 200 mL / 70 cmH$_2$O
= 2.86 mL / cmH$_2$O

In this example, the tubing / circuit compliance is 2.86 mL / cmH$_2$O. That is, for every centimeter of water pressure applied to the circuit, the volume of gas delivered to the patient will be decreased by 2.86 mL.

Not all the volume given with each breath is delivered to the patient. Some volume is lost in the circuit due to compression. Calculation of the compressible volume, or tubing loss as it is referred to, may be accomplished by multiplying the tubing compliance by the peak pressure required to deliver a given volume to the patient.

Measured volume: 800 mL

Peak pressure: 25 cmH$_2$O

Tubing compliance: 2.86 mL / cmH$_2$O

Compressible volume
= Peak pressure × Tubing compliance
= 25 cmH$_2$O × 2.86 mL / cmH$_2$O
= 71.5 mL

To determine the actual volume delivered to the patient, the compressible volume must be subtracted from the measured volume. This is the *corrected tidal volume.*

Poiseuille's Law

Mechanical ventilation involves the bulk movement of gas volumes into and out of the lungs. Therefore, the laws governing the behavior of fluids applies. As you recall, Poiseuille's law relates resistance to gas flow to the radius and length of a tube.

When the diameter of an airway decreases, a significant increase in resistance results. This reduction in diameter can occur because of obstruction from secretions, herniation of the cuff, kinking of the artificial airway or other causes. If the radius of the airway is reduced by 1/2 of the original radius, resistance to gas flow increases a full 16 times. Therefore, a higher pressure must be used to deliver a given volume in a given time.

MEASUREMENT OF GAS FLOW AND PRESSURE

Various devices and methods are used by ventilator manufacturers to measure gas flow and pressure. Many devices are relatively simple; others are quite complex. An understanding of the various methods of measurement is important in understanding the characteristics and monitoring abilities of the different ventilators.

Strain Gauge Pressure Transducer

One way to measure pressure and flow is to use a *strain gauge pressure transducer* (Figure 6-1). A strain gauge pressure transducer con-

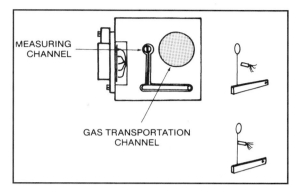

Figure 6-2 *A schematic of the strain gauge flowmeter used on the Siemens Medical Systems 900C ventilator. (Courtesy of Siemens Medical Systems, Inc., Danvers, MA)*

sists of a diaphragm with a strain gauge attached to it, exposed to the area where pressure measurement is desired. The strain gauge is connected by a set of wires to a Wheatstone bridge circuit that is sensitive to a change in resistance.

Pressure exerted on the diaphragm causes the strain gauge to elongate. As the gauge lengthens, the resistance to electrical current increases. This causes the Wheatstone bridge circuit to produce a change in voltage proportional to the pressure applied to the diaphragm. The pressure may be displayed digitally or by an analog gauge.

A strain gauge flow transducer employs a flexible wire with a flag or flat plate on one end. A strain gauge is mounted to the wire in such a way that it is sensitive to bending of the wire. As gas flows past the flag, pressure against it causes the wire to bend or flex. The strain gauge, in turn, flexes, causing a change in electrical resistance. This change then causes a change in voltage. The voltage change is proportional to the gas flow. This type of mechanism is used in the Servo 900C ventilator to measure flow (Figure 6-2).

Vortex Sensor

Vortex sensors, as described in Chapter 5, are also used on some ventilators to directly measure flow. These sensors employ the vortex shedding principle previously described, using ultrasonic energy to detect changes in gas flow (Figure 6-3).

Heated Wire Grid

A wire grid placed in a stream of flowing gas is heated to a constant temperature by a

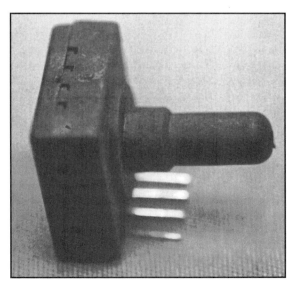

Figure 6-1 *A strain gauge pressure transducer.*

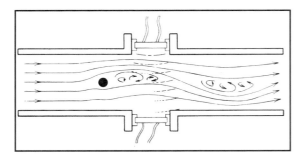

Figure 6-3 *A schematic of a flowmeter using the vortex shedding principle. (Courtesy of Bear Medical Systems, Inc., Riverside, CA)*

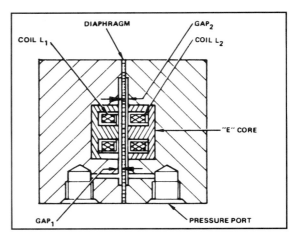

Figure 6-5 *A variable reluctance (magnetic) differential pressure transducer. (Courtesy of Validyne Engineering Corporation, Northridge, CA)*

specially designed circuit. As the gas flows past the grid, it cools the grid by conduction. A temperature sensor detects this change in temperature, and causes the circuit to increase current flow to maintain the constant temperature. Therefore, electrical current flow becomes proportional to gas flow. The flow may be displayed digitally or by using an analog gauge.

Differential Pressure Transducer

A *differential pressure transducer* is a strain gauge–type transducer that compares two pressures by using a diaphragm to separate them (Figure 6-4).

Another means of monitoring pressure changes is to use the principle of magnetism. Movement of a magnetically permeable diaphragm in close proximity to a wire-wound coil will cause changes in reluctance (a measure of magnetic potential difference), by increasing or decreasing the air gap (Figure 6-5). This change in reluctance will alter the induction ratio of an alternating current (AC) bridge circuit. Therefore a change in magnetic flux

causes a change in output voltage from the AC bridge circuit.

By connecting the pressure inputs of a sensitive differential pressure transducer to a resistive type flow transducer (Fleisch pneumotachometer), as shown in Figure 6-6, one can accurately measure flow. The pneumotachometer consists of two pressure ports, one proximal and one distal to a resistive element, which is generally a metal screen. The pressure differential between the two pressure ports becomes greater as flow increases. An increase in flow will cause a proportional voltage increase. If sampling time is known, volume also can be measured because the cross sectional area of the transducer is known. This type of system, besides being used in ventila-

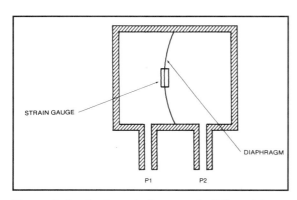

Figure 6-4 *A schematic diagram of a differential pressure transducer. Note the two pressure-measuring ports.*

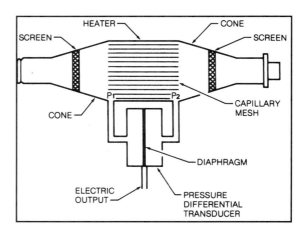

Figure 6-6 *A screen-type pneumotachometer. Note the two pressure ports, one distal and one proximal to the screen.*

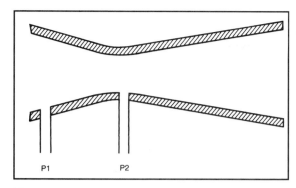

Figure 6-7 *A schematic of a venturi pneumotachometer. Note the pressure port proximal to the restriction and another at the restriction.*

tors, is also used in pulmonary function equipment to measure flow and volume.

Another way to use a differential pressure transducer to measure flow is to connect the two pressure ports to a venturi tube. Pressure is compared before the restriction and at the restriction (Figure 6-7). The pressure differential in this system is proportional to flow.

VALVE OPERATION

Valves are used in mechanical ventilators to control or direct gas flow. Valves operate using different control systems and ways of regulating gas direction and flow. Some valves are automated while others allow the operator to control their function. An understanding of the basic types of valves used in mechanical

ventilators is important in order to understand the capabilities of mechanical ventilators.

Solenoid Valves

Solenoid valves are often used in mechanical ventilators to direct or control main gas flow to the patient. The solenoid valve operates as a simple on-off switch. Solenoid valves may be automated (controlled by an electric timer or microprocessor), manually activated, pressure activated or all three (Figure 6-8).

The valve consists of a gate or plunger, valve seat, electromagnet, diaphragm, spring, and two electrical contacts. The valve is opened when electric current flows through the electromagnet and creates a magnetic field that pulls the plunger open. Conversely, when the current stops, the magnetic field collapses and a spring closes the plunger against its seat.

The current to the electromagnet may be controlled in three different ways. First, an electric timer or microprocessor can send an electric current to the electromagnet, activating it and opening the valve. Second, subambient pressure created by the patient attempting to take a breath will cause the diaphragm to descend, closing an electrical contact which then opens the valve. Lastly, many ventilators allow the operator to deliver a "manual breath" by pushing a button or closing a switch. This causes current to be delivered to the electromagnet, opening the solenoid valve.

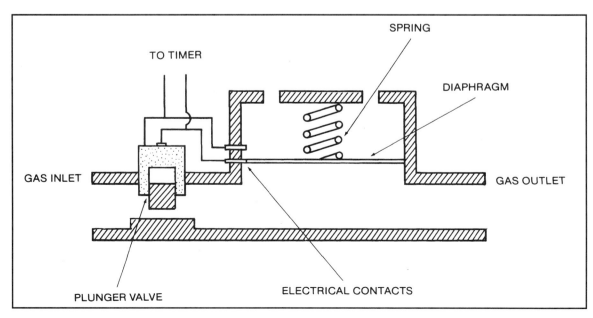

Figure 6-8 *A schematic of a solenoid valve.*

PROPORTIONAL SOLENOID VALVES

Proportional solenoid valves are valves that are able to open in very small increments. The solenoid valve previously described is either fully open or fully closed. Proportional control of gas flow allows ventilator manufacturers to design equipment that better responds to patient needs using microprocessor feedback and control mechanisms.

The term *servo feedback control* is often used to describe the operation of the control systems for these valves. Sensors monitor pressure, flow, and sometimes F_IO_2 inside the ventilator, in the patient circuit, or both. Signals from these sensors are compared to reference values set by the operator who adjusts the controls. Other reference values may be provided by monitoring the patient's respiratory rate, volume, compliance or other physiological parameters. When the measured values from the sensors differ from the reference values, the microprocessor sends signals opening or closing the valves, adjusting the output to more closely match the reference value. This system of monitoring, comparing, and monitoring again, can be repeated by the microprocessor thousands of times each second and is termed a closed feedback loop control system.

Proportional solenoid valves (PSOLs) are incorporated into the design of the Puritan Bennett 7200a ventilator. These valves are microprocessor controlled and have several thousand different positions from fully closed to fully open. These valves regulate flow, volume, pressure, F_IO_2 and waveform in the operation of this ventilator. Signals from the feedback control system open or close the valves in response to changes in the measured values.

Proportional Scissor Valves

Proportional scissor valves are incorporated into the design of the Servo Ventilators manufactured by Siemens Medical Systems. Both valves in the 900C use moveable arms that function like a scissors compressing or opening a rubber tube (Figure 6-9).

Signals from the control system cause the stepper motor to open or close the valve in small intervals or steps. The valve opens or closes at a rate of up to 480 steps per second. Each step results in a change in flow of roughly 10%. Photoelectric cells determine

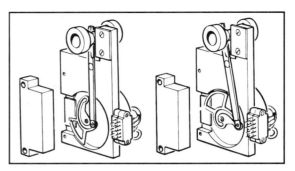

Figure 6-9 *A schematic drawing of the Siemens Medical Systems 900C inspiratory scissor valves. (Courtesy of Siemens Medical Systems, Inc., Danvers, MA)*

whether the valve is fully open or closed. This occurs when a cam obstructs the light path indicating the valve is open in one position and closed in the other.

The expiratory valve illustrated in Figure 6-10 opens by an electromagnet. Signals from the control system cause a fluctuation in current applied to the electromagnet. Depending on the strength of the current, the magnetic field is either strong (fully closing the valve) or weak (partially closing the valve). If no current flows through the magnet, a spring opens the valve. This is a safety feature that will allow the patient to exhale in the event of a power failure.

DEMAND VALVES

Demand valves are specialized valves that respond to a patient's inspiratory efforts (generation of subambient pressures). Unlike solenoid valves that also respond to subambient pressures, demand valves provide a con-

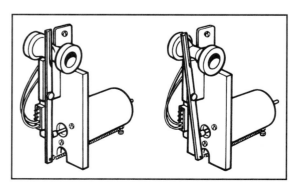

Figure 6-10 *A schematic drawing of the Siemens Medical Systems 900C expiratory scissor valves. (Courtesy Siemens Medical Systems, Inc., Danvers, MA)*

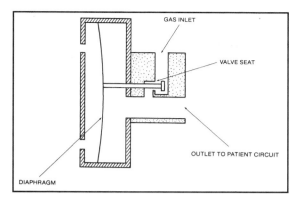

Figure 6-11 *A schematic of a demand valve.*

tinuous flow of gas to the patient when they open. This continuous flow allows the patient to breathe spontaneously, without ventilator assistance (machine breaths or volumes).

A simplified demand valve is illustrated in Figure 6-11. When subambient pressure is communicated to the chamber of the demand valve, the diaphragm distorts, opening the valve. Gas then flows into the patient circuit until pressure in the chamber moves the diaphragm in the opposite direction, closing the valve.

Many ventilators incorporate demand valves which allow the ventilator to operate in Synchronized Intermittent Mandatory Ventilation (SIMV) and Continuous Positive Airway Pressure (CPAP) modes (refer to the "Modes of Ventilation" section in this chapter). The valves allow the ventilator to deliver gas flow in response to the patient's spontaneous efforts.

VENTILATOR CLASSIFICATION

Ventilator technology has evolved since the introduction of mechanical ventilators over thirty years ago. Since that time, a multitude of manufacturers have produced and marketed ventilators of all sizes, descriptions and capabilities. Many manufacturers have coined new terms to describe their ventilators and to accentuate how their product is different from the others. Several different ventilator classification systems may be employed to describe mechanical ventilators. The majority of these systems focus on the differences between ventilators rather than the similarities.

CHATBURN'S CLASSIFICATION SYSTEM

Robert Chatburn has proposed a new way to classify mechanical ventilators based upon related features, physics and engineering. Chatburn's ventilator classification system has been featured in several articles and textbooks. It allows flexibility, as ventilator technology evolves, in contrast to other systems that employ more narrowly defined design principles, or rely to a greater extent on manufacturer's terms.

As ventilator technology evolves over the next decade or more, the flexibility of Chatburn's classification system will be validated. Unfortunately today, not all practitioners, or educators, have adopted this newer classification system. This author feels the system is important enough that it should be included in this text and others which describe ventilator operational characteristics. A student learning about this classification system should refer to the bibliography at the conclusion of this chapter and read Chatburn's original contributions as well as this text.

VENTILATORY WORK

Pulmonary physiologists have described the work ventilatory muscles perform during inspiration and how muscles can actively assist during exhalation. During inspiration, the primary ventilatory muscles cause the size (volume) of the thoracic cage to increase, overcoming the elastic forces of the lungs and thorax, and the resistance of the airways. As the volume of the thoracic cage increases, intrapleural pressure becomes more negative, resulting in lung expansion as the visceral pleura expand with the parietal pleura. Gas flows from the atmosphere, into the lungs, as a result of the transairway pressure. During expiration, the muscles of inspiration relax. The elastic forces of the lung and thorax cause the chest to decrease in volume. Exhalation occurs as a result of the greater pressure at the alveolus when compared to atmospheric pressure. All of this muscle activity, to overcome the elastic and resistance properties of the lungs and thorax, requires energy and work.

The work that the muscles and/or the ventilator must perform is proportional to the pressure required for inspiration multiplied by the tidal volume. The pressure required to deliver the tidal volume is referred to as the "load" either the muscles or the ventilator must work against. There is an elastic load (proportional to volume and inversely proportional to compliance) and a resistance load (proportional to airway resistance and inspiratory flow). These variables are related by the equation of motion for the respiratory system:

Muscle Pressure + Ventilator Pressure = Volume\Compliance + (Resistance)(Flow)

Compliance is defined as a change in volume divided by a change in pressure, which is a measure of the elastic forces of the lungs and thorax. Flow, as defined earlier, is a unit of volume divided by a unit of time. Resistance is the force that must be overcome to move gas through the conducting airways, which is best described by Poiseuille's law.

A mechanical ventilator is simply a machine or device that can fully or partially substitute for the ventilatory work accomplished by the patient's muscles. If the patient's ventilatory muscles contribute no work (sedation, paralysis, etc.), the mechanical ventilator provides full ventilatory support. If the patient's muscles are able to sustain all of the patient's ventilatory requirements, no support is provided by the machine and ventilatory support is zero. Between the two extremes, partial support can be provided by the mechanical ventilator in assisting the ventilatory muscles.

INPUT POWER

Mechanical ventilators may be first classified as to the power source that is utilized to provide the energy required to support the patient's ventilation. As described earlier, ventilation requires work and therefore, energy.

Pneumatically powered ventilators use compressed gas as an energy source for their operation. Medical gases are anhydrous, and oil free at a pressure of 50 psi. Examples of ventilators that utilize pneumatic power include the Bennett PR-2, Bird Mark 7, Percussionaire IPV, Monaghan 225/SIMV and the Percussionaire VDR.

Ventilators may also be electrically powered, utilizing 120 volt, 60 Hz alternating current or 12 volt direct current for a power source. The electrical power can be used to run electric motors to drive pistons, compressors or other mechanical devices which generate gas flow. An example of an electrically powered ventilator include the Emerson 3-MV,

Aequitron Medical LP-10, Bear Medical Systems Bear 33, and the Puritan Bennett 2801 Companion.

A ventilator may also be powered by a combination of both pneumatic and electric power sources. Many third-generation ventilators require both an electrical (for microprocessor control systems) and a pneumatic power source. These ventilators include the Bear 1000, Hamilton Veolar, Puritan Bennett 7200ae and many other third-generation ventilators.

DRIVE MECHANISM

The drive mechanism is the system utilized by the ventilator to transmit or convert the input power to useful ventilatory work. The type of drive mechanism determines the characteristic flow and pressure patterns each ventilator produces. The use of microprocessors and proportional solenoid valves allows current generation ventilators to produce a variety of user selected inspiratory flow or pressure patterns. An understanding of the different drive mechanisms will allow you to apply a ventilator more effectively in the clinical environment. Drive mechanisms include pistons, bellows, reducing valves and pneumatic circuits.

Piston Drive Mechanism

An electrically driven piston, with an inspiratory one-way valve, can be used to generate a pressure gradient to drive a ventilator (Figure 6-12). During the back stroke of the piston, gas enters the cylinder through the one-way valve. When the piston travels in the opposite direction, a second one-way valve opens, delivering the compressed gas to the patient.

Pistons are usually electrically powered. However, they may be rotary or linear driven. Figure 6-13 compares a linear driven and a rotary driven piston. Output waveforms, which are discussed later in this chapter, vary depending upon how the piston is driven.

Bellows Drive Mechanism

Ventilators may also use a bellows to compress the gas for delivery to the patient (Figure 6-14). A bellows may be compressed by a spring, a weight or by gas pressure if it is in a sealed chamber. A one-way valve admits gas to the bellows expanding it. When it is compressed, the one-way valve closes, causing gas delivery to the patient.

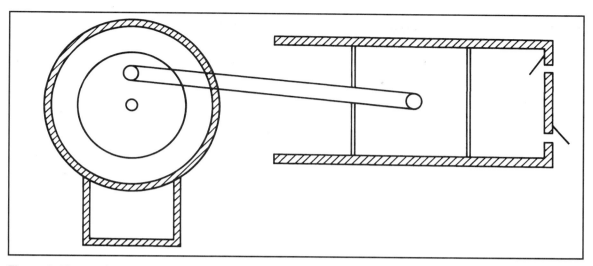

Figure 6-12 *A schematic diagram of a rotary driven piston drive mechanism for a mechanical ventilator.*

Reducing Valve Drive Mechanism

A reducing valve may be used to drive a ventilator providing enough of a pressure gradient to cause ventilation. The Bennett PR-2 is one example of a ventilator that uses a reducing valve. (The PR-2 and its drive mechanism were discussed in Chapter 3.)

Microprocessor-Controlled Pneumatic Drive Mechanisms

Although, technically speaking, both pistons and bellows are pneumatic systems, a separate classification is required for the newer ventilators, which use proportional solenoid valves and microprocessor controls. Current generation ventilators use programmed algorithms in the microprocessors to open and close the solenoid valves to mimic virtually any flow or pressure wave pattern. Furthermore, with advances in clinical medicine, the microprocessors can be reprogrammed to deliver new patterns that may not yet be described in the literature. Ventilator manufacturers, using microprocessors and the associated proportional solenoid valves, have a greater flexibility in designing and updating ventilator technology.

CONTROL CIRCUIT

The control circuit is the system that governs, or controls, the ventilator drive mecha-

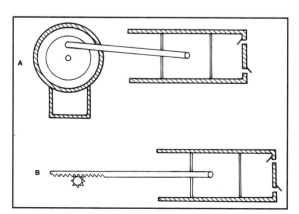

Figure 6-13 *A comparison between (A) a rotary driven piston and (B) a linear driven piston drive mechanism for a mechanical ventilator.*

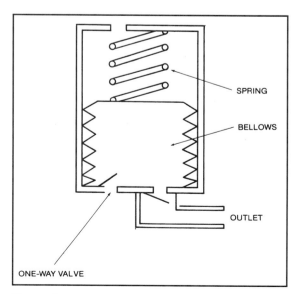

Figure 6-14 *A schematic diagram of a bellows drive mechanism for a mechanical ventilator.*

nism or output control valve. The control circuit is the system that is responsible for the characteristic output waveforms which will be discussed later in this chapter. Control circuits may be classified as open or closed loop control circuits, mechanical, pneumatic, fluidic, electric and electronic.

An open loop control circuit is one where the desired output is selected and the ventilator achieves the desired output without any further input from the clinician or the ventilator itself.

A closed loop control circuit is one where the desired output is selected and then the ventilator measures a specific parameter or variable (flow, pressure, or volume) continuously, and the input is constantly adjusted to match the desired output. This type of control circuit may also be referred to as servo controlled.

Mechanical

Mechanical control circuits employ simple machines such as levers, pulleys, or cams to control the drive mechanism. Early mechanical ventilators utilized these systems to control their outputs. Being mechanical, some of these control systems were very durable but lack flexibility by being an open loop type control system.

Pneumatic

Pneumatic devices can be utilized as control circuits. These devices include valves, nozzles, ducted ejectors, and diaphragms. The IPPB ventilators and the Percussionaire IPV and VDR ventilators all utilize pneumatic control circuits.

FLUIDICS

Fluidics is the application of gas flow and pressure to control the direction of other gas flows and to perform logic functions. As you will learn, moving gases can be used to alter the direction of another gas flow. The logic functions of fluidics have their origin in digital electronics. Fluidic elements, just like digital electronic gates, control their outputs according to the inputs received. By combining fluidic elements in a specific way, a ventilator can be designed that operates in ways similar to other ventilators that are electronically controlled. The Monaghan 225 is an example of a ventilator that is purely pneumatically powered and pneumatically controlled.

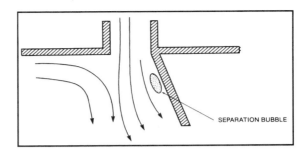

Figure 6-15 *A schematic illustrating the Coanda effect.*

Functional Characteristics of Fluidic Elements

Although control and logic operations differ among fluidic elements, all elements have certain similarities. These similarities include the *Coanda effect,* that the element is either mono- or bi-stable, and the way that the output may be described using a truth table.

Coanda Effect

If gas exits a jet at a high velocity adjacent to a wall (Figure 6-15), the gas flow will attach to one of the adjacent walls. This occurs because of the formation of a separation bubble. An area of reduced lateral pressure is formed around the fast moving gas. The separation bubble forms between the wall and the gas stream. Until the flow is interrupted or other forces cause it to be deflected, it will remain attached to the wall.

Fluidic elements use a flow splitter located beside adjacent walls to control the direction of flow and to perform logic functions (Figure 6-16). An element may either be mono-stable (attaching to one specific wall, unless acted upon) or bi-stable (having no preference for either wall).

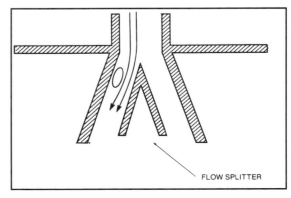

Figure 6-16 *A schematic diagram illustrating a fluidic flow splitter.*

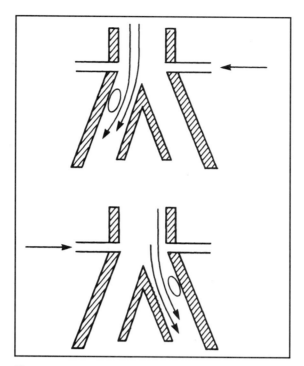

Figure 6-17 *A schematic diagram illustrating beam deflection as a result of a control input.*

The phenomenon of *beam deflection* occurs as a result of a control input. If a control signal (pressure) is applied at port C1 (Figure 6-17), the gas jet or beam will be deflected to the opposite channel or port 02. This of course will result in a change in the output of the device. If the device is bi-stable, the flow will remain attached to the new wall. If it is mono-stable, when the control signal is removed, it will reattach to the original wall.

Fluidic Nomenclature

As stated earlier, the nomenclature used to describe fluid elements has its roots in digital electronics. The terms used to describe a fluidic element and its truth table have a corresponding element with equivalent logic in an electrical component. The names may seem unusual for medical devices, but the technology first began with early work in digital electronics, specifically computer technology.

Truth tables are based on the fact that an electronic component has essentially two functions or positions. Like a light bulb it is either on or it is off. Electronic inputs control the output of these devices, turning them on or off. If a digital element is on, it is assigned a value of one in the truth table. If it is off, it is assigned a value of zero. Similar truth tables are constructed to describe the operation of fluidic ele-

ments. Boolean algebra and binary, hexadecimal and octal codes are used by engineers to combine elements to perform a useful function.

Operation and Logic of Fluidic Elements

In this section the operation of the fluidic elements, their truth tables, and the application of the element in ventilator design will be discussed. The elements include the flip-flop, and/nand, or/nor, back pressure switch, Schmidt trigger and the proportional amplifier.

Flip-Flop

The flip-flop element is a bi-stable device that may be applied as a control valve to control the phase of ventilation (inspiration or expiration). Figure 6-18 is a schematic of a flip-flop valve. Notice that the valve has two control inputs (C1 and C2). Application of a jet of gas to either port will cause the gas flow or beam to be deflected to the other opposite wall, causing a change of output to 01 or 02. Depending upon the control input, C1 or C2 will have a logic value of one. This is shown in the following truth table (Table 6-1). Since the element is bi-stable, it is said to have a memory. It will remain in the attached position (output 01 or 02), until a control input changes its position.

And/Nand

The and/nand gate is a mono-stable element with two control ports (Figure 6-19). The

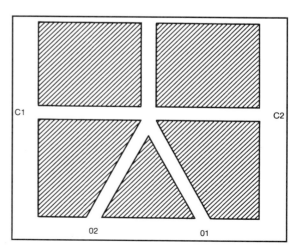

Figure 6-18 *A schematic diagram of a flip-flop fluidic element.*

TABLE 6-1 Flip Flop Truth Table

CONTROL PORTS		OUTPUT	
C1	C2	01	02
1	0	1	0
0	0	1	0
0	1	0	1
0	0	0	1

TABLE 6-2 And/Nand Truth Table

CONTROL PORTS		OUTPUT	
C1	C2	01	02
0	0	0	1
1	0	0	1
0	1	0	1
1	1	1	0

stable position or output for this element is 02. An application of a control signal to port C1 or C2 will not cause beam deflection. This is because the control signal simply exits the other control port. If a control signal is applied at both C1 and C2, then beam deflection will occur, resulting in the logic value of one at 01. The Monaghan ventilator uses these elements to power the mushroom exhalation valve in the ventilator circuit.

The truth table for the and/nand gate is shown in Table 6-2. As you can see by studying the truth table, a control input at both C1 and C2 is required to cause a change in the output logic from 02 to 01.

Or/Nor Gate

Like the and/nand gate, the or/nor gate is a mono-stable device. Unlike the and/nand gate, application of a control input at either C1 or C2 will cause beam deflection (Figure 6-20). In the Monaghan 225, the or/nor logic is com-

bined with other element outputs to control the exhalation valve in concert with the flip-flop element.

The truth table for an or/nor gate with two control inputs is shown in Table 6-3. As the table illustrates, application of a control signal at either control port or both results in a change from the mono-stable condition (output 02) to the output 01.

Back Pressure Switch

The back pressure switch is a mono-stable element that requires the diversion of some of the main gas flow powering it to cause the logic to change. A restriction distal to the control port channel causes some of the flow to be diverted (Figure 6-21). If the control port C1 is blocked, pressure builds because of a restriction between the outlet of the control port and the point where the beam is deflected. This restriction acts to amplify the diverted flow. When enough pressure builds, beam de-

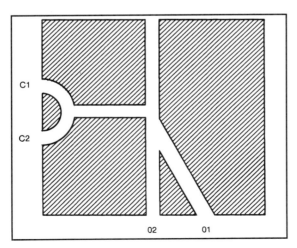

Figure 6-19 *A schematic diagram of an and/nand fluidic element.*

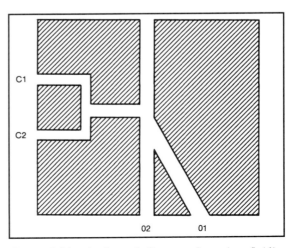

Figure 6-20 *A schematic diagram of an or/nor fluidic element.*

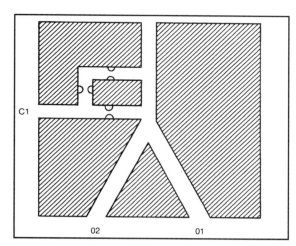

Figure 6-21 *A schematic diagram of a back pressure switch fluidic element.*

flection occurs, changing the output to 01. Blockage of the control port is usually electronically controlled rather than pneumatically controlled. The logic for this element is shown in Table 6-4.

By studying the table, you can see that only if the control port is blocked will the logic change from 02 to 01. Once the control port is opened again, the element resumes its output at 02.

Proportional Amplifier

A proportional amplifier is a device with two opposing control ports C1 and C2 (Figure 6-22). Gas can exit the element through both outputs 01 and 02 simultaneously. The signal strength from each control port determines where and how strong the output is. If the signal from C1 is greater than that from C2, 01 will have the greater portion of the flow passing through it. An advantage of the proportional amplifier is its ability to boost the control signal gain or level. Typically these de-

TABLE 6-4 Truth Table for the Back Pressure Switch

CONTROL PORT	OUTPUT	
C1	01	02
0	0	1
1	1	0

vices will boost the signal strength by a factor between five to seven times. If these devices are connected in series, signal strength may be amplified dramatically. For example, if three proportional amplifiers are connected in series, each having a gain of 5, total signal strength will be boosted 125 times ($5 \times 5 \times 5$)!

Schmidt Trigger

The Schmidt trigger is an element that is commonly used to sense negative or positive pressure changes. Although only one element is shown in Figure 6-23, it is actually composed of three proportional amplifiers and two flip-flop elements. If the inputs from the control ports C1 and C2 are equal, equal amounts of gas exit both 01 and 02. If the C2 signal becomes greater than the C1 signal, the logic changes to the 02 output and vice versa. The total output from the element is considered to be the difference between 01 and 02. The proportional amplifiers incorporated in this fluidically integrated circuit allow small pressure changes to be sensed and cause the original small signal to change the logic of the device.

TABLE 6-3 Or/Nor Truth Table

CONTROL PORTS		OUTPUT	
C1	C2	01	02
0	0	0	1
0	1	1	0
1	0	1	0
1	1	1	0

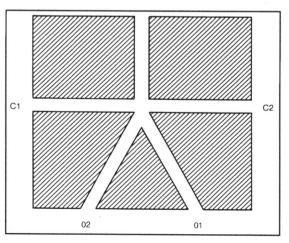

Figure 6-22 *A schematic diagram of a proportional amplifier fluidic element.*

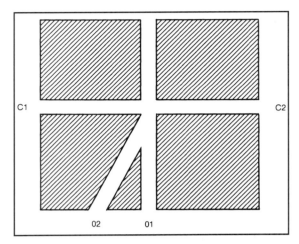

Figure 6-23 *A schematic diagram illustrating a Schmidt trigger fluidic element.*

Electric

Electric control circuits utilize simple switches to control the drive mechanism. Some home care ventilators control tidal volume delivery using electric switches to control the travel limit of the piston that drives the ventilator. The Emerson 3-MV ventilator uses two microswitches to control the inspiratory and expiratory time.

Electronic

Electronic devices such as resistors, diodes, transistors, integrated circuits and microprocessors can be used to provide sophisticated

levels of control over the drive mechanisms of contemporary ventilators. Electronic control systems provide greater flexibility but often at the expense of complexity.

CONTROL VARIABLES

When providing ventilatory support, the mechanical ventilator can control four primary variables during inspiration. These four variables are volume, pressure, flow and time. Figure 6-24 illustrates an algorithm which can be applied to determine which variable the ventilator is controlling.

Pressure Controller

A ventilator is classified as a pressure controller if the ventilator controls the transrespiratory system pressure (airway pressure minus body surface pressure). Further classification of a ventilator, as a positive or negative pressure ventilator, depends upon whether the airway pressure rises above baseline (positive) or body surface pressure is lowered below baseline (negative).

A positive pressure ventilator applies pressure inside the chest to expand it. This type of ventilator requires the use of a tight-fitting mask, or more commonly, an artificial airway. A pressure greater than atmospheric pressure is applied to the lungs, causing them to expand (Figure 6-25). Once positive pressure is no longer applied, the patient is allowed to exhale passively to ambient pressure. Exhalation

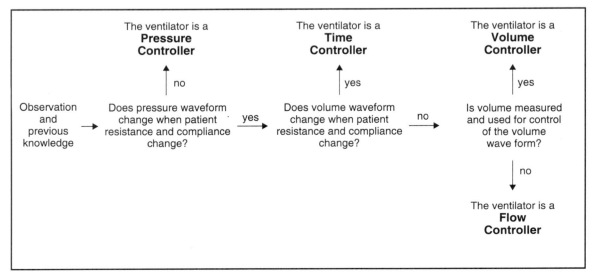

Figure 6-24 *Criteria for determining the control variable during a ventilator-assisted inspiration. (From R.L. Chatburn, Respiratory Care, Vol. 36, No. 10, 1991. Used by permission)*

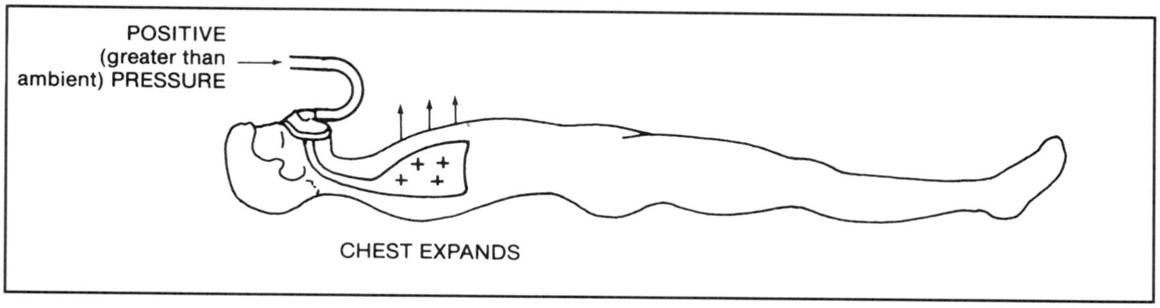

POSITIVE
(greater than
ambient) PRESSURE

CHEST EXPANDS

Figure 6-25   *A schematic diagram illustrating positive pressure ventilation.*

occurs because of the pressure differential between the lungs and the atmosphere and through the elastic recoil of the lungs and thorax. This is the type of ventilator most commonly used today.

Negative pressure ventilators apply subatmospheric pressure outside of the chest to inflate the lungs. The negative pressure causes the chest wall to expand, and the pressure difference between the lungs and the atmosphere causes air to flow into the lungs (Figure 6-26). Once negative pressure is no longer applied, the patient is allowed to exhale passively to ambient pressure. Positive pressure may also be applied to further assist the patient during exhalation.

Regardless of whether a ventilator is classified as positive or negative pressure, the lungs expand as a result of the positive transrespiratory system pressures generated. It is the transrespiratory pressure gradient that largely determines the depth or volume of inspiration. An ideal pressure controller is unaffected by changes in the patient's compliance or resistance. That is, the pressure level which is delivered to the patient will not vary in spite of changes in patient compliance or resistance.

Volume Controller

To be classified as a volume controller, volume must be measured and used as a feedback signal to control the output (volume) delivered. A volume controller allows pressure to vary with changes in resistance and compliance, while volume delivery remains constant.

Volume controllers can measure volume by the displacement of the piston, or bellows, which serves as the ventilator's drive mechanism. If the displacement of the bellows, or piston, is controlled, volume therefore is also controlled. Two examples of this type of ventilator, discussed later in the text, are the Bennett MA-1 and MA-2+2 and the Emerson 3-MV. The Bennett ventilators control bellows displacement while the Emerson 3-MV controls piston displacement. Another way to control volume is to measure flow and turn it into a volume signal electronically.

Flow Controllers

Flow controllers allow pressure to vary with changes in the patient's compliance and resistance while directly measuring and controlling flow. Flow may be measured by vortex sensors, heated wire grids, venturi pneumotachometers, strain gauge flow sensors and other devices. What is important is that the ventilator directly measures flow and uses the flow signal as a feedback signal to control its output.

Many ventilators are incorrectly classified

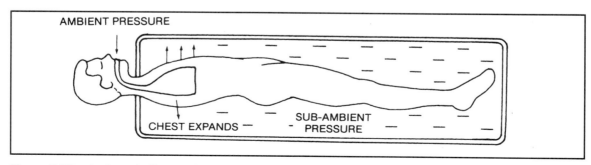

Figure 6-26   *A schematic diagram illustrating negative pressure ventilation.*

as "volume ventilators." Even though a tidal volume is set or displayed, many ventilators measure flow and then derive volume from the flow measurement (volume = flow × time). However, if a ventilator is operated in pressure support, or pressure control mode, the ventilator then becomes a pressure controller, since pressure is the variable which is measured and controlled.

Time Controllers

Time controllers are ventilators that measure and control inspiratory and expiratory time. These ventilators allow pressure and volume to vary with changes in pulmonary compliance and resistance. Since neither pressure nor volume is directly measured or used, as a control signal, time (inspiratory, expiratory or both) remains the only variable that may be controlled.

PHASE VARIABLES

A ventilator supported breath may be divided into four distinct phases; (1) the change from expiration to inspiration, (2) inspiration, (3) the change from inspiration to expiration, and (4) expiration. More detail can be learned by studying what occurs to the four variables (pressure, volume, flow, and time) during these phases. When the variable is examined during a particular phase, it is termed a phase variable.

Trigger Variable

The trigger variable is the variable which determines the start of inspiration (Figure 6-27). Pressure, volume, flow or time may be measured by the ventilator and used as a variable to initiate inspiration. Most ventilators use time or pressure as trigger variables.

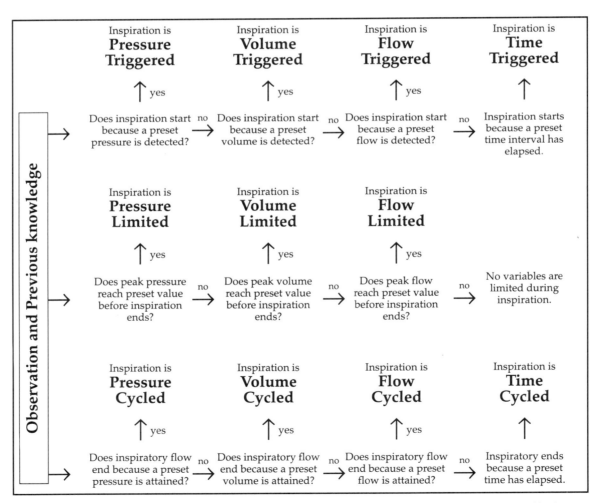

Figure 6-27 *Criteria for determining the phase variables during a ventilator-assisted breath. (From R.L. Chatburn, Respiratory Care, Vol. 36, No. 10, 1991. Used by permission)*

Some third-generation ventilators measure flow. When the patient's inspiratory flow reaches a specific value, a ventilator supported breath is delivered. Flow triggering has been shown to be more sensitive and responsive to a patient's efforts than pressure triggering.

One infant ventilator (Sechrist IV-100) uses inductive plethysmography to initiate a ventilator supported breath. When the infant's chest expands, a small electrical signal is generated between two chest leads, which is commonly used to monitor the infant's respiratory rate. The ventilator is interfaced to the respiratory rate monitor, and inspiratory triggering occurs when the signal is detected by the ventilator. This type of triggering is much faster and responsive than pressure or flow triggering, since it is directly measuring the infant's inspiratory efforts or excursions.

How hard the patient must work to initiate, or trigger, a breath is termed the ventilator sensitivity. If the ventilator is made more sensitive to the patient's efforts (pressure, flow, or volume), it is easier for the patient to trigger a breath. The converse, is also true.

Limit Variables

During a ventilator supported breath, volume, pressure and flow all rise above their respective baseline values. Inspiratory time is defined as the time interval between the start of inspiratory flow and the beginning of expiratory flow. If one or more variables (pressure, flow or volume), is not allowed to rise above a preset value during the inspiratory time, it is termed a limit variable. Note that in this definition, inspiration does not end when the variable reaches its preset value. The breath delivery continues, but the variable is held at the fixed, preset value. Figure 6-27 provides a useful algorithm for determining the limit variable during the inspiratory phase.

Cycle Variable

Inspiration ends when a specific variable (pressure, flow, volume or time) is reached. This variable must be measured by the ventilator and used as a feedback signal to end inspiratory flow delivery, which then allows exhalation to begin (Figure 6-27).

Again it is easy to make false assumptions regarding many ventilators by classifying them as volume cycled. Most newer ventilators measure flow, and are flow controllers.

Since flow is measured and used as a feedback signal for gas delivery, volume becomes a function of flow and time (volume = flow × time). Therefore, these ventilators are really time cycled, rather than "volume cycled." Inspiration ends because a preset time interval has passed, and volume has not been directly measured.

Baseline Variable

Expiratory time is defined as the interval between the start of expiratory flow and the beginning of inspiratory flow. This is also termed the expiratory phase. The variable which is controlled during the expiratory phase or expiratory time is termed the baseline variable. Most commonly, pressure is controlled during the expiratory phase.

Applications of Positive End Expiratory Pressure (PEEP) and Continuous Positive Airway Pressure (CPAP) are used to increase the Functional Residual Capacity (FRC), to improve gas distribution and oxygenation. These pressures, when applied during exhalation, maintain the lungs in a partially inflated state. This helps to prevent alveolar collapse, recruit previously collapsed alveoli and distend those alveoli which are already patent. PEEP and CPAP pressures must be titrated carefully, monitoring hemodynamic functions, blood gases or oximetry and compliance, to achieve the greatest benefit with the least amount of detrimental side effects.

Conditional Variable

Conditional variables are defined as patterns of variables which are controlled by the ventilator during the ventilatory cycle. Early ventilators such as the Puritan Bennett MA-1, used relatively simple conditional variables (volume cycled, pressure limited, pressure triggered, and PEEP). Newer third-generation microprocessor controlled ventilators, such as the Puritan Bennett 7200ae, are capable of delivering complex ventilatory patterns. Figure 6-28 summarizes the ventilator classification system as described to this point.

OUTPUT WAVEFORMS

Output waveforms are graphical representations of the control or phase variables in relation to time. Output waveforms are typically presented in the order of pressure, volume and flow. The ventilator determines the shape of the control variable, while the other two are

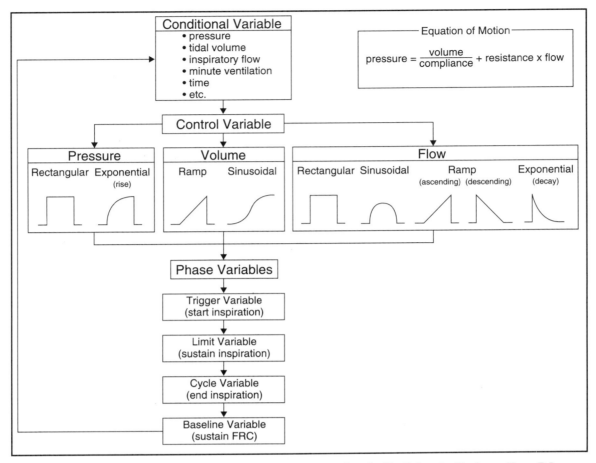

Figure 6-28 *A summary of the ventilator classification system as described by Robert L. Chatburn. (From R.L. Chatburn, Respiratory Care, Vol. 37, No. 9, 1992. Used by permission)*

dependent upon the patient's compliance and resistance. Convention dictates that flow values above the horizontal axis are inspiratory, while flow below the horizontal axis is expiratory. This corresponds to pressure and flow values rising above the horizontal axis for inspiration and falling back to the baseline during expiration. The ideal waveforms are represented in Figure 6-29.

Careful observation and assessment of waveforms during mechanical ventilation can provide useful information for the clinician. Waveforms can assist the clinician in the detection of inadvertent PEEP, the patient's ventilatory work, resistance and compliance changes as well as many other events or changes. Some ventilators are able to present pressure versus volume waveforms to assist in minimizing the patient's work of breathing. Still other manufacturers can present flow versus volume waveforms, to aid in the assessment of bronchodilator therapy during mechanical ventilation and the assessment of airway obstruction.

As waveforms become widely used, their usefulness will approach that of the electrocardiogram (ECG) tracing in the assessment of the heart.

Pressure Waveforms

Pressure waveforms include rectangular, exponential, sinusoidal and oscillating (Figure 6-30). Each of these waveforms would have these characteristic shapes, providing that pressure is the control variable. The descriptors used to describe each waveform is based upon their respective shapes.

The rectangular waveform is characterized by a near instantaneous rise to a peak pressure value which is held to the start of exhalation. During expiration, the pressure rapidly drops to baseline.

The exponential waveform is depicted by a more gradual increase in pressure when compared with the rectangular waveform. This type of waveform is common in some infant

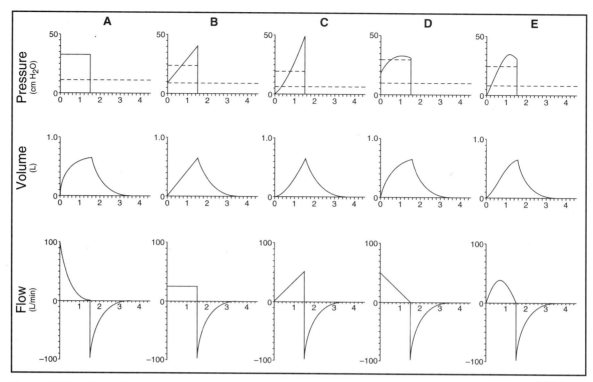

Figure 6-29 *Theoretical output waveforms for (A) pressure controlled inspiration with rectangular pressure waveform, identical to flow-controlled inspiration with an exponential-decay flow waveform; (B) flow-controlled inspiration with rectangular flow waveform, identical to volume-controlled inspiration with an ascending-ramp flow waveform; (C) flow-controlled inspiration with an ascending-ramp flow waveform; (D) flow-controlled inspiration with a descending-ramp flow waveform; and (E) flow-controlled inspiration with a sinusoidal flow waveform. The short dashed lines represent mean inspiration pressure, while the longer dashed lines denote mean airway pressure (assuming zero end-expiratory pressure). For the rectangular pressure waveform in (A), the mean inspiratory pressure is the same as the peak inspiratory pressure. These output waveforms were created by (1) defining the control waveform (e.g., an ascending-ramp flow waveform is specified as flow = constant × time) and specifying that tidal volume equals 644 mL (about 9 mL/kg for a normal adult); (2) specifying the desired values for resistance and compliance (for these waveforms, compliance = 20 mL/cm H₂O and resistance = 20 cm H₂O/L/sec, according to ANSI recommendations); (3) substituting the above information into the equation of motion; and (4) using a computer to solve the equation for pressure, volume and flow and plotting the results against time. (From R.L. Chatburn, Respiratory Care, Vol. 36, No. 10, 1991. Used by permission)*

ventilators and has become an option on some adult ventilators. Ventilator settings such as flow and inspiratory time regulate how steep the waveform rises toward peak inspiratory pressure.

The sinusoidal waveform resembles one half of a sine wave (the positive portion.). Sinusoidal waveforms are characteristically produced by ventilators having a rotary-driven piston drive mechanism (Figure 6-31). Ventilators using this drive mechanism include the Emerson 3-MV, Lifecare PLV-100, Bear 33, Puritan Bennett 2801 Companion and the Aequitron Medical LP-10.

The oscillating waveform is usually produced by a high frequency ventilator, such as the Infrasonics Star. The waveform is unique, in that negative (subambient) pressures may be generated if the average pressure, or mean pressure, is near zero (ambient).

Volume Waveforms

Volume waveforms can be classified into two types, (1) ascending ramp and (2) sinusoidal. The ascending ramp wave form is produced by a constant (i.e., rectangular) inspiratory flow pattern. The shape is characterized by a linear rise to the peak inspiratory pressure value. Sinusoidal volume waveforms are produced by ventilators that have a rotary-driven piston drive mechanism (Figure 6-32). Ventilators using this drive mechanism include the Emerson 3-MV, Lifecare PLV-100, Bear 33, Puritan Bennett 2801 Companion and the Aequitron Medical LP-10.

Flow Waveforms

The types of flow waveforms are shown in Figure 6-33. The waveforms include rectangular, ramp (ascending and descending) and sinusoidal.

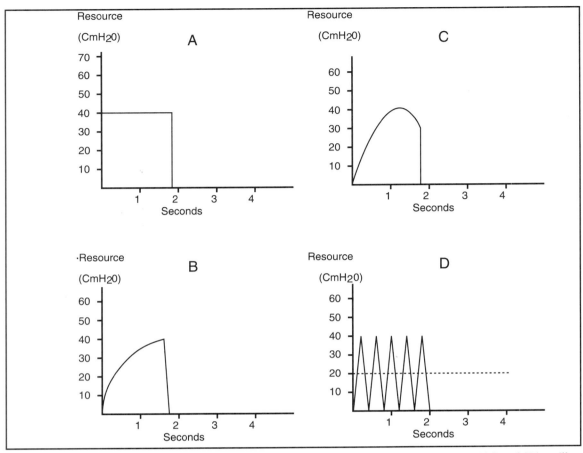

Figure 6-30 *The four types of pressure waveforms: (A) rectangular, (B) exponential, (C) sinusoidal, and (D) oscillating.*

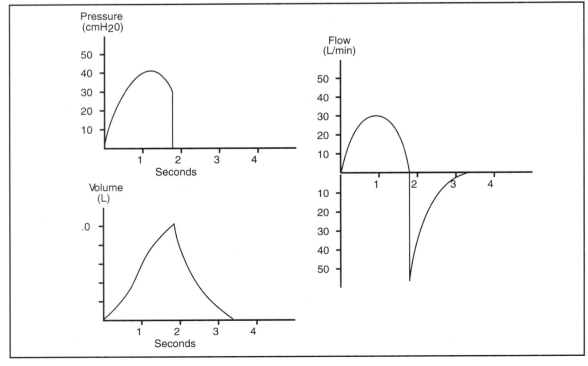

Figure 6-31 *The sinusoidal pressure waveform illustrated with the corresponding volume and flow waveforms. This type of pattern is typical of a rotary-driven piston drive mechanism.*

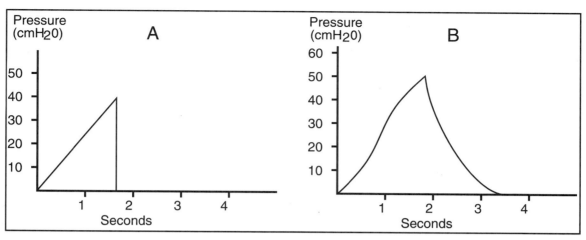

Figure 6-32 *The two types of volume waveforms: (A) ascending ramp and (B) sinusoidal.*

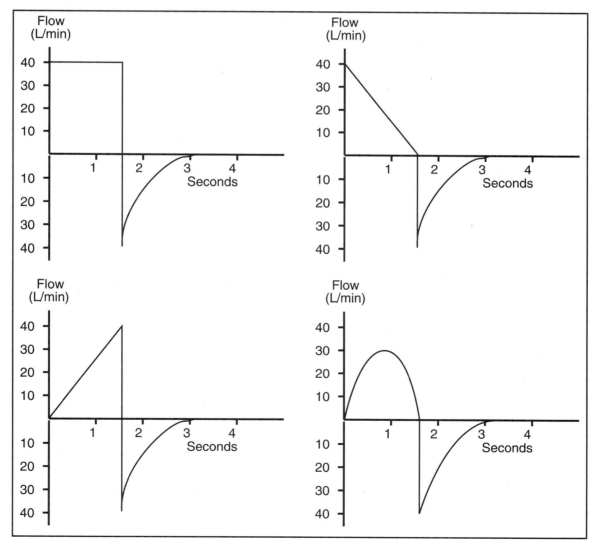

Figure 6-33 *The four types of flow waveforms: (A) rectangular, (B) ascending ramp, (C) descending ramp, and (D) sinusoidal.*

The rectangular waveform is produced when volume is the control variable and the output is an ascending ramp. The flow waveform (a derivative of the volume waveform with respect to time) assumes the characteristic rectangular shape.

The ramp waveform can either be ascending or descending (Figure 6-33). If flow rises as the breath is delivered, it is termed ascending ramp. If flow falls during the ventilator supported breath, it is called descending ramp.

The sinusoidal waveform, as described earlier and illustrated in Figure 6-32B, resembles the positive portion of a sine wave. It is generated by a rotary driven piston drive mechanism.

PATIENT CIRCUIT

The ventilator circuit may be classified as a single or double circuit. A single circuit is one in which the gas that drives the ventilator is the same gas that is delivered to the patient (Figure 6-34A). A double circuit uses an independent gas source in the drive mechanism, while a separate gas source is delivered to the patient (6-34B).

The patient's ventilator circuit also has an effect on the output of the ventilator during supported breaths. The circuit (tubing) has its own characteristic compliance and the gas, as it flows through the circuit, becomes compressed. Therefore, if one were to measure control or phase variables, or waveforms, at the airway, they would be different than if measured at the ventilator.

The volume delivered to the patient may be calculated from the following equation:

Volume delivery =

$$\frac{1}{1 + \dfrac{C_{pc}}{C_{rs}}} \text{ (volume setting on ventilator)}$$

where C_{pc} is the compliance of the patient circuit (tubing compliance) and C_{rs} is the compliance of the patient's lungs and thorax. As the compliance of the ventilator circuit increases when compared to the patient, volume delivery to the patient decreases.

Tubing compliance may be calculated using the following formula:

$$C_{pc} = \frac{V_{T\text{-set}}}{P_{plateau} - EEP}$$

where $V_{T\text{-set}}$ is the set tidal volume delivered through the ventilator circuit and $P_{plateau}$ is the plateau pressure and EEP is the end expiratory pressure.

Washout time refers to the time necessary for a change in F_IO_2 to stabilize at the patient's airway. For example, if a patient is being ventilated at an F_IO_2 of 0.30 and you change the F_IO_2 to 1.0 in order to hyperoxygenate before suctioning, it may take several minutes before 100% oxygen is delivered to the airway. Washout time depends upon the ventilator settings

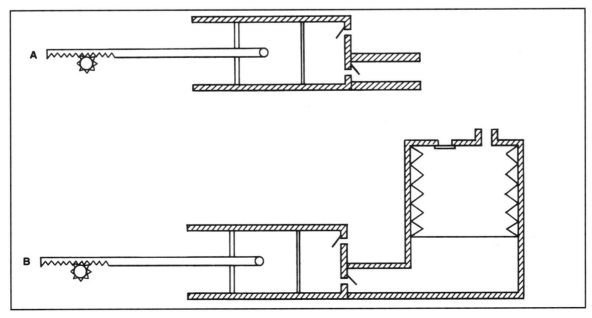

Figure 6-34 *A schematic representation of (A) a single and (B) a double circuit ventilator.*

(rate and tidal volume), length of the ventilator circuit, and whether or not the ventilator has a large internal volume (reservoir, accumulator, bellows, etc.).

Positive End Expiratory Pressure (PEEP)

As you recall from earlier in this chapter, PEEP is the application of positive pressure during the expiratory phase. Before ventilators were designed that incorporated PEEP systems into their circuitry, PEEP was added by placing a device on the expiratory limb of the patient circuit. These devices include water seals, water columns, Boeringer valves, and Downs' valves, and magnetic valves.

Water Column

A *water column* is the simplest and most easily understood PEEP device (Figure 6-35). A water seal consists of a large jar filled with water.

The expiratory limb of the circuit is immersed into the water to the desired level of PEEP. If 10 cmH$_2$O of PEEP is the clinical goal, the expiratory limb is submerged 10 cm below the level of the water. The patient, when exhaling, must first overcome the positive pressure from the water.

The advantages of this system are (1) simplicity and (2) cost. Disadvantages include (1) PEEP changes with evaporation, (2) personnel may spill the water, and (3) rapidly flowing gas splashes the water and creates a mess.

Water-Weighted Diaphragm

The Emerson water column is illustrated in Figure 6-36. The exhaled gas from the patient's circuit is directed against a diaphragm at the base of a water column. Water above the diaphragm provides the positive end expiratory pressure.

Advantages of this system include its

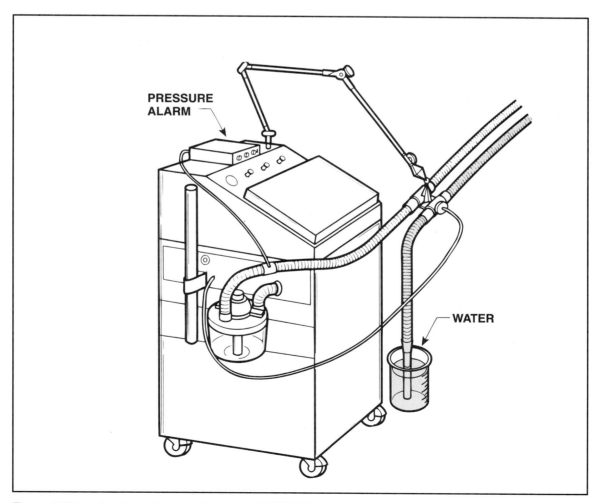

Figure 6-35 *A functional diagram of a water seal PEEP/CPAP system.*

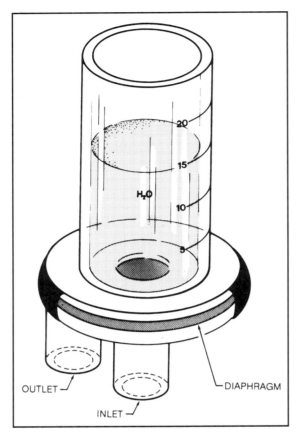

Figure 6-36 *A functional diagram of the Emerson Water Column PEEP/CPAP generator.*

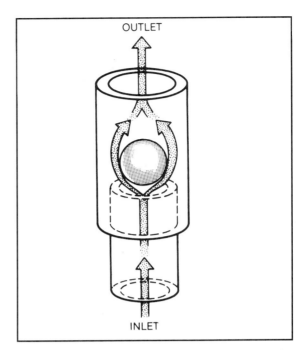

Figure 6-37 *A schematic drawing of a Boeringer valve PEEP/CPAP generation device.*

smaller size and the fact that exhaled gas passing through it does not cause water to splash. Problems due to evaporation are less due to the smaller surface area of the water column. The water column also may be mounted on the ventilator, so that the likelihood of water spills is lessened.

Boeringer Valves

Boeringer valves are specially designed valves with a weighted ball (Figure 6-37). The weight of the ball determines the PEEP level. When the valve is placed on the expiratory limb, the patient's exhaled gas must overcome the pressure exerted by gravity's attraction on the ball, creating the PEEP level.

Advantages include the lack of problems associated with a water type system and its compact size. The disadvantage is that PEEP pressures may be less than desired, or even lost entirely, if the valve is not absolutely vertical.

Downs' Valves

Downs' valves are one example of spring-loaded PEEP valves. The Downs' valve is a

fixed value PEEP valve. Other spring-type valves are adjustable. Figure 6-38 is an illustration of a Downs' valve. Exhaled gas passing the diaphragm must overcome spring tension, thus creating the PEEP. The Downs' valve has the advantage of being small, inexpensive and capable of being used in any position without altering PEEP levels.

Magnetic Valves

Magnetic valves utilize a permanent magnet and a ferrous metal diaphragm (Figure

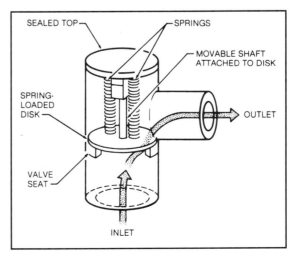

Figure 6-38 *A schematic of a Downs' CPAP/PEEP valve.*

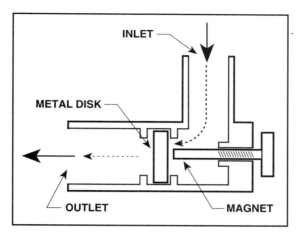

Figure 6-39 *A schematic drawing of a magnetic CPAP/PEEP valve.*

6-39). The threaded barrel of the valve allows the position of the magnet to change in relation to the diaphragm, varying the amount of magnetic attraction between them. As magnet attraction increases, more pressure must be generated to overcome it, increasing the positive pressure within the circuit, creating PEEP.

Intermittent Mandatory Ventilation (IMV) Systems

Long before current-generation ventilators offered SIMV as a feature, these systems were added externally to the ventilator circuits. The disadvantage of external IMV systems is that, since they are not synchronized with the patient, it is possible to deliver a mandatory breath following the patient's spontaneous breath (breath stacking). IMV systems may be divided into open and closed IMV systems.

Open IMV System

In this system, a blender or oxygen mixer powers a heated nebulizer (Figure 6-40). Gas from the nebulizer flows to an aerosol T (Brigg's adapter) and a reservoir of large-bore tubing open to the atmosphere (hence the open system name). Gas is then conducted to a one-way valve attached to the inspiratory limb of the patient circuit. When the patient inhales, the one-way valve opens in response to the pressure change and gas flows to the

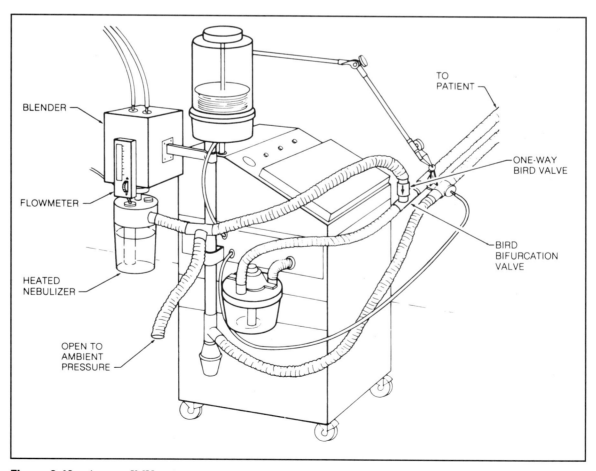

Figure 6-40 *An open IMV system.*

patient's lungs. During a mandatory breath, positive pressure closes the one-way valve, causing the breath to be delivered to the patient.

Closed IMV System

A closed IMV system is shown in Figure 6-41. This may also be referred to as an IMV "H" valve. An oxygen blender mixes air and oxygen to the desired F_IO_2 and the gas is conducted to a nipple that supplies flow to a 4 to 5 liter reservoir bag. Gas flows from the reservoir bag through a one-way valve to the ventilator's humidifier. The humidifier warms and humidifies the inspired gas going to the patient. When the patient initiates an inspiratory effort, the one-way valve opens in response to the pressure change, delivering gas. During a mandatory breath, the positive pressure in the ventilator circuit closes the one-way valve, causing gas from the ventilator to be delivered to the patient.

Continuous Positive Airway Pressure (CPAP) Systems

CPAP systems may be free standing or incorporated into the new generation's ventilator systems. A free-standing CPAP system is shown in Figure 6-42. The oxygen blender mixes the gases to the desired F_IO_2. Gas is then conducted through a humidifier (others may be substituted for the Cascade shown), which warms and humidifies it. The gas then is directed to two places: a reservoir bag and positive pressure device and the patient. The reservoir bag typically has a 3 to 5 liter capacity and provides a large reserve in the event the patient has an instantaneously high flow or volume demand. The positive pressure device may be any of the PEEP devices described earlier. The patient limb of the circuit consists of a Rudolph valve (Figure 6-43), which is a unidirectional valve composed of two one-way valves in series and another positive pressure PEEP device. It is important to note that the pressures of both PEEP devices must be

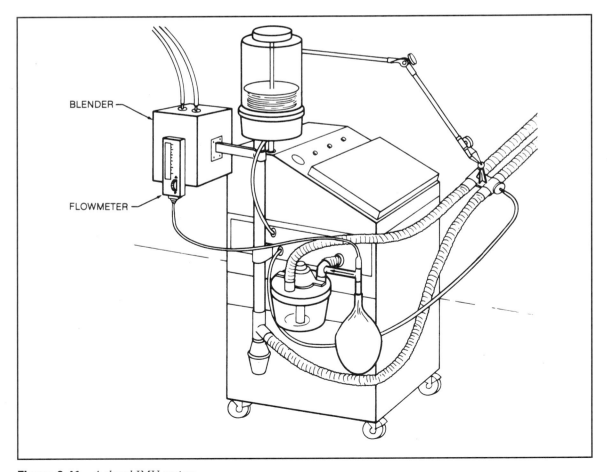

Figure 6-41 *A closed IMV system.*

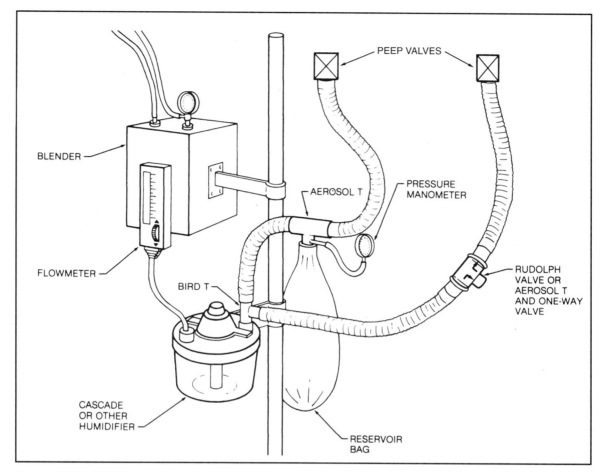

Figure 6-42 *A CPAP system.*

equal; otherwise a pressure differential will exist, resulting in undesirable gas flow.

CPAP with IMV

A circuit may be constructed to provide CPAP during the spontaneous ventilation portion of IMV and PEEP during the mandatory breaths (Figure 6-44). The CPAP side functions identically to the CPAP system described above. The gas from the CPAP system is deliv-ered to the inspiratory limb of the patient circuit through a one-way valve. The ventilator circuit incorporates a PEEP device on the expiratory limb of the circuit. Both the PEEP device and the CPAP pressure device must be of equal value.

When the patient inhales spontaneously, gas is drawn from the CPAP system at a pressure greater than ambient. During exhalation, the one-way valve closes, and the exhaled gas passes through the PEEP valve on the expira-

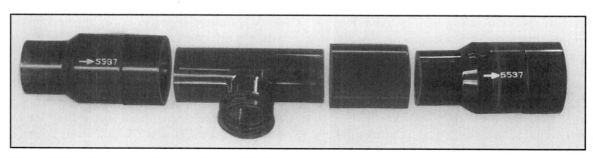

Figure 6-43 *A one-way valve assembly for a CPAP system.*

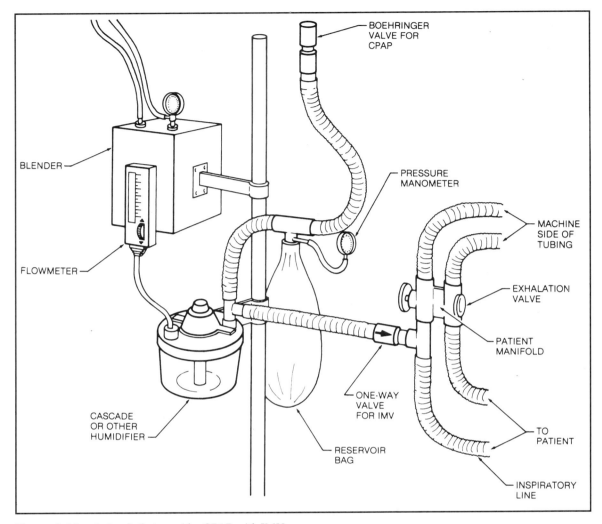

Figure 6-44 *A circuit that provides CPAP with IMV.*

tory limb, maintaining positive pressure. During the mandatory portion of the IMV, the system functions identically to a ventilator with a PEEP device added to the expiratory limb of the circuit.

ALARM SYSTEMS

Alarm systems are designed to alert the clinician to events. Day and MacIntyre have defined an event as any condition that requires clinician awareness or action. As the complexity of mechanical ventilators has increased, so have the number and complexity of the alarm systems. Technical events are those events limited to the performance of the ventilator, while patient events are those relating to the patient's condition. Alarms can be visual, audible or both, depending upon the seriousness of the event.

Input Power Alarms

Input power alarms can be further classified as to loss of electrical or pneumatic power.

Loss of electrical power usually results in the ventilator activating a backup alarm, which is battery powered. Most battery backup alarms are powered by rechargeable nickel cadmium batteries, which are recharged when alternating current power is available. When commercial power is lost, the backup batteries activate audible and visual alarms.

Loss of either air or oxygen pneumatic sources will result in a technical event alarm. If either input pressure falls below a specified value from 50 psi, the alarm will result. Some alarms are electronic (BEAR 1000, BEAR I, II and III, Puritan Bennett 7200ae), while others are pneumatic read alarms such as those employed in oxygen blenders.

Control Circuit Alarms

Control circuit alarms alert the clinician to settings or parameters that are not within acceptable ranges or specifications, or that the ventilator has failed some part of a self-diagnostic test. In the event of an incompatible setting or parameter, the clinician is allowed the opportunity to change the input to one that is compatible. A failure of a ventilator self-diagnostic test may render the ventilator inoperative, with a message displayed to the clinician indicating that failure has occurred.

Output Alarms

Output alarms can be further subdivided into pressure, volume, flow, time, inspiratory and expiratory gas.

Pressure alarms include high/low peak, mean and baseline airway pressures. High and low values may be set for each of these output parameters, to alert the clinician to changes in the patient's physiological status. Additionally, an alarm may be provided to detect failure of the airway pressure to return to the baseline valve. This could be caused by airway obstructions, circuit obstructions or ventilator malfunctions.

Volume alarms include high/low exhaled tidal volumes for both ventilator supported breaths and spontaneous breaths. Low volumes may result from sedation (spontaneous volumes), disconnection, or apnea (spontaneous volumes).

Flow alarms are limited to exhaled minute volume. High and low values may be set on some ventilators to alert the clinician to changes in the patient's minute ventilation.

Time alarms include high/low frequency or rate, excessive or inadequate inspiratory time, and excessive or inadequate expiratory time. High/low ventilatory rate alarms alert the clinician to changes in the patient's ventilatory rate. Inspiratory and expiratory time alarms may alert the practitioner to circuit obstructions or malfunctions, changes in gas distribution or inappropriate ventilator settings.

Inspired gas alarms alert the clinician to changes in oxygen concentration or gas temperature. Some ventilators incorporate an oxygen analyzer to detect changes in F_IO_2. High/low alarms alert the clinician to these changes. Inspired gas temperature may be controlled by a servo controlled humidifier or monitored by an independent ventilator temperature alarm. High/low temperature alarms can alert the clinician to changes in the inspiratory gas temperature.

Exhaled oxygen tension or end tidal carbon dioxide tension can be monitored and high/low alarms can be servoed to the exhaled gas monitoring system. These monitors can assist the clinician in determining the V_D/V_T, gas exchange and determining the respiratory exchange ratio (R).

MODES OF VENTILATION

Ventilators operate in different ways to provide support to patients in respiratory failure. Not all patients require full ventilatory support. The availability of different modes of ventilation allows the practitioner to adjust the level of support to meet a given patient's needs. The next section of this chapter will describe the various modes of mechanical ventilation and classify them according to the system described by Robert Chatburn.

Continuous Mandatory Ventilation (CMV)

As the name implies, continuous mandatory ventilation (CMV) supports a patient in respiratory failure (Figure 6-45). The ventilator determines when and how much gas is given. The ventilator initiates inspiration and the inspiratory phase is terminated based on volume, pressure, time or flow. In CMV, the patient is unable to initiate inspiration. All the patient's spontaneous efforts are ignored by the ventilator. This mode should only be used if a patient is apneic or if ventilation is suppressed by the use of drugs such as Pavulon. Any attempt to use control mode on a patient with spontaneous ventilator efforts may result in asynchronous ventilation and an increase in the work of breathing.

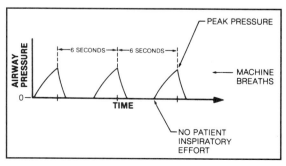

Figure 6-45 *A graphical representation of Continuous Mandatory Ventilation (CMV).*

CMV is only classified according to what occurs during the mandatory breaths, since no spontaneous ventilation is permitted. The control variables may be pressure, volume, or flow, the trigger variable is time, the limit variable may be pressure, volume or flow, the cycle variable may be time, pressure, volume or flow, and there are no conditional variables. Table 6-5 compares CMV with the other ventilator modes currently available.

Assist/Control

The *assist/control* allows the patient to initiate a breath (Figure 6-46). These ventilators have a sensitivity or assist system that will respond to the patient's inspiratory effort by opening the main solenoid valve, delivering a breath. If the patient fails to initiate a breath, the ventilator functions automatically as in CMV, and ventilates the patient. This backup rate guarantees that the patient will receive an adequate minute ventilation to support their physiological needs. Note that when pressure falls below baseline pressure, the ventilator initiates inspiration. Besides being pressure triggered as shown in Figure 6-46, this mode may also be volume or flow triggered, depending upon what ventilator is being used (manufacturer specific).

This mode of ventilation is only classified during mandatory portion, since spontaneous breathing without ventilatory support is not permitted. Control variables may be pressure, volume or flow. Trigger variables may be time, pressure, volume or flow. Limit variables may be pressure, volume or flow. Cycle variables may be time, pressure, volume or flow. Table 6-5 compares assist/control with other mechanical ventilation modes.

Assisted Mechanical Ventilation (AMV)

Assisted mechanical ventilation is a variation of assist/control in which there is no set respiratory rate. All breaths are patient-triggered, with pressure, flow, volume as the trigger variable. Since no breaths are guaranteed as in assist/control, the patient's respiratory drive must be intact or hypoventilation and hypercarbia will result.

This mode is classified in the following way. Control variables may be pressure, volume or flow. Trigger variables may be pressure, volume or flow. Cycle variables may be time, pressure, volume or flow. Table 6-5 compares the AMV classification with other ventilator modes.

Intermittent Mandatory Ventilation (IMV) and Synchronized Intermittent Mandatory Ventilation (SIMV)

IMV and SIMV will be considered together even though slight differences exist in the way each functions. Both IMV and SIMV modes allow the patient to breathe spontaneously between ventilator breaths (mandatory breaths). When spontaneously breathing, the patient determines his or her own rate and tidal volume (Figure 6-47). The ventilator rate or mandatory rate ensures that, should the patient fail to breathe enough, the ventilator will provide the ventilatory support needed.

Most newer models of ventilators functioning in the SIMV modes rely on demand valve systems to provide the gas flow required by the patient. The patient's spontaneous efforts open the demand valve and gas flows into the circuit to the patient.

When IMV was first described and used on adults, the circuit was added externally to the ventilator (this will be described later in the "Special Ventilatory Procedures" section). In

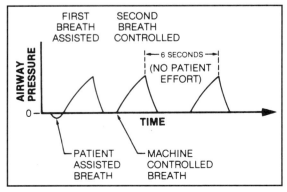

Figure 6-46 *A graphical representation of Assist/Control ventilation.*

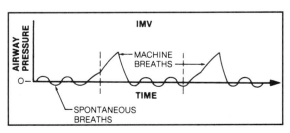

Figure 6-47 *A graphical representation of SIMV ventilation.*

this configuration, it is possible for the ventilator to deliver a breath after the patient has just taken one spontaneously. This is referred to as stacking breaths. Breath stacking results in unusually large tidal volumes and higher than normal peak airway pressures. However, research showed that most patients synchronized themselves with the ventilator.

SIMV eliminates breath stacking by synchronizing the mandatory breaths so that they are not delivered on top of a spontaneous breath. This is typically accomplished through the sensitivity controls of the ventilator. When a spontaneous effort is first sensed, the ventilator will deliver a mandatory breath.

Continuous Positive Airway Pressure (CPAP)

Continuous Positive Airway Pressure (CPAP) is the application of continuous positive pressure during both inspiration and expiration during spontaneous ventilation. The patient breathes at his/her own rate, tidal volume and frequency. CPAP pressures increase the patient's FRC, improving gas exchange. No ventilator (machine) support is provided in terms of guaranteed tidal volumes or respiratory rates. During CPAP, baseline pressure is always greater than ambient pressure (Figure 6-48).

Since CPAP is purely a spontaneous mode, only that portion is classified. The control variable is pressure (set CPAP pressure above ambient pressure). The trigger variable may be pressure, volume or flow. The limit variable and the cycle variable are both pressure (Table 6-5).

Pressure Controlled Ventilation (PCV)

Pressure Controlled Ventilation (PCV) is a form of continuous mandatory ventilation in which all breaths are pressure limited and time cycled. All ventilation is provided by the mechanical ventilator.

Pressure controlled ventilation may be provided during CMV as described above or also utilized in conjunction with IMV or SIMV. When employed in conjunction with these modes, the mandatory breaths (machine) are all pressure controlled, time triggered, pressure limited and time cycled. The spontaneous breaths are pressure controlled, pressure volume or flow triggered, pressure limited and

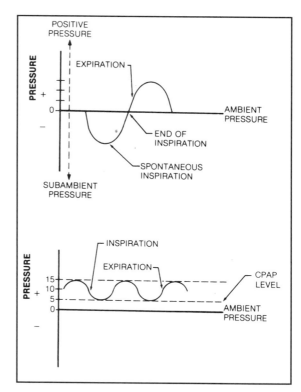

Figure 6-48 *A graphical representation of CPAP.*

pressure cycled. Table 6-5 compares the classification of PCV-IMV and PCV-SIMV with the other modes of ventilation.

Pressure Controlled, Inverse Ratio Ventilation (PCIRV)

Pressure Controlled, Inverse Ratio Ventilation (PCIRV) is a form of PCV in which no patient triggered breaths are permitted. Additionally, the inspiratory time is longer than the expiratory time (inverse ratio), resulting in I:E ratios varying between 4:1 and 1:1.1. The inverse I:E ratio results in gas trapping, which causes an increase in the baseline pressure above ambient pressure.

PCIRV is classified as a pressure controlled, time triggered, pressure limited, time cycled mode of ventilation (Table 6-5). The feature that distinguishes it from PCV is the inverse I:E ratio.

Airway Pressure Release Ventilation (APRV)

Airway Pressure Release Ventilation (APRV) combines two separate levels of CPAP pressures. The patient may breathe spontaneously from both CPAP levels. The higher CPAP level provides for volume aug-

Table 6-5 Expanded Classification of Modes of Ventilator Operation

MODE	MANDATORY BREATH				SPONTANEOUS BREATH					CONTROL LOGIC	
	CONTROL	TRIGGER	LIMIT	CYCLE	CONTROL	TRIGGER	LIMIT	CYCLE	SUPPORTED	CONDITIONAL VARIABLE	ACTION
CMV*	Pressure, volume, or flow	Time	Pressure, volume, or flow	Time, pressure, volume, or flow	—	—	—	—	—	—	—
A/C	Pressure, volume, or flow	Time, pressure, volume, or flow	Pressure, volume, or flow	Time, pressure, volume, or flow	—	—	—	—	—	Time or patient effort	Machine-to-patient triggered
AMV	Pressure, volume, or flow	Pressure, volume, or flow	Pressure, volume, or flow	Time, pressure, volume, or flow	—	—	—	—	—	—	—
IMV	Pressure, volume, or flow	Time	Pressure, volume, or flow	Time, pressure, volume, or flow	Pressure	Pressure, volume, or flow	Pressure	Pressure	No	—	—
SIMV	Pressure, volume, or flow	Time, pressure, volume, or flow	Pressure, volume, or flow	Time, pressure, volume, or flow	Pressure	Pressure, volume, or flow	Pressure	Pressure	No	Time or patient effort	Machine-to-patient triggered
CPAP	—	—	—	—	Pressure	Pressure, volume, or flow	Pressure	Pressure	No	—	—
PCV	Pressure	Time	Pressure	Time	—	—	—	—	—	—	—
PC-IMV	Pressure	Time	Pressure	Time	Pressure	Pressure, volume, or flow	Pressure	Pressure	No	—	—

(continues)

Table 6-5 Expanded Classification of Modes of Ventilator Operation (continued)

MODE	MANDATORY BREATH				SPONTANEOUS BREATH					CONTROL LOGIC	
	CONTROL	TRIGGER	LIMIT	CYCLE	CONTROL	TRIGGER	LIMIT	CYCLE	SUPPORTED	CONDITIONAL VARIABLE	ACTION
PC-SIMV	Pressure	Time, pressure, volume, or flow	Pressure	Time	Pressure	Pressure, volume, or flow	Pressure	Pressure	No	Time or patient effort	Machine-to-patient triggered
PCIRV	Pressure	Time	Pressure	Time	Pressure						
APRV	Pressure	Time or pressure	Pressure	Time	Pressure	Pressure, volume, or flow	Pressure	Pressure	No	Time or patient effort	Machine-to-patient triggered
PSV	—	—	—	—	Pressure	Pressure, volume, or flow	Pressure	Volume	Yes		
MMV	Volume or flow	Time	Volume or flow	Time, volume, or flow	Pressure	Pressure, volume, or flow	Pressure	Pressure or volume	Yes*	Minute ventilation, time	Spontaneous to-mandatory breath
VAPS	Flow	Time or pressure	Flow	Time or volume	Pressure	Pressure or flow	Pressure	Flow	Yes*	Tidal volume	Pressure-to-volume control
BiPAP	Pressure	Time	Pressure	Time	Pressure	Pressure	Pressure	Pressure	No	—	—

*CMV = continuous mandatory ventilation; NA = not applicable; A/C = assist/control; AMV = assisted mechanical ventilation; IMV = intermittent mandatory ventilation; SIMV = synchronized mandatory ventilation; CPAP = continuous positive airway pressure; PCV = pressure-controlled ventilation; PC-IMV = pressure-controlled IMV; PCIRV = PC inverse-ratio ventilation; APRV = airway pressure release ventilation; PSV = pressure support ventilation; MMV = mandatory minute ventilation; VAPS = volume-assisted pressure support; BiPAP = bilevel positive airway pressure.

Source: "Technical description and classification of modes of ventilator operation" by R. D. Branson and R. L. Chatburn, Respiratory Care, September 1992, Vol. 37, No. 9, p. 1029. (Copyright 1992 Daedalus Enterprises, Inc. Adapted with permission).

mentation during the patient's spontaneous breathing. Periodically, pressure is dropped to the lower CPAP level, reducing mean airway pressure. The expiratory time is kept short, to minimize the loss of FRC. Often, the I:E ratio is inverse as in PCIRV. The time spent at each different CPAP level is adjustable. In this mode, the mandatory (machine) breaths are those in which the pressure rises to the higher CPAP level.

Mandatory breaths in APRV are classified as Pressure controlled, time or pressure triggered, pressure limited and time cycled. The spontaneous breaths (lower CPAP level) are classified as pressured controlled, pressure, volume or flow triggered, pressure limited, and pressure cycled (Table 6-5).

BiPAP® (Bilevel Positive Airway Pressure)

BiPAP® is a trademark of Respironics, Inc. BiPAP® is another form of APRV except that pressure support (described later in this section) can be provided concurrently with the spontaneous ventilation. The clinician sets two pressure levels for BiPAP®, one pressure for inspiration—Inspiratory Positive Airway Pressure (IPAP)—and one for expiration—Expiratory Positive Airway Pressure (EPAP). If pressure support is delivered (mandatory breaths), they are time triggered and pressure limited.

BiPAP®'s mandatory breaths are classified as pressure controlled, time triggered, pressure limited and time cycled. The spontaneous breaths are pressure controlled, pressure triggered, pressure limited and pressure cycled (Table 6-5).

Pressure Support Ventilation (PSV)

Pressure support ventilation provides pressure augmentation during spontaneous breathing. The breath may be pressure, flow or volume triggered. Once triggered, a set pressure is delivered above baseline to augment the patient's spontaneous tidal volume. The breath ends when the delivered flow drops to a percentage of the peak inspiratory flow (typically 25%). The patient then determines their rate, inspiratory time and volume.

Pressure support is classified as pressure controlled, pressure, volume or flow triggered, pressure limited and volume cycled. Table 6-5 compares pressure support with other modes of ventilation.

Mandatory Minute Ventilation (MMV)

Mandatory Minute Ventilation (MMV) automatically adjusts minute ventilation based upon the patient's spontaneous ventilation. The practitioner selects the minute ventilation that is desired for the patient and adjusts the ventilator's tidal volume and flow to accomplish it. If the patient's spontaneous ventilation meets or exceeds the set mandatory ventilation, no supported breaths are delivered. If the patient's spontaneous ventilation falls below the set mandatory ventilation level, supported breaths are given by the ventilator to ensure that the desired minute ventilation is met (at the set tidal volume and flow rate). Some ventilators accomplish the MMV minute volume using pressure support rather than mandatory breaths. This mode is helpful during weaning, when a patient may become fatigued and not breathe enough spontaneously to sustain physiological needs.

MMV's mandatory breaths are classified as volume or flow controlled, time triggered, volume or flow limited, and time, volume or flow cycled. The spontaneous breaths are pressure controlled, pressure, volume or flow triggered, pressure limited and volume cycled. Table 6-5 compares MMV with the other modes of ventilation.

Volume Assisted Pressure Support (VAPS)

Volume Assisted Pressure Support (VAPS) is a form of pressure support that assures that the patient will receive a specific tidal volume during pressure supported breaths. If the patient's pressure supported volume falls below minimum tidal volume desired by the clinician, flow is held constant, allowing pressure to rise until the desired volume has been delivered.

With VAPS, a given breath may be either a flow-controlled, mandatory breath (i.e., flow limited and volume cycled) or a pressure-controlled, spontaneous breath (i.e., pressure limited, flow cycled) depending on the relative values of the ventilator settings (i.e., pressure limit, flow limit and tidal volume) and patient effort. Table 6-5 compares VAPS with the other modes of ventilation.

CLINICAL CORNER

Flow and Pressure Measurement Equipment

1. You are called to check a patient on a BEAR 2 ventilator. The low tidal volume alarm intermittently sounds while you are monitoring the patient. What could you check or do to correct the situation?

PEEP/CPAP and IMV Equipment

1. The ventilator your home care company uses does not have provisions for PEEP. How can you set up the ventilator to provide the 10 cmH₂O PEEP the patient needs?
2. You need to supply PEEP for an intubated patient with a self-inflating manual resuscitator while you transport the patient from CT to the ICU. How will you do this using a manual resuscitator?
3. You need to provide IMV for a patient's home care ventilator. The ventilator does not have IMV as a built-in feature. How can you provide it?

Self-Assessment Quiz

1. Poiseuille's law is significant in mechanical ventilation and affects:
   I. Gas flow through artificial airways.
   II. Gas flow through patient circuits.
   III. Driving pressure.
   IV. Resistance.
   a. I only
   b. I and II
   c. I and III
   d. II and III
   e. I, II, III, and IV

2. Strain gauge pressure transducers may be used to measure:
   I. Circuit pressures.
   II. Blood pressure.
   III. Central venous pressure.
   IV. Intracranial pressure.
   a. I only
   b. I and II
   c. II and III
   d. I, II and III
   e. I, II, III, and IV

3. A vortex shedding spirometer measures flow by using:
   a. A differential pressure transducer.
   b. A strain gauge.
   c. A venturi tube.
   d. Ultrasonic waves.
   e. A resistive element.

4. In contrast to a solenoid valve, a proportional solenoid valve:
   I. Is either open or closed.
   II. Easily responds to patient effort.
   III. Opens in discrete intervals.
   IV. Is often under microprocessor control.

a. I only
b. I and II
c. II and III
d. I, III, and IV
e. III and IV

5. *Ventilator drive mechanism* refers to:
   a. The power source for the ventilator.
   b. The system used to convert the input power to ventilatory work.
   c. The system used to control rate and tidal volume.
   d. The gas pressure powering the ventilator.
   e. The controls on the ventilator.

6. Physics defines work as force times distance. The equivalent ventilatory work performed by the muscles of inspiration is:
   a. Volume divided by compliance plus resistance times flow.
   b. Pressure times compliance.
   c. Pressure times volume.
   d. Resistance times compliance.

7. If a ventilator is a volume controller:
   I. A constant volume is delivered each breath.
   II. Volume must be measured.
   III. Flow is measured and used to control flow waveform.
   IV. The breath ends when a preset time is reached.
   a. I
   b. I and II
   c. I and III
   d. III and IV

8. A cycling variable is:
   a. The variable measured and used to begin inspiration.
   b. The variable measured and used to end inspiration.
   c. The variable measured and used to control inspiration.
   d. The variable measured and used during expiration.

9. A trigger variable is:
   a. The variable measured and used to begin inspiration.
   b. The variable measured and used to end inspiration.
   c. The variable measured and used to control inspiration.
   d. The variable measured and used during expiration.

10. Which of the following can be control variables?
    I. Pressure.
    II. Volume.
    III. Flow.
    IV. Time.
    a. I
    b. I and II
    c. I, II and III
    d. I, II, III and IV

11. Which of the following can be trigger variables?
    I. Pressure.
    II. Volume.
    III. Flow.
    IV. Time.
    a. I
    b. I and II
    c. I, II and III
    d. I, II, III and IV

12. The difference between a limit variable and a cycle variable is:
    I. Inspiration does not end when the limit is met.
    II. The limit variable is not allowed to rise above a preset level.
    III. Inspiration ends and an alarm sounds.
    IV. The variable is only measured during expiration.
    a. I
    b. I and II
    c. II and III
    d. III and IV

13. Expiratory time is defined as:
    a. The time between the start of inspiratory flow to the start of expiratory flow.
    b. The time between the start of expiratory flow and the start of inspiratory flow.
    c. The ratio of inspiratory to expiratory time.
    d. The time when baseline pressure is zero.

14. Types of pressure waveforms include:
    I. Rectangular.
    II. Exponential.
    III. Sinusoidal.
    IV. Oscillating.
    a. I
    b. I and II
    c. I, II, and III
    d. I, II, III and IV

15. Types of flow waveforms include:
    I. Rectangular.
    II. Ramp.
    III. Sinusoidal.
    IV. Oscillating.
    a. I
    b. I and II
    c. I, II, and III
    d. I, II, III and IV

16. Ventilator washout time refers to:
    a. The time required clean the ventilator following use.
    b. The time it takes gas to flow through the circuit.
    c. The amount of time before an F_iO_2 change reaches a stable value.
    d. The time necessary to exhale the tidal volume.

17. A single circuit ventilator:
    a. Has one gas source which drives the ventilator and is delivered to the patient.
    b. Has only one tube from the ventialtor to the patient.
    c. Uses one exhalation valve.
    d. Takes less time to clean than a double circuit ventilator.

18. Which of the following are PEEP devices?
    I. Downs' valve.
    II. Water column.
    III. Magnetic valve.
    IV. Boeringer valve.
    a. I
    b. I and II
    c. I, II and III
    d. I, II, III and IV

19. Input power alarms include:
    I. Loss of electrical power.
    II. Failure of a self-diagnostic test.
    III. Loss of pneumatic power.
    IV. Low delivered tidal volume.

a. I and II
b. I and III
c. II and III
d. III and IV

20. Output alarms include:
    I. Failure of self-diagnostic test.
    II. Low delivered tidal volume.
    III. Loss of pneumatic power.
    IV. Flow alarms.
    a. I and II
    b. II and III
    c. II and IV
    d. III and IV

21. Which of the following are true regarding Pressure Controlled Ventilation (PCV)?
    I. Can be employed during CMV, IMV or SIMV.
    II. Pressure is the control variable.
    III. Pressure is the limit variable.
    IV. Volume or flow may be the trigger variable.
    a. I
    b. I and II
    c. I, II, and III
    d. I, II, III and IV

22. Which of the following are true regarding CPAP?
    I. Pressure is the control variable.
    II. Pressure or flow may be the trigger variable.
    III. Pressure is the limit variable.
    IV. Pressure is the cycle variable.
    a. I
    b. I and II
    c. I, II and III
    d. I, II, III and IV

23. A mode of ventilation that allows spontaneous breathing but guarantees a minimum minute ventilation is:
    a. CMV.
    b. Assist/control.
    c. SIMV.
    d. Pressure support.
    e. MMV.

24. A mode of ventilation that augments spontaneous ventilation with a constant positive pressure is:
    a. CMV.
    b. Assist/control.
    c. SIMV.
    d. Pressure support.
    e. MMV.

25. A mode of ventilation that delivers mandatory breaths irrespective of patient effort is:
    a. CMV.
    b. Assist/control.
    c. SIMV.
    d. Pressure support.
    e. MMV.

26. Fluidic logic operates using:
    a. Bernoulli's principle.
    b. Venturi's principle.
    c. The Coanda effect.

    d. Electronic elements.

    e. Volume displacement.

27. A fluidic element commonly used to control the cycling of a ventilator between inspiration and expiration is:

    a. A back pressure switch.

    b. A flip/flop.

    c. A Schmidt trigger.

    d. An or/nor.

    e. An and/nand.

28. A fluidic element often used to sense a patient's inspiratory effort is:

    a. A back pressure switch.

    b. A flip/flop.

    c. A Schmidt trigger.

    d. An or/nor.

    e. An and/nand.

29. Truth tables are used to:

    a. Describe the logic of the fluidic element.

    b. Determine a component's stable state.

    c. Determine when it is off.

    d. Combine one element with another.

    e. All of the above.

30. What fluidic element does the Sechrist IV-100B use to initiate inspiration?

    a. A back pressure switch.

    b. A flip-flop.

    c. A Schmidt trigger.

    d. An or/nor.

    e. An and/nand.

Selected Bibliography

Aequitron Medical, Inc., *LP-6 Volume Ventilator Reference Manual*, Minneapolis, MN, 1987.

Albert, Richard K., "Non-Respiratory Effects of Positive End-Expiratory Pressure," *Respiratory Care*, Vol. 33, No. 6, pp. 464–471, 1988.

Banner, Michael J., "Expiratory Positive-Pressure Valves: Flow Resistance and Work of Breathing," *Respiratory Care*, Vol. 32, No. 6, pp. 431-439, 1987.

Bear Medical Systems, *Bear 33 Volume Ventilator Clinical Instruction Manual, Part Number 50000-10133*, Riverside, CA, 1984.

Bear Medical Systems, *Instruction Manual, Bear 5*, P/N 50000-10700, Riverside, CA, 1983.

Bear Medical Systems, *Instruction Manual, Bourns Adult Volume Ventilator (Bear I)*, P/N 5000-10500, Riverside, CA, 1977.

Bear Medical Systems, *Instruction Manual, Bourns Infant Pressure Ventilator* (Model BP 200), P/N 50000-10200, Riverside, CA.

Bird Products Corporation, *V.I.P. Bird Infant-Pediatric Ventilator Instruction Manual, Part Number L1194*, Palm Springs, CA, 1991.

Branson, Richard D., and Chatburn, Robert L., "Technical Description and Classification of Modes of Ventilator Operation," *Respiratory Care*, Vol. 37, No. 9, pp. 1026–1044, 1992.

Chatburn, Robert L., "A New System for Understanding Mechanical Ventilators," *Respiratory Care*, Vol. 36, No. 10, pp. 1123–1155, 1991.

Chatburn, Robert L., "Classification of Mechanical Ventilators," *Respiratory Care*, Vol. 37, No. 9, pp. 1009–1025, 1992.

Corning Fluidic Products, *Fluidic Industrial Control Modules*, P/N EPD EBR-3, Corning, NY, 1971.

Demers, Robert, et al., "Use of the Concept of Ventilator Compliance in the Determination of Static Total Compliance," *Respiratory Care*, Vol. 26, No. 7, pp. 664–648, 1981.

Dupuis, Yvon, *Ventilators: Theory and Clinical Application*, 2nd Ed., C. V. Mosby Company, 1992.

East, Thomas D., "What Makes Noninvasive Monitoring Tick? A Review of Basic Engineering Principles," *Respiratory Care*, Vol. 35, No. 6, pp. 500–519, 1990.

Eubanks, David H., and Roger C. Bone, *Comprehensive Respiratory Care*, C. V. Mosby Company, 1985.

Gambro Engstrom, *Engstrom Erica Reference Manual*, P/N 56-10937-32, Bromma, Sweden, 1984.

Henry, William C., et al., "A Comparison of the Oxygen Cost of Breathing between a Continuous-Flow CPAP System and a Demand-Flow CPAP System," *Respiratory Care*, Vol. 28, No. 10, pp. 1273–1281, 1983.

Kacmarek, Robert M., et al., "Technical Aspects of Positive End-Expiratory Pressure (PEEP): Part I. Physics of PEEP Devices," *Respiratory Care*, Vol. 27, No. 12, pp. 1479–1489, 1982.

Lifecare, *Lifecare PLV-100 Operating Manual*, Lafayette, CO, 1985.

Maxwell, Christopher, et al., "A Modification of the Bennett MA-1 Ventilator to Permit On-Demand Flow and Exhaled Volume Monitoring during Continuous Flow IMV with PEEP," *Respiratory Care*, Vol. 25, No. 9, pp. 941–943, 1980.

McPherson, S., *Respiratory Home Care Equipment*, Daedalus Enterprises, Inc., 1988.

McPherson, S., *Respiratory Therapy Equipment*, C. V. Mosby Company, 1985.

Monaghan, *Fluidics and Monaghan Volume Ventilators*, P/N 66007-02, Littleton, CO, 1976.

Monaghan, *Monaghan 225 Volume Ventilator Operator's Manual: Questions and Answers*, 13929-01 5m, Littleton, CO, 1975.

Pierson, David J., "Maximum Ventilatory Capabilities of Four Current-Generation Mechanical Ventilators," *Respiratory Care*, Vol. 31, No. 11, pp. 1054–1058, 1986.

Puritan Bennett Corporation, *Companion 2800 Portable Volume Ventilator Clinician Guide*, Boulder, CO, 1986.

Puritan Bennett Corporation, *7200 Microprocessor Ventilator Operator's Manual*, 31002, Santa Monica, CA, 1984.

Puritan Bennett Corporation, *Supplementary 7200a Microprocessor Ventilator Operator's Manual*, 20268, Santa Monica, CA, 1985.

Sassoon, Catherine S. H., "Inspiratory Work of Breathing on Flow-By and Demand-Flow Continuous Positive Airway Pressure," *Critical Care Medicine*, Vol. 17, No. 11, pp. 1108–1114, 1989.

Sechrist Industries, Inc., *Operational Instructions and Routine Maintenance, Infant Ventilator Model IV-100B*, P/N 100006, Anaheim, CA, 1986.

Siemens-Elema, *Servo Ventilator 900C Operating Manual*, P/N 69 78 761 E313E, Solona, Sweden, 1984.

Siemens-Elema, *Servo Ventilator Training Instructions*, P/N 69 79 066 E315E, Solona, Sweden, 1982.

Smith, Richard K., "Respiratory Applications of Fluidics," *Respiratory Therapy*, Vol. 3, No. 3, pp. 29–32, 1973.

Spearman, Charles B., et al., "The New Generation of Mechanical Ventilators," *Respiratory Care*, Vol. 32, No. 6, pp. 403–418, 1987.

Stock, M. Christine, and John B. Downs, "Airway Pressure Release Ventilation: A New Approach to Ventilatory Support during Acute Lung Injury," *Respiratory Care*, Vol. 32, No. 7, pp. 517–524, 1987.

Stoller, James K., "Respiratory Effects of Positive End-Expiratory Pressure," *Respiratory Care*, Vol. 33, No. 6, pp. 454–463, 1988.

CHAPTER 7

ADULT ACUTE CARE VENTILATORS: VENTILATORS HAVING VOLUME AS A CONTROL VARIABLE

INTRODUCTION

Chapter 6 described the ventilator classification system developed by Robert Chatburn. According to the classification system, ventilators can be classified according to their input power, drive mechanism (power conversion or transmission), control scheme, output, and alarm systems. In this chapter and the remaining chapters, the control variable has been chosen as a means to distinguish ventilators from one another as well as to group ventilators with common traits together.

Use of the input power and drive mechanism can be quite broad and all encompassing. Using these criteria for classification would include too many ventilators in one particular group and not allow sufficient differences to distinguish one from another. The same would be true by using output or alarm systems as a means to classify the various ventilators.

Classifying ventilators by their control variable will group smaller numbers of ventilators together while allowing sufficient detail to be added to the phase variables, output, and alarm systems to distinguish one ventilator from another's capabilities and control circuitry.

OBJECTIVES

After completing this chapter, the student will be able to accomplish the following objectives:

- Explain what is meant by the control variable and how specifically a ventilator can be classified as having volume as a control variable.
- For the ventilators described in this chapter, apply Chatburn's classification system and classify them according to:

— Input power
— Drive mechanism
— Control scheme
— Output
— Alarm systems
- Describe how to assemble and troubleshoot the following ventilators:
— Emerson 3MV-IMV
— Monaghan 225/SIMV
— Puritan Bennett MA-1 and MA-2+2

THE CONTROL VARIABLE

During a ventilator-supported breath, a mechanical ventilator can control one of the following variables: pressure, volume, flow or time. In order for a ventilator to be classified as controlling one of these variables, two conditions must be met. First that variable must be measured and second it must be used as feedback to control the ventilator's output. Therefore, for a ventilator to be classified as a volume controller, volume must be measured and used as feedback to control the ventilator's output.

EMERSON 3MV-IMV VENTILATOR

Power Input

The Emerson 3MV-IMV ventilator is electrically powered, using 120 volt, 60 Hz alternating current as a power source (Figure 7-1). The electrical power provides energy to drive the motor and piston (drive mechanism) and also to power the control circuitry.

The gas supply system consists of two Thorpe tube flowmeters (air and oxygen) that are adjusted using two needle valves (mixing valve). Gas flows from the mixing valve to two 5 liter reservoir bags. One bag supplies gas to the piston (left-hand bag), and the other supplies gas to the patient during spontaneous ventilation (right-hand bag). During spontaneous ventilation, the 3MV-IMV ventilator provides a continuous gas flow.

The humidification system consists of a simple heated passover humidifier (a modified pressure cooker) and a tube filled with copper mesh. The copper mesh inhibits bacterial growth in the tubing. Humidity is absorbed by evaporation, and the heating element improves efficiency. A humidifier control varies the current applied to the humidifier heater, using a simple rheostat.

Drive Mechanism

The 3MV-IMV ventilator employs a rotary-driven piston drive mechanism. (Rotary-driven piston drive mechanisms were discussed in Chapter 6.) Adjustment of the tidal volume is performed by rotating a handwheel on the upper right-hand side of the ventilator (Figure 7-1). Rotating the handwheel accomplishes two tasks. The first is that the piston's connecting rod is moved closer to, or farther from, the pivot point in the drive mechanism. The closer the connecting rod is to the pivot point, the lower the stroke volume of the piston will be. The farther the connecting rod is from the pivot point, the greater the tidal volume delivery will be. Tidal volume ranges from 0 to 2000 mL. The second task is that the tidal volume display indicator moves, showing the change in volume.

Control Circuit

The control circuit on the 3MV-IMV is both electrical and mechanical. The mechanical por-

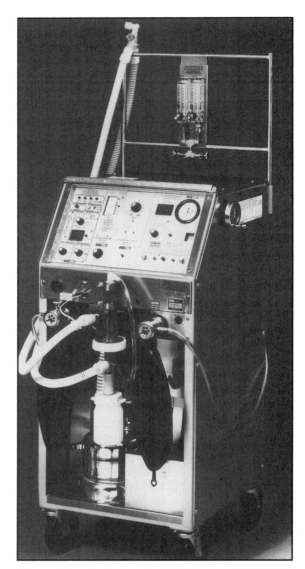

Figure 7-1 *A photograph of the Emerson 3MV-IMV ventilator. (Courtesy of J. H. Emerson Company, Cambridge, MA)*

tion consists of the variable pivot point, controlling tidal volume delivery as described earlier.

Respiratory rate is controlled by using two respiratory rate controls. One control establishes the total cycle time for each breath (inspiratory time + expiratory time), while the other sets only the inspiratory time.

The total cycle time control is a thumb wheel located adjacent to the pressure manometer (Figure 7-1). Adjusting the thumb wheel sets the desired cycle time for each mandatory breath rate. For example, setting the control to 3.0 seconds would establish a mandatory rate of 20 breaths per minute (60 seconds / 3.0 seconds = 20).

The inspiratory time control establishes the speed of the motor, which controls the speed of the piston. Settings are available from one to five seconds. The expiratory time is the difference between the total cycle time and the inspiratory time (total cycle time – inspiratory time = expiratory time). Two microswitches control when the inspiratory time setting is active (Figure 7-2A).

Control Variables

The Emerson 3MV-IMV ventilator is a volume controller when the pressure limit is not reached during the inspiratory phase. If the pressure limit is reached, the pop off valve opens (Figure 7-2B), venting excess pressure to the atmosphere. When the pop off valve

opens, the ventilator is a pressure controller rather than a volume controller.

Phase Variables
Trigger Variable

The trigger variable used by the Emerson 3MV-IMV is time. As described earlier, total cycle time and inspiratory time are adjusted by the practitioner. Inspiratory times may be adjusted between 1 and 5 seconds, and cycle times can be adjusted between 2.3 seconds and 5 minutes. This gives a respiratory rate range of 1 breath every 5 minutes to 26 breaths per minute.

An optional pediatric control module may be added to provide increased respiratory

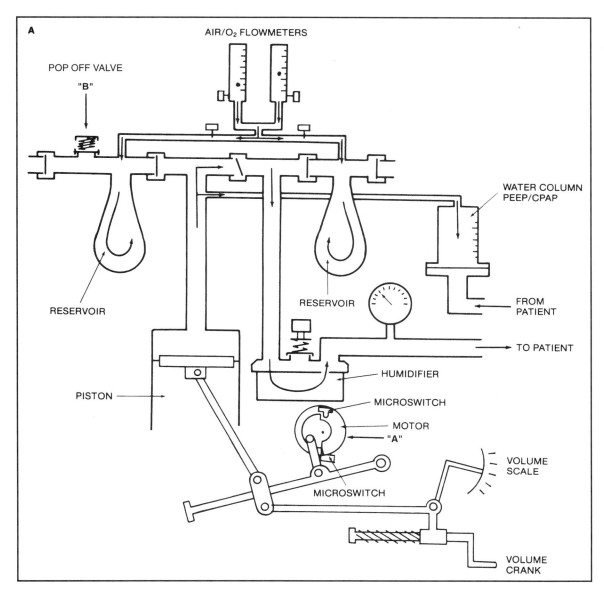

Figure 7-2A *A schematic diagram of the Emerson 3MV pneumatic system. Mandatory breath.*

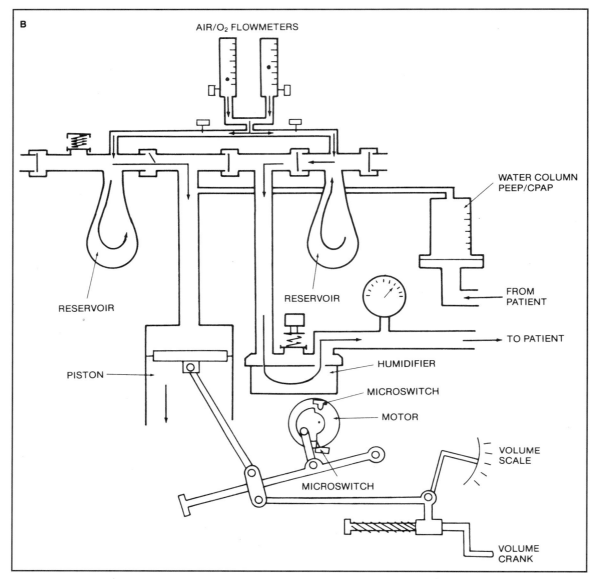

Figure 7-2B *Spontaneous breath.*

rates. When using the pediatric module, inspiratory times are adjustable between 0.5 and 2.5 seconds. The pediatric module allows respiratory rates of up to 45 breaths per minute. The ventilator may also be manually triggered by the clinician.

Limit Variable

The 3MV-IMV ventilator may be pressure limited by adjustment of the Peak/Max Pressure control. If the pressure control is set to a pressure lower than what would normally be attained during a ventilator supported breath, excess pressure (above control setting) will be vented to the atmosphere. As described earlier, when operated in this mode the ventilator is a pressure controller.

Cycling Variable

Besides being a volume controller (or pressure controller if the pressure limit is reached), the 3MV-IMV ventilator is also volume cycled. That is, inspiration ends following delivery of a set volume.

If the ventilator is operating as a pressure controller, inspiration ends following a preset time interval (inspiratory time). Therefore, when operated this way the ventilator becomes pressure limited and time cycled.

Baseline Variable

The baseline variable can be controlled by using the external Emerson water column (water weighted diaphragm) to add PEEP/

TABLE 7-1 Emerson 3MV-IMV Monitors

Pressure manometer
Pump operation lamp
Humidifier operation lamp
Main power lamp
Inspired tidal volume indicator

CPAP. Baseline pressures are adjustable from 0 to 25 cmH$_2$O above ambient pressure using the standard water column.

Output

The Emerson 3MV-IMV, having a rotary driven piston drive mechanism, delivers a sinusoidal flow and volume waveform during ventilator supported breaths. These waveforms were discussed in Chapter 6 (Figure 6-31).

Output monitors include pressure (analog manometer) and a tidal volume display window. Electric lamps illuminate to verify the operation of the pump, humidifier, and main electrical power (Table 7-1).

Alarms
Input Power

If the electrical power is lost, the Emerson 3MV-IMV will activate an audible alarm.

Control Circuit Alarms

A normal cycle alarm is provided to alert the practitioner if the pressure does not reach the set value (0.0–90 cmH$_2$O) within a specified time window (1 second to 5 minutes).

Output Alarms

High and low pressure alarms are provided to alert the practitioner to disconnects

TABLE 7-2: Emerson 3MV-IMV Alarms

Cycle failure
PEEP failure
High pressure (20–140 cmH$_2$O)
Low pressure (–5 to 25 cmH$_2$O)
Alarm disable
Power failure
Cycling alarm

or pressure limit conditions. The high pressure alarm is adjustable from 20 to 140 cmH$_2$O and the low pressure alarm is adjustable from –5 to 25 cmH$_2$O.

A cycle failure (apnea) alarm will also alert the practitioner to apneic intervals. A PEEP Fail alarm will activate if PEEP pressure is lost. The alarms are summarized in Table 7-2.

Control Interaction

The most significant control interaction is the relationship between inspiratory and expiratory time on the ventilatory rate. Flow rate becomes a function of inspiratory time and the tidal volume that is set (piston stroke). Flow rate is not adjustable. Careful adjustment and monitoring are essential with the Emerson 3MV-IMV ventilator, as with all ventilators, for effective clinical application.

Modes of Ventilation

During normal operation, the Emerson 3MV-IMV ventilator operates in a continuous flow IMV mode, allowing spontaneous ventilation interspersed with ventilator supported breaths. The supported breaths are time triggered, pressure limited and volume cycled. The mandatory supported breaths may also be time triggered, pressure limited and time cycled, as described earlier. Table 7-3 summarizes the Emerson 3MV-IMV ventilator specifications.

TABLE 7-3: Emerson 3MV-IMV Ventilator Specifications

Tidal Volume	0–2000 mL
Respiratory Rate	1 breath every 5 minutes to 26 breaths/min
Rate (pediatric)	Up to 45 breaths/min
Inspiratory Time	1 to 5 seconds
Cycle Time	2.3 seconds to 5 minutes
Maximum Pressure	160 cmH$_2$O
PEEP	0.0–25 cmH$_2$O

ASSEMBLY AND TROUBLESHOOTING

Assembly—Emerson 3MV-IMV

The following is a suggested assembly guide for the Emerson 3MV-IMV ventilator.

1. Connect the power cord to a 120 volt, 60 Hz grounded electrical outlet.

2. Attach the circuit to the water trap and to the ventilator outlet.

3. Fill the humidifier and turn the humidifier control to the desired temperature range. Once operating, monitor the inspired gas temperature.

4. Fill the PEEP/CPAP column to the desired level.

5. Adjust the piston stroke to the desired volume by turning the crank and observing the tidal volume indicator.

6. Adjust the oxygen concentration to the desired level.

7. Turn on the pump and set the mandatory breath cycle time and the inspiratory cycle time.

Troubleshooting

ALG 7-1 presents a troubleshooting flowchart for the Emerson 3MV-IMV ventilator.

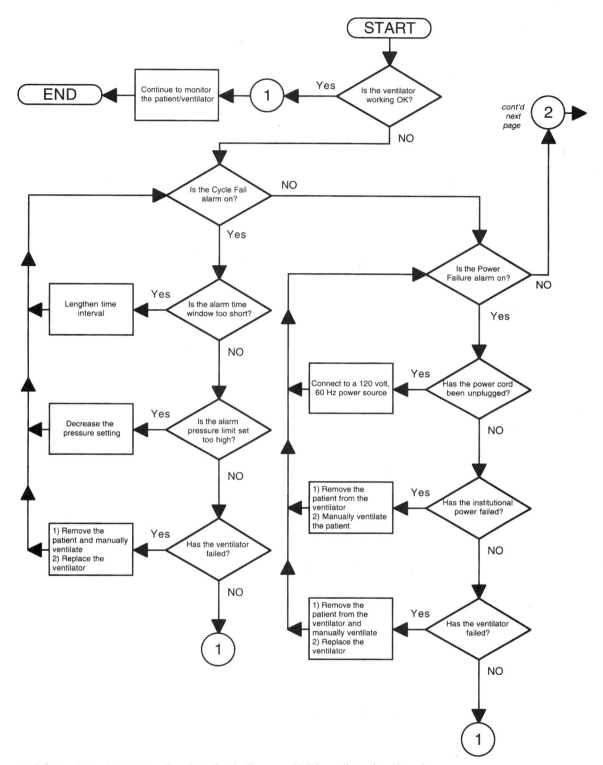

ALG 7-1 *A troubleshooting flowchart for the Emerson 3MV ventilator (continues).*

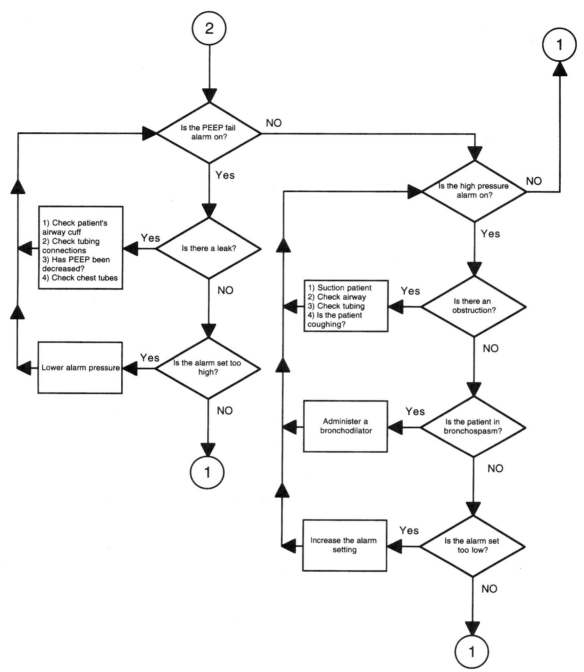

ALG 7-1 *(continued)*

MONAGHAN 225/SIMV VENTILATOR

Power Input

The Monaghan 225/SIMV ventilator is a pneumatically powered and fluidically controlled ventilator (Figure 7-3A and B). The power sources required to operate the ventilator are a 50 psi air and oxygen medical gas source.

Drive Mechanism

The drive mechanism of the 225/SIMV ventilator is the 50 psi gas source. The incoming gas passes through a fluid amplifier (Figure 7-4) and then is directed through the flow rate control and into the bellows canister. The gas admitted to the bellows canister pressurizes it, causing the contents of the bellows to be emptied, delivering gas to the patient.

Control Scheme
Control Circuit

The Monaghan 225/SIMV ventilator is unique in that it is entirely fluid controlled. Various fluidic elements are used for regulation of control, phase, and output variables as well as alarm systems. Each control system

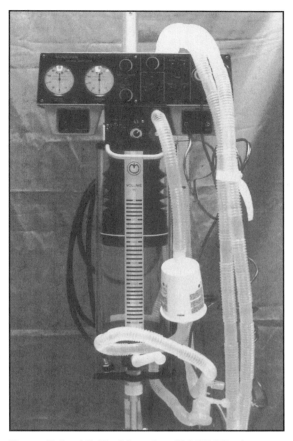

Figure 7-3 *(A) The Monaghan 225/SIMV volume ventilator (continues).*

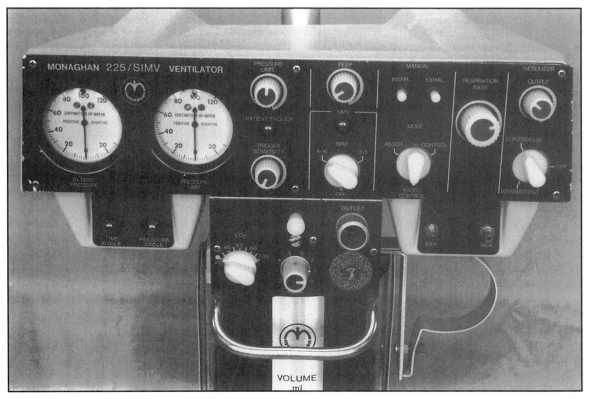

Figure 7-3 *(continued) (B) The Monaghan 225/SIMV control panel.*

and its components will be discussed as the classification of the ventilator is further developed.

Control Variable

The control variable for the 225/SIMV is volume. Tidal volume is controlled by turning a crank at the base of the bellows canister, which causes the bottom of the bellows to rise or fall. The outside of the bellows canister is calibrated in liters, indicating the volume contained in the bellows. The volume of the bellows contents determines tidal volume delivery. When the bellows reaches the top of the canister, a control port is occluded, sending a control signal to the master flip flop, terminating the inspiratory phase. Volume is adjustable from 0 to 3,000 mL.

Phase Variables
Trigger Variables

The trigger variables of the 225/SIMV are pressure, time and manual triggering. The trigger sensitivity control establishes the effort required by the patient to initiate inspiration during assist/control and SIMV modes. Sensitivity may be adjusted from autocycling to a –10 cmH$_2$O. The sensitivity system employs a Schmidt trigger in its operation (Figure 7-4).

Although a Schmidt trigger is represented schematically with one symbol, it is, in reality, a series of fluidic elements. The Schmidt trigger in the Monaghan 225/SIMV is composed of three proportional amplifiers and three flip flop gates. The Schmidt trigger senses patient effort, amplifies it, and ultimately sends a control signal to initiate inspiration.

Subambient pressure from the patient circuit is applied to the control-port of the patient trigger circuit (Figure 7-4). If enough subambient pressure is generated, the patient trigger switches output from 4R to 2R. The new output is used as a control input for the master flip-flop, changing from expiration to inspiration.

Adjustment of the sensitivity control

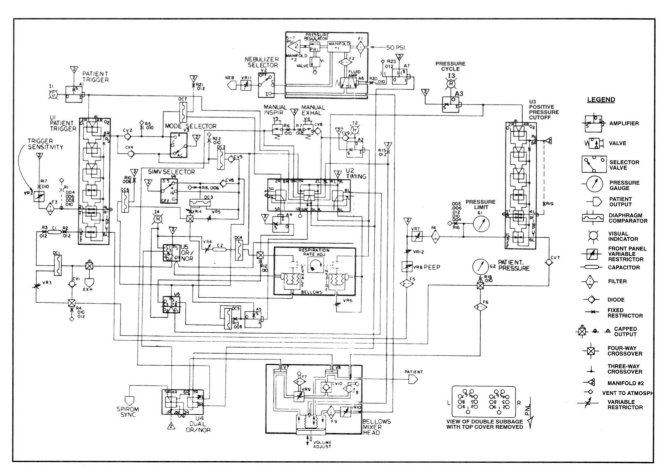

Figure 7-4 *A schematic of the Monaghan 225/SIMV pneumatic system. (Courtesy of Monaghan Medical Corporation, Platsburgh, NY.)*

causes a needle valve to be opened or closed. Flow through the needle valve provides a reference signal to the second element in the patient trigger system. Flow from the needle valve is directed just opposite, from the subambient pressure input from the patient. Increased flow, from the sensitivity control, causes beam deflection toward the subambient input, therefore making it easier for the patient to initiate a breath.

In the absence of any spontaneous effort, the ventilator is time triggered. The rate control determines the frequency of ventilator assisted breaths. The rate control determines the length of expiratory time. (This is discussed in the section on the cycle variable.)

The ventilator may also be manually triggered by depressing the manual inspiration button on the control panel. When depressed, a control signal is applied to the master flip-flop, initiating inspiration.

Limit Variable

Flow is the limit variable for the 225/SIMV ventilator. The flow rate control at the base of the bellows canister is a needle valve. Adjustment of the control regulates the flow of gas into the bellows canister. Flow rates are adjustable between near zero to 100 L/min.

Cycle Variable

There are several cycling variables for the Monaghan 225/SIMV ventilator. These include pressure, volume, and time.

Pressure

The ventilator is pressure cycled when the inspiratory pressure reaches the pressure set on the pressure limit control. The pressure limit control operates during CMV, assist/control and the mandatory breaths during SIMV. When the pressure limit is reached, inspiration is terminated.

This control operates using a device similar to the sensitivity control. A control signal (pressure from the patient circuit) provides a control input to a Schmidt trigger (Figure 7-5). If sufficient pressure is generated in the circuit, output changes, resulting in a control input to the master flip-flop. Output from the master flip-flop changes from 5L to 6R, ending inspiration.

Adjustment of the pressure limit control changes the position of a needle valve. Flow from the needle valve is directed opposite the control input signal (pressure in the patient circuit). Since in this case flow opposes the pressure signal, an increase in flow from the pressure limit control causes the ventilator to pressure limit (lower pressure) sooner.

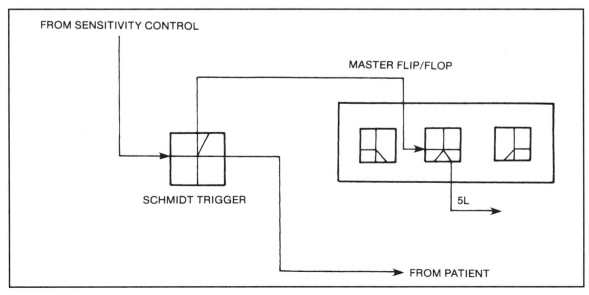

Figure 7-5 *A schematic of the Monaghan 225/SIMV assist/sensitivity system.*

Volume

Volume cycling occurs when the volume of the bellows is adjusted using the tidal volume control (crank) at the base of the bellows. This system was discussed earlier in the control variable section on this ventilator.

Time

The ventilator can be time cycled if inspiration is completed before the bellows reaches its control port at the top of the bellows canister. This is accomplished through a pneumatic timing device.

During inspiration, a small bellows (right-hand bellows, Figure 7-6) is filled by the output of the flip-flop gate to the right of the master flip-flop. Flow into the bellows chamber occurs at a constant rate since gas is admitted through a fixed orifice. Inspiratory time becomes a function of the distance the bellows travels before contacting the control port at the top of the bellows compartment. Adjustment of the rate control causes the control port sensor to be moved closer or further from the bellows, increasing or decreasing inspiratory time.

The length of the expiratory time is controlled in a similar way. The small, left-hand bellows (Figure 7-7) is filled by gas from the U5 or/nor gate. Gas from the or/nor gate fills the bellows through a fixed orifice, similar to the right-hand bellows described earlier.

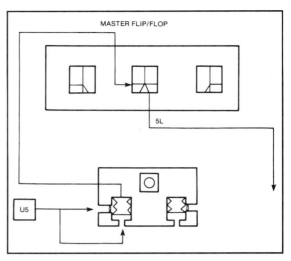

Figure 7-7 *A schematic of the Monaghan 225/SIMV timing mechanism during the expiratory phase.*

When the bellows contacts its control port, a signal is sent to the master flip-flop changing the output to 5L, beginning inspiration. Adjustment of the control port is also accomplished by adjustment of the rate control.

Baseline Variable

The baseline variable the ventilator controls is pressure (PEEP). Baseline pressure is adjustable from 0 to 20 cmH₂O. The PEEP control is a needle valve. The PEEP control is supplied with gas pressure between 5 and 7 psi. Gas pressure is applied to a four-way crossover valve and to a resistance element that vents most of the pressure to the atmosphere (Figure 7-4). Output from the resistive element is conducted to the sensitivity system (to reference the sensitivity to PEEP pressure) and to the exhalation valve to achieve the desired PEEP level. Functionally, as the needle valve is opened, more gas flow goes to the exhalation valve, increasing its pressure and increasing the PEEP pressure above ambient pressure.

Conditional Variables

Two conditional variables are employed during SIMV ventilation: pressure and time. During spontaneous ventilation, the exhalation valve is not pressurized, so gas is delivered to the patient in a flow-by fashion. Subambient pressure, generated by the patient through the assist system, causes gas to be delivered from the bellows. Since gas is deliv-

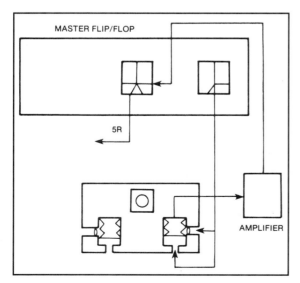

Figure 7-6 *Once the touch sensor closes contact, a signal is sent to the fluidic amplifier A2. The output from the fluidic amplifier changes the output of the master flip flop from 5L to 5R, terminating inspiration.*

ered under a slight pressure, the patient will not draw room air in through the patient circuit from the exhalation valve. Once the left-hand exhalation time bellows reaches its touch sensor, the next patient effort (pressure) will trigger a mandatory breath. The variable between mandatory breaths is time, which is determined by the rate control adjusting the position of the control port on the expiration time bellows.

Output
Output Waveforms

The Monaghan 225/SIMV delivers a rectangular flow and exponential pressure waveform. These waveforms were discussed in Chapter 6 and are illustrated in Figures 6-29 and 6-30, pp. 351–352.

Output Monitors

The ventilator has several output monitors including pressure, pressure cycle, time cycle, and tidal volume. The pressure in the patient circuit is displayed on an analog pressure gauge on the front panel of the ventilator. When the ventilator pressure cycles, a pressure cycle visual indicator changes color. (A colored lid covers the indicator window when pressure is applied to it.) The time cycle indicator changes color when the ventilator is time cycled and not volume cycled. It is an indicator similar in design to the pressure cycle indicator. The tidal volume is monitored by viewing the position of the bellows in relation to the calibration marks on the bellows canister.

Alarm Systems

The Monaghan 225/SIMV does not incorporate any audible alarms in its monitoring/alarm systems. The visual monitors were discussed in the previous section. An external pressure disconnect alarm is frequently added to alert the practitioner to any patient disconnect situations.

Modes of Ventilation

With the 225/SIMV ventilator, when operating in the CMV mode (Control), all breaths are time triggered, volume cycled and pressure limited. If the inspiratory pressure reaches the setting on the pressure limit control prior to delivery of the full tidal volume, the breath is then time triggered and pressure

cycled. The ventilator supported breath may also be time cycled if the inspiratory time ends prior to the delivery of the set tidal volume, as described earlier.

During assist/control all breaths are pressure or time triggered, pressure limited and volume cycled. Similar circumstances, as described above, could result in either pressure or time cycling in lieu of volume cycling.

During SIMV, the mandatory breaths are pressure triggered, pressure limited and volume cycled. The spontaneous breaths are pressure triggered, pressure limited and pressure cycled.

Control Interactions

A significant control interaction is the relationship of the flow rate, tidal volume and the respiratory rate on the inspiratory time. While inverse ratios are not possible, ratios as low as 1:1 may occur. When delivering large volumes, it is important to increase the flow rate to prevent the ventilator from time cycling.

Although the sensitivity system attempts to compensate for PEEP levels, full compensation does not occur. At high levels of PEEP (20 cmH$_2$O), the patient may need to generate inspiratory pressure of up to 4 cmH$_2$O below PEEP to initiate inspiration. Careful observation of the manometer is important to minimize the work of breathing when using higher levels of PEEP. Table 7-4 summarizes the capabilities of the Monaghan 225/SIMV.

TABLE 7-4: Monaghan 225/SIMV Ventilator

Tidal Volume	0–3000 mL
Respiratory Rate	6–60 Breaths/minute
Expiratory Time	0.5–7.5 Seconds
Flow Rate	0.0–100 L/minute
Maximum Pressure	100 cmH$_2$O
PEEP	0.0–25 cmH$_2$O
Sensitivity	Autocycling –10.0 cmH$_2$O
Oxygen (F$_1$O$_2$)	.21–1.00
Modes	CMV, Assist/Control, SIMV

ASSEMBLY AND TROUBLESHOOTING

Assembly—Monaghan 225/SIMV

To assemble the Monaghan 225/SIMV for use, follow the suggested assembly guide.

1. Connect the high pressure gas lines to 50 psi oxygen and air sources.

2. Assemble and fill the humidifier. Since many humidifiers may be used, specific assembly instructions will not be included here.

3. Connect a bacteria filter to the ventilator outlet using an appropriate adapter.

4. Connect the humidifier inlet to the bacteria filter using a length of large-bore tubing.

5. Connect the inspiratory limb of the patient circuit to the outlet of the humidifier.

6. Connect the exhalation valve tubing to the exhalation valve nipple on the ventilator.

7. If the use of an in-line nebulizer is desired, connect its drive line to the nebulizer nipple on the ventilator.

8. Pressure test the ventilator circuit.

Troubleshooting

ALG 7-2 illustrates a flowchart for troubleshooting the Monaghan 225/SIMV ventilator.

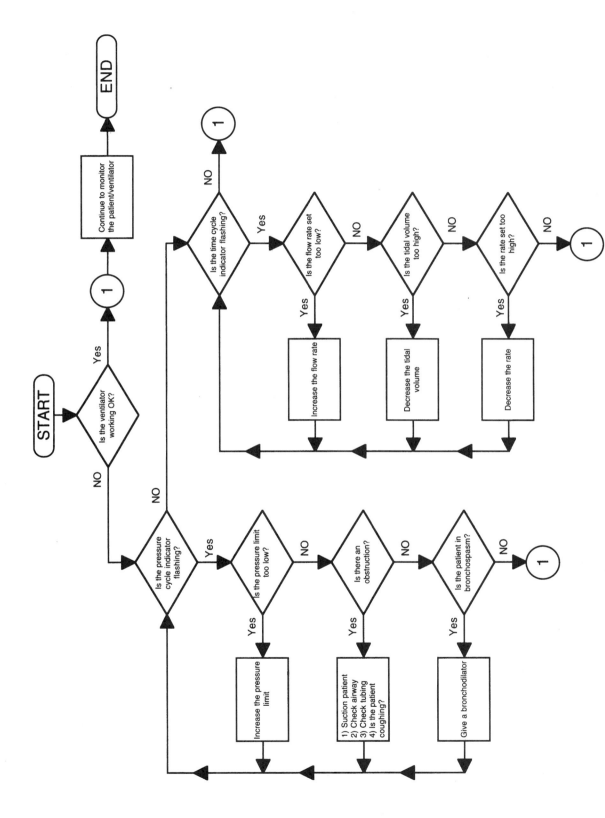

ALG 7-2 *A troubleshooting flowchart for the Monaghan 225/SIMV volume ventilator.*

PURITAN BENNETT MA-1 AND MA-2+2 VENTILATORS

The Puritan Bennett MA-1 and MA-2+2 ventilators are similar and therefore will be discussed together. When the two ventilators differ, the differences will be presented and discussed. Both ventilators are electrically powered, electronically controlled, double circuit ventilators which are volume controllers. The MA-2+2 (Figure 7-8) was released in 1982, later than the 1965 MA-1 (Figure 7-9), and has CMV, assist/control, IMV, CPAP and PEEP capabilities. The MA-1 is limited to CMV and assist/control and has an optional PEEP attachment.

Power Input

The input power which operates the ventilators is electricity, 120 volt, 60Hz alternating current. This electrical energy powers the control circuitry and the compressor motor, which provides compressed air for the pneumatic circuit.

Pneumatic power is provided by a medical gas source, 50 psi oxygen and 50 psi air (may be used in lieu of the internal compressor on the MA-2+2). When an external 50 psi air

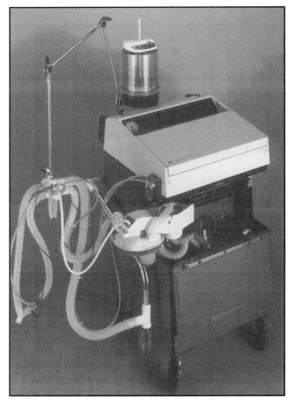

Figure 7-8 *(A) The Puritan Bennett MA-2+2 volume ventilator. (Courtesy of Puritan Bennett Corporation, Carlsbad, CA) (continues)*

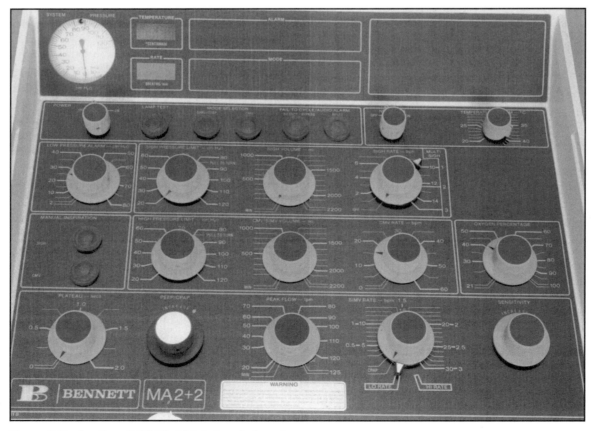

Figure 7-8 *(continued) (B) The MA-2+2 control panel.*

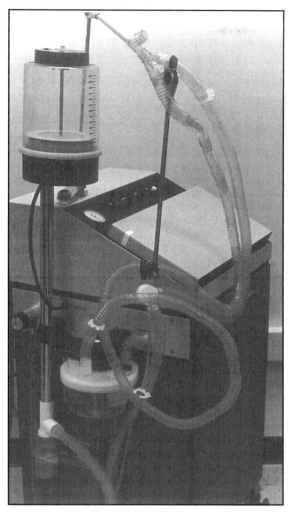

Figure 7-9 *(A) The Puritan Bennett MA-1 volume ventilator. (continues)*

source is employed with the MA-2+2, the internal compressor is inoperative. The pneumatic gas supply is reduced from 50 psi to about 7 psi by an internal reducing valve.

The oxygen, after leaving the pressure reducing valve, is directed to a solenoid valve which is opened only when the oxygen percent control is set above 21%. The oxygen then enters an accumulator which further reduces the pressure to between 1.85 and 2.1 cmH₂O.

Oxygen and air are blended together by means of a proportioning valve (Figure 7-10). The oxygen percentage control rotates a shutter across a valve with three ports: a common port, an oxygen port and an air port. The position of the shutter varies the F₁O₂ by changing the relative amount of air and oxygen admitted.

Drive Mechanism

The drive mechanism for both ventilators is an air powered venturi. Flow from the com-

pressor or air supply line, at about 6 psi, drives the venturi jet. Gas flow from the venturi is used to compress a bellows (secondary patient circuit) to deliver the volume to the patient.

Gas flow to the venturi is controlled by the main solenoid valve. During inspiration, gas is routed to the venturi, causing the bellows to be compressed. During expiration, the gas is vented to the atmosphere.

The MA-2+2 has a microswitch within the bellows chamber at the top. If the bellows reaches the top of the chamber (exhausting all gas), it will automatically return to the bottom position, refilling it. After a ventilator supported breath delivery, the bellows will automatically reset to the bottom of the chamber.

Control Variables

The MA-1 and MA-2 are both volume controllers. The gas delivered to the patient comes from an internal bellows. Volume delivery from the bellows is controlled by a potentiometer feedback system.

The tidal volume control itself is a potentiometer. (A potentiometer is a variable electrical resistor, much like the volume control on a radio.) The potentiometer is used to establish a reference value (resistance) that is used by an electronic circuit card.

Attached to the base of the bellows is a fine wire (Figure 7-11). As the bellows empties, wire is unwound from a spool. A bellows potentiometer is turned as the wire unwinds from the spool, changing its resistance value.

The circuit card compares the reference potentiometer (volume control) with the bellows potentiometer. When the values are equal, the main solenoid stops flow to the venturi, ending inspiration.

Phase Variables
Trigger Variable
Pressure

The trigger variable for both the MA-1 and MA-2+2 is pressure. The MA-1 utilizes pressure triggering during assist/control, while the MA-2+2 uses pressure triggering for assist/control, IMV, and CPAP. The trigger variable is controlled by the sensitivity control.

The sensitivity control functions as a patient effort control. The sensitivity may be adjusted between –0.1 and –10 cmH₂O subambient pressure.

The sensitivity control for the MA-1 adjusts the position between two electrical contacts,

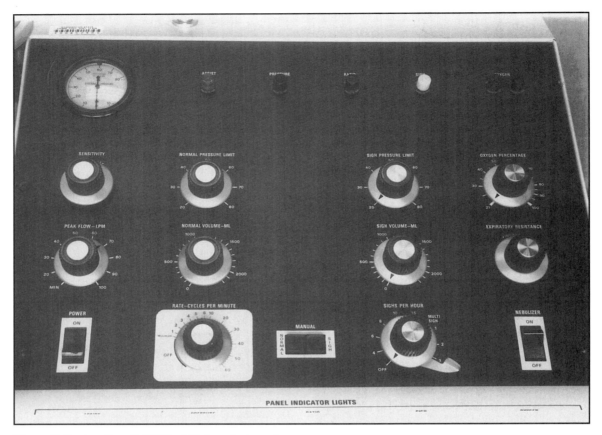

Figure 7-9 *(continued) (B) The MA-1 control panel.*

with one contact attached to a diaphragm (Figure 7-12). When electrical contact is broken, an electrical signal opens the main solenoid valve to the venturi, driving the bellows. When the contacts are near one another, more subambient pressure must be generated to separate them; therefore, the ventilator is less sensitive. IF PEEP is applied, using the optional PEEP valve (externally), the sensitivity control must be readjusted to account for the elevated baseline pressure. Failure to do so will mean that the patient will have to generate sufficient subambient pressures to overcome the sensitivity level *plus the PEEP level.* The sensitivity system in the MA-1 is not PEEP compensated.

The MA-2+2 sensitivity system uses the

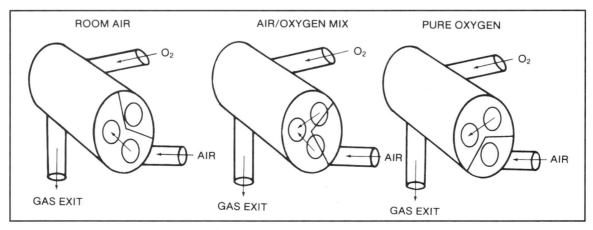

Figure 7-10 *A schematic diagram of the Puritan Bennett MA-1 oxygen proportioning valve.*

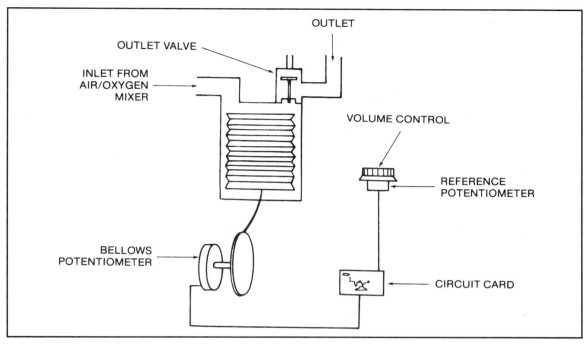

Figure 7-11 *A schematic diagram of the Puritan Bennett MA-1 tidal volume measuring system.*

PEEP system to pressurize the chamber containing the diaphragm. Therefore PEEP pressures and the pressure above the diaphragm are the same. This in effect compensates for the PEEP pressure so that addition of PEEP will not increase the sensitivity.

Time

When the sensitivity is "dialed out" so that it does not function, the ventilators operate in CMV. Any patient effort (subambient pressure) will fail to trigger a breath. Under these circumstances the ventilators are time triggered. A ventilator supported breath is delivered after a specific time interval has passed.

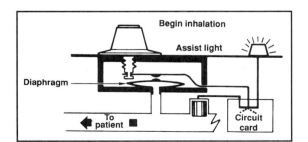

Figure 7-12 *A schematic diagram of the Puritan Bennett MA-1 sensitivity system. (Courtesy of Puritan Bennett Corporation, Carlsbad, CA)*

If the sensitivity is correctly set and no spontaneous effort (pressure) is detected, the ventilators will also be time triggered as described above.

When time triggered, the rate control determines when breaths are delivered. The rate control is an electric timer. Each minute is divided by the value set on the rate control. This interval includes both inspiration and expiration. For example, if a rate of 12 is set on the rate control, 60 seconds would be divided by 12, establishing a breath every 5 seconds. Every 5 seconds a signal (electrical) is sent to the main solenoid, opening it, which begins inspiration.

The MA-2+2 has two independent rate mechanisms; one functions in the CMV and assist/control modes and the other during IMV. The rate control for the CMV and assist/control modes functions identically to the MA-1 rate control. The IMV rate control, however, is different. The off position provides CPAP mode. With the rate switch in the low position, rates of between 0.3 and 3 breaths per minute are available, and in the high position breaths of between 3 and 30 breaths per minute are available.

Manual

Both ventilators may become manually triggered if the practitioner depresses either the manual button for normal breath delivery or sigh breath delivery.

Limit Variables

Volume

The ventilators can be volume limited if the expiratory resistance control is set at its maximum setting. Under these conditions there is a slight inspiratory pause prior to exhalation.

The expiratory resistance control adjusts the amount of resistance the patient encounters during exhalation. Physiologically, it applies back pressure to the lungs, similar to the way a COPD patient exhales through pursed lips.

When the expiratory resistance control is increased, gas from the exhalation valve is diverted through two restricted orifices that retard exhalation (Figure 7-13). When fully closed, a slight inspiratory pause occurs before the exhalation valve begins to empty. This occurs because there is a time lag as the pressure drops across both restricted orifices.

Flow

The ventilators can be flow limited if the peak flow setting is low and the patient's compliance is high and their resistance is low, presenting a small workload for the ventilator. Under these circumstances, flow will reach a constant level during the inspiratory phase.

When the ventilators are operated using higher flow rates and the patient's resistance increases and compliance worsens, the flow will actually taper. The waveform resembles a descending ramp. The drive mechanism does not have sufficient power to overcome high ventilator workloads without tapering the inspiratory flow.

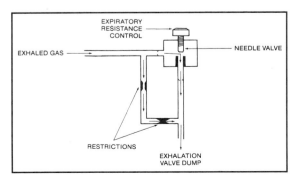

Figure 7-13 *A schematic diagram of the Puritan Bennett expiratory retard system.*

Cycle Variables

Pressure

The ventilators are pressure cycled if the inspiratory pressure reaches the pressure set on the pressure limit control (normal pressure limit or sigh pressure limit). The pressure limit control determines the maximum pressure that can build in the patient circuit during inspiration. Pressure limits may be adjusted between 20 and 80 cmH₂O (MA-1) or 20 and 120 cmH₂O (MA-2+2).

Pressure from the patient circuit is conducted to a diaphragm, displacing it. Adjustment of the control moves an electrical contact closer or further from the diaphragm, increasing or decreasing the limit. When the contacts are further apart, more pressure must build to raise the diaphragm higher in order to make electrical contact. Once the pressure limit has been reached, the main solenoid switches to the expiratory position while simultaneously a visual and audible alarm sounds. Under these circumstances, the ventilators are pressure cycled.

Volume

During supported breaths, both ventilators are volume cycled if the entire tidal volume is delivered. The tidal volume regulation was discussed earlier under the section describing control variables.

Time

The ventilators operate under time cycling when the expiratory resistance control is set to a maximum, resulting in an inspiratory hold. The expiratory resistance control was described in the previous section discussing phase variables.

The MA-2+2 may also be time cycled when the plateau control is used. This control only operates in the CMV mode. Inspiratory plateaus occur following volume delivery and vary from zero to two seconds. Adjustment of the control causes the plateau solenoid to delay the opening of the exhalation valve. As long as the valve remains closed, gas is held in the lungs and exhalation is prevented. Inspiration therefore becomes time cycled.

Baseline Variable

The baseline variable for both ventilators is pressure. The MA-1 uses an external PEEP attachment, while the MA-2+2 has built in PEEP capability.

The MA-1 PEEP attachment is a plug-in valve that attaches to the side of the ventilator adjacent to where the spirometer pole attaches. The PEEP valve is a single stage adjustable reducing valve, which creates PEEP. PEEP pressures are changed by adjusting the spring tension within the PEEP valve and verifying PEEP pressures using the manometer (adjustable between 0 and 15 cmH$_2$O). PEEP pressures are applied to the exhalation valve, creating a threshold resistance to exhalation.

The MA-2+2 PEEP system uses air pressure from either the bellows or the regulator (external air source). This pressure is conducted to the PEEP control. Functionally, the PEEP control is a needle valve. The output from the PEEP control is channeled to a venturi. Flow from the venturi is applied to the exhalation valve partially closing it, generating a threshold resistance. The PEEP pressure builds in the circuit to the same level at which the exhalation valve diaphragm is pressurized.

Conditional Variables
Time

During sigh mode ventilation, time is the conditional variable the ventilators monitor to determine which ventilatory pattern to deliver. During normal ventilator supported breaths, they are volume controlled, pressure triggered, pressure limited and volume cycled. When sigh mode is active, sigh rate, sighs per hour, sigh volume and sigh pressure limits must be set.

The sighs per hour time window is monitored. Each hour may be divided into time periods lasting 4 to 15 minutes. That is, every 4 to 15 minutes the ventilator switches to sigh mode. Once the sigh mode becomes active, the ventilator delivers one to three sigh breaths. Under these circumstances, the conditional variable becomes time.

The sigh system is used to deliver larger tidal volumes periodically, mimicking a normal sigh. The sigh volume and sigh pressure limit control function identically to the normal volume and normal pressure limit controls.

When the MA-2+2 operates in the IMV mode, time and pressure become the conditional variables. The IMV rate control determines the frequency at which ventilator supported breaths are delivered. If the time window has not closed (spontaneous breathing), the patient is free to breathe spontaneously from the gas supply system. If the window closes (ventilator supported breath), the next patient effort sensed (pressure) will result in a mandatory breath delivery.

Output
Output Waveforms

As described earlier, under low ventilator workloads (low resistance and high compliance), the ventilators deliver a rectangular flow pattern (Figure 6-29). When ventilator work increases (high resistance and low compliance), the flow pattern becomes a descending ramp waveform.

Control Interactions

As discussed earlier, on the MA-1 it is important to know how PEEP affects the sensitivity. Addition of PEEP requires the readjustment of the sensitivity control.

Another interaction to remember with both ventilators is the relationship of the ventilatory rate, peak flow, and tidal volume to the inspiratory time. If high volume or high respiratory rates are required, peak flow must be increased or inverse I:E ratios may occur. The I:E ratio limit system, however, will not prevent inverse ratio ventilation—it merely alerts you to the fact that it is occurring.

Monitoring Systems

Several monitors exist on the MA-1 and MA-2+2 to assist the clinician in monitoring the patient/ventilator system. Features of these monitors are summarized in Table 7-5.

TABLE 7-5: MA-1 and MA-2+2 Monitors

	MA-1	MA-2+2
Circuit Pressure	x	x
Sigh Breath Delivery	x	x
Volume Monitoring Spirometer	x	x
Assisted Breath Monitor	x	x
Oxygen Pressure Light	x	x
Circuit Temperature		x
Breaths per Minute		x
Mode Display		x
Oxygen Percentage		x

Alarm Systems
Input Power

Oxygen Supply   The MA-1 and MA-2+2 both incorporate an alarm to alert the clinician to oxygen supply failure. In the event of inlet pressure loss, both an audible and visual alarm are activated. This alarm is not an oxygen percentage alarm, rather it is a pressure sensor.

Control Circuit Alarms

Inverse I:E Ratio

Both the MA-1 and MA-2+2 have an inverse I:E ratio alarm. In the event that the I:E ratio becomes greater than 1:1, an audible and visual alarm will sound (visual only on the MA-1). This alarm is active during CMV and sigh breaths (MA-1) and CMV, sigh and mandatory breaths during IMV (MA-2+2).

Failure to Cycle

MA-2+2 has a failure to cycle alarm. This audible and visual alarm is activated if the electrical power is switched on and the ventilator fails to cycle into inspiration within 20 seconds.

Output Alarms
Pressure

Both ventilators have a high pressure alarm. If the circuit pressure exceeds the pressure setting on the pressure limit control (normal or sigh), inspiration will be terminated and both audible and visual alarms will be activated.

TABLE 7-6: Alarm Systems

	MA-1	MA-2+2
Input Power		
Oxygen Pressure	x	x
Control Circuit		
Inverse I:E Ratio	x	x
Failure to Cycle	x	x
Output		
High Pressure (Pressure Limit)	x	x
Low Pressure		x
Volume (Monitoring Spirometer)	x	x
Temperature		x

The MA-2+2 also incorporates a low pressure alarm. In the event circuit pressure drops 5 cmH_2O below baseline, or does not reach a clinician-set pressure 10 cmH_2O above baseline, both audible and visual alarms will result.

Volume

Both ventilators incorporate a volume alarm into the monitoring spirometer. The alarm is battery operated and has both audible and visual indicators. If the set volume is not reached by the bellows within the specified time, both audible and visual alarms will result.

TABLE 7-7: Ventilator Capabilities

	MA-1	MA-2+2
Volume	0–2,200 ml	0–2,200 ml
Pressure	20–80 cmH_2O	20–80 cmH_2O
Rate	6–60 breaths/min	0–60 breaths/min
Peak Flow	15–100 L/min	15–125 L/min
PEEP	0–15 cmH_2O	0–45 cmH_2O
Sensitivity	−0.1– −10 cmH_2O	Autocycle– −8 cmH_2O
F_IO_2	0.21–1.0	0.21–1.0

Temperature

If the inspired gas exceeds the temperature set by the clinician or if the humidifier malfunctions, this audible and visual alarm will be activated. This feature is only available on the MA-2+2.

Table 7-6 compares the alarm systems of the MA-1 and the MA-2+2, and Table 7-7 compares the two ventilators' capabilities.

Summary

The classification and operation of the MA-1 and MA-2+2 ventilators have been presented together, while the differences between each have been discussed. Table 7-8 further demonstrates the differences between the ventilators by examining and comparing their respective classifications.

ASSEMBLY AND TROUBLESHOOTING

Assembly—MA-1 and MA-2+2

To prepare the MA-1 and MA-2+2 for use, complete this suggested assembly guide.

1. Open the door on the front of the ventilator and attach a bacteria filter to the side of the ventilator using the provided clamp.

2. Connect the inlet of the bacteria filter to the ventilator outlet using a length of large bore tubing and close the door.

3. Assemble the Cascade humidifier and attach it to the heater on the side of the ventilator.

4. Connect the Cascade humidifier inlet to the bacteria filter outlet with the Bennett angled connector or a six-inch length of large-bore tubing.

5. Attach the patient circuit to the support arm.

6. Connect the inspiratory limb to the humidifier outlet. Attach the expiratory limb to the collection jar at the base of the spirometer pole. The MA-2+2 has a temperature probe that will need to be placed on the inspiratory limb of the circuit, near the patient wye.

7. Connect the exhalation valve to the exhalation nipple on the side of the ventilator. Connect the nebulizer drive line to the nebulizer nipple on the side of the ventilator.

8. Assemble the spirometer and attach it to the top of the spirometer pole. Connect the dump valve line to the spirometer nipple on the side of the ventilator.

9. The MA-2+2 will have a proximal airway line from the patient wye that will need to be connected to the proximal airway water trap on the side of the ventilator.

10. Connect the oxygen (or oxygen and air for the MA-2+2) to a 50 psi source.

11. Connect the power cord to a 120 volt, 60 Hz outlet.

12. Pressure test the ventilator.

Troubleshooting

ALG 7-3 is a flowchart to assist you in troubleshooting the MA-1 and MA-2+2 ventilators.

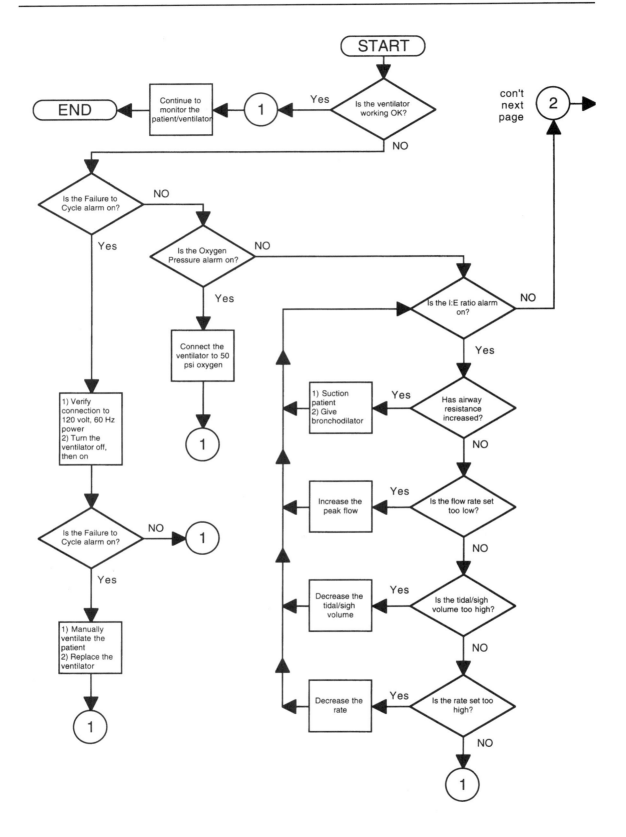

ALG 7-3 *A troubleshooting flowchart for the Puritan Bennett MA-1 and MA-2+2 volume ventilators. (continues)*

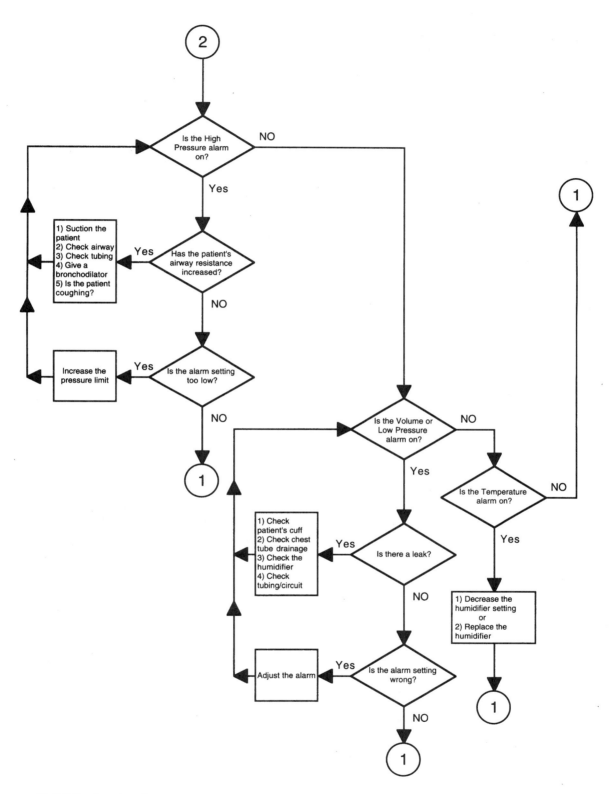

ALG 7-3 *(continued)*

TABLE 7-8: Classification of Volume Controllers

VENTILATOR	INPUT POWER	CIRCUIT	DRIVE MECHANISM	CONTROL MECHANISM	CONTROL VARIABLE	TRIGGER VARIABLE	LIMIT VARIABLE	CYCLING VARIABLE	ALARMS
Emerson 3MV	Electric	Double	Piston	Mechanical Electrical	V/P	T	P	V/T	I/CC/P
Monaghan 225/SIMV	Pneumatic	Double	Bellows	Fluidic	V	P/T/M	F	P/V/T	P/V/T
Puritan Bennett									
MA-1	Electric	Double	Bellows	Electronic	V	P/T/M	V/F	P/V/T	I/CC/P/V
MA-2+2	Electric	Double	Bellows	Electronic	V	P/T/M	V/F	P/V/T	I/CC/P/V/TP

P — Pressure, T — Time, F — Flow, CC — Control Circuit, V — Volume, M — Manual, I — Input Power, TP — Temperature.

CLINICAL CORNER

Emerson 3MV-IMV Ventilator

1. You have set the inspiratory time control for 2 seconds and the cycle time control for 6 seconds. What is the ventilatory rate, and what is the I:E ratio?
2. The PEEP Fail alarm goes on for a patient who is on 10 cmH₂O of PEEP. Describe how you would troubleshoot the alarm.

Monaghan 225/SIMV Ventilator

1. You are called to assess a patient who is being ventilated by a Monaghan 225/SIMV ventilator. The time cycle indicator is flashing, and the patient is in obvious discomfort. What should you do in this situation?

2. You are monitoring a patient on a Monaghan 225/SIMV ventilator. The patient is on 7 cmH₂O PEEP. The pressure manometer reaches zero before the start of each breath. What should you do in this situation?

Puritan Bennett MA-1 and MA-2 + 2 Ventilators

1. You are monitoring a patient on an MA-1 ventilator. Following the delivery of each breath, the bellows on the monitoring spirometer slowly collapses. The attending nurse expresses concern. What should you do?
2. The Low Pressure alarm is sounding on an MA-2+2 ventilator. Discuss the items you should check when troubleshooting this situation.

Self-Assessment Quiz

1. What is the input power for the Emerson 3MV ventilator?
   a. Electrical.
   b. Pneumatic.
   c. Mechanical.
   d. a and b.

2. The drive mechanism for the Emerson 3MV consists of:
   a. A bellows.
   b. A fluidic circuit.
   c. A rotary driven piston.
   d. A venturi ejector.

3. The control circuit of the Emerson 3MV consists of:
   I. Electrical.
   II. Mechanical.
   III. Pneumatic.
   IV. Fluidic.
   a. I
   b. I and II
   c. I and III
   d. III and IV

4. The control variables of the Emerson 3MV are:
   I. Pressure.
   II. Volume.
   III. Flow.
   IV. Time.
   a. I and II
   b. II and III
   c. III and IV
   d. II and IV

5. The limit variable for the Emerson 3MV is:
   a. Pressure.
   b. Volume.
   c. Flow.
   d. Time.

6. The cycling variables for the Emerson 3MV are:
   I. Pressure.
   II. Volume.
   III. Flow.
   IV. Time.
   a. I and II
   b. II and III
   c. III and IV
   d. II and IV

7. The Emerson 3MV is capable of delivering up to 25 cmH$_2$O of PEEP. This variable is termed the:
   a. Control variable.
   b. Limit variable.
   c. Cycling variable.
   d. Baseline variable.

8. The output characteristics of the Emerson 3MV ventilator consist of:
   a. Sinusoidal pressure, volume and flow waveform.
   b. Rectangular flow waveform.
   c. Rectangular volume waveform.
   d. Exponential pressure waveform.

9. Maximum tidal volume delivery for the Emerson 3MV is:
   a. 2000 mL.
   b. 2200 mL.
   c. 3000 mL.
   d. 3500 mL.

10. Maximum pressure delivery for the Emerson 3MV is:
    a. 80 cmH$_2$O.
    b. 100 cmH$_2$O.
    c. 120 cmH$_2$O.
    d. 160 cmH$_2$O.

11. What is the input power for the Monaghan 225/SIMV ventilator?
    a. Electrical.
    b. Pneumatic.
    c. Mechanical.
    d. a and b.

12. The drive mechanism for the Monaghan 225/SIMV consists of:
    a. A bellows.
    b. A fluidic circuit.
    c. A rotary driven piston.
    d. A venturi ejector.

13. The control circuit of the Monaghan 225/SIMV consists of:
    I. Electrical.
    II. Mechanical.
    III. Pneumatic.
    IV. Fluidic.
    a. I
    b. I and II
    c. I and IV

d. III and IV

14. The control variable of the Monaghan 225/SIMV is:
    a. Pressure.
    b. Volume.
    c. Flow.
    d. Time.

15. The limit variable for the Monaghan 225/SIMV is:
    a. Pressure.
    b. Volume.
    c. Flow.
    d. Time.

16. The cycling variables for the Monaghan 225/SIMV are:
    I. Pressure.
    II. Volume.
    III. Flow.
    IV. Time.
    a. I and II
    b. I, II and IV
    c. III and IV
    d. II and IV

17. Conditional variables for the Monaghan 225/SIMV include:
    I. Pressure.
    II. Volume.
    III. Flow.
    IV. Time.
    a. I
    b. I and IV
    c. I and II
    d. II and IV

18. The output waveforms for the Monaghan 225/SIMV are:
    I. Sinusoidal pressure, volume and flow waveform.
    II. Rectangular flow waveform.
    III. Rectangular volume waveform.
    IV. Exponential pressure waveform.
    a. I
    b. II
    c. II and IV
    d. III and IV

19. Modes of ventilation for the Monaghan 225/SIMV include:
    I. CMV.
    II. Assist/Control.
    III. SIMV.
    IV. Pressure support.
    a. I
    b. I and II
    c. I, II and III
    d. I, II, III and IV

20. What is the input power for the Puritan Bennett MA-1 ventilator?
    a. Electrical.
    b. Pneumatic.
    c. Mechanical.
    d. a and b.

21. The drive mechanism for the Puritan Bennett MA-1 and MA-2+2 consists of:

    a. A bellows.
    b. A fluidic circuit.
    c. A rotary-driven piston.
    d. A venturi ejector.

22. The control circuit of the Puritan Bennett MA-2+2 consists of which element(s):
    I. Electronic.
    II. Mechanical.
    III. Pneumatic.
    IV. Fluidic.
    a. I
    b. I and II
    c. I and III
    d. III and IV

23. The control variable of the Puritan Bennett MA-1 and MA-2+2 ventilators is:
    a. Pressure.
    b. Volume.
    c. Flow.
    d. Time.

24. The trigger variable(s) for the Puritan Bennett MA-1 and MA-2+2 is (are):
    I. Pressure.
    II. Volume.
    III. Flow.
    IV. Time.
    V. Manual.
    a. I
    b. I and II
    c. I, IV and V
    d. II and IV

25. The cycling variables for the Puritan Bennett MA-1 are:
    I. Pressure.
    II. Volume.
    III. Flow.
    IV. Time.
    a. I and II
    b. I, II and IV
    c. III and IV
    d. II and IV

26. Conditional variables for the Puritan Bennett MA-1 and MA-2+2 include:
    I. Pressure.
    II. Volume.
    III. Flow.
    IV. Time.
    a. I
    b. I and II
    c. II and III
    d. IV

27. The output waveforms (under low ventilator workloads) for the Puritan Bennett MA-1 and MA-2+2 are:
    I. Sinusoidal pressure, volume and flow waveforms.
    II. Rectangular flow waveform.
    III. Rectangular volume waveform.
    IV. Exponential pressure waveform.
    a. I
    b. II
    c. II and IV

d. III and IV

28. Under conditions of reduced compliance and increased resistance, the Puritan Bennett MA-1 delivers what type of output waveform?
    a. Sinusoidal pressure, volume and flow waveforms.
    b. Rectangular flow waveform.
    c. Rectangular volume waveform.
    d. Descending ramp waveform.

29. Which of the following controls affect the I:E ratio when using the Puritan Bennett MA-1 and MA-2+2?
    I. Tidal volume.
    II. Peak flow.
    III. Rate.
    IV. Oxygen percentage.
    a. I
    b. I and II
    c. I, II and III
    d. I, II, III and IV

30. Which of the following alarms are included on the Puritan Bennett MA-1?
    I. Pressure.
    II. Failure to cycle.
    III. Oxygen pressure.
    IV. Temperature.
    a. I
    b. I and II
    c. I, II, and III
    d. I, II, III and IV

Selected Bibliography

Branson, Richard D., and Robert L. Chatburn, "Technical Description and Classification of Modes of Ventilator Operation," *Respiratory Care,* Vol. 37, No. 9, pp. 1026–1044, 1992.

Chatburn, Robert L., "A New System for Understanding Mechanical Ventilators," *Respiratory Care,* Vol. 36, No. 10, pp. 1123–1155, 1991.

Chatburn, Robert L., "Classification of Mechanical Ventilators," *Respiratory Care,* Vol. 37, No. 9, pp. 1009–1025, 1992.

Corning Fluidic Products, *Fluidic Industrial Control Modules,* P/N EPD EBR-3, Corning, NY, 1971.

Dupis, Yvon, *Ventilators: Theory and Clinical Application,* 2nd Ed., Mosby-Yearbook, 1992.

Floyd, Thomas L., *Digital Fundamentals,* 3rd Ed., Charles E. Merrill Publishing Company, 1986.

Monaghan, *Monaghan 225 Volume Ventilator Operator's Manual: Questions and Answers,* Form 13929-01 5m, Littleton, CO, 1975.

Monaghan, *Fluidics and Monaghan Volume Ventilators,* Form P/N 66007-02, Littleton, CO, 1976.

Pierson, David J., "Maximum Ventilator Capabilities of Four Current-Generation Mechanical Ventilators," *Respiratory Care,* Vol. 31, No. 11, pp. 1054–1058, 1986.

Smith, Richard K., "Respiratory Applications of Fluidics," *Respiratory Therapy,* Vol. 3, No. 3, pp. 29–32, 1973.

CHAPTER 8

ADULT ACUTE CARE VENTILATORS: VENTILATORS HAVING FLOW AND PRESSURE CONTROL VARIABLES

INTRODUCTION

Chapter 7 described the adult acute care ventilators employing volume as a control variable. This chapter will describe the adult acute care ventilators that utilize flow and pressure as the control variables.

As discussed in Chapter 6, for a variable (pressure, volume, flow, or time) to be classified as a control variable, certain conditions must be met. Those conditions are that (1) the variable must be measured, (2) the variable must be used as a feedback signal to control the ventilator's output. The group of ventilators discussed in this chapter directly measure the delivered flow or pressure and use this signal to modify and control the ventilator's output. Pressure becomes a control variable when the ventilators are operated in the CPAP or pressure support modes.

OBJECTIVES

After completing this chapter, the student will accomplish the following objectives:
- Explain what is meant by the term *control variable* and how a specific ventilator may be classified as having flow or pressure as a control variable.
- For the ventilators described in this chapter, apply Chatburn's classification system and classify them according to:
  — Power Input
  — Drive mechanism
  — Control scheme
  — Output
  — Alarm systems
- Describe how to assemble and troubleshoot the following ventilators:

— BEAR Medical Systems, Inc., BEAR 1, 2, 3, 5, and 1000
— Bird Products Corporation 8400ST®*i*
— Bird Products Corporation, TBird® AVS
— Dräger, Evita 4
— Hamilton Medical, Veolar
— Infrasonics, Adult Star
— Newport Medical Instruments, Wave
— Puritan Bennett Corporation, 7200ae
— Nellcor Puritan Bennett, 840
— Siemens-Elema Servo 900C and Servo 300

THE CONTROL VARIABLE

During a ventilator-supported breath, a mechanical ventilator can control one of the following variables: pressure, volume, flow or time. In order for a ventilator to be classified as controlling one of these variables, two conditions must be met. First, that variable must be measured, and second it must be used as feedback to control the ventilator's output. Therefore, for a ventilator to be classified as a flow or pressure controller, flow or pressure must be measured and used as a signal to control the output from the ventilator. The ventilators discussed in this chapter meet these criteria and are classified as either a flow or pressure controller.

BEAR MEDICAL SYSTEMS, BEAR 1, 2, AND 3

The BEAR 1, 2 and 3 ventilators are similar to one another and therefore will be discussed together (Figures 8-1A, 8-1B, 8-2A, 8-2B, 8-3A, and 8-3B). When differences occur, they will be presented and compared.

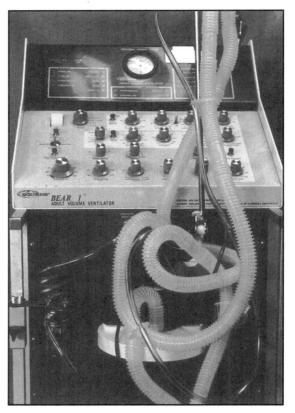

Figure 8-1A *A photograph of the BEAR 1 volume ventilator.*

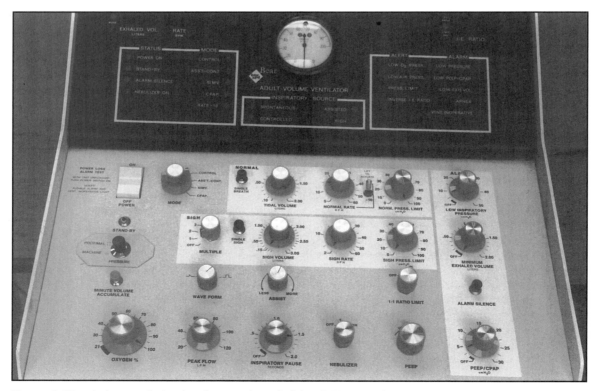

Figure 8-1B *A photograph showing the control panel of the BEAR 1 ventilator.*

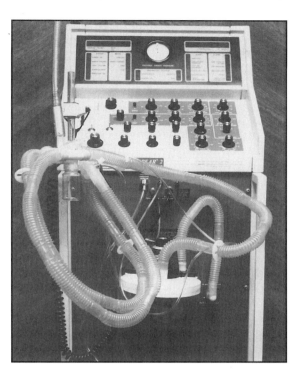

Figure 8-2A *A photograph of the BEAR 2 volume ventilator.*

Power Input

The BEAR ventilators are both pneumatically powered and electronically controlled. Alternating electric current at 120 volts, 60 Hz, is utilized to control the electronic control circuitry. The ventilator also relies on a pneumatic gas source (30 to 100 psi) for oxygen and air. If compressed medical air is not available, an internal compressor will provide air (10 to 11.2 psi) to the blender.

Drive Mechanism

The pneumatic drive mechanism reduces the line pressure of the incoming gas to between 10 and 11 psi. Once the incoming pressure has been reduced, air and oxygen are mixed in the blender to the desired F_IO_2. Gas exiting the blender is reduced in pressure once again to between 1 and 3 psi by the waveform control and the peak flow control.

The waveform control is a variable orifice distal to the main solenoid valve. When set at the square wave position, 3.2 psi is provided

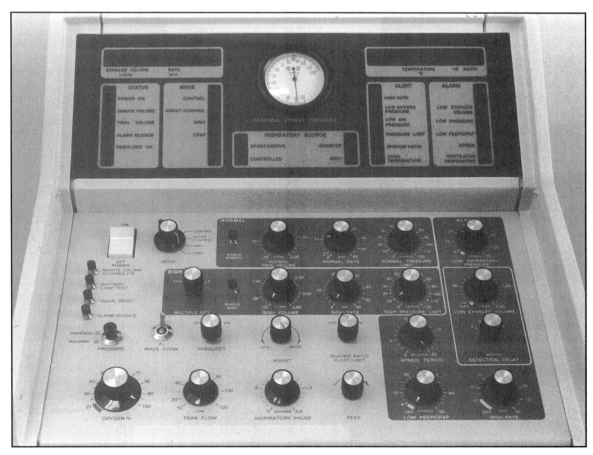

Figure 8-2B *A photograph showing the control panel of the BEAR 2 ventilator.*

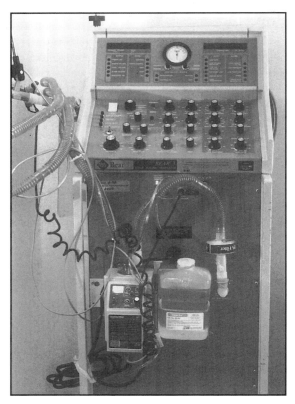

Figure 8-3A *A photograph of the BEAR 3 volume ventilator.*

to the inlet of the variable orifice when the main solenoid valve has opened. Depending upon the patient's airway resistance and compliance, a pressure drop occurs across the waveform control valve. If the airway resistance is low and compliance is high, a higher flow will result through the valve since the pressure drop is low. Conversely, if the patient's airway resistance is high and compliance is low, a greater pressure drop will result and flow through the valve will be decreased. In the square wave setting, the drop in peak flow can be as high as 20% if the back pressure in the circuit reaches 100 cmH$_2$O.

Adjustment of the waveform control valve to the tapered position results in a further reduction in the delivered flow, tapering it. In the taper position, drive pressure through the variable orifice valve is reduced to 1.8 psi. At this lower drive pressure, changes in resistance and compliance (circuit back pressure) will cause a more dramatic reduction in delivered flow. The waveform control on the BEAR 1 is infinitely variable between the square and tapered settings. The BEAR 1 and 3 waveform controls are two position switches (50% taper or square).

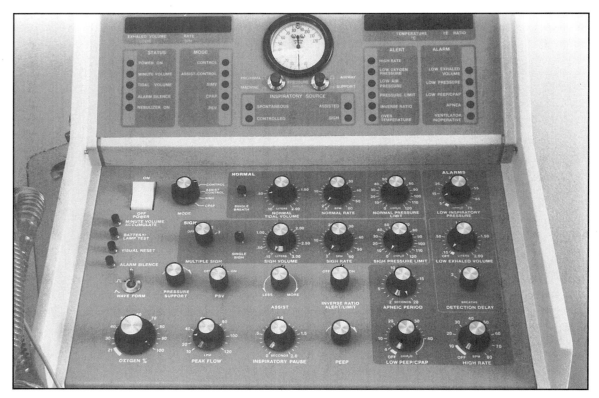

Figure 8-3B *A photograph showing the control panel of the BEAR 3 ventilator.*

The flow rate control determines the peak flow delivered during a ventilator-supported breath (Control, Assist Control and the mandatory portion of SIMV). It is also a variable orifice operating in tandem with the waveform control valve. Adjustment of the waveform control valve opens or closes the peak flow control valve to maintain the desired peak inspiratory flow rate.

Control Circuit

The BEAR 1, 2, and 3 utilize pneumatic and electronic devices in their control circuitry. During spontaneous modes of ventilation (SIMV and CPAP), a pneumatic demand valve (Figure 8-4) opens in response to a pressure drop in the patient circuit (below PEEP). Once fully opened, flow rates of up to 100 L/min can be provided to meet the patient's inspiratory needs.

The assist transducer is a thermistor which measures flow output from the demand valve. A constant current is applied to the small thermistor bead, heating it to a constant temperature. When gas flows across the thermistor, cooling it, a voltage drop occurs. During the mandatory portion of SIMV, when a voltage drop is sensed by the assist transducer, a signal is sent to the main solenoid valve, delivering a mandatory breath, synchronizing the mandatory breath with the patient's spontaneous efforts. The assist transducer is also used during SIMV and CPAP to detect spontaneous breaths. When a voltage drop occurs, the ventilators activate the spontaneous light, and the breath rate reflects the combined ventilatory rate (ventilator and patient).

During Assist/Control operation, the assist sensitivity can be set by adjusting the flow threshold of the assist transducer. In its most sensitive position, approximately 10 ml, or -1 cmH_2O below PEEP, must be generated to trigger a mandatory breath. In its least sensitive position, 70 ml, or -5 cmH_2O below PEEP, is required to trigger a mandatory breath.

During control mode, an electronic solenoid locks out the demand valve (lockout solenoid). Once locked out, gas flow to the patient circuit is solely controlled by the main solenoid valve and the electronic timing circuitry (rate control).

Volume delivery is controlled by a flow transducer located at the output of the ventilator. The delivered volume is determined by the integration of flow during the inspiratory time. Hence, volume is determined indirectly as a function of flow, and these ventilators are classified as flow controllers. The measured volume is compared to a reference signal (tidal volume control) and when the signals match, the main solenoid closes, ceasing mandatory gas delivery from the ventilator.

Pressure is measured by a pressure transducer near the ventilator outlet (BEAR 1). The BEAR 2 and 3 measure pressure using the proximal airway line. The pressure transducer converts gas pressure to an electronic signal which is utilized in the alarm system and the pressure limit systems for normal and sigh breath delivery.

PEEP pressure is controlled by the application of pressure to the exhalation valve in the patient circuit and the demand valve. Pressure is generated by a venturi inside the ventilator. Pressure from the venturi is conducted to the reference side of the demand valve (so that application of PEEP will not affect the sensitivity) and to the exhalation valve (Figure 8-4). The pressure applied to the exhalation valve closes it slightly during the expiratory phase, which maintains pressure in the circuit and the patient's lungs.

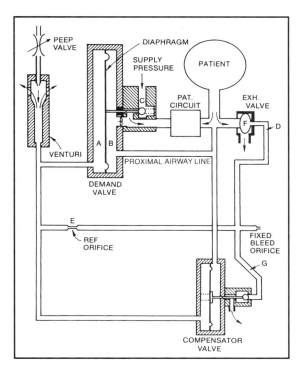

Figure 8-4 *A schematic drawing illustrating the BEAR demand valve. (Courtesy BEAR Medical Systems, Inc., Riverside, CA)*

Control Variables

As described earlier, during Assist/Control, Control and the mandatory portion of SIMV, the BEAR 1, 2 and 3 function as flow controllers. Flow is measured by a vortex shedding transducer located near the outlet of the ventilator. Its signal is compared to a reference setting (tidal volume or sigh volume controls) and used to control the ventilator's output. Volume is measured directly as a function of flow over time.

During CPAP (BEAR 1, 2 and 3), and Pressure Support (BEAR 3), pressure is measured and used as a feedback signal to control the ventilator output via the demand valve. During these modes, inspiratory flow varies to maintain the set CPAP or pressure support level.

Phase Variables
Trigger Variable

The trigger variables for the BEAR 1, 2, and 3 can be pressure/flow, time or manual. The assist transducer senses flow as a result of the opening of the demand valve (pressure). Therefore, the ventilator is neither purely pressure or purely flow triggered, but rather a combination of both.

Time triggering occurs when inspiration begins following a set time interval (rate control). This may occur during Control, Assist/Control and SIMV modes.

Manual triggering can occur with all three ventilators by depressing the single breath control or manual sigh control, delivering a single mandatory breath (normal or sigh).

Limit Variables

The limit variables for the BEAR ventilators include pressure, volume and flow. The ventilators become pressure limited when they are operated in the spontaneous modes (SIMV, CPAP and pressure support). The demand valve in these modes limits inspiratory pressures to the settings adjusted on the PEEP/CPAP control or the pressure support control. The demand valve maintains the pressure level by varying flow and is capable of providing up to 100 L/min (BEAR 1), and 120 L/min (BEAR 2 and 3).

Volume becomes a limit variable when the inspiratory pause control is set to a value greater than zero. Under these conditions, the inspired volume is held until the pause time has elapsed. Inspiratory pause is adjustable between 0 and 2 seconds. Once the inspira-

tory pause time has elapsed, the ventilator ends inspiration. Therefore, volume becomes the limit variable (volume is not allowed to exceed a preset value, and inspiration has not been terminated).

The ventilators become flow limited when operated in the rectangular waveform. When the waveform control is set in this position, inspiratory flow is limited to the value set on the peak flow control (adjustable between 20 and 120 L/min).

Cycle Variables

The cycle variables for the BEAR ventilators include pressure, flow (BEAR 3), and time. Pressure becomes a cycling variable if the pressure limit, or sigh pressure limit controls are set below the peak inspiratory pressure level during mandatory breaths (Control, Assist/Control or mandatory portion of SIMV). The ventilators are also pressure cycled during SIMV and CPAP when the demand valve opens and closes in response to pressure gradients. The BEAR 3 becomes flow cycled during pressure support. In this mode, inspiratory flow is measured and monitored. When the inspiratory flow drops to 25% of the peak flow value, the pressure supported breath is terminated.

Baseline Variable

The baseline variable for the BEAR ventilators is pressure. Pressure is controlled during CPAP and PEEP to maintain a positive pressure in the airway. CPAP/PEEP pressures are controlled by adjusting a needle valve which regulates flow through a venturi. The output from the venturi is applied to the exhalation valve in the patient circuit and also to the demand valve, so that the demand valve is pressure compensated for CPAP/PEEP pressures. Baseline pressure is adjustable from zero to 30 cmH$_2$O (BEAR 1) and zero to 50 cmH$_2$O (BEAR 2 and 3).

Conditional Variables
Time

Time becomes a conditional variable during sigh delivery. During normal tidal volume delivery, the ventilator breaths flow controlled, pressure, time or manually triggered, and pressure or time cycled. During sigh delivery, each hour may be divided into windows lasting between 1 and 30 minutes. That is, every 1 to 30 minutes, the ventilator switches to sigh mode and the sigh controls become active. Once activated, the ventilator will deliver between one and three breaths. Under these circumstances, the conditional variable is time.

Time and Pressure

Time and pressure become conditional variables during SIMV mode. The rate control determines the frequency of mandatory breath delivery during SIMV mode. The rate control is essentially an electronic timer, delivering a breath at specified time intervals. Between mandatory breath delivery, the patient opens and closes the demand valve as a result of pressure fluctuations in the patient circuit. As the spontaneous breathing window closes, the ventilator senses the next inspiration (assist transducer) and activates the main solenoid valve, delivering a mandatory breath.

Output Waveforms

The BEAR ventilators can deliver either a rectangular or descending ramp flow waveform output. In the rectangular position under conditions of low resistance and high compliance, the output waveform is rectangular. As resistance increases and compliance decreases, the flow waveform can taper as much as 20%.

When set in the descending ramp waveform position, less driving pressure is available (1.8 psi), resulting in a more drastic tapering of the rectangular flow waveform output due to changes in the patient's resistance or compliance.

The BEAR 1 is infinitely variable between the rectangular and the descending ramp flow waveform positions. The BEAR 2 and 3 can be selected between each setting, but an adjustable output is not possible.

Control Interactions

The tidal volume and flow rate controls can have a profound effect upon inspiratory time. As tidal volume is increased, inspiratory time is also increased (unless compensated for by increasing the peak flow). A decrease in the peak flow rate control will have the same effect. If I:E ratios of 1:2 or greater are desired, adjustment of the tidal volume, rate and peak flows must be manipulated correctly.

If inverse I:E ratio ventilation is desired, the BEAR ventilators can be adjusted to pro-

vide it. To ventilate a patient using inverse ratios, the 1:1 ratio limit control must be turned off and the controls adjusted to achieve an I:E ratio greater than 1:1.

Monitoring and Alarm Systems
Monitoring Systems

Several monitors are available to assist the practitioner in patient management. Three BEAR monitors are described in Table 8-1.

Alarm Systems
Input Power

The BEAR ventilators have three input power alarms: for loss of electrical power, loss of oxygen pressure and loss of air pressure. In the event air pressure is lost, a built-in compressor will be activated, and it will supply the pneumatic pressure required to operate the blender and other systems. These alarms are both visual and audible. The loss of electric power alarm is battery powered and operates from a bank of rechargeable nickel cadmium batteries.

TABLE 8-1: BEAR Ventilator Monitors

	BEAR 1	BEAR 2	BEAR 3
Exhaled Volume	X	X	X
Rate	X	X	X
Status Indication	X	X	X
Mode Display	X	X	X
Pressure Manometer	X	X	X
Spontaneous Breath Monitor	X	X	X
Assisted Breath Monitor	X	X	X
Controlled Breath Monitor	X	X	X
Sigh Breath Monitor	X	X	X
Alert Display	X	X	X
Alarm Display	X	X	X
1:1 Limit Off Display	X		
I:E Ratio	X	X	X
Temperature		X	X

Control Circuit Alarms

Inverse I:E Ratio

The I:E ratio limit control, when activated, prevents patient ventilation at a ratio of greater than 1:1. It works by monitoring the inspiratory and expiratory time. In the control mode, if the inspiratory time equals 50% of the total ventilatory cycle, the main solenoid closes, ending inspiration. If inspiration is terminated, the ventilator then functions as a time cycled ventilator.

If the control is off, a light illuminates on the control panel and inverse I:E ratio ventilation is possible. Each time a breath is delivered at an inverse I:E ratio, an indicator light will illuminate.

Ventilator Inoperative

The ventilator inoperative alarm will be activated on the BEAR ventilators during conditions of adequate power and gas pressure if an internal malfunction in the volume control circuitry is detected. If electric power and gas pressure are adequate and the alarm is activated, the ventilator must be removed from use and alternative ventilation for the patient must be provided.

Output Alarms

Pressure

High peak pressure alarms are available on the BEAR ventilators. These alarms may be adjusted between 0 and 100 cmH$_2$O (BEAR 1) and 0 and 120 cmH$_2$O (BEAR 2 and 3). When pressure in the patient circuit reaches the reference setting on the normal pressure limit or sigh pressure limit controls, inspiration is terminated and visual and audible alarms are activated. Pressure is measured by a pressure transducer near the outlet of the ventilator (BEAR 1, referenced to machine pressure) or at the proximal airway (BEAR 2 and 3). To adjust the alarm, it is necessary to depress the proximal/machine pressure switch to measure the machine pressure and properly reference the alarm (BEAR 1).

ASSEMBLY AND TROUBLESHOOTING

Assembly—BEAR 1, BEAR 2, BEAR 3

The following is a suggested guide for the assembly of the BEAR 1, BEAR 2 and BEAR 3 ventilators:

1. Using a universal rubber adapter, connect the bacterial filter to the ventilator outlet.

2. Humidifier assembly:
   a. Assemble the humidifier and connect it to its heating element on the front of the ventilator. Since many popular humidifiers may be adapted for use on this ventilator, specific instructions are not included here.
   b. Attach a short piece of large bore tubing between the bacteria filter and the humidifier inlet.

3. Assemble the circuit as shown in Figure 8-5. The BEAR circuit requires that the temperature probe be placed close to the proximal airway.

4. Attach the inspiratory limb of the circuit to the humidifier outlet.

5. Attach the ¼-inch diameter proximal airway line to the external condenser assembly (BEAR 1) or proximal line filter (BEAR 2 and 3).

6. Attach the exhalation valve drive line to the exhalation valve nipple on the front of the ventilator.

7. Attach the vortex sensing tube to the expiratory limb of the circuit at the manifold, distal to the exhalation valve.

8. Connect the air (if available) and oxygen inlets to 50 psi medical gas sources.

9. Connect the power cord to a 120 volt, 60 Hz power source.

10. Pressure test the ventilator in accordance with the manufacturer's recommendations.

Troubleshooting

Refer to the troubleshooting algorithms found at the end of this chapter.

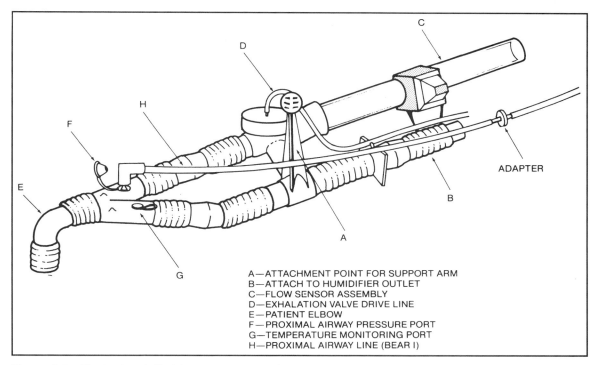

A—ATTACHMENT POINT FOR SUPPORT ARM
B—ATTACH TO HUMIDIFIER OUTLET
C—FLOW SENSOR ASSEMBLY
D—EXHALATION VALVE DRIVE LINE
E—PATIENT ELBOW
F—PROXIMAL AIRWAY PRESSURE PORT
G—TEMPERATURE MONITORING PORT
H—PROXIMAL AIRWAY LINE (BEAR I)

Figure 8-5 *The BEAR Medical Systems BEAR 1 volume ventilator circuit.*

Low inspiratory pressure alarms are also available on the BEAR ventilators. They function in a similar way to the high peak pressure alarms. Settings are adjustable between 0 and 50 cmH$_2$O (BEAR 1) and 0 and 75 cmH$_2$O (BEAR 2 and 3).

Baseline pressure alarms are available to alert the practitioner to loss of baseline (PEEP/CPAP) pressures. The alarm is adjustable to between 0 and 30 cmH$_2$O (BEAR 1) and 0 and 50 cmH$_2$O (BEAR 2 and 3).

Volume

Low tidal volume alarms are included on the BEAR ventilators. Exhaled tidal volume is measured by an external flow sensor located on the patient circuit's expiratory limb. The alarm is adjustable between 0 and 2 liters. If the exhaled volume falls below the threshold set on the alarm for three consecutive breaths, both visual and audible alarms are activated.

Apnea

The apnea alarm alerts the practitioner to absence of ventilation (spontaneous or mechanical). The alarm is activated if no breaths are sensed over a 20-second interval. The BEAR 2 and 3 have an adjustable apneic period alarm (same function as the apnea alarm). The alarm is adjustable between a 2- and a 20-second interval.

High Ventilatory Rate

The BEAR 2 and 3 ventilators have a high ventilatory rate alarm to alert the practitioner of high ventilatory rates. The alarm is adjustable between 10 and 80 breaths per minute.

Table 8-2 compares the alarm systems of the BEAR 1, 2 and 3 ventilators, and Table 8-3 compares their capabilities.

BEAR MEDICAL SYSTEMS, BEAR 5

The BEAR Medical Systems BEAR 5 is a microprocessor-controlled pediatric and adult ventilator. The microprocessor controller and the Cathode Ray Tube (CRT) display/monitor provide a flexible machine capable of ventilating a variety of patients (Figures 8-6 and 8-7).

The BEAR 5 is classified as a flow and pressure controller. Flow is measured and used as a feedback signal to control the stepper motor valves to regulate volume delivery. The ventilator operates as a pressure controller during CPAP and pressure support modes.

TABLE 8-2: BEAR 1, 2, and 3 Alarm Systems

	BEAR 1	BEAR 2	BEAR 3
Input Power			
Oxygen Pressure	X	X	X
Air Pressure	X	X	X
Electric Power	X	X	X
Control Circuit			
Inverse I:E ratio	X	X	X
Ventilator Inop.	X	X	X
Output			
High Pressure	X	X	X
Low Pressure	X	X	X
Low Baseline Pressure	X	X	X
Low Tidal Volume	X	X	X
Apnea	X	X	X
High Ventilatory Rate		X	X

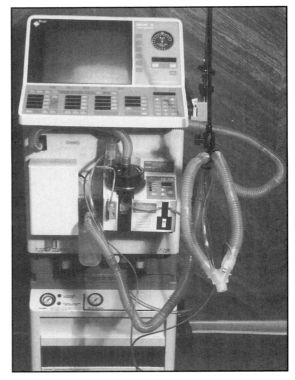

Figure 8-6 *A photograph of the BEAR 5 volume ventilator.*

Power Input

Power to run the microprocessor control circuitry and the stepper motor control system is provided by 115 volt, 60 Hz electrical power. The pneumatic system is powered by 50 psi air and oxygen. If 50 psi medical air is not available, the built-in compressor may be used to supply the gas needed to operate the ventilator.

Drive Mechanism

The pneumatic drive mechanism (Figure 8-8) reduces the line pressure of the incoming

TABLE 8-3: BEAR 1, 2, and 3 Ventilator Capabilities

	BEAR 1	BEAR 2	BEAR 3
Modes	CMV, Assist CMV, SIMV, CPAP	CMV, Assist CMV, SIMV, CPAP	CMV, Assist CMV, SIMV, CPAP, Pressure Support
Volume	0-2200 mL	0 - 2200 mL	0 - 2200 mL
Pressure	0 - 100 cmH$_2$O	0 - 120 cmH$_2$O	0 - 120 cmH$_2$O
Rate	0 - 60	0 - 60	0 - 60
Peak Flow	0 - 120 L/min	0 - 120 L/min	0 - 120 L/min
PEEP/CPAP	0 - 30 cmH$_2$O	0 - 50 cmH$_2$O	0 - 50 cmH$_2$O
Sigh Volume	150 - 3000 mL	150 - 3000 mL	150 - 3000 mL
Insp. Pause	0 - 2 seconds	0 - 2 seconds	0 - 2 seconds
F$_1$O$_2$	.21 - 1.0	.21 - 1.0	.21 - 1.0

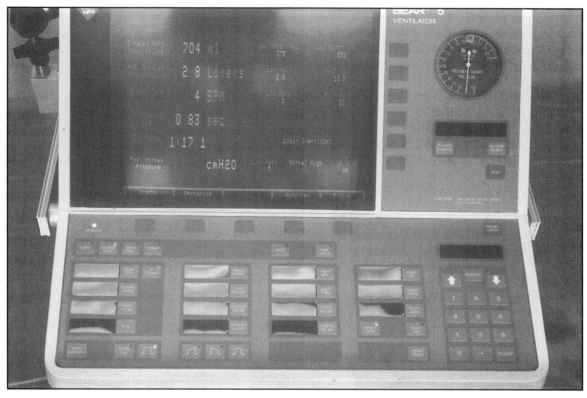

Figure 8-7 *A photograph showing the control panel of the BEAR 5 ventilator.*

gas to 18.2 psi (±.1 psi) by means of the air regulator and the O_2 relay. The gas pressures and temperatures are closely matched to enhance the accuracy of the blending system. Gas flows from these pressure-controlling elements to the oxygen blender.

The oxygen blender is a type of proportioning valve that mixes the oxygen and air. Signals from the microprocessor control a stepper motor that controls the position of the proportioning valve. Gas then exits the blender to an accumulator.

The accumulator is a reservoir with a volume of 3.6 liters. The accumulator helps to minimize instantaneous flow demands from the blender. It also functions as a mixing chamber enhancing oxygen stability and enables the ventilator to meet instantaneous flow demands of up to 150 L/min.

Control Circuit

The BEAR 5 ventilator uses a microprocessor and a stepper motor–controlled flow control valve to regulate flow output from the ventilator. This system, operating in conjunction with an internal vortex flow transducer, regulates gas flow during bias flow, continu-

ous flow, demand flow, and during ventilator supported breaths. The vortex flow sensor measures flow and uses it as a feedback signal to the microprocessor, controlling the position of the stepper motor and regulating the output from the flow control valve. A temperature sensor located proximal to the vortex flow sensor measures temperature, allowing the ventilator to deliver gas at BTPS, assuming the gas is 100% saturated with water vapor when delivered to the patient.

This system also allows delivery of tidal volumes, which are compensated for the volume compressed in the patient circuit. The circuit compliance factor may be entered into the microprocessor, which will automatically compensate the delivered volume, correcting for volume lost due to compression in the patient circuit.

Output waveforms include rectangular, ascending and descending ramp, and sinusoidal waveforms. All of these waveforms are possible through microprocessor control of the stepper motor in the flow control valve.

Pressure is controlled by the pilot pressure control/exhalation valve system. The pilot pressure control valve is also controlled by a

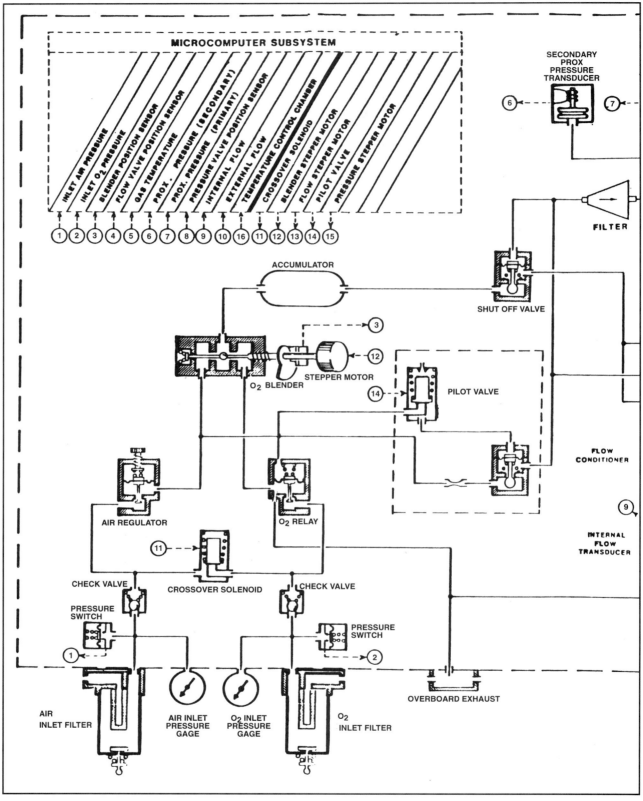

Figure 8-8 *A schematic diagram of the BEAR 5 pneumatic system. (Courtesy BEAR Medical Systems, Inc., Riverside, CA)*
(continues)

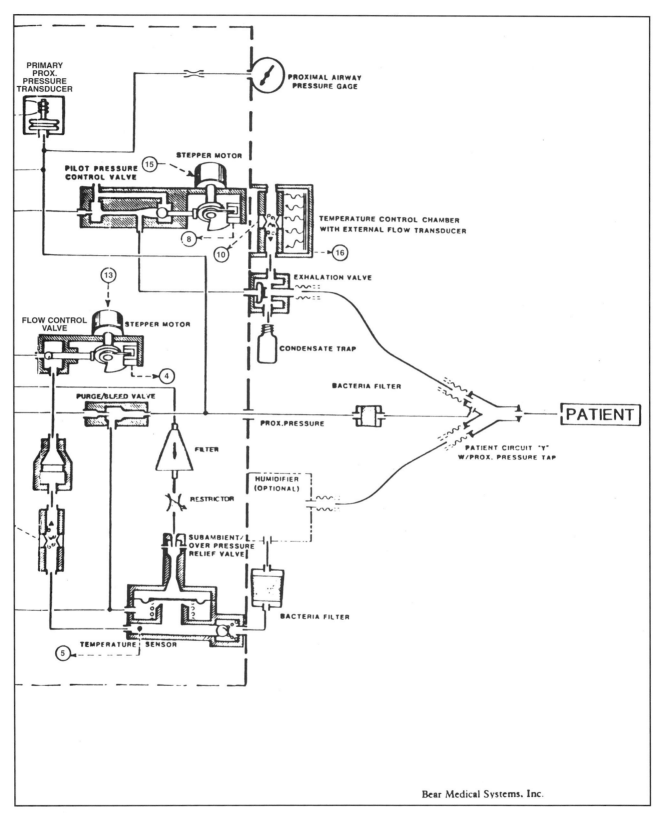

Figure 8-8 *(continued)*

stepper motor receiving signals from the microprocessor. Pressure is sensed by a proximal pressure transducer and is used to provide a feedback signal to the microprocessor. Output from the pilot pressure control valve is directed to the exhalation valve diaphragm, which controls the pressure in the patient circuit. The application of PEEP/CPAP is also controlled through this system.

Control Variables

As described earlier, during CMV (Control), Assist CMV (Assist/Control) and the mandatory portions of SIMV, the ventilator operates as a flow controller. Flow is measured by a vortex sensor downstream from the flow control valve. Its output is used as a feedback signal to the microprocessor, controlling the operation of the flow control valve. The tidal volume setting and sigh volume setting provide a reference signal and are used to servo the flow control valve. Volume delivery is determined directly as a function of flow and time by the microprocessor.

During CPAP and pressure support and time cycled ventilation, inspiratory pressure is regulated by the flow control valve described earlier. Pressure sensed by the proximal pressure transducer is used as feedback to adjust flow to the circuit to maintain the desired pressure. Any excess pressure is vented through the exhalation valve. When operated in these modes, the ventilator becomes a pressure controller.

Phase Variables
Trigger Variable

Inspiration may be pressure, time or manually triggered. The ventilator is pressure triggered when the pressure in the patient circuit drops to the level set on the assist sensitivity control. Pressure in the patient circuit will fall below baseline pressure when the patient initiates a breath. Sensitivity levels between 0.5 and 5.0 cmH$_2$O subbaseline may be selected. Pressure is sensed by the proximal pressure transducer, located in the ventilator.

The ventilator is time triggered when no patient effort is sensed by the microprocessor through the Assist/Sensitivity system or when operating in CMV mode. The setting on the normal rate control determines the time interval (respiratory rate) for ventilator assisted breaths. Rate may be set between 0.5 and 150 breaths per minute. After the set time interval

has passed, a ventilator supported breath will be initiated.

The ventilator may also be manually cycled by the practitioner by depressing the manual breath or sigh control.

Limit Variables

The BEAR 5 may be pressure, volume or flow limited. The ventilator is pressure limited during the spontaneous breaths in the pressure support and CPAP modes. The flow control valve, operating in conjunction with the pilot pressure control valve, will maintain the desired pressure in the patient circuit. During pressure support, pressure support levels may be adjusted between 0 and 72 cmH$_2$O. During PEEP and CPAP, pressures are adjustable between 0 and 50 cmH$_2$O.

The ventilator becomes volume limited any time the inspiratory pause control is set for a time greater than zero. Under these conditions, the inspired volume is held until the pause time has elapsed. Inspiratory pause is adjustable between 0 and 2 seconds. Once the inspiratory pause time has elapsed, the ventilator ends inspiration. Therefore, volume becomes the limit variable (volume is not allowed to exceed a preset value and inspiration has not been terminated). Under these conditions, volume becomes the limit variable since the delivered volume is always reached prior to the termination of the breath.

The ventilator is flow limited during flow controlled breaths. Under these circumstances, flow is limited to the setting on the peak flow control. Peak inspiratory flow is adjustable between 5 and 150 L/min.

Cycle Variables

The BEAR 5 ventilator can be pressure, flow, or time cycled. The ventilator becomes pressure cycled if the proximal airway pressure exceeds the value set on the high peak normal or sigh pressure alarm setting. If this pressure level is reached prior to delivery of the mandatory breath, both an audible and visual alarm will sound and inspiration will be terminated.

The ventilator becomes flow cycled during pressure support mode. During pressure support, the ventilator assisted breath is terminated when inspiratory flow falls to a value less than 25% of the peak inspiratory flow required to maintain the pressure support level.

Time cycling occurs when the ventilator is

time cycled and pressure controlled. Inspiration ends when the inspiratory time has elapsed. Inspiratory times are adjustable between 0.1 and 3.0 seconds. Time is also a cycling variable when the inspiratory pause control is adjusted greater than zero. Inspiration is terminated following the set inspiratory pause (time).

Baseline Variables

The baseline variable for the BEAR 5 is pressure. Baseline pressure may be adjusted during PEEP and CPAP between 0 and 50 cmH$_2$O.

Conditional Variables
Time

Time becomes a conditional variable during sigh delivery. Normal ventilator supported breaths are flow controlled, pressure triggered, and pressure or time cycled. During sigh delivery, each hour may be divided into windows lasting between 1 and 30 minutes. That is, every 1 to 30 minutes, the ventilator switches to sigh mode and the sigh controls become active. Once activated, the ventilator will deliver between one and three breaths. Under these circumstances, the conditional variable is time.

Time and Pressure

Time and pressure become conditional variables during SIMV mode. The rate control determines the frequency of mandatory breath delivery during SIMV mode. The rate control is essentially an electronic timer, delivering a breath at specified time intervals. Between mandatory breath delivery, the patient breathes through the flow/volume/demand control subsystem. The ventilator measures proximal airway pressure to determine if the patient is attempting to initiate a breath. In response to the pressure change, the patient is able to draw gas spontaneously through the flow control valve to meet their inspiratory needs. Flow may be provided on a demand basis or by a continuous flow of gas of between 5 and 40 L/min baseline flow.

Time and Volume

Time and volume become conditional variables during AMV ventilation. A set minimum exhaled volume is established by the practitioner. Should the patient fail to meet this minute volume, the ventilator will deliver breaths at a rate equal to the minimum minute

volume setting divided by the set tidal volume. Apnea results in time triggered ventilation. Flow becomes the conditional variable because the BEAR 5 measures flow and determines volume directly as a function of flow and time.

Output Waveforms
Pressure

The BEAR 5 can deliver a rectangular pressure waveform when operated using time-cycled or pressure-supported ventilation. Under these circumstances, pressure rises rapidly to a constant value where it remains through the delivery of the breath. At the termination of inspiration, pressure falls to the baseline value.

Flow

The flow output waveform capabilities of the BEAR 5 include rectangular, ascending and descending ramp, and sinusoidal. As described earlier, these waveforms can be accurately reproduced by the feedback system between the internal vortex flow transducer, the microprocessor and the stepper motor driven flow control valve.

Alarms
Input Power Alarms

The input power alarms include loss of electrical and loss of pneumatic power. In the event of a loss of electrical power, a battery powered alarm will be activated both visually and audibly. During a loss of electrical power, the power LED on the upper left corner of the control panel will not be illuminated.

If the oxygen line pressure falls below 27 psi, an audible and visual alarm will be activated. In the event that air pressure falls below 27 psi and electric power is still available, the compressor will be activated to compensate for the loss of air pressure. The compressor's power switch must be in the ON position, and the compressor must be connected to a 115 volt, 60 Hz electrical outlet for the compressor to act as a backup system for the piped medical air system.

Control Circuit Alarms

The control circuit alarms include ventilator inoperative settings, incompatible settings and inverse I:E ratio alarms. The ventilator inoperative alarm may indicate the following cor-

ASSEMBLY AND TROUBLESHOOTING

Assembly—BEAR 5

Although the BEAR 5 is a complex ventilator, circuit assembly is very easy. The following is a suggested assembly guide.

1. Attach the high pressure hoses to an oxygen and air source. If no source of 50 psi air is available and the ventilator is equipped with the optional compressor, no air supply is required.

2. Verify that the exhalation valve assembly is secured well to its slide mount. Screw the collection jar into place and tighten it.

3. Place the vortex flow tube into its holder in the temperature control chamber and connect the external flow sensors to the flow tube.

4. Attach the crossover flow tube between the vortex sensor and the exhalation valve. Then close the door to the temperature control chamber.

5. Attach the collector vial to the exhalation valve filter and close its door.

6. Assemble and fill the humidifier and attach it to the front of the ventilator. Many different humidifiers may be adapted to the BEAR 5, so specific assembly instructions will not be included here.

7. Assemble the adult circuit, verifying the integrity of connections at the proximal airway port, patient wye and temperature probe ports.

8. Connect the main flow bacteria filter between the ventilator outlet and the humidifier. Attach the adult circuit to the outlet of the humidifier and the exhalation limb to the collection jar proximal to the temperature control chamber.

9. Connect the power cord to a suitable 120 volt, 60 Hz outlet.

Troubleshooting

Refer to the troubleshooting algorithms found at the end of this chapter.

rectable situations: (1) the patient circuit has become kinked (expiratory limb or proximal airway line), (2) the temperature control chamber door is open (TCC Door Open/TCC Temp Low), or (3) an improperly installed external flow sensor (Ext. Flow Sensor). The practitioner should attempt to correct these conditions and disable the ventilator inoperative alarm. If the alarm cannot be silenced or cannot be traced to these situations, an internal problem has been detected and the ventilator should be removed from service.

An alarm will alert the practitioner to settings which are not compatible. For example, if a tidal volume of 3000 is entered, an "E" will appear at the left of the key pad display and "Available Range 50 to 2000" will appear on the CRT display.

The inverse I:E ratio alarm is enabled if the 1:1 ratio limit is activated by the practitioner. If activated, the ventilator will terminate inspiration if the I:E ratio reaches 1:1. If the ratio limit is overridden, I:E ratios of less than 1:1 may be used up to a maximum of a 3:1 I:E ratio.

Output Alarms
Pressure

Pressure output alarms include high and low peak, high and low baseline, and high and low mean pressures. The high and low peak airway pressure alarms are adjustable between 0.0 and 140 cmH_2O except during time cycled ventilation, when it is adjustable between 0.0 and 80 cmH_2O. Mean airway pressure alarms are adjustable between 0.0 and 75 cmH_2O. Baseline pressure alarms may be set between 0.0 and 55 cmH_2O.

Volume

A low exhaled tidal volume is available for both mandatory breaths and spontaneous breaths. The alarm parameters are adjustable between 30 and 2000 mL for both mandatory and spontaneous alarms.

Flow

A low exhaled minute volume alarm may be adjusted between 0.3 and 40.0 L/min. A

TABLE 8-4: BEAR 5 Alarm Systems

ALARM	CONDITION/SETTINGS
Input Power	
Oxygen Pressure	<27 psi
Air Pressure	<27 psi
Electric Power	Loss of 115 volt, 60 Hz power
Control Circuit	
Ventilator Inoperative	Correctable:
	Kinked patient circuit
	Temperature Control Chamber door open
	External Flow Sensor installed wrong
	Not Correctable:
	Internal malfunction detected
Incompatible Settings	Practitioner selected settings not compatible with the ventilator's capabilities
I:E Ratio	I:E ratio less than 1:1 if the ratio limit is enabled
Output Alarms	
High Airway Pressure	0.0–140 cmH₂O
Low Airway Pressure	0.0–140 cmH₂O
High Baseline Pressure	0.0–55 cmH₂O
Low Baseline Pressure	0.0–55 cmH₂O
High Mean Airway Pres.	0.0–75 cmH₂O
Low Mean Airway Pres.	0.0–75 cmH₂O
Low Exhaled Tidal Vol.	30–2000 mL
(Spontaneous)	30–2000 mL
High Minute Volume	1.0–80 L/min
Low Minute Volume	0.3–40 L/min
High Breath Rate	3–155 breaths per minute (BPM)
(Time Cycled Vent.)	0–155 BPM
High Insp. Time	0.10–3.2 seconds
Low Insp. Time	0.01–3.0 seconds

high exhaled minute volume alarm can be adjusted between 1.0 and 80.0 L/min.

Time

A high and low ventilatory rate alarm can be set between 3 and 155 breaths per minute. During time cycled ventilation, the alarm is adjustable between 0.0 and 155 breaths per minute.

A high and low inspiratory time alarm is available when operating the BEAR 5 in time cycled ventilation. The low inspiratory time is adjustable between 0.05 and 3.00 seconds and the high inspiratory time alarm is adjustable between 0.10 and 3.2 seconds.

Table 8-4 illustrates the BEAR 5 alarm systems and Table 8-5 illustrates its capabilities.

BEAR MEDICAL SYSTEMS BEAR 1000

The BEAR Medical Systems BEAR 1000 is a microprocessor controlled pediatric and adult

TABLE 8-5: BEAR 5 Ventilator Capabilities

Modes	CMV, Assist CMV, SIMV/IMV, CPAP, AMV (MMV), Time Cycle, Pressure Support
Volume	50–2000 mL
Pressure	0.0–150 cmH₂O
Rate	0.0–150 BPM
Peak Flow	5–150 L/min
PEEP/CPAP	0.0–50 cmH₂O
Sigh Volume	65–3000 mL
Insp. Pause	0.0–2.0 seconds
F₁O₂	0.21–1.00

ventilator (Figures 8-9 and 8-10). The microprocessor controller allows operator flexibility and the ability to upgrade the ventilator to meet future needs.

The BEAR 1000 is classified as a pressure controller. During volume delivery (Assist CMV and the mandatory portion of SIMV), pressure is measured and used as a feedback signal controlling the ventilator's output. Flow and volume are determined indirectly as a function of pressure (differential pressure across the flow control valve). During CPAP, pressure control and pressure support, pressure is also measured and used to control the output of the flow control valve.

Power Input

Power to run the microprocessor control circuitry and the stepper motor control system is provided by 120 volt, 60 Hz electrical power. The pneumatic system is powered by 50 psi air and oxygen. If 50 psi medical air is not available, a built-in compressor may be used to supply the gas needed to operate the ventilator.

Drive Mechanism

The pneumatic drive mechanism (Figure 8-11) reduces the line pressure of the incoming gas to 18.0 psi (±.1 psi) by means of the air regulator and the O₂ relay. The gas pressures and temperatures are closely matched to enhance the accuracy of the blending system. In the event medical air or oxygen pressure is lost (<27.5 psi), a crossover solenoid opens, divert-

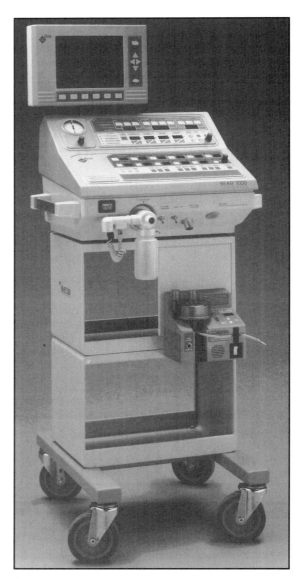

Figure 8-9 *A photograph of the BEAR 1000 volume ventilator. (Courtesy BEAR Medical Systems, Inc., Riverside, CA)*

ing the remaining high pressure gas to the air regulator. Under these circumstances, the F₁O₂ delivered is 1.0 or 0.21, depending upon which gas was lost. Gas flows from these pressure controlling elements to the oxygen blender.

The oxygen blender is a type of proportioning valve that mixes the oxygen and air. Signals from the microprocessor control a stepper motor that regulates the opening and closing of the proportioning valve. Gas then exits the blender to an accumulator.

The accumulator is a reservoir with a volume of 3.5 liters at 10.0 to 18.0 psi, depending upon flow demands. The accumulator helps to minimize instantaneous flow demands from

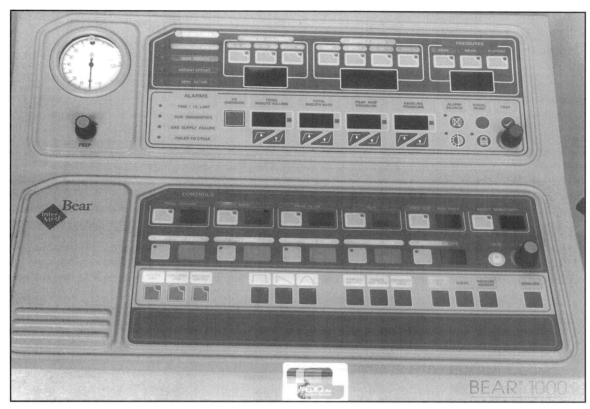

Figure 8-10 *A photograph showing the control panel of the BEAR 1000 ventilator.*

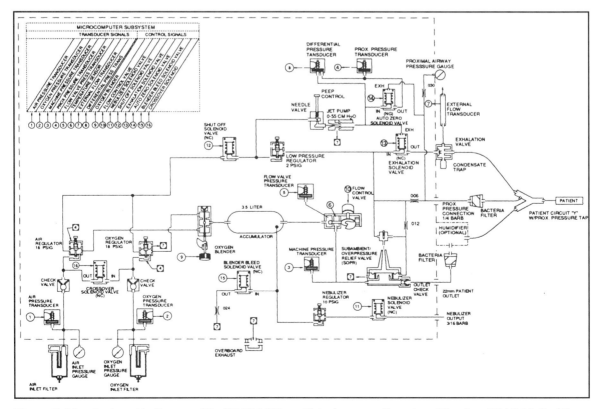

Figure 8-11 *A schematic diagram of the BEAR 1000 ventilator's pneumatic system. (Courtesy BEAR Medical Systems, Inc., Riverside, CA)*

the blender. The accumulator also functions as a mixing chamber enhancing oxygen stability. The accumulator also enables the ventilator to meet instantaneous flow demands of over 200 L/min.

Control Circuit

The BEAR 1000 ventilator uses a microprocessor and a stepper motor–driven flow control valve to regulate flow output from the ventilator. This system operates in conjunction with two pressure transducers, one located at the inlet and the other located at the outlet of the flow control valve. When the valve is open, a pressure difference will exist between the flow control valve inlet and outlet. This pressure is proportional to flow at the present position of the flow control valve. The microprocessor logic uses reference values established by the tidal volume, peak flow and waveform control settings to establish an initial flow signal to the flow control valve. Once the valve is opened, signals from the pressure transducers are used to ensure that flow delivery matches the ventilator settings for tidal volume delivery. Tidal volume delivery becomes a function of time and flow, with flow being determined as a function of the pressure differential across the flow control valve and the valve's position. Technically, the ventilator is really a pressure controller when delivering mandatory breaths, since pressure is measured and used as a signal to regulate the output from the flow control valve.

This system also allows delivery of tidal volumes which are compensated for the volume compressed in the patient circuit. The circuit compliance factor may be entered into the microprocessor which will automatically compensate the delivered volume, correcting for volume lost due to compression in the patient circuit.

Output waveforms include rectangular, descending ramp, and sinusoidal waveforms. All of these waveforms are possible through microprocessor control of the stepper motor in the flow control valve.

Pressure must be measured and controlled during pressure controlled ventilation, pressure support and pressure augmentation. Pressure in the patient circuit is regulated by the feedback from the proximal pressure transducer via adjustment of flow from the flow control valve and the low pressure control system regulating the exhalation valve. Reference signals from the pressure support/

inspiratory pressure, inspiratory time and the PEEP controls are used as inputs to the microprocessor. The flow control valve is opened providing sufficient flow to maintain the proximal airway pressure established by these controls. Pressure controlled breath delivery ceases based upon the inspiratory time set by the practitioner. PEEP regulation is accomplished through the low pressure control system. Gas supplied from the PEEP control needle valve and the jet pump are directed through the exhalation solenoid valve to the exhalation diaphragm, regulating PEEP pressure in the patient circuit.

Control Variables

As described earlier, the control variable used by the BEAR 1000 ventilator is pressure. Differential pressure measured across the flow control valve is used to regulate the valve during tidal volume delivery during mandatory breaths. Pressure is also the control variable during PEEP/CPAP, pressure controlled ventilation, pressure support, and pressure augmentation.

Phase Variables
Trigger Variables

The trigger variables for the BEAR 1000 include pressure, flow, time and manual variables. When inspiratory pressure falls below the threshold established by the assist sensitivity control, the ventilator will initiate a breath. The assist sensitivity may be set between 0.2 and 5.0 cmH$_2$O below baseline pressure by the practitioner.

Flow becomes a trigger variable when flow triggering is established by adjusting base flow and flow trigger (sensitivity) levels. Base flow is adjustable between 5 and 20 L/min. The flow trigger may be set between 1 and 15 L/min. When the flow transducer senses that flow has dropped below the trigger level, a breath is given.

Time becomes a trigger variable during assist CMV, SIMV and pressure control if no inspiratory effort (pressure drop) is sensed by the ventilator. If the patient does not trigger a breath, the ventilator will deliver a mandatory breath at the set breath rate. This is also true during pressure control ventilation.

The ventilator may be manually triggered by the practitioner depressing the manual breath key on the control panel. When depressed, the ventilator will deliver a volume controlled breath (assist/CMV, SIMV and CPAP) or a pressure controlled breath during pressure control mode.

Limit Variables

The limit variables of the BEAR 1000 include pressure, volume and flow. Pressure becomes a limit variable during SIMV (with PEEP applied), CPAP, pressure support, pressure augmentation and pressure control ventilation. Under these conditions, the ventilator will augment flow to maintain the desired pressure level. PEEP/CPAP pressures are adjustable between 0.0 and 50.0 cmH2O. Pressure support is adjustable between 0.0 and 80.0 cmH2O.

Volume becomes a limit variable when the inspiratory pause control is adjusted greater than zero. Inspiratory pause may be adjusted between 0.0 and 2.0 seconds. When activated, a volume breath is delivered and held until the set inspiratory pause time period has elapsed.

Flow becomes a limit variable when the rectangular waveform output is selected during assist/CMV or during sigh breath delivery. When selected, the rectangular waveform output limits flow during inspiration to the setting established on the peak flow control. Peak flow is adjustable between 10 and 150 L/min.

Cycle Variables

Cycle variables for the BEAR 1000 include pressure, volume flow and time. Pressure becomes a cycle variable if the inspiratory pressure reaches the setting on the peak inspiratory pressure control. Peak inspiratory pressure may be adjusted between 0 and 120 cmH2O. When the pressure limit is reached, inspiration is terminated and both audible and visual alarms are activated.

Volume becomes a cycle variable during sigh breath delivery. When selected, a sigh breath will be given every 100th breath. The sigh volume delivered will be 150% of the normal tidal volume setting. Sigh breath delivery cannot be used during pressure control ventilation. During assist CMV and the mandatory portion of SIMV, the ventilator is also volume cycled. The control circuit uses the pressure drop across the flow control valve and its position to determine volume. The breath ends once the volume delivery is complete.

Flow becomes a cycle variable during pressure support ventilation. Inspiration is ter-minated when inspiratory flow falls to approximately 30% of the peak inspiratory flow. Once flow decays to this point, pressure falls to the baseline value. During pressure augmentation if the patient requires additional gas flow beyond the set tidal volume, the ventilator also becomes flow cycled.

Time becomes a cycle variable during pressure control ventilation. In this mode, a constant pressure is applied until the time set on the inspiratory time control has been reached. The trigger variable during pressure control is also time, which is established by the rate control. Time is also a cycle variable when the inspiratory pause control is set greater than zero. Inspiration is terminated after the inspiratory pause time has elapsed (0.0 to 2.0 seconds).

Baseline Variable

PEEP/CPAP pressures are adjustable between 0 and 50 cmH2O. Baseline pressures are increased above ambient by the exhalation solenoid partially closing the exhalation valve.

Conditional Variables
Time

Time becomes a conditional variable during sigh delivery. During normal ventilator supported breaths, they are pressure controlled, pressure triggered, pressure or time cycled. During sigh delivery, a sigh breath will be given every 100th breath.

Time and Pressure

Time and pressure become conditional variables during SIMV mode. The rate control determines the frequency of mandatory breath delivery during SIMV mode. The rate control is essentially an electronic timer, delivering a breath at specified time intervals. Between mandatory breath delivery, the patient breathes through the flow control valve subsystem. The ventilator measures proximal airway pressure to determine if the patient is attempting to initiate a breath. In response to the pressure change, the patient is able to draw gas spontaneously through the flow control valve to meet inspiratory needs.

Time and Volume

Time and volume become conditional variables during MMV (Mandatory Minute Ventilation). A set minimum exhaled volume is established by the practitioner. Should the patient fail to meet this minute volume, the ven-

ASSEMBLY AND TROUBLESHOOTING

Assembly—BEAR 1000

To prepare the BEAR 1000 for use, follow this suggested assembly guide:

1. Attach the high pressure hoses to an oxygen and air source. If no source of 50 psi air is available and the ventilator is equipped with the optional compressor, no air supply is required.

2. Exhalation valve assembly:

   a. Insert the small end of the exhalation valve into the exhalation valve diaphragm and secure it by turning the retaining nut until it stops over the end of the diaphragm.

   b. Pull out on the diaphragm inflating it.

   c. Occlude the end of the exhalation valve and press on the diaphragm to ensure it remains inflated and is secured properly.

3. Insert the assembled exhalation valve into its seat on the ventilator and attach the condensate jar to the exhalation valve by inserting it over the valve and rotating the assembly counterclockwise.

4. Install the external flow sensor assembly to the outlet of the condensate jar, and attach its coiled cable to it.

5. Assemble and fill the humidifier, and attach it to the front of the ventilator. Many different humidifiers may be adapted to the BEAR 1000, so specific assembly instructions will not be included here.

6. Assemble the adult circuit, verifying the integrity of connections at the proximal airway port, patient wye and temperature probe ports.

7. Connect the main flow bacteria filter between the ventilator outlet and the humidifier. Attach the adult circuit to the outlet of the humidifier and the exhalation limb to the condensate jar.

8. Connect the power cord to a suitable 115 volt, 60 Hz outlet.

Troubleshooting

Refer to the troubleshooting algorithms found at the end of this chapter.

---

tilator will deliver breaths at a rate equal to the minimum minute volume setting divided by the set tidal volume. Apnea results in time triggered ventilation. Flow becomes the conditional variable because the BEAR 1000 measures flow and determines volume indirectly as a function of flow and time.

Output Waveforms
Pressure

The pressure output of the BEAR 1000 ventilator may be rectangular or adjustable. The rectangular waveform output occurs when the ventilator is operating in the pressure support and pressure control modes. In these modes, pressure rises sharply to the level set on the pressure support/inspiratory pressure control.

The pressure waveform may be adjusted by using the pressure slope control. When employed, the pressure can be adjusted to rise slowly or quickly to its peak value.

Volume

Volume output is an ascending ramp when the ventilator is operated with the flow output in the rectangular waveform setting. Under these conditions, the volume gradually increases in a linear fashion as pressure increases.

Flow

The flow output of the BEAR 1000 may be adjusted between rectangular, descending ramp and sinusoidal outputs. The stepper motor–driven flow control valve, in combination with the microprocessor and pressure feed back system, enables the ventilator to accurately reproduce these flow output waveforms.

Alarms
Input Power

Input power alarms on the BEAR 1000 include loss of electrical and pneumatic power.

When electrical power is lost, the failed-to-cycle alarm will be activated for a minimum of 5 minutes or until power is restored. A nickel cadmium battery pack powers the audible and visual alarm, independent of the 115 volts, 60 Hz power for the ventilator.

If air or oxygen pressure falls below 27.5 psi, the gas supply failure alarm will be activated. Both audible and visual alarms will be activated when this condition exists.

Control Circuit Alarms

Control circuit alarms on the BEAR 1000 include failure to cycle and time/I:E limit. The

TABLE 8-6: BEAR 1000 Alarms

ALARM	CONDITION/SETTINGS
Input Power	
Oxygen Pressure	< 27.5 psi
Air Pressure	< 27.5 psi
Electric Power	Loss of 120 volt, 60 Hz power
Control Circuit	
Failed to Cycle	Internal Faults Detected
Time/I:E Limit	Inspiratory time exceeds 5 seconds plus inspiratory pause or I:E ratio exceeds the limit set.
Output Alarms	
High Airway Pressure	0.0–120 cmH$_2$O
Low Airway Pressure	3.0–99 cmH$_2$O
High Baseline Pressure	0.0–50 cmH$_2$O
Low Baseline Pressure	0.0–50 cmH$_2$O
High Minute Volume	0.0–80 L/min
Low Minute Volume	0.0–50 L/min
High Breath Rate	0–155 BPM
Low Breath Rate	3–90 BPM

failed-to-cycle alarm is activated when power is lost or an internal fault is found when the microprocessor conducts its diagnostics routine. The time/I:E limit alarm is activated if the practitioner has set an improper tidal volume, rate and peak flow, and inspiratory pause settings. The alarm will also activate if the inspiratory time exceeds 5 seconds plus pause time or if the I:E ratio exceeds the set limit.

Output Alarms
Pressure

The BEAR 1000 incorporates high and low peak pressure and high and low baseline pressure alarms. The high peak pressure alarm is adjustable between 0.0 and 120 cmH$_2$O and the low peak pressure alarm is adjustable between 3 and 99 cmH$_2$O. The high and low baseline pressure alarms are adjustable between 0.0 and 50 cmH$_2$O.

Flow

High and low minute volume alarms are incorporated into the BEAR 1000. The low minute volume alarm is adjustable between 0.0 and 50 L/min. The high minute volume alarm is adjustable between 0.0 and 80 L/min.

Time

Adjustable high and low breath rate alarms are also incorporated into the BEAR 1000 ventilator. The low breath rate alarm is adjustable between 3 and 99 breaths per minute. The high breath rate alarm can be adjusted between 0 and 155 breaths per minute.

Table 8-6 summarizes the BEAR 1000 ventilator alarm systems, and Table 8-7 summarizes its capabilities.

BIRD PRODUCTS CORPORATION 8400ST®*i*

The Bird Products Corporation's 8400ST®*i* volume ventilator is a pneumatically powered, microprocessor controlled ventilator which is capable of ventilating a wide spectrum of patients (Figures 8-12, 8-13). The microprocessor, in conjunction with the flow control valve and electronically controlled exhalation valve, gives the ventilator a high degree of flexibility.

Power Input

Power to run the microprocessor control circuitry and the stepper motor control system

TABLE 8-7: BEAR 1000 Ventilator Capabilities

Modes	Assist CMV, SIMV/CPAP, Pressure Support, MMV, Pressure Control, and Pressure Augmentation.
Volume	10–2,000 mL
Min. Minute Volume	0.0–50 L/min
Pressure	0.0–120 cmH₂O
Press. Support	0.0–80 cmH₂O
Rate	0.0–120 BPM
Peak Flow	5–150 L/min
PEEP/CPAP	0.0–50 cmH₂O
Sigh Volume	150% of Tidal Volume
Insp. Pause	0.0–2.0 seconds
Insp. Time	0.1–5.0 seconds
F₁O₂	0.21–1.0

is provided by alternating 120 volt, 60 Hz electrical power or 16 volt DC power. The pneumatic system is powered by 50 psi air and oxygen. The oxygen and air must be mixed using an external blender such as the Bird 3800™ MicroBlender.

Control Circuit

Gas from the blender enters the ventilator and passes though a coalescing filter which removes both liquid and solid particles from the compressed gas source (Figure 8-14). The gas then passes through a relief valve (100 psi) and into a 1.1 liter accumulator. The accumulator functions as a reservoir to provide gas to meet high instantaneous flow demands. From the accumulator, the gas is reduced in pressure to 20 psi by a reducing valve (regulator).

The 8400ST®i ventilator uses a microprocessor and a stepper motor–driven flow control valve to regulate flow output from the ventilator. The valve is supplied with gas at a pressure of 20 psi from the reducing valve.

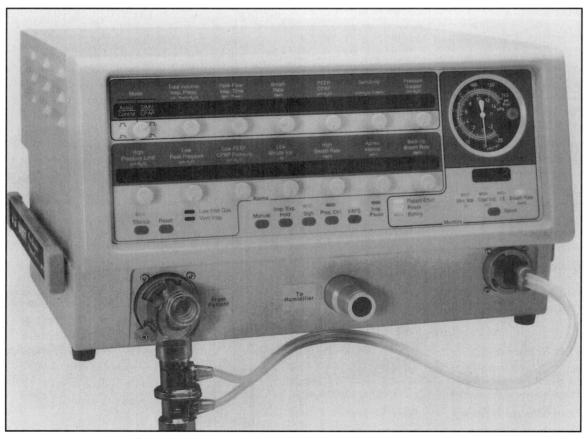

Figure 8-12 *A photograph of the Bird Medical Products Corporation 8400ST volume ventilator. (Courtesy Bird Products Corporation, Palm Springs, CA)*

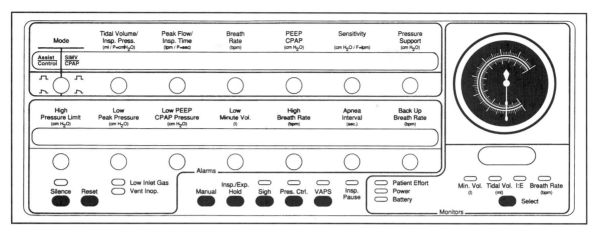

Figure 8-13 *A drawing showing the control panel of the Bird 8400ST ventilator. (Courtesy Bird Products Corporation, Palm Springs, CA)*

Between the reducing valve and the flow control valve is a 200 mL pulsation dampener. Since the valve can instantaneously demand more gas flow, the pulsation dampener helps to reduce pressure fluctuations and act as a buffer between the reducing valve and the flow control valve.

The way the 8400ST®*i* determines flow from the flow control valve is based upon valve position. An optical sensor detects the valve's position. Gas flow exiting the valve is sonic up to a back pressure of 210 cmH$_2$O (3 psi). Mass flow from the flow control valve is unchanged up to back pressures of 210 cmH$_2$O down

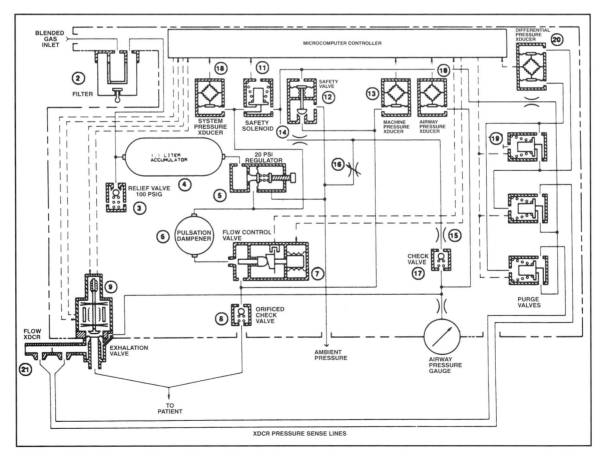

Figure 8-14 *A schematic drawing showing the Bird 8400ST ventilator's pneumatic system. (Courtesy Bird Products Corporation, Palm Springs, CA)*

stream (patient circuit). Therefore, flow from the valve is directly proportional to how far the valve has opened. The microprocessor uses an algorithm to determine flow based upon the feedback from the optical sensor, which senses valve position. Although flow is not directly measured, valve position is directly proportional to flow. Output from the flow control valve varies from 0.0 to 120 L/min in 1 L/min increments, or steps, of resolution.

Pressure must be measured and controlled during pressure control, pressure support and PEEP/CPAP. Pressure in the patient circuit is regulated by the dynamic exhalation valve, flow control valve and the airway pressure transducer. Feedback from the transducer determines the output (flow) from the flow control valve required to maintain a given level of pressure support during inspiration. The exhalation valve changes position, partially closing, and when provided with flow from the flow control valve can maintain the desired level of PEEP/CPAP, acting as a threshold resister.

Control Variables

The control variables for the 8400ST®*i* are flow and pressure. Flow is the control variable during volume breath delivery (Control, Assist/Control and SIMV). When a volume breath is delivered, volume is determined as a function of flow and time. As stated earlier, flow is not directly measured but is a linear function of valve position.

Pressure becomes the control variable during pressure control, CPAP and pressure support. Pressure is measured by the airway pressure transducer and is used by the microprocessor to determine output from the flow control valve and position of the exhalation valve.

Phase Variables
Trigger Variables

The trigger variables of the 8400ST®*i* include pressure, flow, time and manual. Pressure becomes a trigger variable when the patient inhales, reducing pressure in the circuit below the reference level set on the sensitivity control. Sensitivity may be adjusted between 1.0 and 20 cmH$_2$O below baseline pressure. Pressure operates as a trigger variable for mandatory breaths during assist control, SIMV and pressure support.

Flow is a trigger variable when the special flow triggering flow sensor has been installed. Once installed, a bias flow of 10 L/min flows through the patient circuit. Sensitivity levels of between 1 and 10 L/min threshold may be set using the sensitivity control. Once the flow threshold has been detected, inspiration is triggered.

Time is a trigger variable during control, assist control, and SIMV when no spontaneous breaths occur. Breath delivery is based upon the rate control (time) and is adjustable between 0 and 80 breaths per minute.

The ventilator may also be manually triggered by depressing the manual breath button. When depressed, the ventilator initiates a controlled breath at the tidal volume, waveform and peak flow or inspiratory pressure, and inspiratory time (for pressure control breaths) set on the control panel.

Limit Variables

The limit variables include pressure, volume and flow. Pressure becomes the limit variable during SIMV (with PEEP/CPAP), CPAP, pressure control, and pressure support modes. The demand flow system (flow control valve, exhalation valve and airway pressure transducer) maintains pressure in the patient circuit at the desired level. PEEP/CPAP is adjustable between 0.0 and 30 cmH$_2$O. Pressure support may be adjusted between 0.0 and 50 cmH$_2$O.

Volume becomes a limit variable when the inspiratory hold button is depressed. When depressed, inspiration will be held following breath delivery until the button is released or 6 seconds have elapsed. The inspiratory hold button facilitates the measurement of static inspiratory pressure in the patient circuit, since both the flow control valve and the exhalation valve are held in the closed position.

Flow is the limit variable when the rectangular inspiratory flow waveform is selected. Flow is adjustable between 10 and 120 L/min. The flow delivery is limited to the value set on the peak flow control.

Cycle Variables

The cycle variables include pressure, flow and time. Pressure becomes the cycle variable when inspiratory pressure reaches the pressure set on the high peak pressure control. The high peak pressure is adjustable between 1 and 140 cmH$_2$O. When the pressure limit is reached, inspiratory flow is stopped and both audible and visual alarms are activated.

Flow becomes the cycle variable during pressure support. When inspiratory flow decays to 25% of the peak inspiratory flow, breath delivery stops. When the ventilator is flow triggered in CPAP mode (flow support), inspiration is also flow cycled.

Time becomes the cycle variable during mandatory breath delivery. The microprocessor determines volume as a function of flow and inspiratory time. Once the appropriate inspiratory time has been reached, based upon peak flow and tidal volume settings or inspiratory time setting (pressure control), breath delivery ceases.

Baseline Variable

PEEP/CPAP pressures are adjustable between 0.0 and 30 cmH$_2$O. As described earlier, the dynamic exhalation valve acts as a threshold resistor, creating the PEEP/CPAP pressure.

Conditional Variables
Time

Time becomes a conditional variable during sigh delivery. During normal ventilator supported breaths, they are flow controlled, pressure or flow triggered, pressure flow or time cycled. During sigh delivery, a sigh breath will be given every 100th breath equal to 150% of the tidal volume set on the tidal volume control. Sigh breath delivery is available during all modes of ventilation except pressure control.

Time and Pressure

Time and pressure become conditional variables during SIMV mode. The rate control determines the frequency of mandatory breath delivery during SIMV mode. The rate control is essentially an electronic timer, delivering a breath at specified time intervals. Between mandatory breath delivery the patient breathes through the flow control valve demand system. The ventilator measures proximal airway pressure to determine if the patient is attempting to initiate a breath. In response to the pressure change, the patient is able to draw gas spontaneously through the flow control valve to meet their inspiratory needs.

Output Waveforms
Pressure

Pressure waveform output is rectangular. This waveform occurs during pressure sup-

port and pressure control. During pressure support, pressure rises rapidly to the pressure support level and is maintained there until flow decays to 25% of the peak inspiratory flow value. During pressure control, pressure rises rapidly to the inspiratory pressure level and is maintained there until the inspiratory time has elapsed.

Flow

The flow output may be selected between rectangular and decelerating ramp waveforms. The waveform is selected using the mode control switch.

Alarms
Input Power

In the event of electrical power failure, the "Ventilator Inoperative" LED will be illuminated and an audible warning will be activated. This alarm is battery powered and operates independently from the 120 volt, 60 Hz electrical power.

The low inlet gas alarm is activated whenever system gas pressure drops below 16 psi for 1 second. The alarm is both audible and visual. Loss of system pressure can occur from loss of supply pressure, clogged inlet filter or a reducing valve malfunction.

Control Circuit Alarms

Control circuit alarms include ventilator inoperative, sensor disconnect and I:E alarms. The ventilator inoperative alarm will be activated in the event that an internal system failure has been detected by the microprocessor.

The sensor disconnect alarm is both an audible and a visual alarm. This alarm is activated if the flow sensor becomes disconnected during ventilator operation.

The I:E ratio LED will flash every time a breath is delivered in an inverse I:E ratio. The flashing will stop once settings are adjusted such that inverse I:E ratio ventilation has ceased.

Output Alarms
Pressure

High and low peak pressure alarms are available on the 8400ST®i ventilator. The high peak pressure alarm is adjustable between 1 and 140 cmH$_2$O. The low peak pressure alarm is adjustable between 2 and 140 cmH$_2$O.

ASSEMBLY AND TROUBLESHOOTING

Assembly—Bird 8400ST®*i*

1. Attach a 90° elbow adapter to the outlet of the ventilator and connect the ventilator outlet to a bacteria filter with a short length of large-bore tubing.

2. Connect the opposite end of the bacteria filter to the humidifier.

3. Since many humidifiers may be used with the 8400ST®*i*, specific assembly instructions will not be included here.

4. Exhalation valve assembly:

   a. Install the exhalation valve diaphragm by inserting it onto its seat on the ventilator.

   b. Install the exhalation valve body onto the ventilator.

5. Connect the inspiratory limb of patient circuit to the outlet of the humidifier and the expiratory limb to the exhalation valve assembly.

6. Connect the flow transducer assembly to the outlet of the exhalation valve, and connect the male end into the female receptacle on the lower right front of the ventilator.

7. Check all tubing connections and pressure test the ventilator circuit.

8. Connect the power cord to a 120 volt, 60 Hz source.

Troubleshooting

Refer to the troubleshooting algorithms found at the end of this chapter.

TABLE 8-8: 8400ST®*i* Alarms

ALARM	CONDITION/SETTINGS
Input Power	
System pressure	< 16 psi for one minute
Electric Power	Loss of 120 volt, 60 Hz power
Control Circuit	
Ventilator Inoperative	System failure detected
I:E ratio	Inverse ratio ventilation
Output Alarms	
High Airway Pressure	1.0–140 cmH$_2$O
Low Airway Pressure	2.0–140 cmH$_2$O
Low Baseline Pressure	–20–30 cmH$_2$O
Low Minute Volume	0.0–60.0 L/min
High Breath Rate	3–150 BPM
Apnea	10–60 seconds

A low baseline pressure alarm will alert the practitioner to loss of PEEP/CPAP pressures. The alarm is adjustable between –20 and 30 cmH$_2$O. The subambient pressure setting may be used to detect inspiratory efforts on a patient who was previously being ventilated in the control mode.

Flow

A low minute ventilation alarm may be set between 0.0 and 60.0 L/min. The alarm may be used for all modes of ventilation, alerting the practitioner to hypoventilation.

Time

A high breath rate alarm may be set to alert the practitioner to tachypnea. The alarm is adjustable between 3 and 150 breaths per minute.

An apnea interval alarm may be adjusted between 10 and 60 seconds, alerting the practitioner to periods of patient apnea.

Table 8-8 illustrates the Bird 8400ST®*i* alarms, and Table 8-9 illustrates its capabilities.

BIRD PRODUCTS CORPORATION, TBIRD® AVS VENTILATOR

The Bird Products Corporation's TBird® Advanced Ventilatory System (AVS) ventilator

TABLE 8-9: 8400ST®*i* Ventilator Capabilities

Modes	Control, Assist/Control, SIMV, Flow Support (flow triggering), Pressure Support, Volume Assured Pressure Support, Pressure Control, CPAP, SIGH
Volume	50–2,000 mL
Pressure	0.5–100 cmH₂O
Press. Support	0.0–50 cmH₂O
Rate	0–80 BPM
Insp. Time	0.1–9.8 seconds
Peak Flow	5–120 L/min
PEEP/CPAP	0.0–30 cmH₂O
Sigh Volume	150% of Tidal Volume
Insp. Hold	up to 6 seconds
Insp. Pause	0.0–2.0 seconds
F₁O₂	0.21–1.0

is designed to meet the needs of acute care patients (Figure 8-15). The TBird® AVS is an electrically and pneumatically powered ventilator, which is microprocessor controlled. The ventilator's microprocessor control system, when combined with its pressure and flow sensors, provides a flexible system capable of caring for a wide variety of patients.

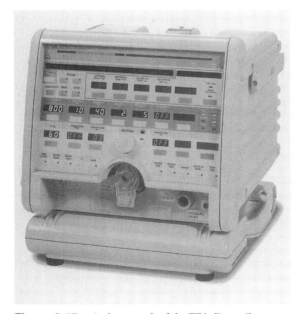

Figure 8-15 *A photograph of the TBird® ventilator. (Courtesy Bird Products Corporation, Palm Springs, CA)*

Power Input

Electrical power supplies the microprocessor control system, the drive mechanism and the various pressure and flow sensors of the TBird® AVS ventilator. Power is selectable between 120 v, 60 Hz AC and 220 v, 60 Hz AC; internal battery; or external 48V DC battery. Power may be selected by means of a switch located on the rear of the ventilator.

Pneumatic power for the ventilator is supplied by an oxygen source between 40 and 60 psi. Two DISS fittings on the rear of the ventilator are provided for the attachment of oxygen sources. In the event a clinician wishes to transfer from piped wall oxygen to a cylinder, the cylinder may be connected before interruption of the wall oxygen, thus providing a seamless transition between the two sources.

Drive Mechanism

Once gas enters the ventilator, it passes through check valves and into the blender system (Figure 8-16). The blender consists of five solenoids with a fixed orifice at each output. The microprocessor determines which and how many solenoids are required to be opened to add the required oxygen to the accumulator/diffuser.

Ambient air passes through a filter (Figure 8-16) and into the accumulator/diffuser. The accumulator/diffuser functions to initially mix the two gases (oxygen and air) and acts as a baffling device to muffle the noise of the high-speed turbine.

The drive mechanism of the TBird® AVS is a small pneumatic turbine capable of providing near-instantaneous flows with a rapid response time. Gas from the accumulator/diffuser passes through a filter silencer to the turbine. The turbine rapidly compresses the blended gas and provides the instantaneous flow demands needed by the patient. The turbine further homogenates the mixture of air and oxygen through its operation. Gas exiting the turbine passes through another silencer, which muffles the turbine noise.

Control Circuit

The control circuit of the TBird® AVS ventilator consists of a turbine differential pressure transducer, an exhalation differential pressure transducer, an electrodynamic exhalation valve and the microprocessor.

The turbine differential pressure transducer monitors the pressure drop across the

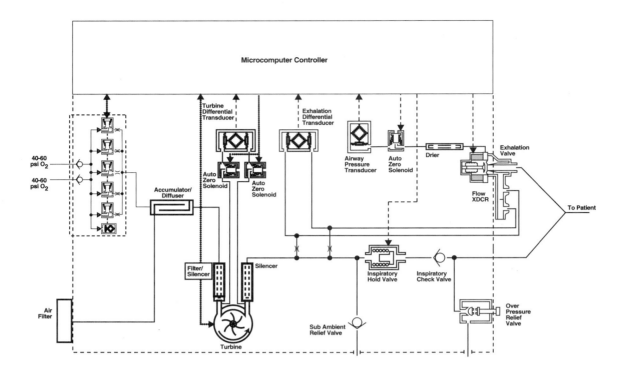

Figure 8-16 *A schematic drawing showing the TBird® ventilator's pneumatic system. (Courtesy Bird Products Corporation, Palm Springs, CA)*

turbine (Figure 8-16). The differential pressure, combined with the speed of the turbine, is used by the microprocessor to precisely regulate the turbine's output. An optical sensor detects the turbine's speed, providing feedback to the microprocessor.

The exhalation differential pressure transducer provides a flow signal to the microprocessor, which reflects what is being exhaled by the patient (Figure 8-16). The body of the expiratory flow transducer has a variable orifice element in the center. The flexible element bends as flow increases, creating a pressure drop across the two ports, which is sensed by the pressure transducer.

The electrodynamic exhalation valve is used to regulate PEEP/CPAP pressures, and it closes during mandatory breaths. The valve consists of a high-energy permanent magnet with a suspended coil, which is energized with current. As current is applied to the coil, it is drawn into the core of the valve, closing it.

Control Variable

The control variable for the TBird® AVS is pressure. Differential pressure is detected across the turbine and is used to regulate its output. The microprocessor integrates turbine speed (optically sensed) and the pressure differential to precisely regulate the flow and pressure provided by the turbine drive mechanism.

Phase Variables
Trigger Variables

The trigger variables of the TBird® AVS are flow, time and manual triggering. During flow-triggered operation, the clinician sets a base flow through the patient circuit. Base flows are adjustable between 10 and 20 L/min. The flow sensitivity is then set; and it is adjustable between 1 and 8 L/min.

Time triggering occurs during mandatory breaths and is a function of the breath rate control, which may be set between 2 and 80 breaths per minute (BPM). When the appropriate time interval has passed, the exhalation valve closes and the ventilator provides a mandatory breath.

The TBird® AVS may be manually triggered by the clinician depressing the manual breath button located at the lower left of the control panel. Depressing this button delivers a volume or pressure controlled breath, depending upon the breath type selected.

Limit Variables

The limit variables of the TBird® AVS include pressure, volume and flow. Pressure becomes the limit variable during SIMV (with PEEP/CPAP, CPAP, pressure control and pressure support ventilation. When the TBird® AVS is operating in these modes, pressure is measured and maintained at a consistent level during breath delivery. PEEP/CPAP pressure may be adjusted between 0 AND 30 cmH$_2$O. Pressure control and pressure support may be adjusted between 1 to 100 cmH$_2$O and 1 to 60 cmH$_2$O, respectively.

Volume becomes a limit variable when inspiratory pause is selected. Inspiratory pause may be adjusted between 0 and 2.0 seconds. When inspiratory pause is selected, the inspiratory hold valve closes in conjunction with the exhalation valve, holding the breath in the patient's lungs for the set time interval (Figure 8-16). Under these conditions, volume becomes limited during the inspiratory phase.

Flow becomes a limit variable when the Square Waveform button is depressed and the ventilator is set for volume controlled ventilation (rate, tidal volume, and peak flow). Peak flow is adjustable between 10 and 140 L/min. The inspiratory flow limit becomes the value selected using the peak flow control.

Cycle Variables

The cycle variables for the TBird® AVS include pressure, flow and time. Pressure becomes a cycle variable when inspiratory pressure reaches the value set on the high pressure limit control. This control is adjustable between 5 and 120 cmH$_2$O. When the high pressure limit is reached, inspiration is terminated and exhalation begins, and both audible and visual alarms are activated.

Flow is the cycling variable during pressure support. When inspiratory flow decays to 25% of the peak inspiratory flow value, the breath is terminated and the patient is allowed to exhale. If the flow is slow to decay during inspiration, the breath will be terminated after 3 seconds or breath periods, whichever occurs first.

Time is a cycle variable during mandatory breath delivery. The microprocessor determines volume as a function of flow and inspiratory time. Once the desired time has been met, the breath is terminated.

Conditional Variables
Time

Time becomes a conditional variable during sigh breath delivery. During sigh breath deliver, a sigh breath is delivered every 100 breaths, which is equal to 150% of the set tidal volume. Sigh breaths may be used in all modes of ventilation.

Time and Pressure

Time and pressure become conditional variables during SIMV mode. The rate control determines the frequency of mandatory breath delivery during SIMV move. The rate control is essentially an electronic timer, delivering a breath at a specified time intervals. Between periods of mandatory breath delivery the patient can obtain spontaneous breaths (pressure support or pure spontaneous) through the ventilator's gas delivery system.

Output Waveforms
Pressure

Pressure waveform output is rectangular. This output waveform occurs during pressure support and pressure control. During these modes, pressure rises rapidly and plateaus at the set pressure level until exhalation begins.

Flow

The flow wave form may be toggled between rectangular (square) and decelerating during volume controlled breath delivery. This is accomplished by selecting or not selecting the Square Waveform button on the lower left of the control panel.

Alarms
Input Power

The input power alarms consist of electrical power and gas pressure alarms. In the event that AC power is interrupted, the ventilator switches to battery backup power without interrupting ventilation and an audible alarm sounds, while simultaneously the internal battery indicator is illuminated. In the event that the internal or external batteries are low on power, both audible and visual alarms will result.

When the oxygen inlet pressure is less than 35 psi and the oxygen percentage control is set to greater than 21%, both audible and visual alarms will be activated. Remember, the

ASSEMBLY AND TROUBLESHOOTING

Assembly TBird® AVS

1. Exhalation valve assembly: Install the exhalation valve diaphragm and the exhalation valve body into the ventilator. When correctly installed, you will hear a click as it seats into the correct position.

2. Attach a 90° elbow adapter to the ventilator outlet and secure a bacteria filter to it. Connect the ventilator to a heated humidifier using a short length of 22-mm diameter, large-bore tubing.

3. Connect the inspiratory limb from the outlet of the humidifier to the patient wye and the expiratory limb of the circuit to the exhalation valve assembly. The use of water traps in both the inspiratory and expiratory limbs of the circuit is recommended.

4. Connect the ventilator to a 50 psi oxygen source.

5. Connect the power cord to a suitable AC power outlet.

Troubleshooting

Refer to the troubleshooting algorithm found at the end of this chapter.

TBird® AVS may be powered by two independent oxygen sources, and when thus connected, one source can serve as a backup for the other.

Control Circuit

The control circuit alarm consists of internal operations, circuit fault and EEPROM failure alert. All of these alarms are part of the ventilator's self-testing and troubleshooting systems. In the event these alarms are triggered, you should discontinue use of the ventilator and contact a certified Bird service technician or have the unit checked by a suitable biomedical repair facility.

The flow sensor alarm will sound if a flow sensor is not detected by the ventilator. In this case, check to ensure that the exhalation valve body is correctly seated in its receptable or replace it with a new one.

Output Alarms
Pressure

Pressure alarms consist of high and low pressure alarms. The high pressure limit alarm may be set at between 5 and 120 cmH$_2$O. The low pressure alarm alerts the practitioner to decreased inspiratory pressures and is adjustable between 2 and 60 cmH$_2$O.

Flow

A low minute ventilation alarm may be set between 0.1 and 99.9 mL. The alarm may be used in all modes to alert the clinician to hypoventilation.

Time

The ventilator incorporates a high breath rate and an apnea alarm. The high breath rate alarm is adjustable between 2 and 150 breaths per minute.

The apnea alarm alerts the clinician to apneic periods. The alarm interval may be adjusted from 10 to 60 seconds. If a breath is not detected within the set time window, the ventilator will auomatically switch to backup ventilation. Table 8-10 illustrates the Bird Products Corporation TBird® AVS alarm, and Table 8-11 illustrates its capabilities.

DRÄGER, EVITA 4 INTENSIVE CARE VENTILATOR

The Dräger, Inc., Evita 4 intensive care ventilator is a microprocessor-controlled ventilator intended for intensive care use for adults and pediatric patients having a body weight of at least 3 kg (Figure 8-17). The ventilator is

Table 8-10: TBird® AVS Alarms

ALARM	CONDITION
Input Power	
Battery On	AC power failure
Low Battery	Internal battery power is low
Ext Battery	External battery power is low
Control Circuit	
Circuit Fault	Kinked or occluded breathing circuit
EEPROM Fault	EEPROM fails to accept a new value.
Vent Inop	Internal ventilator fault has been detected
Output Alarms	
High Pressure	5–120 cmH$_2$O
Low Pressure	2–60 cmH$_2$O
Low Minute Volume	0.1–99.9 mL/min
High Breath Rate	3–150 breaths per minute
Apnea	10–60 seconds

Table 8-11: TBird® AVS Ventilator Capabilities

Modes	Volume control, pressure control, assist/control, SIMV, plus Pressure Support, CPAP, SIGH
Volume	50–2,000 mL
Pressure	5–100 cmH$_2$O
Pressure support	1–60 cmH$_2$O
Rate	2–80 breaths per minute
Inspiratory time	0.3–10 seconds
Peak flow	10–140 L/min
Sigh volume	150% of tidal volume
Inspiratory pause	0.0–2.0 seconds
F$_I$O$_2$	0.21–1.00

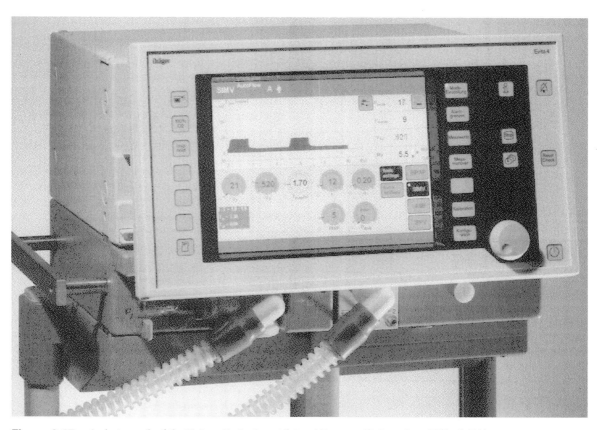

Figure 8-17 *A photograph of the Dräger Evita 4 ventilator. (Courtesy Dräger, Inc., Telford, PA)*

very flexible, having both pressure and volume controlled ventilation with a good monitoring and alarm package to facilitate its application in the care of critically ill patients.

Power Input

The Evita 4 requires both electrical and pneumatic power for its operation. Electric power may be provided by 120 v, 60 Hz or 220 v, 60 Hz AC power, or the unit may be powered by a 12 or 24 V DC external battery. Electrical power is used for the microprocessor control system and the various pressure and flow monitoring and display systems.

Both air and oxygen supplies are required for the Evita 4 ventilator. DISS fittings are located on the rear of the ventilator and gas pressures should range between 43.5 and 87 psi (maximum), with the standard of 50 psi being the preferred pressure.

Gases enter the rear of the ventilator and each type (air and oxygen) passes through a filter and into the mixing unit (Figure 8-18). A gauge pressure transducer monitors the incoming line pressure before the gas line pressure before the gas enters solenoid valves, which accurately blend the air and oxygen to the desired percentage.

Control Circuit

The control circuit consists of the microprocessor, the flow control valve, a differential pressure transducer and the exhalation valve (Figure 8-18). Differential pressure measured across the flow control valve is proportional to the flow-out of the ventilator. The microprocessor integrates flow over time to determine the delivered volume.

The exhalation valve is used to regulate pressure during the PEEP/CPAP and pressure

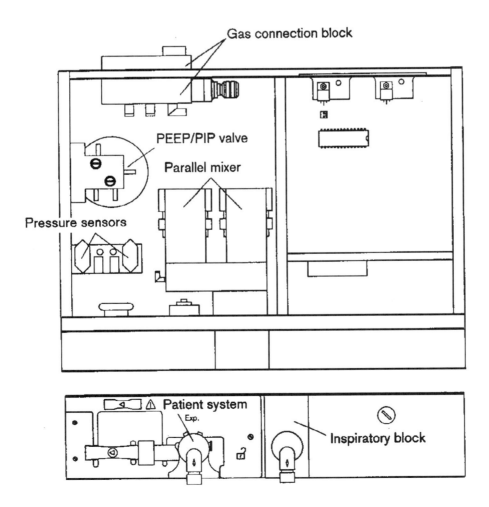

Figure 8-18 *A schematic drawing showing the Evita 4 ventilator's pneumatic system. (Courtesy Dräger, Inc., Telford, PA)*

ventilation modes. Partial closure of the valve creates pressure in the circuit and a pressure transducer provides a feedback signal to the microprocessor, which then regulates the output of the flow control valve.

In the event of gas supply or electrical power failure, ambient air may be drawn in through a port and filter to provide gas to the patient. The check valve prevents gas from the ventilator's pneumatic system from escaping to ambient pressure.

Control Variables

The control variables for the Evita 4 ventilator are flow and pressure. Flow is a control variable during the volume control modes. As described earlier, the ventilator integrates flow over time to determine volume delivery.

Pressure is the control variable during pressure-controlled ventilation, pressure support and PEEP/CPAP. The exhalation valve partially closes the patient circuit, which permits pressure to build and be regulated by the microprocessor and flow control valve system.

Phase Variables
Trigger Variable

Trigger variables for the Evita 4 ventilator include flow, time and manual triggering. Flow is the trigger variables for the Evita 4 ventilator. Flow triggering is adjustable between 1 and 15 L/min and is available during all breath modes.

Time triggering occurs during mandatory breath delivery in the absence of a patient-initiated breath. When the ventilator is time triggered, breath delivery is governed by the breath rate control, which may be adjusted from 0 to 100 breaths per minute.

Manual triggering occurs when the clinician depresses the manual breath button is depressed. When selected, a manual breath is delivered in all modes except for CPAP without pressure support.

Limit Variables

The limit variables for the Evita 4 ventilator include pressure and flow. Pressure becomes a limit variable during CPAP, pressure control and pressure support modes of ventilation. The inspiration unit (gas flow delivery system) maintains an appropriate flow to provide the constant pressure required in the circuit.

Flow becomes a limit variable during volume controlled breaths when the ventilator is

delivering a square wave flow pattern. Inspiratory flow is adjustable between 6 and 120 L/min.

Cycle Variables

The cycle variables for the ventilator include pressure, flow and time. Pressure becomes the cycling variable when inspiratory pressure reaches the level set on the inspiratory pressure limit control. The peak pressure limit may be adjusted between 0 and 100 cmH$_2$O. When the pressure limit is reached, inspiration is terminated and both audible and visual alarms result.

Flow is a cycling variable during pressure support, during which, if inspiratory flow tapers to 25% of the peak inspiratory flow value, the inspiratory phase is terminated. If the flow is slow to decay, the breath will automatically end after 4 seconds have elapsed.

Time is a cycle variable during mandatory breath delivery. The microprocessor determines what inspiratory time is required for a specific volume to be delivered, or ends the breath based upon the inspiratory time setting (during pressure-controlled ventilation).

Baseline Variable

The baseline variable for the Evita 4 ventilator is pressure. PEEP/CPAP pressures may be adjusted between 0 and 35 cmH$_2$O. As described earlier, the exhalation valve functions as a threshold resistor, creating pressure in the circuit.

Conditional Variables
Time and Flow

Time and pressure become conditional variables during SIMV mode. The rate control determines the frequency of mandatory breath delivery. The rat control is essentially an electronic timer, which determines mandatory breaths at specific time intervals. Between mandatory breaths, the ventilator monitors flow to determine whether the patient is initiating a spontaneous breath. The gas delivery system responds to the patient's efforts, providing gas for spontaneous ventilation and synchronizing mandatory breaths.

Output Waveforms
Pressure

The pressure output is rectangular during pressure support and pressure control ventilation modes. During these modes, pressure rises rapidly to the set pressure value and is held there until exhalation begins.

Flow

Flow output can be rectangular (square), during volume breath delivery, or decelerating, during pressure-controlled breath delivery.

Alarms
Input Power

The input power alarms include electrical power failure and gas supply failure (air and oxygen). In the event that AC electrical power is lost, audible and visual alarms will sound. The Evita 4 ventilator can operate for about 10 minutes on internal battery power if the optional 12/24 V DC battery pack is installed. In the event of either gas or air pressure loss, both audible and visual alarms will result. If the line pressure falls below 43.5 psi (air or oxygen), the alarm will be triggered.

Control Circuit

The Evita 4 ventilator control circuit alarms include Check Settings, Device Failure, Expiratory Valve Inop (inoperative), Fan Failure, Flow Measurement Inop, Flow Sensor, Failure to Cycle, and Loss of Data. The ventilator, through the microprocessor, constantly evaluates and verifies the function of many key components required for safety during ventilator operation. The Check Settings alarm occurs if there is a power interruption while alarms or settings are being entered. To correct the alarm, check the settings and then reset the alarm.

A device failure alarm is triggered if the microprocessor detects the failure of a critical internal component. When this occurs, disconnect the ventilator, provide an alternate means of ventilatory support for the patient and remove the unit from service.

The Expiratory Valve Inop alarm occurs if the valve is not properly seated, the flow sensor is defective or not calibrated, or the expiratory valve is defective. Make sure the valve is correctly installed, calibrate the flow sensor and/or replace the exhalation valve to correct the alarm.

A Fan Failure alarm occurs if the internal fan ceases to function. Discontinue using the ventilator, provide an alternate means of sup-

porting the patient and remove the unit from service.

The Flow Measurement Inop alarm occurs if the ventilator fails to detect flow through the flow sensor. Usually this occurs with a flow sensor failure. Discontinue using the ventilator, provide an alternate means of supporting the patient and remove the unit from service.

The Flow Sensor alarm occurs if the sensor is not seated properly. Disconnect the sensor and reinstall it, making certain it is fully inserted in the rubber tip of the exhalation valve.

A Failure to Cycle alarm can occur if the ventilator fails to deliver a breath or the microprocessor detects a critical fault in the control system. If this alarm occurs, first check the peak pressure settings to verify that they are correct. If the alarm persists, discontinue use of the ventilator and remove it from service.

If the internal lithium battery becomes fully discharged, a Loss of Data alarm will result. Discontinue using the ventilator, provide an alternate means of supporting the patient and remove the unit from service.

Output Alarms
Pressure

The Evita 4 ventilator pressure alarms include High and Low Airway Pressure and High PEEP or Baseline Pressure. The High Airway Pressure alarm is adjustable between 10 and 100 cmH$_2$O.

The Low Airway Pressure alarm is linked to the PEEP control setting. In the event of a circuit or cuff leak that drops the baseline pressure, the Low Airway Pressure alarm will sound to alert the clinician of the event. The High PEEP alarm is also nonadjustable and is linked to the PEEP control setting. In the event the expiratory circuit or exhalation valve becomes obstructed, raising the baseline pressure, this alarm will alert the clinician to the event.

Volume

The Evita 4 ventilator includes an adjustable High Tidal Volume alarm and a nonadjustable Low Tidal Volume alarm. The High Tidal Volume alarm is adjustable between 30 and 4000 ml. The Low Tidal Volume alarm is linked to the tidal volume setting and, like the Low PEEP alarm, it alerts the clinician to cuff or circuit leaks.

ASSEMBLY AND TROUBLESHOOTING

Assembly—Dräger Evita 4

1. Install the exhalation valve:
   a. Tilt the control panel upward for better access to the valve set and flow sensor fittings.
   b. Push the valve assembly into its receptacle. Check to ensure it is seated by gently pulling on the exhalation port.
   c. Connect a flow sensor by pushing it into place, ensuring that it is seated on the rubber lip of the exhalation valve.

2. Install an O_2 sensor capsule:
   a. Turn the exhalation port to the left.
   b. Use a coin or a large screw driver to remove the protective cover.
   c. Loosen the two thumb screws and open the sensor chamber.
   d. Install a new sensor capsule and replace the chamber cover and protective plate.

3. Turn the ventilator outlet port to the right and install a bacteria filter.

4. Assemble the patient circuit:
   a. Connect the bacteria filter to a heated humidifier with a short length of 22-min, large-diameter tubing.
   b. Connect the inspiratory limb of the patient circuit to the outlet of the humidifier, and the opposite end to the patient wye.
   c. Connect the expiratory limb to the exhalation port.
   d. It is recommended that water traps be used on both the inspiratory and expiratory limbs of the circuit.
   e. Connect the humidifier temperature probe to the port on the airway.
   f. If Pet CO_2 monitoring is desired, install the sensor between the patient wye and the patient's airway.

5. Connect 50 psi air and oxygen supplies to their respective DISS fittings on the rear of the ventilator.

6. Connect the electrical supply cord to an appropriate AC outlet.

Troubleshooting

Refer to the troubleshooting algorithms found at the end of this chapter.

Flow

Both High and Low-Minute Ventilation alarms are available on the Evita 4 ventilator. The High-Minute Ventilation alarm may be set between 0.5 and 41 L/min, and the Low-Minute alarm, between 0 and 40 L/min. These alarms may be used in all modes.

Time

The High Rate alarm is adjustable between 5 and 120 breaths per minute. The High Rate alarm serves to alert the clinician to tachypneic events. An Apnea alarm also alerts the clinician to apneic events. The apnea alarm is adjustable between 15 and 60 seconds.

Inspired Gas

The inspired gas alarm consists of High and Low F_IO_2 alarms. The alarm limits are not adjustable but are based upon the F_IO_2 settings. If the F_IO_2 is 0.60 or less, the alarm will automatically be set for ±4%, and if the F_IO_2 is greater than 0.60, the limits will automatically be set for ±6%.

Expired Gas

The Evita 4 ventilator also incorporates an Exhaled CO_2 monitor and alarm. Alarm limits are available for both Upper and Lower PetCO_2. The upper limit is adjustable between 0 and 100 mmHg, while the lower limit is adjustable between 0 and 99 mmHg.

Table 8-12 summarizes the Dräger Evita 4 alarms, and Table 8-13 summarizes its capabilities.

Table 8-12: Dräger Evita 4 Alarms

ALARM	CONDITION/SETTINGS
Input Power	
Air supply low	Air pressure less than 43.5 psi
Oxygen supply low	Oxygen pressure less than 43.5 psi
Electrical power failure	Loss of AC power
Control Circuit	
Check settings	Power interruption during entry
Device failure	Internal fault/system failure detected
Exp valve inop	Valve not seated, flow sensor not calibrated or expiratory valve failure
Fan failure	Failure of internal fan
Flow measurement inop	Flow sensor defective or flow measurement defect
Flow sensor	Flow sensor not seated correctly
Failure to cycle	Incorrect peak pressure settings or internal failure
Loss of data	Lithium battery fully discharged
Output Alarms	
High airway pressure	10–100 cmH_2O
Low airway pressure	Automatic
High baseline pressure	Automatic
Low baseline pressure	Automatic
High tidal volume	30–4,000 mL
Low tidal volume	Automatic
High breath rate	5–120 BPM
Apnea	15–60 seconds
Inspired Gas	
Oxygen	±4% or ±6%, depending on F_IO_2 setting
Expired Gas	
High PetCO$_2$	0–100 mmHg
Low PetCO$_2$	0–99 mmHg

Table 8-13: Dräger Evita 4 Ventilator Capabilities

Modes	Volume controlled, pressure controlled, SIMV, MMV, pressure support/CPAP, APRV, MMV
Volume	.02–2.0 liters
Pressure	0–80 cmH_2O
Pressure support	0–80 cmH_2O
Rate	0–100 / min
Insp. time	0.1–10 seconds
Peak flow	6–120 L/min
PEEP/CPAP	0–35 cmH_2O
Insp. hold	15 seconds
F_IO_2	0.21–1.0

HAMILTON MEDICAL, VEOLAR

Hamilton Medical, Inc., markets the Veolar ventilator, which is another example of a pneumatically powered, microprocessor controlled flow controller (Figures 8-19, 8-20). The microprocessor, when combined with appropriate flow and pressure sensors, can provide a flexible feedback control system allowing a variety of modes, monitors and alarms.

Power Input

Power to run the microprocessor control circuitry is provided by 115 volt, 60 Hz electrical power. The pneumatic system is powered by 50 psi source of medical air and oxygen.

Drive Mechanism

The pneumatic drive mechanism (Figure 8-21) reduces the line pressure of the incoming gas to 22 psi by means of the air and oxygen reducing valves. The gas pressures are closely matched to enhance the accuracy of the blending system. Gas flows from these pressure controlling elements to the oxygen blender.

The oxygen blender is a type of proportion-

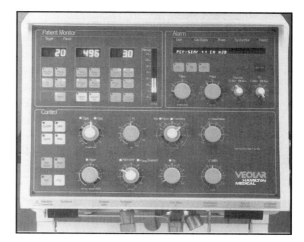

Figure 8-20 *A photograph showing the Veolar ventilator's control panel. (Courtesy Hamilton Medical, Reno, NV)*

ing valve that mixes the oxygen and air. Gas then exits the blender to another reducing valve, which holds a constant pressure of 350 cmH_2O. The gas flows from the second reducing valve to a tank or reservoir. When pressurized to 350 cmH_2O, the reservoir volume is close to 8 liters. The large reservoir serves as a buffer when high flow demands are made on the ventilator. A safety popoff valve set at 400 cmH_2O provides a margin of safety if excessive pressures build in the pneumatic circuit, protecting the patient.

If rapid changes in F_IO_2 are required, the flush control button may be depressed and held. When held down, 60 L/min of gas flows through the reservoir, quickly expelling the gas and facilitating a more rapid change in oxygen concentration.

Control Circuit

The Veolar uses a microprocessor and an electrodynamic flow control valve to regulate flow output from the ventilator. The flow control valve is a plunger type valve, which is electromagnetically controlled. A potentiometer measures the actual valve opening, ensuring precise and virtual instantaneous control. This system operates in conjunction with a differential pressure transducer. When the valve is open, a pressure difference will exist between the flow control valve inlet and outlet. This pressure differential is proportional to flow. The microprocessor has programmed into its memory the resistance the valve has at various positions. This resistance will cause a

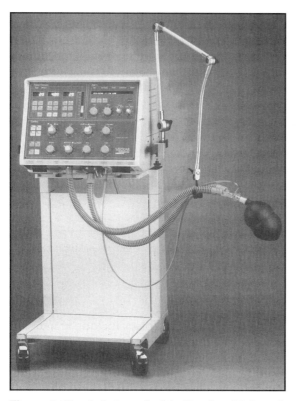

Figure 8-19 *A photograph of the Hamilton Veolar volume ventilator. (Courtesy Hamilton Medical, Reno, NV)*

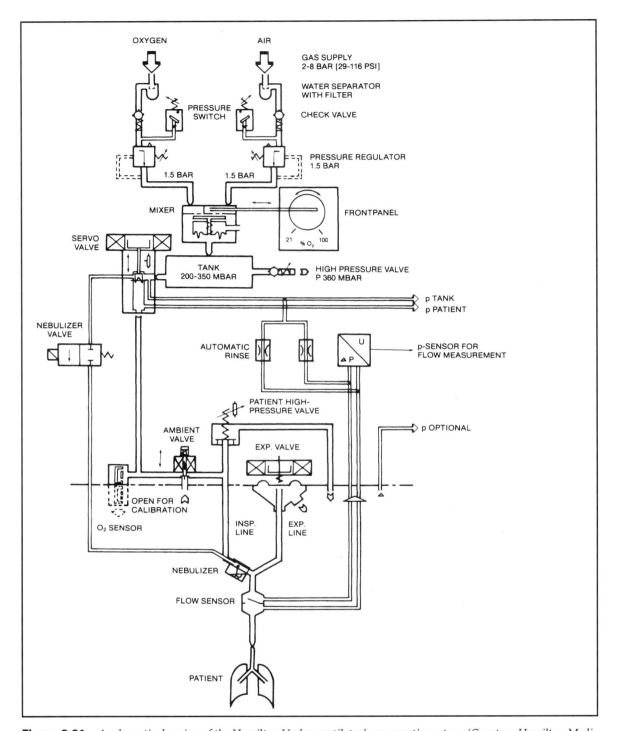

Figure 8-21 *A schematic drawing of the Hamilton Veolar ventilator's pneumatic system. (Courtesy Hamilton Medical, Reno, NV)*

pressure drop that is proportional to gas flow. Volume delivery becomes a function of inspiratory flow and time. Technically, the ventilator is really a pressure controller when delivering mandatory breaths, since pressure is measured and used as a signal to regulate the output from the flow control valve.

Flow output waveforms include rectangular, ascending and descending ramp and sinusoidal waveforms. All of these waveforms are possible through microprocessor control of the flow control valve.

The exhalation valve is an electronically controlled valve. The dynamic motor is actually an electromagnetic device. During inspiration, the plunger valve closes, causing gas to flow into the patient circuit and into the patient's lungs. During expiration, the motor opens the exhalation valve and the patient exhales. The valve also determines PEEP levels, partially closing to maintain pressure in the patient circuit.

Control Variables

As described earlier, the control variable used by the Hamilton Veolar ventilator is pressure. Differential pressure, measured across the flow control valve, is used to regulate the valve during tidal volume delivery during mandatory breaths. Pressure is also the control variable during PEEP/CPAP, and pressure support.

Phase Variables
Trigger Variables

The trigger variables for the Hamilton Veolar include pressure, time and manual variables. Pressure is used as a trigger variable for demand breaths during assist/CMV, SIMV, and pressure support. When inspiratory pressure falls below the threshold established by the trigger sensitivity control, the ventilator will initiate a breath. The trigger sensitivity may be set between 1.0 and 15.0 cmH_2O below baseline pressure by the practitioner or turned off.

Time becomes a trigger variable during assist CMV if no inspiratory effort (pressure drop) is sensed by the ventilator. If the patient does not trigger a breath, the ventilator will deliver a mandatory breath at the set tidal volume and rate. Respiratory rates are adjustable between 5 and 60 breaths per minute (CMV) or 0.5 and 30 breaths per minute (SIMV).

The ventilator may be manually triggered by the practitioner depressing the mandatory breath key on the control panel. When depressed, the ventilator will deliver a volume controlled breath (Assist/CMV, SIMV and CPAP).

Limit Variables

The limit variables of the Hamilton Veolar include pressure, volume and flow. Pressure becomes a limit variable during SIMV (with PEEP applied), MMV, CPAP, and pressure support. Under these conditions, the ventilator will augment flow to maintain the desired pressure level. PEEP/CPAP pressures are adjustable between 0.0 and 50.0 cmH_2O. Pressure support is adjustable between 0.0 and 100 cmH_2O.

Volume becomes a limit variable when the inspiratory pause is adjusted to greater than zero. Inspiratory pause may be activated when the inspiratory and expiratory time controls are separated. The difference between them becomes the inspiratory pause. When activated, a volume breath is delivered and held until the set inspiratory pause time period has elapsed.

Flow becomes a limit variable during mandatory breaths. Flow rate is a function of the tidal volume, respiratory rate and inspiratory time percent, and waveform control settings. Flow is variable between 0 and 180 L/min.

Cycle Variables

Cycle variables for the Hamilton Veolar include pressure, flow and time. Pressure becomes a cycle variable if the inspiratory pressure reaches the setting on the maximum inspiratory pressure control. Peak inspiratory pressure may be adjusted between 10 and 110 cmH_2O. When the pressure limit is reached, inspiration is terminated and both audible and visual alarms are activated.

Flow becomes a cycle variable during pressure support ventilation. Inspiration is terminated when inspiratory flow falls to approximately 25% of the peak inspiratory flow. Once flow decays to this point, pressure falls to the baseline value.

Time becomes a cycle variable when inspiratory pause has been adjusted. Inspiratory pause may be activated when the inspiratory and expiratory time controls are separated. If inspiratory pause has been activated, inspiration will be terminated when the pause time has elapsed.

Baseline Variable

PEEP/CPAP pressure is generated by the electrodynamic exhalation valve partially closing during inspiration, creating the PEEP/CPAP pressure. PEEP/CPAP pressures are adjustable between 0.0 and 50 cmH_2O.

Output Waveforms
Pressure

The Hamilton Veolar can deliver a rectangular pressure waveform during MMV mode and also during pressure support (SIMV or spontaneous modes). Under these conditions,

ASSEMBLY AND TROUBLESHOOTING

Assembly—Hamilton Veolar Ventilator

To assemble the Hamilton Veolar, follow this suggested assembly guide.

1. Connect high pressure hoses to a 50 psi medical air and oxygen source.

2. Connect the power cord to a 120 volt, 60 Hz outlet.

3. Attach a bacteria filter to the ventilator outlet.

4. Connect the humidifier inlet to the bacteria filter using large bore tubing. Since a variety of humidifiers may be used with this ventilator, specific instructions will not be included here.

5. Connect the inspiratory limb of the circuit to the outlet of the humidifier. Attach the expiratory limb to the exhalation valve fitting.

6. Connect the proximal airway line to the proximal airway fitting on the ventilator.

Troubleshooting

Refer to the troubleshooting algorithms found at the end of this chapter.

---

pressure rises rapidly and is held until inspiration is terminated.

Flow

The flow output waveform capabilities of the Veolar include rectangular, ascending and descending ramp, and sinusoidal. As described earlier, these waveforms can be accurately reproduced by the feedback system between the internal differential pressure transducer, the microprocessor and the electrodynamic flow control valve.

Alarms
Input Power

In the event of electrical power failure, the "Power" LED will be illuminated and an audible warning will be activated. This alarm is powered by a rechargeable battery and operates independently from the 120 volts, 60 Hz electrical power.

The low inlet gas alarm is activated whenever system gas pressure drops below 29 psi. The alarm is both audible and visual. An alarm will also alert the practitioner if the reservoir pressure falls below 200 cmH$_2$O.

Control Circuit Alarms

Control circuit alarms include ventilator malfunction and user (incompatible settings) problems. The ventilator malfunction alarm will be activated in the event that an internal system failure has been detected by the microprocessor.

The user (incompatible settings) alarm will be activated if the practitioner adjusts the controls such that they are out of range for the ventilator.

Output Alarms
Pressure

High and low peak pressure alarms are available on the Veolar ventilator. The high peak pressure alarm is adjustable between 10 and 120 cmH$_2$O. The loss of PEEP pressure alarm is not adjustable and activates when pressure falls 3 cmH$_2$O below the set baseline pressure.

Flow

A low minute ventilation alarm may be set between 0.2 and 50 L/min. The alarm may be used for all modes of ventilation, alerting the practitioner to hypoventilation.

Time

A high breath rate alarm may be set to alert the practitioner to tachypnea. The alarm is adjustable between 10 to 70 breaths per minute.

An apnea interval alarm alerts the practitioner to periods of patient apnea. The alarm is not adjustable and becomes active when no flow has been detected through the flow sen-

TABLE 8-14: Hamilton Veolar Alarms

ALARM	CONDITION/SETTINGS
Input Power	
Gas Supply Pressure	< 29 psi
Power	Loss of 120 volt, 60 Hz power
Control Circuit	
Dysfunction	System failure detected
User	Incompatible settings
Output Alarms	
High Airway Pressure	10 0–120 cmH$_2$O
Loss of PEEP	3.0 cmH$_2$O below baseline
Low Minute Volume	0.2–50 L/min
High Breath Rate	10–70 BPM
Apnea	15–20 seconds
Inspired Gas	High/Low Oxygen Tension (18–103%)

TABLE 8-15: Hamilton Veolar Ventilator Capabilities

Modes	CMV, Spontaneous (CPAP), SIMV, Pressure Control, MMV, Pressure Support
Volume	20–2,000 ml
Pressure	0.0–120 cmH$_2$O
Press. Support	0.0–100 cmH$_2$O
Rate	5–60 BPM
I:E	1:4 to 4:1
Peak Flow	Up to 180 L/min (not adjustable)
PEEP/CPAP	0.0–50 cmH$_2$O
MMV	1–25 L/min
Insp. Pause	Difference between Insp. and Exp. Time (0.0–3.0 seconds)
F$_I$O$_2$	0.21–1.0

sor during the past 15 seconds. A failure-to-cycle alarm is activated if no flow has been detected through the flow control valve over the past 20 seconds.

Inspired Gas

An oxygen alarm is incorporated into the ventilator to facilitate patient management. If the oxygen concentration is lower or higher than the adjusted oxygen concentration (range of 18–103%), a high/low oxygen alarm will alert the practitioner to the condition.

Table 8-14 illustrates the Hamilton Veolar alarms, and Table 8-15 illustrates its capabilities.

INFRASONICS, ADULT STAR

The Adult Star, marketed by Infrasonics, Inc., is another example of a pneumatically powered, microprocessor controlled flow controller (Figures 8-22, 8-23). The microprocessor system, when combined with appropriate

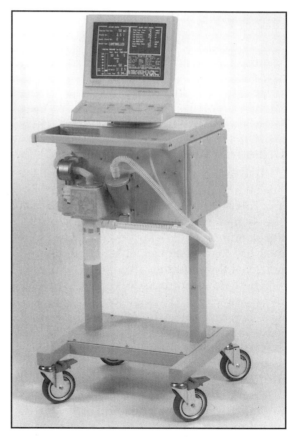

Figure 8-22 *A photograph of Infrasonics, Inc., Adult Star ventilator. (Courtesy Infrasonics, Inc., San Diego, CA)*

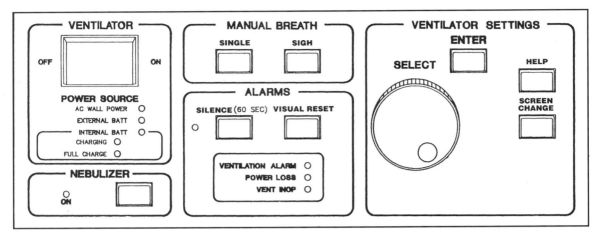

Figure 8-23 *A drawing showing the Adult Star control panel. (Courtesy Infrasonics, Inc., San Diego, CA)*

flow and pressure sensors, can provide a flexible feedback control system allowing a variety of modes, monitors and alarms. The Adult Star incorporates the use of 5 microprocessors in the control system design architecture.

Power Input

Power to run the microprocessor control circuitry is provided by an internal 12-volt battery which is continually charged by 120 volt, 60 Hz electrical power. The pneumatic system is powered by 50 psi source of medical air and oxygen. If 50 psi medical air is not available, an internal compressor can provide the air source to power the ventilator.

Drive Mechanism

Two reducing valves (air and oxygen) reduce the 50 psi line pressure to between 6.5 and 7.5 psi (Figure 8-24). The gas pressures are closely matched, to enhance the accuracy of the blending system. Gas flows from these pressure controlling elements to paired proportional flow control valves.

These flow control valves control the inspiratory waveform, oxygen concentration, volume, and inspiratory flow. The flow control valves are microprocessor controlled solenoid valves capable of opening and closing in discrete steps in response to the signals from the microprocessor.

From the flow control valves, gas flows through a screen type pneumotachometer which measures the inspiratory flow providing feedback to the microprocessor. Pressure drop across the screen elements is proportional to flow through the pneumotachometer.

Gas flows from the pneumotachometer into the patient circuit.

A small internal compressor can be used to power a small volume nebulizer in the patient circuit. Gas powering the compressor is removed from the patient circuit just distal to the flow control valves and is then added back into the circuit through the nebulizer. This system prevents variation of tidal volume and changes in F_IO_2 when the nebulizer is operated.

Control Circuit

As described earlier, the Adult Star uses two microprocessors and two proportional flow control valves to regulate output from the ventilator. This system operates in conjunction with a screen pneumotachometer and a differential pressure transducer to measure flow. When the flow control valves are open, a pressure difference will exist across the individual control valve orifice. This pressure differential is proportional to flow. The two microprocessors (one for each valve) use the flow signal as a feedback system to control the proportional solenoid valves regulating oxygen concentration, inspiratory waveforms, flow rates and volume delivery. Flow output is verified by a screen pneumotachometer.

Flow output waveforms include rectangular, ascending and descending ramp, and sinusoidal waveforms. All of these waveforms are possible through microprocessor control of the flow control valves.

The exhalation valve is a large surface diaphragm valve which is pneumatically controlled. During inspiration, the valve closes, causing gas to flow into the patient circuit and into the patient's lungs. During expiration, the valve opens and the patient exhales. The valve also determines PEEP levels, partially closing to maintain pressure in the patient circuit. Distal to the exhalation valve is an expiratory flow pneumotachometer, similar to the inspiratory flow pneumotachometer. This flow system senses expiratory flow rates and indirectly determines exhaled volumes for the display and alarm systems.

Control Variables

As described earlier, the control variable used by the Adult Star ventilator is flow. Differential pressure, measured across the individual flow control valves, is used to regulate the position of the flow control valves regulating tidal volume delivery during mandatory breaths. Proximal airway pressure is also the control variable during PEEP/CPAP and pressure support.

Phase Variables
Trigger Variables

The trigger variables for the Infrasonics Adult Star include pressure, time and manual variables. Pressure is used as a trigger variable for demand breaths during assist/CMV, SIMV, and pressure support. When inspiratory pressure falls below the threshold established by the sensitivity control, the ventilator will initiate a breath. The sensitivity may be set between 0.5 and 20.0 cmH$_2$O below baseline pressure by the practitioner.

Time becomes a trigger variable during assist CMV if no inspiratory effort (pressure drop) is sensed by the ventilator. If the patient does not trigger a breath, the ventilator will deliver a mandatory breath at the set tidal volume, peak flow and rate established by the practitioner.

The ventilator may be manually triggered by the practitioner depressing the manual breath button on the control panel. When depressed, the ventilator will deliver a volume controlled breath (assist/CMV, SIMV and CPAP). When in pressure controlled ventilation, a pressure controlled breath is delivered when the manual breath button is depressed.

Limit Variables

The limit variables of the Adult Star include pressure, volume and flow. Pressure becomes a limit variable during SIMV (with PEEP applied), CPAP, pressure support and pressure control. Under these conditions, the ventilator will augment flow to maintain the desired pressure level. PEEP/CPAP pressures are adjustable between 0.0 and 30.0 cmH$_2$O. The Adult Star is available with 0 to 50 cmH$_2$O of PEEP/CPAP as an option. Pressure support is adjustable between 0.0 and 70 cmH$_2$O.

Volume becomes a limit variable when the inspiratory pause is adjusted greater than zero. Inspiratory pause may be adjusted between 0.0 and 2.0 seconds. When activated, a volume breath is delivered and held until the set inspiratory pause time period has elapsed.

Flow becomes a limit variable when the rectangular waveform output is selected during assist/CMV. When selected, the rectangular waveform output limits flow during inspiration to the flow rate set on the peak flow control. Peak inspiratory flow is adjustable between 10 and 120 L/min.

Cycle Variables

Cycle variables for the Adult Star include pressure, flow and time. Pressure becomes a cycle variable if the inspiratory pressure reaches the setting on the high inspiratory pressure control. Inspiratory pressure limits may be adjusted between 10 and 120 cmH$_2$O. When the pressure limit is reached, inspiration is terminated and both audible and visual alarms are activated.

Flow becomes a cycle variable during pressure support ventilation. Inspiration is terminated when inspiratory flow falls to 4 L/min. Once flow decays to this point, pressure falls to the baseline value. Inspiration is also terminated during pressure support ventilation if pressure reaches 3 cmH$_2$O greater than the pressure support setting plus PEEP or if 3.5 seconds of inspiratory time has elapsed.

Time becomes a cycle variable when inspiratory pause has been adjusted. If inspiratory pause has been activated, inspiration will be terminated when the pause time has elapsed.

Baseline Variables

The baseline variable for the Adult Star is pressure. Baseline pressure is adjustable between 0 and 30 cmH$_2$O or optionally available between 0 and 50 cmH$_2$O. As described earlier, PEEP/CPAP pressure is generated by the exhalation valve partially closing during expiration.

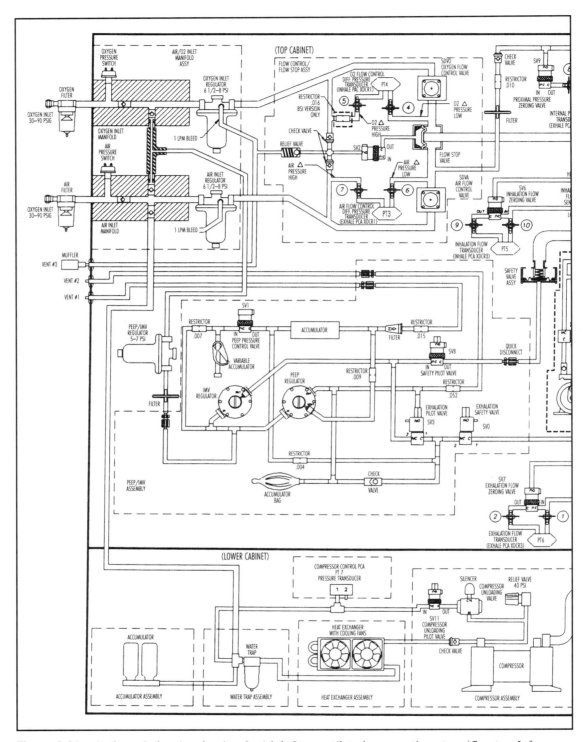

Figure 8-24 *A schematic drawing showing the Adult Star ventilator's pneumatic system. (Courtesy Infrasonics, Inc., San Diego, CA) (continues)*

Output Waveforms
Pressure

The Infrasonics Adult Star can deliver a rectangular pressure waveform when the flow to the ventilator is operated in pressure support and pressure control ventilation. Under these circumstances, pressure rises rapidly to a constant value where it remains through the delivery of the breath. At the termination of inspiration, pressure falls to the baseline value.

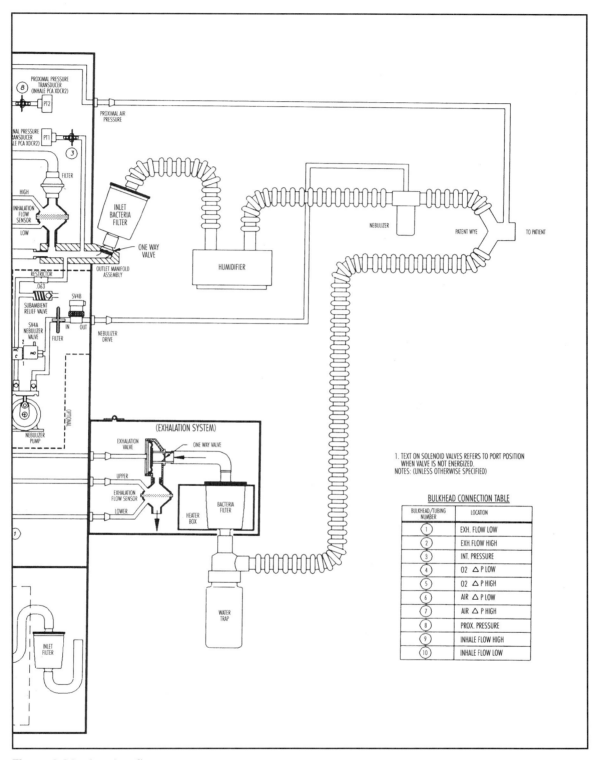

Figure 8-24 *(continued)*

Flow

The flow output waveform capabilities of the ventilator include rectangular, ascending and descending ramp, and sinusoidal. As described earlier, these waveforms can be accurately reproduced by the feedback system between the internal flow transducer, the microprocessor and the proportional flow control valves.

ASSEMBLY AND TROUBLESHOOTING

Assembly—Infrasonics Adult Star

To assemble the Infrasonics Adult Star, follow this suggested assembly guide.

1. Connect high-pressure hoses to a 50 psi medical air and oxygen source.

2. Connect the power cord to a 120 volt, 60 Hz outlet.

3. Attach an inspiratory and expiratory bacteria filter into their respective receptacles.

4. Connect the humidifier inlet to the inspiratory bacteria filter using large bore tubing. Since a variety of humidifiers may be used with this ventilator, specific instructions will not be included here.

5. Connect the inspiratory limb of the circuit to the outlet of the humidifier. Attach the expiratory limb to the exhalation water trap and expiratory bacterial filter fitting.

6. Connect the proximal airway line to the proximal airway fitting on the ventilator.

Troubleshooting

Refer to the troubleshooting algorithms found at the end of this chapter.

Alarms
Input Power Alarms

The input power alarms include loss of electrical and loss of pneumatic power. In the event of a loss of electrical power, a red LED will be illuminated, and the ventilator will continue to operate since it is powered by the battery at all times. The battery backup will operate the ventilator for up to 30 minutes without AC power. If the internal battery voltage drops to 10.9 volts for more than 15 seconds, the low battery alarm will be activated. If voltage drops further to 10.0 volts for 5 seconds, a ventilator inoperative condition will result.

If the oxygen line pressure falls below 26 psi, an audible and visual alarm will be activated. In the event that air pressure falls below 26 psi and electric power is still available, the compressor will be activated to compensate for the loss of air pressure. Should the air compressor fail to deliver at least 16 psi, a low air pressure result will occur, and the ventilator will automatically switch to 100% oxygen.

Control Circuit Alarms

The control circuit alarms include ventilator inoperative, insufficient inspiration and exhalation time. The ventilator inoperative alarm may indicate the following situations: detection of an internal malfunction and loss of electrical power (with an internal battery charge of less than 10.0 volts).

An alarm will alert the practitioner if inspiratory or expiratory times are not sufficient. If inspiratory time is less than 0.24 seconds the insufficient inspiration time alarm will be activated. If expiratory time is less than 0.20 seconds, or 0.26 seconds for pressure support, the insufficient exhalation time alarm will be activated.

Output Alarms
Pressure

Pressure output alarms include high and low peak and low baseline. The high inspiratory pressure alarm is adjustable between 10.0 and 120 cmH$_2$O. Low inspiratory pressure may be set between 3 and 60 cmH$_2$O. Baseline pressure alarms may be set between 0.0 and 30 cmH$_2$O (0 to 50 cmH$_2$O optionally).

Volume

Low mechanical volume and low spontaneous volume alarms are available for both mandatory breaths and spontaneous breaths. The mechanical volume alarm parameters are adjustable between 0.0 and 2,500 mL for both mandatory and spontaneous alarms.

Flow

A low exhaled minute volume alarm may be adjusted between 0.0 and 60.0

L/min. In the event that the patient's exhaled minute volume falls below the threshold parameter, audible and visual alarm will be activated.

Time

A high ventilatory rate alarm can be set between 0 and 90 breaths per minute. In the event that the patient's respiratory rate exceeds the established threshold, both an audible and visual alarm will result.

Table 8-16 illustrates the Infrasonics Adult Star alarm systems, and Table 8-17 illustrates its capabilities.

TABLE 8-16: Adult Star Alarm Systems

ALARM	CONDITION/SETTINGS
Input Power	
Oxygen Pressure	< 26 psi
Air Pressure	< 26 psi or < 16 psi from compressor
Electric Power	Loss of 120 volt, 60 Hz power
	Battery power less than 10.0 volts
Control Circuit	
Ventilator Inoperative	Internal malfunction detected
Insuf. Insp. Time	Insp. time less than 0.250 seconds
Insuf. Exp. Time	Exp. time less than 0.20 seconds
Output Alarms	
High Airway Pressure	10.0–120 cmH$_2$O
Low Airway Pressure	3.0–60 cmH$_2$O
Low Baseline Pressure	0.0–30 cmH$_2$O
Low Exhaled Tidal Vol.	0.0–2,500 mL
(Spontaneous)	0.0–2,500 mL
Low Minute Volume	0.0–60 L/min
High Breath Rate	0–90 BPM

TABLE 8-17: Adult Star Ventilator Capabilities

Modes	Assist/Control, SIMV, Pressure Support, Pressure Control, CPAP
Volume	100–2,500 mL (50–2,500 ml with optional pediatric ventilation)
Pressure	0.0–120 cmH$_2$O
Press. Support	0.0–70 cmH$_2$O
Rate	0.5–80 BPM (0.5 to 120 BPM with optional pediatric ventilation)
Peak Flow	10–120 L/min (machine); 10–160 L/min Spontaneous, Pressure Support and Pressure Control
PEEP/CPAP	0.0–30 cmH$_2$O
Sigh Volume	100–2,500 mL (50–2,500 ml with pediatric ventilation option)
Sigh Rate	0 to 20 sighs per hour (SPH)
Multiple Sighs	1–3 sighs
Insp. Pause	0.0 to 2.0 seconds
Sensitivity	0.5 to 20 below baseline pressure
F$_I$O$_2$	0.21 to 1.0

NEWPORT MEDICAL INSTRUMENTS, WAVE

Newport Medical Instruments, Inc., manufactures and distributes the Newport Wave ventilator (Figures 8-25, 8-26). The ventilator is a pneumatically powered and microprocessor-controlled flow and pressure controller. Flow is utilized by the microprocessor to control the ventilator's output.

Power Input

Power to run the microprocessor control circuitry is provided by 120 volt, 60 Hz (220 volt, 60 Hz switchable) electrical power. The pneumatic system is powered by 50 psi source of medical air and oxygen.

Drive Mechanism

The 50 psi air and oxygen source gas enters the ventilator's blender where the two gases

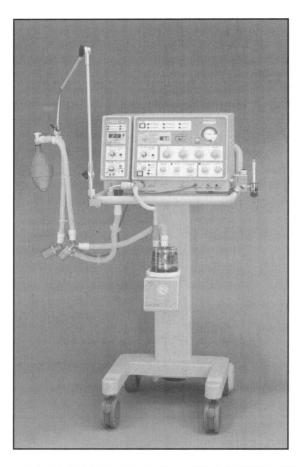

are mixed to the desired F_IO_2 level (Figure 8-27). Gas exits the blender at 28 psi, where it flows to an accumulator tank. The accumulator functions as a reservoir to meet high patient flow demands and also as a mixing chamber to further stabilize the oxygen concentration. The volume of the accumulator tank is 1 liter at a pressure of 2 atmospheres.

Control Circuit

Gas exits the accumulator through a filter and into a servoid metering valve. The servoid valve is an electrodynamic valve, which is controlled by the microprocessor. Gas flowing from the servoid valve passes through a laminar flow element with pressure taps proximal and distal to it. Feedback signals from a differential pressure transducer provide flow information to the microprocessor to regulate inspiratory flow. Hence, the ventilator is a

Figure 8-25 *A photograph of Newport Medical Instruments E200 Wave ventilator. (Courtesy Newport Medical Instruments, Inc., Costa Mesa, CA)*

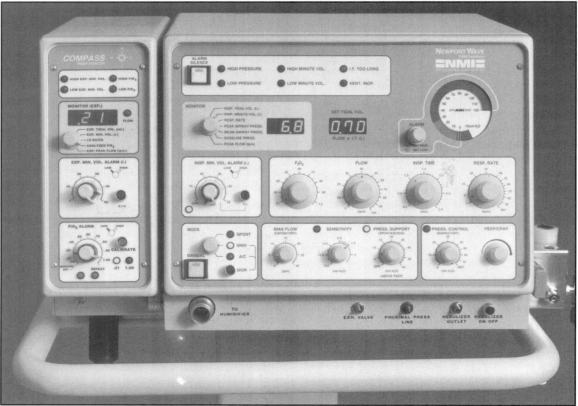

Figure 8-26 *A photograph of the E200 Wave ventilator's control panel. (Courtesy Newport Medical Instruments, Inc., Costa Mesa, CA)*

flow controller. The flow output waveform for the Wave ventilator is a rectangular waveform. During pressure control ventilation, proximal airway pressure is used as a feedback signal to the microprocessor which adjusts flow output to regulate the pressure.

The exhalation valve diaphragm is pneumatically actuated. During inspiration the valve closes, causing gas to flow into the patient circuit and into the patient's lungs. During expiration the valve opens and the patient exhales. The valve also determines PEEP levels, partially closing to maintain pressure in the patient circuit.

Control Variables

The control variables used by the Newport Wave ventilator are flow and pressure. Flow becomes the control variable during mandatory volume delivery, volume controlled assist/control and SIMV ventilation. During pressure controlled assist/control and pressure support, pressure becomes the control variable.

Phase Variables
Trigger Variables

The trigger variables for the Newport Wave ventilator include pressure, time and manual variables. Pressure is used as a trigger variable for demand breaths during volume controlled assist/control, SIMV, sigh breath delivery, pressure control, and pressure support. When inspiratory pressure falls below the threshold established by the assist sensitivity control, the ventilator will initiate a breath. The sensitivity may be set between 0.0 and 5.0 cmH$_2$O below baseline pressure by the practitioner.

Time becomes a trigger variable if no inspiratory effort (pressure drop) is sensed by the ventilator (volume- or pressure-controlled ventilation). If the patient does not trigger a breath, the ventilator will deliver a mandatory breath at the established rate, inspiratory time and peak flow, and pressure (pressure-control ventilation).

The ventilator may be manually triggered by the practitioner depressing the manual breath button on the control panel. When depressed, a mandatory breath will be delivered (volume- or pressure-controlled).

Limit Variables

The limit variables of the Newport Wave include pressure, volume and flow. Pressure becomes a limit variable during pressure controlled ventilation. During pressure control, inspiratory pressure reaches a preset limit and is held there until the inspiratory time has passed. During volume controlled ventilation, it is also possible to pressure limit the ventilator. This is accomplished by setting the pneumatic pressure relief valve to a level that is lower than the peak inspiratory pressure. Peak inspiratory pressure is a function of inspiratory time and flow rate settings. The pneumatic pressure relief valve is adjustable between 0.0 and 120 cmH$_2$O.

Volume becomes a limit variable when the inspiratory pause control is active. Inspiratory pause may be adjusted between 10, 20, or 30% of the cycle time. When activated, a volume breath is delivered and held until the set inspiratory pause time period has elapsed. This is only available during volume controlled assist/control and the mandatory portions of SIMV.

Flow becomes a limit variable during volume controlled assist/control, the mandatory portion of volume controlled SIMV or during sigh breath delivery. When a rectangular waveform output is delivered, flow during inspiration is limited to the setting established on the peak flow control. Peak flow is adjustable between 1 and 100 L/min.

Cycle Variables

Cycle variables for the Newport Wave ventilator include pressure, flow and time. Pressure becomes a cycle variable if the inspiratory pressure reaches the setting on the high pressure alarm control or the automatic high pressure alarm during pressure controlled or pressure support ventilation. The peak inspiratory pressure alarm may be adjusted between 10 and 120 cmH$_2$O. When the pressure limit is reached, inspiration is terminated and both audible and visual alarms are activated.

Flow becomes a cycle variable during pressure support ventilation. Inspiration is terminated when inspiratory flow falls to a value determined by the following formula: K × Peak Flow$^{0.6}$ × Elapsed Time, where K equals a constant. A pressure supported breath is also terminated when tidal volume exceeds 4 L, when peak pressure reaches 2 cmH$_2$O over pressure support level or when inspiratory time exceeds 3 seconds.

Time becomes a cycle variable during pressure control ventilation. In this mode, a constant pressure is applied until the time set on

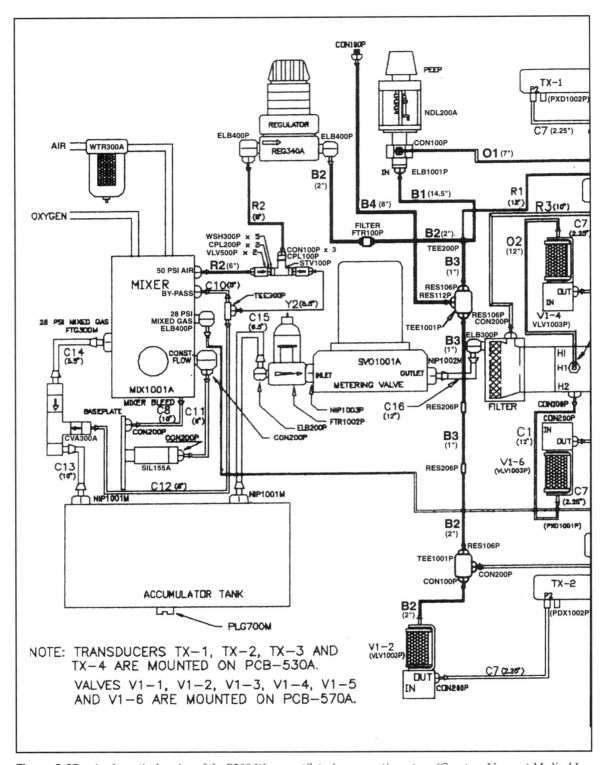

Figure 8-27 *A schematic drawing of the E200 Wave ventilator's pneumatic system. (Courtesy Newport Medical Instruments, Inc., Costa Mesa, CA) (continues)*

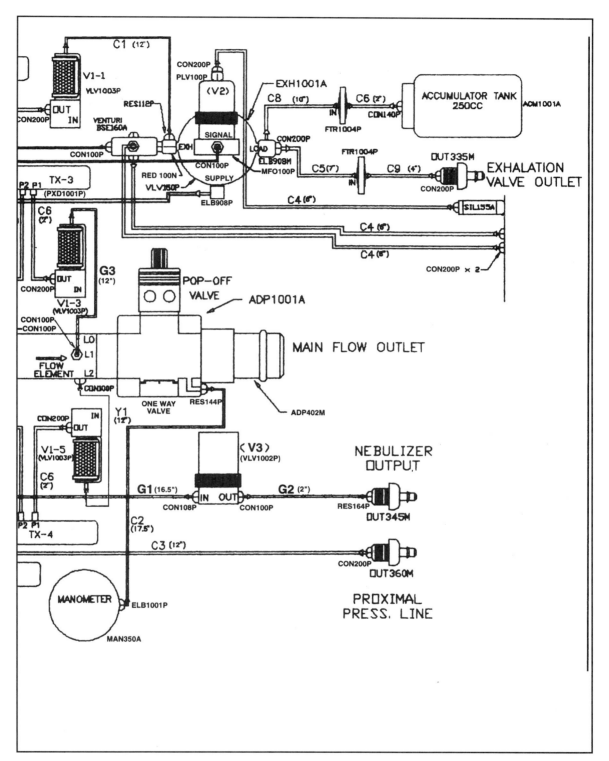

Figure 8-27 *(continued)*

the inspiratory time control has been reached. Inspiratory times are adjustable between 0.1 and 3.0 seconds. Time may also be a cycle variable in pressure support if the inspiratory time exceeds 3 seconds.

Baseline Variable

The ventilator is capable of delivering PEEP/CPAP pressures. PEEP/CPAP pressures are adjustable between 0 and 45 cmH$_2$O. Baseline pressures are elevated in the patient circuit by the exhalation valve partially closing, acting as a threshold resistor.

Conditional Variables
Time

Time becomes a conditional variable during sigh delivery. During normal ventilator supported breaths, they are flow or pressure controlled; pressure or time triggered; pressure, volume or flow limited; pressure, time or flow cycled. During a sigh delivery, a sigh breath will be given every 100th breath. A sigh volume of 150% of the tidal volume is delivered by extending the inspiratory time by 1.5 times the chosen setting.

Time and Pressure

Time and pressure become conditional variables during SIMV mode. The rate control determines the frequency of mandatory breath delivery during SIMV mode. The rate control is essentially an electronic timer, delivering a breath at specified time intervals. Between mandatory breath delivery the patient breathes through the flow control valve. The ventilator measures proximal airway pressure, or distal endotracheal tube pressure, to determine if the patient is attempting to initiate a breath. In response to the pressure change, the patient is able to draw gas spontaneously through the flow control valve to meet inspiratory needs.

Output Waveforms
Pressure

During pressure controlled ventilation, the pressure waveform is a combination of rectangular and exponential. The waveform diminishes (ramps) as the pressure in the airway approaches the pressure control level. If inspiratory time is short, inspiratory pressure may never reach the pressure control level.

Flow

The flow wave for output of the ventilator is a rectangular waveform output during volume controlled ventilation. This occurs providing that the peak inspiratory pressure is less than the setting on the pressure control adjustment.

During pressure controlled ventilation, the flow waveform is a descending ramp. With the exhalation valve closed during inspiration, the ramped flow pattern prevents pressure from increasing above the set pressure limit.

Alarms
Input Power Alarms

The input power alarms include loss of electrical and loss of pneumatic power. In the event of a loss of electrical power, an audible alarm will be activated for a minimum of 10 minutes.

If the oxygen or air line pressure falls below 32 psi, an audible alarm will be activated.

Control Circuit Alarms

The control circuit alarms include ventilator inoperative and inverse I:E ratio. The ventilator inoperative alarm indicates detection of an internal malfunction.

An I:E ratio alarm is available to alert the practitioner to long inspiratory times. The alarm is selectable between two positions, 1:1 and 3:1. The ventilator is capable of delivering inverse I:E ratios of up to 3:1 if the alarm is set at the 3:1 position. Once inspiratory time exceeds 75% of the ventilatory cycle, the ventilator will automatically terminate inspiration. If the ratio limit alarm is limited to an I:E ratio of 1:1 and the inspiratory time exceeds 50% of the ventilatory cycle, the alarm condition will result, terminating inspiration.

Output Alarms
Pressure

Pressure output alarms include high and low peak pressure alarms. The high inspiratory pressure alarm is adjustable between 5.0 and 120 cmH$_2$O. Low inspiratory pressure may be set between 0.3 and 110 cmH$_2$O.

Flow

A high and low inspiratory minute volume alarm is available on the Newport Wave. The

ASSEMBLY AND TROUBLESHOOTING

Assembly—Newport Wave Ventilator

To assemble the Newport Wave ventilator, follow this suggested assembly guide.

1. Connect high pressure hoses to a 50 psi medical air and oxygen source.

2. Connect the power cord to a 120 volt, 60 Hz (220 volt, 60 Hz selectable) outlet.

3. Attach an inspiratory bacteria filter to the ventilator outlet.

4. Connect the humidifier inlet to the inspiratory bacteria filter using large-bore tubing (adult) or pediatric tubing. Since a variety of humidifiers may be used with this ventilator, specific instructions will not be included here.

5. Connect the inspiratory limb of the circuit to the outlet of the humidifier. Attach the expiratory limb to the exhalation valve fitting.

6. Connect the exhalation valve to the exhalation valve nipple on the front of the ventilator.

7. Connect the proximal airway line to the proximal airway fitting on the ventilator.

Troubleshooting

Refer to the troubleshooting algorithms found at the end of this chapter.

TABLE 8-18: Newport Wave Ventilator Alarm Systems

ALARM	CONDITION/SETTINGS
Input Power	
Oxygen Pressure	< 32 psi
Air Pressure	< 32 psi
Electric Power	Loss of 120 volt, 60 Hz (220 volt, 60 Hz) power
Control Circuit	
Ventilator Inoperative	Internal malfunction detected
I:E Ratio	Insp. time > 75% of cycle time (3:1)
	Insp. time > 50% of cycle time (1:1)
Output Alarms	
High Airway Pressure	10.0–120 cmH$_2$O
Low Airway Pressure	3.0–99 cmH$_2$O
Low Minute Volume	0.0–49 L/min
High Minute Volume	0.0 50 L/min BPM

high inspiratory minute volume alarm is adjustable between 0 to 50 and 0 to 5 L/min. The low inspiratory minute volume alarm is adjustable between 0.0 and 49 L/min.

Table 8-18 illustrates the Newport Wave ventilator's alarm systems, and Table 8-19 illustrates its capabilities.

PURITAN BENNETT CORPORATION, 7200ae

The Puritan Bennett 7200ae is a pneumatically driven, electrically powered, microprocessor-controlled ventilator (Figure 8-28, 8-29). A single pneumatic circuit drives the ventilator while microprocessor control provides control, assist/control, SIMV, PEEP/CPAP, pressure support and pressure control in either assist/control or SIMV. All breath types may be pressure or flow triggered.

Power Input

Power to run the microprocessor control circuitry is provided by 120 volt, 60 Hz electrical power. The pneumatic system is powered by 35 to 100 psi source of medical air and oxygen. If compressed medical air is not available, an optional internal compressor in the pedestal will provide an air source to power the pneumatic system.

TABLE 8-19: Newport Wave Ventilator Capabilities

Modes	Volume Controlled Ventilation
	Assist/Control (with or without bias flow)
	SIMV (with or without bias flow or pressure support)
	Pressure Controlled Ventilation
	Assist/Control (with or without bias flow)
	SIMV (with or without pressure support or bias flow)
	Spontaneous Modes
	Pressure support (with or without bias flow)
Volume	10–2,000 mL
Pressure	0.0–120 cmH$_2$O
Press. Support	0.0–60 cmH$_2$O
Press. Control	0.0–80 cmH$_2$O
Rate	0–100 BPM
Peak Flow	1 to 100 L/min (Machine);
	1 to 160 L/min (Spontaneous)
Bias Flow	0.0–30 L/min
Insp. Time	0.1–3.0 seconds
PEEP/CPAP	0.0–45 cmH$_2$O
Sigh Volume	150% of tidal volume
Sigh Rate	Every 100th breath
Insp. Pause	10, 20 or 30%
Sensitivity	0.0 to 5 cmH$_2$O below baseline pressure
F$_I$O$_2$	0.21 to 1.0

Drive Mechanism

The pneumatic drive mechanism (Figure 8-30) reduces the line pressure of the incoming gas to 10 psi by means of the air and oxygen reducing valves. A crossover solenoid connects the air and oxygen supply so in the event air pressure is lost, the ventilator will still operate using oxygen. Gases are conducted through flow and temperature transducers before they reach the proportional solenoid valves (PSOLs were discussed in Chapter 6.).

Control Circuit

The 7200ae uses a microprocessor, two flow transducers, two temperature transducers, a pressure transducer, and two PSOL valves to regulate flow output from the ventilator. The PSOLs regulate F$_I$O$_2$, inspiratory flow, pressure, and volume delivery.

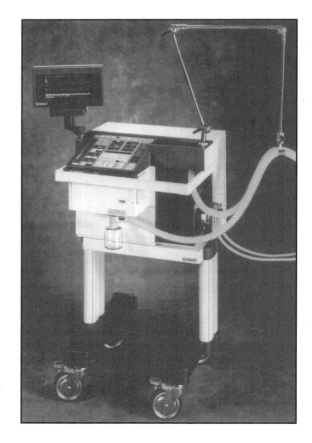

Figure 8-28 *A photograph of the Puritan Bennett 7200ae ventilator. (Courtesy of Puritan-Bennett Corporation, Carlsbad, CA, Puritan-Bennett® and the 7200® series ventilatory system)*

Figure 8-29 *A photograph of the Puritan Bennett 7200ae control panel. (Courtesy of Puritan-Bennett Corporation, Carlsbad, CA. Puritan-Bennett,® and the 7200® series ventilatory system)*

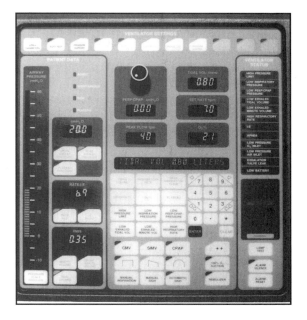

Gases are conducted through flow and temperature transducers before they reach the PSOLs. The purpose of the flow and temperature transducers is to provide feedback to the microprocessor. The microprocessor constantly monitors the flow and temperature transducers (air and oxygen) during the inspiratory phase. The opening of the PSOLs is adjusted to establish the exact volume, flow, F_IO_2, flow pattern and mode, as set by the practitioner using the keyboard.

Gas flows from the PSOLs to the patient outlet, passing through a safety check valve. Output from the PSOLs also is conducted to an absolute pressure transducer. This transducer provides feedback to the microprocessor, monitoring ambient pressures to correct for varying gas densities.

The exhalation valve is powered by diversion of some of the gas pressure from the patient circuit. When the solenoid is open, the exhalation valve diaphragm is pressurized, closing it. Gas flow from the PSOLs is then directed into the patient's lungs. The exhalation valve also plays an important role in the regulation of PEEP/CPAP pressures.

Activation of the PEEP/CPAP control knob causes gas to be delivered from the PEEP/CPAP solenoid to the PEEP/CPAP regulator (control adjustment). Pressure from the regulator powers a venturi. Flow from the venturi is directed against the exhalation valve diaphragm, pressurizing it. The partially pressurized diaphragm maintains pressure within the circuit equal to the pressure applied to it. PEEP/CPAP may be adjusted between 0 and 45 cmH$_2$O.

During the expiratory phase, the microprocessor sends signals to the PSOLs closing them. When the PSOLs have closed, all gas flow to the patient ceases. Simultaneously, a signal is sent to the exhalation pilot control solenoid, which switches to the output position and allows the exhalation valve to depressurize. Gas behind the exhalation valve exits the ventilator and the valve opens.

The patient's exhaled air passes through a heated bacteria filter before entering the expiratory flow sensor. This removes contaminant from the exhaled air and warms it to above body temperature. Particulate water is removed; only water vapor will pass through the filter system. The exhaled gas then flows through a temperature and flow transducer that measures exhaled gas temperature and flow. The exhaled gas is then allowed to vent to the atmosphere.

Flow output wave forms include rectangular, descending ramp, and sinusoidal wave forms. All of these wave forms are possible through microprocessor control of the pneumatic system.

Control Variables

The control variable for the 7200ae can be either flow or pressure. Inspiratory flow is measured by the two flow transducers proximal to the air and oxygen PSOLs. Flow is used as a control variable during control, assist/control and the mandatory portions of SIMV for volume delivered breaths. In these modes volume becomes a derivative of flow (flow multiplied by inspiratory time).

Pressure is also the control variable during the inspiratory phase of PEEP/CPAP, pressure support, and pressure control delivery. Pressure is monitored by the expiratory pressure transducer, and flow output from the PSOLs is adjusted to maintain the desired pressure levels.

Phase Variables
Trigger Variables

The trigger variables of the Puritan Bennett 7200ae include pressure, flow, time and manual. Pressure becomes a trigger variable when the patient inhales, reducing pressure in the circuit below the reference level set on the sensitivity control. Sensitivity may be adjusted between 0.5 and 20 cmH$_2$O below baseline pressure. Pressure operates as a trigger vari-

able for all breaths during control assist/control, SIMV, pressure support, and pressure control modes.

Flow becomes a trigger variable when flow-by has been selected (Option 50). When selected the practitioner enters the desired base flow (bias flow) between 5 and 20 L/min. Following base flow entry, the practitioner must enter the flow sensitivity, which is adjustable between 1 and 15 L/min. This flow sensitivity is the drop in returned flow to the expiratory sensor, used as a threshold to detect a breath. Once the established flow threshold (flow sensitivity) has been sensed by the microprocessor, the PSOLs open to deliver a breath.

Time is a trigger variable during control, assist control, and SIMV, when no spontaneous efforts occur. Breath delivery is based

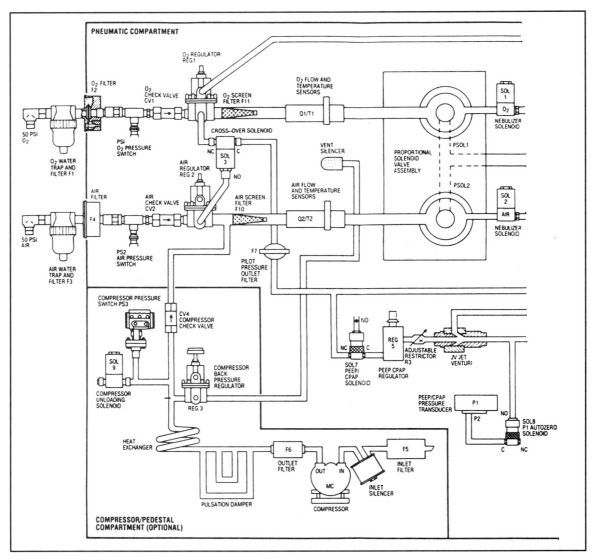

Figure 8-30 *A schematic diagram of the Puritan Bennett 7200ae ventilator pneumatic system. (Courtesy Puritan Bennett Corporation, Carlsbad, CA) (continues)*

upon the respiratory rate setting (time).

The ventilator may also be manually triggered by depressing the manual inspiration key. When depressed, the ventilator initiates a controlled breath at the tidal volume, waveform and peak flow set in volume controlled ventilation or at the pressure level and inspiratory time in pressure controlled ventilation.

Limit Variables

The limit variables include pressure, volume and flow. Pressure becomes the limit variable during the spontaneous breaths when in SIMV (with PEEP/CPAP added), CPAP, pressure control, and pressure support modes. The pneumatic system will maintain the desired pressure in the patient circuit as adjusted by the practitioner. PEEP/CPAP is adjustable between 0.0 and 45 cmH$_2$O, pressure support may be adjusted between 0.0 and 70 cmH$_2$O, and pressure control may be set between 5 and 100 cmH$_2$O.

Volume becomes a limit variable when inspiratory hold has been selected by the practitioner. When selected, inspiratory hold may be adjusted between 0.0 and 2.0 seconds. The ventilator will deliver a breath and it will be held following breath delivery until the set time interval has elapsed.

Flow is the limit variable when the ventilator delivers mandatory flow-controlled breaths. Flow is adjustable between 10 and 120 L/min. The flow delivery is limited to the value set on the peak flow control.

Cycle Variables

The cycle variables include pressure, flow and time. Pressure becomes the cycle variable

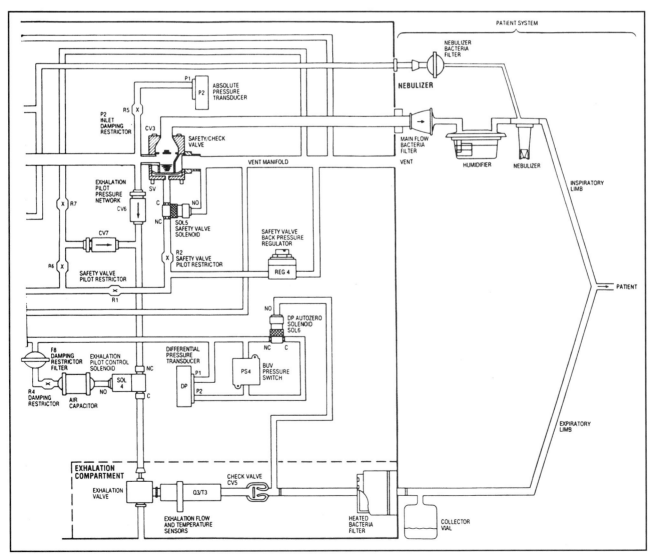

Figure 8-30 *(continued)*

when inspiratory pressure reaches the pressure set on the high pressure limit alarm. The high pressure limit is adjustable between 10 and 120 cmH$_2$O. When the pressure limit is reached, inspiratory flow is stopped and both audible and visual alarms are activated.

Flow becomes the cycle variable during pressure support. When inspiratory flow decays to 5 L/min, or inspiratory pressure falls to 1.5 cmH$_2$O above the set pressure, breath delivery stops.

Time becomes the cycle variable during mandatory breath delivery. The microprocessor determines volume as a function of flow and inspiratory time. Once the appropriate inspiratory time has been reached, based upon peak flow , flow waveform and tidal volume settings, breath delivery ceases. If pressure support fails to cycle off (in the event of a leak), the breath will terminate after 5 seconds.

Baseline Variables

The baseline variable for the Puritan Bennett 7200ae is pressure. PEEP/CPAP pressures are adjustable between 0 and 45 cmH$_2$O. As described earlier, baseline pressure is created by the exhalation valve partially closing during exhalation.

Conditional Variables
Time

Time becomes a conditional variable during sigh delivery. During normal ventilator supported breaths, they are flow or pressure controlled, pressure or flow triggered, pressure, flow, or time cycled. During sigh delivery, sigh volumes may be adjusted between 10 and 2,500 ml at a rate of 1 to 15 sighs per hour, with sigh multiples between 1 and 3. The sigh breaths have their own high pressure limit, which is adjustable between 10 and 120 cmH$_2$O.

Time and Pressure or Time and Flow

Time and pressure become conditional variables during the SIMV mode. The rate control determines the frequency of mandatory breath delivery during SIMV mode. The rate control is essentially an electronic timer, allowing time window for the patient to trigger a breath or delivering a breath at specified time intervals if no efforts are detected. Between mandatory breath delivery, the patient breathes through the ventilator's pneumatic system. The ventilator measures pressure to determine if the patient is attempting to initiate a breath. In response to the pressure change, the patient is able to draw gas spontaneously through the pneumatic system to meet inspiratory needs.

Time and flow become conditional variables during SIMV when flow-by has been selected. The microprocessor senses inspiratory effort using flow rather than pressure. In response to a patient effort, the PSOLs open, attempting to maintain the desired PEEP/CPAP pressure established by the practitioner.

Output Waveforms
Pressure

The pressure output of the 7200ae ventilator is rectangular when the ventilator is operating in the pressure support and pressure control modes. In these modes, pressure rises sharply to the level set by the practitioner. Pressure is maintained until flow reaches approximately 5 L/min, or in pressure control when the set inspiratory time has lapsed.

Flow

The flow output of the 7200ae may be adjusted between rectangular, descending ramp and sinusoidal outputs in volume control ventilation. The PSOL valves, in combination with the microprocessor and feedback control system, enable the ventilator to accurately reproduce these flow output waveforms.

Alarms
Input Power

Input power alarms on the 7200ae include loss of electrical and pneumatic power. When electrical power is lost, an audible alarm will sound and the safety valve will open. A nicad battery pack powers the audible and visual alarm, independent of the 120 volt, 60 Hz power for the ventilator. If power is restored or the On/Off switch is turned off, the alarm will cease.

If air or oxygen pressure falls below 35 psi, the low air or O$_2$ pressure alarm will be activated. Both audible and visual alarms will be activated when this condition exists.

Control Circuit Alarms

Control circuit alarms on the 7200ae include ventilator inoperative, incompatible settings, and I:E limit. The ventilator inoperative alarm is activated when the microprocessor conducts its diagnostics routine and an internal fault is found in the pneumatic delivery section. If the fault is in the microprocessor alone, the "Back Up Ventilator" alarm sounds and the patient is ventilated with an analog circuit at factory preset parameters. The incompatible settings alarm occurs when the practitioner attempts to enter a value falling outside of established parameters for that control. It is an audible alarm in which four short beep tones are given to alert the practitioner. The visual-only I:E limit alert is activated if the practitioner has set a tidal volume, rate and peak flow and inspiratory pause settings which result in an inspiratory time exceeding 50% of the cycle time.

Output Alarms

Pressure

The 7200ae incorporates high and low inspiratory pressure alarms, and a low baseline pressure alarm. The high peak pressure alarm is adjustable between 10.0 and 120 cmH$_2$O and the low peak pressure alarm is adjustable between 3 and 99 cmH$_2$O. The low baseline (PEEP/CPAP) pressure alarm is adjustable between 0.0 and 45 cmH$_2$O.

Volume

A low tidal volume alarm alerts the practitioner to events resulting in the low volume threshold not being met. These could include leaks, patient disconnects and other problems. The low tidal volume alarm is adjustable between 0 and 2,500 mL.

Flow

A low minute volume alarm is incorporated into the 7200ae. The low minute volume alarm is adjustable between 0.0 and 60 L/min.

Time

An adjustable high respiratory rate alarm is also incorporated into the 7200ae ventilator. The high breath rate alarm can be adjusted between 0 and 70 breaths per minute.

Emergency Modes of Ventilation

There are four emergency modes of ventilation that may become active in the event of gas pressure or other systems failures. These modes include apnea ventilation, disconnect ventilation, backup ventilator and safety valve open.

ASSEMBLY AND TROUBLESHOOTING

Assembly—7200ae

To assemble the 7200ae ventilator for use, complete the following suggested assembly guide.

1. Rotate the filter clamp away from the ventilator housing and install an exhalation bacteria filter into its compartment. Rotate the clamp toward the ventilator, locking the filter into place. Attach a water collection vial to the inlet of the expiratory bacterial filter.

2. Install a bacteria filter to the ventilator's outlet by opening the filter compartment door to the right of the control panel.

3. Assemble the humidifier and connect the humidifier inlet to the bacteria filter with a length of large-bore tubing.

4. Attach the patient circuit to the support arm. Connect the inspiratory limb to the outlet of the humidifier. Attach the expiratory limb to the collection vial connected to the expiratory bacteria filter.

5. Connect the nebulizer in the patient circuit to the nebulizer nipple on the front of the ventilator housing.

6. If a servo controlled humidifier is used, connect the temperature probe to the inlet side of the patient wye.

7. Connect the air and oxygen DISS fittings to 50 psi sources.

8. Connect the power cord to a suitable 120 volt, 60 Hz outlet.

Troubleshooting

Refer to the troubleshooting algorithms found at the end of this chapter.

TABLE 8-20: Operator Selectable Apnea Parameters

Apnea interval	10–60 seconds
Tidal volume	.1–2.5 L
Respiratory rate	.5–70 breaths/min
Peak flow	10–120 L/min
F_iO_2	.21–1.00

Apnea Ventilation

If, during an operator set time interval, the expiratory flow sensor fails to detect a volume greater than 50 mL, the apnea alarm will be activated.

Apnea ventilation is operator selectable, and the parameters are listed in Table 8-20. If the operator fails to adjust the apnea parameters, the following parameters are the default values: apnea interval, 20 seconds; tidal volume, .5L; respiratory rate, 12 breaths/min; peak flow, 45 L/min; oxygen concentration, 100%. The ventilator will revert to apnea ventilation whenever apnea is detected.

If the patient takes two consecutive breaths and exhales to or greater than one half of the delivered tidal volume, the ventilator will reset itself to the previous state of operation.

Disconnect Ventilation

If the proximal airway pressure line (Model 7200) becomes disconnected, if the patient circuit becomes occluded, or the expiratory pressure transducer fails, disconnect ventilation is declared. Disconnect ventilation results in the ventilator reverting to the settings established for apnea ventilation. Sensitivity is not recognized by the feedback control system during disconnect ventilation.

Backup Ventilator (BUV)

The backup ventilator is a backup system that operates independently from the microprocessor. The PSOLs are controlled by analog circuits rather than by the digital microprocessor. In the event of a microprocessor failure, patient ventilation is still possible.

If the microprocessor or the electrical system fails, the backup ventilation emergency mode is activated. Backup ventilator settings are the same as the default values listed under apnea ventilation (the operator may not select the settings), except that the alarm silence and alarm reset are both inoperative,

and the pressure limit is 30 cmH₂O, guaranteeing appropriately small volumes for pediatric patients.

Safety Valve Open

The safety valve circuit opens to allow the patient to breathe unassisted, from ambient air. No PEEP/CPAP is applied, so the patient is also breathing at ambient pressures.

This system is activated if any of the following conditions are met.

- Both air and oxygen supplies are lost.
- The POST (Power On Self-Test) is running.
- A system fault has been detected, resulting in an inability of the the Backup Ventilator circuit to run the pneumatic system.
- Power to the ventilator has been disrupted.

Table 8-21 summarizes the Puritan Bennett 7200ae alarms, and Table 8-22 summarizes its capabilities.

TABLE 8-21: Puritan Bennett 7200ae Ventilator Alarm Systems

ALARM	CONDITION/SETTINGS
Input Power	
Oxygen Pressure	< 35 psi
Air Pressure	< 35 psi
Electric Power	Loss of 120 volt, 60 Hz, power
Control Circuit	
Ventilator Inoperative	Internal malfunction detected
Incompatible Settings	Four "beeps" alerting practitioner to parameters that are out of range
I:E Ratio	Insp. time > 50% of cycle time
Output Alarms	
High Pressure Limit	10.0–120 cmH₂O
Low Inspiratory Pressure	3.0–99 cmH₂O
Low PEEP/CPAP Pressure	0.0–45 cmH₂O
Low Exhaled Minute Vol.	0.0–2.5 L
Low Minute Volume	0.0–60 L/min
High Resp. Rate	0–70 BPM

TABLE 8-22: Puritan Bennett 7200ae Ventilator Capabilities

Modes	CMV (volume controlled), CMV (pressure controlled), SIMV, CPAP, Pressure Support, Flow-By (Flow triggering)
Volume	10–2,500 mL
Pressure	0.0–120 cmH$_2$O
Press. Support	0.0–70 cmH$_2$O
Press. Control	5.0–100 cmH$_2$O
Rate	0.5–70 BPM
Peak Flow	10–120 L/min
Base Flow	5–20 L/min
Flow Sens.	1–15 L/min
Insp. Time	0.2–5.0 seconds
PEEP/CPAP	0.0–45 cmH$_2$O
Sigh Volume	0.10 to 2.5 L
Sigh Rate	1–15/hr
Sigh Multiple	1–3
Insp. Pause	0.0 to 2.0 seconds
Sensitivity	0.5 to 20 cmH$_2$O below baseline pressure
F$_I$O$_2$	0.21 to 1.0

NELLCOR PURITAN BENNETT, 840 VENTILATOR

The Nellcor Puritan Bennett 840 ventilator is a pneumatically driven, electrically powered, microprocessor-controlled ventilator (Figure 8-31A, 8-31B). A single pneumatic circuit drives the ventilator, while microprocessor control provides control, assist/control, SIMV, and pressure support in both volume and pressure controlled ventilation. Breaths may be either time, manual, pressure or flow triggered.

Power Input

Power for the microprocessor control system is provided by AC power, which may be either 120 volts, 60 Hz or 220 volts, 60 Hz AC power. The pneumatic system requires medical-grade air and oxygen between 35 and 100 psi. If medical-grade compressed air is not available, an optional compressor in the pedestal will provide an air source to power the pneumatic system.

Drive Mechanism

Air and oxygen enter the ventilator through DISS fittings on the rear of the ventilator and pass through their respective filters (Figure 8-32, pp. 469–472). Line pressure is re-

duced to 10 psi by means of the air- and oxygen-reducing valves. A crossover solenoid connects the air and oxygen supply so that in the event gas pressure is lost, the remaining gas pressure (air or oxygen) can continue to power the pneumatic system. From the regulators, gas enters the inspiratory module.

Control Circuit

The 840 ventilator uses a microprocessor and the inspiratory control module to regulate flow output from the ventilator (Figure 8-32). The inspiratory module consists of two parallel elements, one for air and the other for oxygen. The inspiratory module consists of two proportional solenoid valves (PSOL valves were discussed in Chapter 6), flow sensors and pressure sensors. The inspiratory modules regulate F$_I$O$_2$, inspiratory flow, pressure and volume delivery. Inspiratory flow and temperature transducers provide feedback to the microprocessor, which precisely regulates the PSOLs, delivering the exact volume, flow, pressure and F$_I$O$_2$ desired by the clinician. Gas flows from the inspiratory modules through a bacteria filter and check valve to the patient circuit.

PEEP/CPAP pressures are regulated by the active electrodynamic exhalation valve. When positive expiratory pressures are desired, the

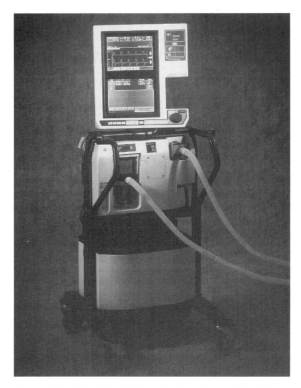

Figure 8-31A *The Nellcor Puritan Bennett 840 Ventilator*

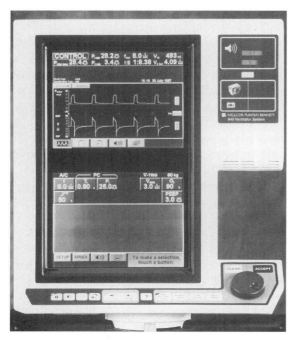

Figure 8-31B *The control panel of the 840*

exhalation valve partially closes, creating a threshold resistor, generating the positive pressure.

Control Variables

The control variables for the Nellcor Puritan Bennett 840 ventilator include flow and pressure. Flow is measured by the two inspiratory flow transducers (air and oxygen) in the inspiratory modules and is used as a feedback signal during volume-controlled breaths for the control, assist/control, and the mandatory portions of SIMV. In these modes, volume delivery is equal to the inspiratory flow multiplied by the inspiratory time.

Pressure is a control variable during PEEP/CPAP, pressure support and pressure-controlled ventilation. Pressure is monitored by the expiratory pressure transducer and used as a feedback signal through the microprocessor, whereby it controls the PSOLs outputs and thus maintains the desired pressure levels.

Phase Variables
Trigger Variables

The Nellcor Puritan Bennett 840 ventilator trigger variables include pressure, flow, time and manual triggering. Pressure triggering may be set between 0.1 and 20 cmH$_2$O below baseline pressure. During inspiration, when the patient inhales, pressure falls in the circuit. When the pressure drop in the circuit equals the sensitivity level, the inspiratory phase begins and gas is delivered to the patient.

Flow triggering may be established by selecting Flow-by™. Flow sensitivity is adjustable between 0.5 and 20 L/min. Base flow and bias flow are not adjustable, but are fixed at a value of 1.5 times the flow sensitivity. For example, if a flow sensitivity of 3 L/min is selected, base flow is automatically set at 4.5 L/min. Once a flow sensitivity is established, when the patient's inspiratory (spontaneous) flow equals the sensitivity value, the inspiratory phase begins and gas is delivered to the patient.

Time triggering occurs during control, assist/control and SIMV provided no spontaneous efforts occur. Breath delivery is based upon the ventilatory rate setting established by the clinician. The rate may be adjusted between 1 and 100 breaths per minute.

Manual trigger may be accomplished by depressing the manual inspiration soft key.

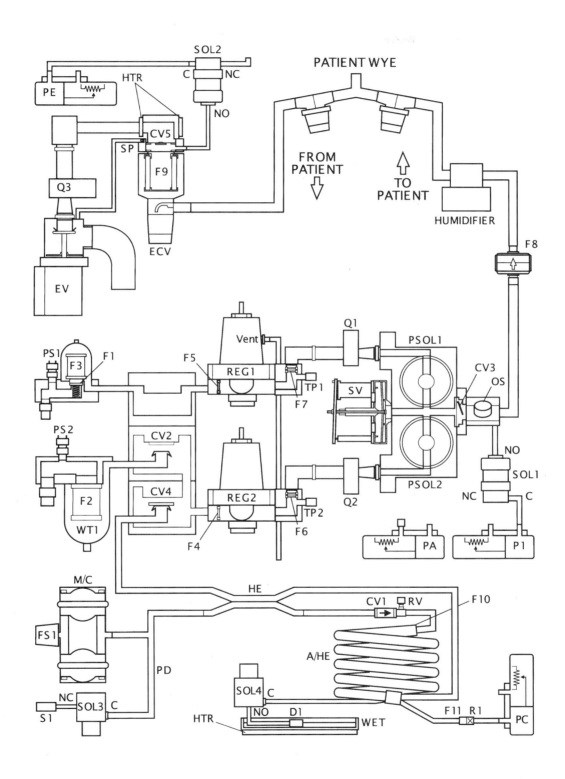

Figure 8-32A *The Nellcor Puritan Bennett, 840 Ventilator (continues)*

Reference designator	Component	Description
	Inspiratory module	
–	Fitting, inlet	Connects external oxygen and air sources to ventilator via hoses. Fittings include diameter index system standard (DISS) (male or female), noninterchangeable screw thread (NIST), Air Liquide, and Sleeved Index System (SIS).
–	Manifold, PSOL/SV	Houses proportional solenoid valves (PSOL1 and PSOL2) and safety valve (SV).
–	Port, inspiratory pressure relief	Bypasses inspiratory check valve to release pressure when an occlusion is present in exhalation circuit while safety valve is open.
CV2 CV4	Check valve, air/compressor	CV2 opens to admit external compressed air and CV4 closes to isolate compressor module. When CV4 opens to allow compressor-supplied compressed air, CV2 closes to prevent compressed air (compressor source) from venting through external air-conditioning components.
CV3	Check valve, inspiratory	Opens to supply inspiratory gas and prevents exhalation flow in reverse direction.
F1	Filter, oxygen impact	Traps particles larger than 65 to 110 μm (microns).
F3 F2	Filter, inlet, oxygen/air	Filters matter greater than 0.3 μm (micron). These filters are part of REG1 or REG2.
F5 F4	Filter, screen, oxygen/air impact	Filters large debris from REG1 and REG2.
F7 F6	Filter, pneumatic noise, oxygen/air	Increases frequency of turbulence to prevent flow sensor tracking. These filters are part of the flow sensor manifold (2 each gas).
OS	Sensor, oxygen (percentage)	Measures partial pressure of oxygen in inspired gas. Range is 21 to 100% O_2.
PA	Pressurer transducer, absolute	Measures atmospheric pressure (psia). Located on inspiration PCB.
PI	Pressure transducer, inspiratory	Measures pressure (psig) at outlet manifold. Located on inspiration PCB.
PS1 PS2	Pressure switch, oxygen/air	Opens when pressure is less than 17 psig (117.2 kPa) nominal. Closes when pressure is greater than 30 psig (206.9 kPa) nominal.
PSOL1 PSOL2	Proportional solenoid valve, oxygen/air	0 to 200 L/min BTPS output (intermittent) or 0 to 180 L/min BTPS output (steady state)
Q1 Q2	Sensor, flow, oxygen/air	Measures oxygen or air flow before PSOL.
REG1 REG2	Regulator, oxygen/air	Reduces input supply pressure (35 to 100 psi, flow up to 200 L/min BTPS) to output pressure (10.5 psi minimum to 11.5 psi maximum).
SOL1	Solenoid, autozero, inspiratory pressure transducer	+6 V, three-way solenoid. Energized (common to normally closed) when transducer is autozeroed. De-energized (common to normally open) all other times.
SV	Safety valve	+24 V actuator. Commanded open (de-energized) at 100 cmH$_2$O, during power on self test (POST), loss of both source gases, or due to ventilator inoperative condition. Energized (closed) all other times.
TP1 TP2	Pressure valve, oxygen/air	Allows measurement of REG1 and REG2 output
WT1	Water trap, air	Houses air inlet filter (F2) and includes a manual drain.
	Patient system	
–	Humidification device (optional)	Humidifies inspired gas.

Figure 8-32B *(continues)*

Reference designator	Component	Description
Patient system (continued)		
–	Wye	Connects inspiration and expiration tubing, forming a closed circuit.
F8	Filter, inspiratory (main flow)	Filters matter greater than 0.3 μm (micron) (nominal) at 100 L/min flow.
WT	Trap, water	Collects excessive water.
Exhalation module		
–	Port, sample, metabolic monitor	Provides a sample port for Nellcor Puritan Bennett 7250 Metabolic Monitor. Future option.
CV5	Check valve, exhalation	Opens during exhalation to let exhaled gas into exhalation system. Prevents rebreathing when safety valve is open.
ECV	Collection vial	Collects water (up to 250 mL) due to condensation in patient circuit.
EV	Exhalation valve	Electronically controlled, electrically operated valve that opens during exhalation, as required to maintain positive end expiratory pressure (PEEP)/continuous positive airway pressure (CPAP). Closed during inspiration.
F9	Filter, expiratory	Filters matter greater than 0.3 μm (micron) (nominal) at 100 L/min flow.
HTR	Heater, exhalation	16 W heater that maintains gas temperature above condensation level.
PE	Pressure transducer, expiratory	Measures pressure (psig) at a port on exhalation PCB.
Q3	Sensor, exhalation flow	Measures exhalation flow.
SOL2	Solenoid valve, autozero	+6 V, three-way solenoid valve. Energized (common to normally closed) when transducer is autozeroed. De-energized (common to normally open) all other times.
Compressor module		
A/HE	Accumulator/heat exchanger	Stores and cools compressed air generated by compressor.
CV1	Check valve, compressor accumulator	Prevents accumulator compressed air from venting back through compressor when SOL3 energizes or the compressor is turned off during stand-by operation. Opens to admit compressor output into accumulator to charge or recharge accumulator.
D1	Diffuser, SOL4	Prevents spraying of water when SOL4 is de-energized.
F10	Filter, compressor outlet	Filters matter greater than 0.3 μm (micron).
F11	Filter, compressor pressure transducer.	Protects this pressure transducer.
FS1	Filter, inlet silencer	Acts as silencer for compressor air intake. Provides filtering for compressor air intake.
HE	Heat exchanger	Transfers heat from the motor compressor output gas flow to the accumulator/heat exchanger output gas flow.
HTR	Heater, water evaporative tray	Speeds evaporation of water in WET.
MC	Motor compressor	Compresses gas up to 25 psi.
RV	Relief valve	Opens when accumulator pressure is greater than 30 psi. Protects system from overpressurization if unloading solenoid valve (SOL3) fails.
PC	Pressure transducer, compressor	Measures pressure of accumulator/heat exchanger. Located on compressor PCB.
PD	Pressure damper	Dampens pressure fluctuations from motor compressor.
R1	Restrictor, damper	Dampens pressure to PC.
S1	Silencer	Reduces the sound of venting gas from SOL3.

Figure 8-32B *(continues)*

Reference designator	Component	Description
Compressor module (continued)		
SOL4	Solenoid valve, drain, compressor	+12 V, three-way solenoid valve. When de-energized, drains accumulator condensate from accumulator/heat exchanger.
SOL3	Solenoid valve, unloading, compressor	+12 V, two-way solenoid valve. When energized, ensures compressor does not start against back pressure in the circuit. Also, when energized, vents excessive compressor output.
WET	Water evaporative tray	Holds water due to condensation from the accumulator/heat exchanger.

Figure 8-32B   *(continued)*

When depressed, a manual breath is delivered according to the mandatory settings. The breath may be volume controlled (set tidal volume, inspiratory flow and F_IO_2) or pressure controlled (set inspiratory pressure, inspiratory time and F_IO_2).

Limit Variables

The limit variables for the 840 ventilator include pressure, volume and flow. Pressure becomes a limit variable during the spontaneous breaths when in SIMV (with PEEP/CPAP added), CPAP, pressure control and pressure support modes. In these modes, the pneumatic system will maintain the desired pressure in the circuit as adjusted by the practitioner. PEEP/CPAP pressures may be adjusted between 0.0 and 45 cmH$_2$O. Pressure control levels are adjustable between 5 and 90 cmH$_2$O. Pressure control levels are adjustable between 5 and 90 cmH$_2$O. Pressure support may be adjusted between 0.0 and 70 cmH$_2$O.

Volume becomes a limit variable when an inspiratory hold has been selected by the practitioner. Inspiratory hold is adjustable between 0.0 and 2.0 seconds. When selected, the ventilator will deliver a breath, which will be held following breath delivery until the set time interval has lapsed.

Flow is a limit variable when the ventilator delivers mandatory flow-controlled breaths.

Flow is adjustable between 3 and 150 L/min. If the peak flow delivered is less than that set by the inspiratory flow rate, flow becomes the limit variable.

Cycle Variables

Cycle variables for the 840 ventilator include pressure, flow and time. Pressure becomes a cycle variable when inspiratory pressure exceeds the value set by the high circuit pressure alarm. High pressure limits are adjustable between 7 and 100 cmH$_2$O. When the pressure limit is reached, inspiration is terminated and the expiratory phase begins.

Flow is a cycle variable during spontaneous breaths (with or without pressure support). When inspiratory flow decays to the following value:

$$\text{End-Inspiratory Flow} = \frac{\text{Peak Flow (Expiratory Sensitivity)}}{100}$$

inspiration ends and the expiratory phase begins. Expiratory sensitivity is adjustable between 1 and 45%.

Time becomes a cycle variable during mandatory breath delivery. The microprocessor determines volume as a function of flow and inspiratory time. Once the appropriate inspiratory time has been reached, breath delivery ceases. During pressure-controlled ventilation, inspiratory time becomes a cycle variable and is adjustable between 0.2 and 8.0 seconds.

Baseline Variables

The baseline variable for the Nellcor Puritan Bennett 840 ventilator is pressure. PEEP/CPAP pressures are adjustable between 0 and 45 cmH$_2$O. The ventilator creates baseline pressure by partially closing the electrodynamic exhalation valve during the expiratory phase.

Conditional Variables
Time and Pressure or Time and Flow

Time and pressure or time and flow become conditional variables during the SIMV mode. The rate control determines the frequency of mandatory breath delivery during the SIMV mode. The rate control is an electronic timer, allowing a time window for the patient to trigger a breath or delivering a breath at specified time intervals if no efforts are detected. Between mandatory breath delivery, the patient breathes through the ventilator's pneumatic system. The ventilator measures pressure or flow to determine if the patient is attempting to initiate a breath. In response to the trigger variable's change, the patient is able to draw gas spontaneously through the pneumatic system to meet his or her inspiratory needs.

Output Waveforms
Pressure

The pressure output waveform of the 840 ventilator is rectangular when the ventilator is operating in the pressure support and pressure control modes. In these modes, pressure rises sharply to the present value and is then maintained at that value until the inspiratory phase ends.

Flow

The flow output may be adjusted between rectangular and descending ramp waveforms. The PSOLs, in combination with the microprocessor and feedback control system, enable the ventilator to accurately reproduce these output waveforms.

Alarms
Input Power

Input power alarms include AC power loss, low battery, no air supply and no oxygen supply alrms. The AC power loss alarm is activated when AC power is interrupted or not available. During this time, the ventilator is powered by the backup power source (BPS), which is an internal DC battery. When this occurs, the clinician should check the AC power source, and prepare for alternate ventilation.

The low battery alarm is activated when the BPS has less than 2 minutes of operational time remaining. If AC power is lost and the ventilator is operating on BPS, an alternative means of ventilation should be established.

Air and oxygen alarms are activated if air or oxygen pressure falls to less than 35 psi. Should this occur, an alternate gas source should be established. A compressor inoperative alarm will also alert the user to compressor failure in the event the optional air compressor fails to supply sufficient pressure to power the ventilator.

Control Circuit

Control circuit alarms include device alert and procedure error. The device alert alarm is activated when the ventilator's microprocessor detects an error during a background or POST test. When this condition occurs, an alternate means of ventilation for the patient should be provided.

The procedure error alarm will occur if the patient is connected to the ventilator circuit prior to completion of the startup procedure. You should wait until the POST test is complete before attaching the patient to the circuit.

Output Alarms
Pressure

The 840 ventilator includes high circuit and internal pressure alarms. If the circuit pressure is equal to or greater than the set limit, the high circuit pressure alarm will be activated. When this alarm is activated, the inspiratory phase is terminated and exhalation begins. The high circuit pressure is adjustable between 7 and 100 cmH$_2$O.

When operating the ventilator in volume controlled ventilation, the high internal pressure alarm will be activated if pressure exceeds 100 cmH$_2$o. When this occurs, inspiration is terminated and exhalation begins.

Volume

In the event that the patient's exhaled tidal volumes exceed the upper or lower limits, an alarm will alert the practitioner to the event. The high exhaled tidal volume alarm may be set between 50 and 3000 mL or not used at all (off). A low exhaled tidal volume may be set for both mandatory and spontaneous breaths. These alarms are adjustable between 5 and 2,500 mL.

Flow

The 840 ventilator incorporates high and low minute volume alarms. The low minute volume alarm may be set between 0.05 and 60.0 L/min, while the high minute volume alarm may be set between 0.1 and 99.9 L/min. When the patient exceeds the value set on the alarm, the ventilator will alert the practitioner.

Time

A high respiratory rate alarm is provided to alert the practitioner when the patient has a high ventilatory rate. This alarm is adjustable between 10 and 110 breaths per minute. When the patient exceeds the value set, the alarm condition will result.

Emergency Modes of Ventilation
Apnea Ventilation

If the 840 ventilator fails to detect inspiratory flow during the time interval set by the practitioner, apnea ventilation will be invoked by the ventilator and an apnea alarm will result. Apnea intervals may be selected between 10 and 60 seconds. The clinician may select breath type (pressure or volume controlled), flow pattern and rate, inspiratory pressure, respiratory rate, tidal volume, oxygen percentage, and I:E ratio within the same limits as for nonapnea ventilator settings. If the patient triggers two consecutive breaths and the exhaled volume is at least 50% of the delivered volume, the ventilator will reset itself into the nonapnea ventilation mode.

Safety Ventilation

In the event the practitioner connects the patient prior to completion of the startup procedure, the procedure error alarm will be activated and safety ventilation will be invoked. Safety ventilation is not clinician adjustable and will result in pressure-controlled ventilation using the settings in Table 8-23.

Safety Valve Open

In the event the ventilator detects system faults (which will not prevent it from providing reliable ventilatory support), the ventilator will alarm and enter the safety valve open (SVO) emergency state. During SVO, the safety, exhalation and inspiratory valves are opened, allowing the patient to breath spontaneously from room air. Check valves on both the inspiratory and expiratory circuits minimize the rebreathing of exhaled gas by the patient. The ventilator will display the elapsed time of SVO; it will not display patient data (including waveforms) or detect circuit occlusion or patient disconnect conditions.

Table 8-24 summarizes the Nellcor Puritan Bennett 840 ventilator alarms, and Table 8-25 summarizes its capabilities.

TABLE 8-23: Safety Ventilation Settings

Mode	Pressure controlled, A/C
Inspiratory pressure	10 cmH₂O
Inspiratory time	1.0 seconds
Respiratory rate	16/minute
PEEP	3.0 cmH₂O
Pressure triggered	−2 cmH₂O
Flow acceleration	50%
Oxygen percentage	100%

TABLE 8-24: Nellcor Puritan Bennett 840 Ventilator Alarms

ALARM	CONDITION/SETTINGS
Input Power	
Oxygen	<35 psi
Air	<35 psi
AC Power	Loss of AC power
Low Battery	Less than 2 minutes of operation time remaining
Control Circuit	
Device Alert	A failure of a background or POST test has been detected
Procedure Error	The patient was connected before completion of startup
Output Alarms	
High Insp Pressure	5–90 cmH₂O
High Circuit Pressure	7–100 cmH₂O
High Internal Pressure	100 cmH₂O
High exhaled tidal volume	50–3,000 mL
Low exhaled spont. tidal vol	5–2,500 mL
Low exhaled mandatory vol	5–2,500 mL
High minute volume	0.1–99.9 L/min
Low minute volume	0.05–60.0 L/min
High frequency	10–110 BPM

TABLE 8-25: Nellcor Puritan Bennett 840 Ventilator Capabilities

Modes	CMV (volume or pressure controlled), SIMV, CPAP, pressure support, spontaneous
Volume	25–2,500 ml
Pressure	5–90 cmH$_2$O
Pressure support	0.0–70 cmH$_2$O
Rate	1.0–100 BPM
Peak flow	3–150 L/min
Flow sensitivity	0.5–20 L/min
Pressure sensitivity	0.1–20 cmH$_2$O below base line
Inspiratory time	0.2–8.0 seconds
PEEP/CPAP	0.0–45 cmH$_2$O
Insp. pause	0.0–2.0 seconds
F$_1$O$_2$	0.21–1.0

SIEMENS-ELEMA SERVO 900C

The Siemens-Elema Servo 900C ventilator is a pneumatically powered, electronically controlled single circuit ventilator (Figure 8-33, 8-34). It can function in volume control, volume control + sigh, SIMV, SIMV + Pressure Support, CPAP, pressure control and pressure support modes. It can operate as a pressure or flow controller.

Drive Mechanism

The Servo 900C requires 120 volts, 60 Hz electrical power to run the microprocessor control system. The electrical cord and power switch are both located on the rear of the ventilator.

The Servo 900C does not have an oxygen blender built into its design. Air and oxygen must be mixed externally before entering the ventilator. Currently the manufacturer recommends either the model 960 or 965 blender.

Gas enters the ventilator via a quick-connect fitting. The gas passes through a non-return valve (one-way valve) to an oxygen-sensing cell (Figure 8-35). The oxygen-sensing cell is a polarographic cell forming part of the oxygen-analyzing system. From the sensing cell, the gas passes through a bacteria filter and into the spring-loaded bellows.

The drive mechanism is the pneumatic gas source (50 psi air and oxygen) and the spring-loaded bellows. Spring tension on the bellows may be adjusted between 10 and 120 cmH$_2$O. The gas supply and the spring tension maintain a uniform pressure within the bellows (working pressure). The working pressure is

---

ASSEMBLY AND TROUBLESHOOTING

Assembly—Nellcor Puritan Bennet 840 Ventilator

To assemble the 840 ventilator for use, complete the following suggested assembly guide.

1. Connect the ventilator to an appropriate AC power source (120 volts, 60 Hz, or 200 volts, 60 Hz).

2. Connect the ventilator to 50 psi air and oxygen supplies. If compressed air is not available, the optional air compressor may be used.

3. Lift the exhalation filter latch into the up position, and install the exhalation filter into position. Once positioned, push the latch down.

4. Connect the ventilator outlet to an inspiratory bacteria filter and then connect the outlet of the filter to a heated humidifier using a short length of 22-mm diameter tubing.

5. Connect the inspiratory limb of the circuit to the outlet of the humidifier and the expiratory limb to the exhalation filter assembly.

6. Complete an extended self-test (EST prior to use.

Troubleshooting

Refer to the troubleshooting algorithms found at the end of this chapter.

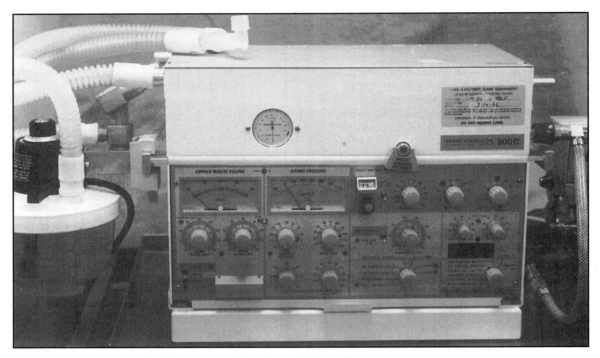

Figure 8-33 *A photograph of the Siemens Elema Servo 900C ventilator.*

displayed on a manometer directly above and between the expired minute volume and airway pressure displays.

Control Circuit

Gas from the bellows flows through a safety valve. The safety valve vents gas from the bellows to the ambient air if pressure exceeds 120 cmH$_2$O or if the bellows overfills.

Gas then flows to a flow transducer and on to the inspiratory proportional scissor valve. The flow transducer consists of a flag in the inspired gas flow that bends or distorts a strain gauge. The strain sensed by the strain gauge

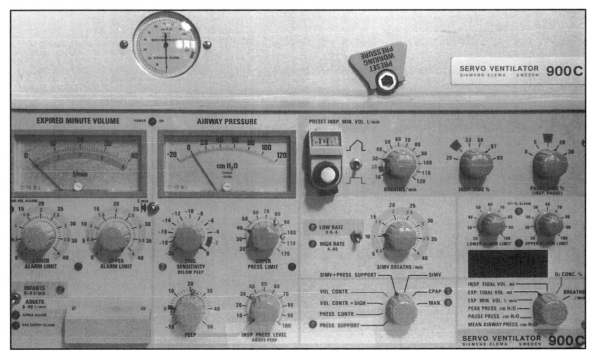

Figure 8-34 *A photograph of the Siemens Medical Systems, Inc., Servo 900C control panel.*

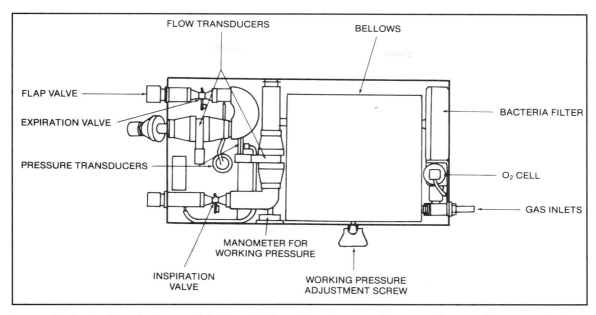

Figure 8-35 *A schematic diagram of the Servo 900C ventilator's pneumatic system. (Courtesy Siemens Medical Systems, Danvers, MA)*

becomes proportional to flow, as described earlier in this section.

The inspiratory proportional valve opens and closes in response to control signals from the electronic control system. The feedback control system consists of the inspiratory flow transducer and a pressure transducer exposed to the inspiratory flow (Figure 8-35). A stepper motor moves in discrete steps or positions in response to signals from the control circuit, opening or closing the valve to match the flow or pressure to the control settings established by the practitioner.

Gas flows from the patient circuit, through an expiratory flow transducer, to an expiratory pressure transducer, and on to the expiratory valve.

The Servo 900C does not have an exhalation valve incorporated into the patient circuit. The expiratory valve is a servo-controlled electromagnetic valve. The control circuit varies the amount of electrical current applied to the valve and therefore controls its opening and closing. (A complete description of the expiratory valve was included in Chapter 6.)

From the expiratory valve, the exhaled gas flows through a one-way flapper valve into the ambient air. The flapper valve is required to prevent backflow into the circuit so that the trigger sensitivity can operate correctly.

PEEP/CPAP pressure is regulated by the expiratory valve. The expiratory valve will remain partially closed during exhalation, main-

taining the desired pressure in the circuit as it acts as a threshold resistor. PEEP/CPAP pressures are adjustable between 0.0 and 50 cmH$_2$O.

Control Variables

As described earlier, the control variable used by the Servo 900C ventilator is flow or pressure. Flow becomes the control variable during mandatory volume delivery, during volume control, volume control + sigh, and the mandatory portion of SIMV ventilation. During these modes of operation, flow is measured and used as a feedback signal to regulate volume delivery (flow multiplied by inspiratory time).

During pressure control and pressure support, pressure becomes the control variable. Pressure is measured and used as a feedback signal to maintain the desired pressure in the patient circuit.

Phase Variables
Trigger Variables

Trigger variables for the Servo 900C include pressure and time triggering. Pressure may be a trigger variable in all modes of ventilation. The trigger threshold is adjusted using the trigger sensitivity control. The sensitivity may be adjusted between 0.0 and 20 cmH$_2$O below baseline pressure.

Time becomes a trigger variable during volume control, the mandatory portions of

SIMV, and pressure control if no inspiratory effort (pressure drop) is sensed by the ventilator. The time interval for triggering is established by the breath rate control. Rates are adjustable between 5 and 120 breaths per minute (volume control and pressure control modes) and .4 to 4 or 4 to 40 breaths per minute in SIMV mode. If the patient does not trigger a breath, the ventilator will deliver a mandatory breath at the established inspiratory time percent and minute volume settings.

Limit Variables

The limit variables of the Servo 900C include pressure, volume and flow. Pressure becomes a limit variable during SIMV (with PEEP applied), CPAP, pressure support, and pressure control ventilation. Under these conditions, the ventilator will augment flow to maintain the desired pressure level. PEEP/CPAP pressures are adjustable between 0.0 and 50.0 cmH₂O. Pressure levels for pressure support and pressure control are adjustable between 0.0 and 100.0 cmH₂O.

Volume becomes a limit variable when the inspiratory pause time percent control is active. Inspiratory pause time percent control may be adjusted between 0 and 30% of the cycle time in increments of 5% (0 to 10% pause time) and 10% (10 to 30% pause time). When activated, a volume breath is delivered and held, until the set inspiratory pause time period has elapsed. This is only available during volume control, pressure control and the mandatory portions of SIMV.

Flow becomes a limit when the rectangular output waveform has been selected. When a rectangular waveform output is delivered, flow during inspiration is limited by the settings established on the minute volume and inspiratory time percent controls.

The inspiratory flow rate is not adjustable on the Servo 900C. Inspiratory flow becomes a function of minute volume and the inspiratory time percent. The ventilator adjusts flow to maintain the desired inspiratory time percent. The inspiratory flow rate may be calculated by multiplying the minute volume by a factor based on the inspiratory time percent. The factors are shown in Table 8-26.

Assume the minute volume is 10 liters per minute and the inspiratory time percent is 25%. The peak inspiratory flow will be 40 liters per minute (4 x 10 L/min).

Alternatively, minute volume may be divided by the inspiratory time percent to calculate the average flow rate. For example, if the minute volume is 12 liters per minute and the inspiratory time percent is 25%, the average flow will be 48 liters per minute.

TABLE 8-26: Flow Rate Calculation Factors

INSPIRATORY TIME (PERCENT)	FACTOR
20%	5
25%	4
33%	3
50%	2
67%	1.5
80%	1.25

Cycle Variables

Cycle variables for the Servo 900C ventilator include pressure, flow, and time. Pressure becomes a cycle variable if the inspiratory pressure reaches the setting on the upper pressure limit control. Peak inspiratory pressure may be adjusted between 16 and 120 cmH₂O. When the pressure limit is reached, inspiration is terminated, and both audible and visual alarms are activated.

Volume becomes a cycle variable during sigh breath delivery. When selected, a sigh breath will be given every 100th breath. The sigh volume delivered will be 200% of the tidal volume (minute volume divided by the breath rate). Sigh breath delivery can not be used during pressure control ventilation.

Flow becomes a cycle variable during pressure support ventilation. Inspiration is terminated when inspiratory flow falls to approximately 25% of the peak inspiratory flow. When inspiratory flow drops to this value, inspiratory pressure support is terminated.

Time becomes a cycle variable during pressure control ventilation. In this mode, a constant pressure is applied until the time set on the inspiratory time percent control has been reached.

Baseline Variable

PEEP/CPAP pressures may be adjusted between 0.0 and 50 cmH₂O. The Servo 900 ventilator creates PEEP/CPAP pressure by partially closing the exhalation valve.

ASSEMBLY AND TROUBLESHOOTING

Assembly—Servo 900C

To assemble the Siemens-Elema Servo 900C for use, complete this suggested assembly guide.

1. Assemble the humidifier and attach it to the side of the ventilator. Fill it with water and connect the inlet of the humidifier to the ventilator outlet. Since many humidifiers may be adapted to this ventilator, assembly instructions will not be included here.

2. Assemble the patient circuit and attach the inspiratory limb to the humidifier outlet and the expiratory limb to the expiration inlet channel.

3. Connect the ventilator to an oxygen blender and the blender supply lines to 50 psi air and oxygen sources.

4. Connect the power cord to a 120 volt, 60 Hz outlet.

5. Adjust the working pressure control to 60 cmH$_2$O.

6. Perform a leak test using the inspiratory pause hold control.

Troubleshooting

The comprehensive monitors and alarms simplify ventilator troubleshooting. Careful assembly and pressure testing will readily identify leaks in the patient circuit.

Other leaks may occur internally. Sources include the valve assemblies (incorrect installation) or the bellows itself. If performance seem sluggish or erratic, check the silicone rubber pinch valves to ensure they were not twisted upon assembly. Also check the exhalation flow transducer screen for obstruction by contamination or condensation from the expiratory limb of the patient circuit.

Refer to the troubleshooting algorithms found at the end of this chapter for further troubleshooting assistance.

Conditional Variables
Time

Time becomes a conditional variable during sigh delivery. During normal ventilator supported breaths, they are pressure controlled, pressure triggered, pressure or time cycled. During sigh delivery, a sigh breath will be given every 100th breath.

Time and Pressure

Time and pressure become conditional variables during SIMV mode. The rate control determines the frequency of mandatory breath delivery during SIMV mode. The rate control is essentially an electronic timer, delivering a breath at specified time intervals. Between mandatory breath delivery, the patient breathes through the flow control valve subsystem. The ventilator measures proximal airway pressure to determine if the patient is attempting to initiate a breath. In response to the pressure change, the patient is able to draw gas spontaneously through the flow control valve to meet inspiratory needs.

Output Waveforms
Pressure

Pressure waveform output is rectangular during pressure control and pressure support. During pressure control and pressure support, pressure rises rapidly to the inspiratory pressure level and is maintained there until the inspiratory time percent value has been reached.

Flow

The flow output may be selected between rectangular and sinusoidal waveforms. The waveform is selected using the waveform toggle switch.

Alarms
Input Power

Input power alarms include gas supply and power failure. The gas supply alarm activated in the event that gas supply is lost or disconnected. This alarm is inactivated if the respiratory rate is greater than 80 BPM and the inspiratory time percent is 20 or 25. The alarm is both visual and audible.

A power failure alarm will sound if the external 120 volt, 60 Hz source fails, and the green power light will go off. The alarm is battery powered and will function for 5 to 10 minutes.

Output Alarms
Pressure

The Servo 900C has an upper pressure limit alarm. The upper pressure limit alarm is adjustable between 16.0 and 120 cmH$_2$O. When the pressure limit is reached, inspiration is terminated and both audible and visual alarms are activated.

Flow

The Servo 900C incorporates both high and low minute ventilation alarms, which rely on the expiratory flow transducer signal to the control system. Lower limits range from 0.0 to 4.0 liters per minute (infants), while the upper limits ranges from 0 to 40 liters per minute (adults).

Time

If no inspiratory pressure drop has been sensed for 15 seconds, this alarm will be activated. The alarm alerts the practitioner to the patient's absence of inspiratory efforts.

Inspired Gas

The Servo 900C has a built-in oxygen analyzer. Alarm limits may be set above and

below the desired F$_I$O$_2$. If those parameters are exceeded, the alarm will be activated.

Table 8-27 summarizes the Servo 900C alarms, and Table 8-28 summarizes its capabilities.

TABLE 8-27: Servo 900C Ventilator Alarm Systems

ALARM	CONDITION/SETTINGS
Input Power	
Gas Supply	Loss of gas supply pressure
Electric Power	Loss of 120 volt, 60 Hz power
Output Alarms	
High Pressure Limit	16.0–120 cmH$_2$O
Low Exhaled Minute Vol.	0.0–4.0 L/min
Low Minute Volume	0.0–40 L/min
Apnea	No pressure trigger or mandatory breath for 15 seconds
Inspired Gas	
Oxygen Percentage	20–100 % oxygen

TABLE 8-28: Servo 900C Ventilator Capabilities

Modes	Volume Control, Volume Control + Sigh, SIMV, SIMV + Pressure Support, Pressure Control, Pressure Support, CPAP
Minute Volume	0.5–40 L/min
Pressure	0.0–120 cmH$_2$O
Press. Support	0.0–100 cmH$_2$O
Press. Control	0.0–100 cmH$_2$O
Rate	5–120 BPM
Insp. Time %	20, 25, 33, 50, 67, or 80%
PEEP/CPAP	0.0–50 cmH$_2$O
Sigh Volume	200% of tidal volume
Sigh Rate	Every 100th breath
Insp. Pause	0, 5, 10, 20 or 30%
Sensitivity	0.0 to 20 cmH$_2$O below baseline pressure
F$_I$O$_2$	0.21 to 1.0

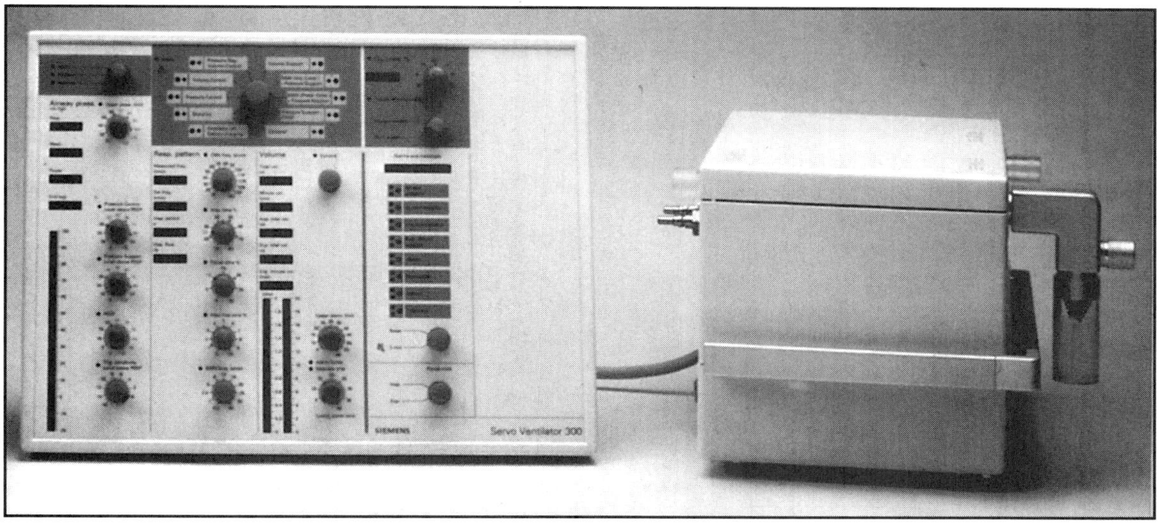

Figure 8-36 *A photograph of the Siemens Medical Systems, Inc., Servo 300 ventilator. (Courtesy Siemens Medical Systems, Electromedical Group, Danvers, MA)*

SIEMENS-ELEMA SERVO 300

The Siemens-Elema Servo 300 ventilator is a pneumatically powered, electronically controlled single circuit ventilator (Figures 8-36 and 8-37). It can function in pressure control, volume control, pressure regulated volume control, volume support, SIMV (pressure control or volume control) + pressure support, and CPAP + pressure support. The ventilator can operate as a pressure or flow controller.

Drive Mechanism

Power to run the microprocessor control circuitry is provided by 120 volt, 60 Hz electrical power. The pneumatic system is powered by 50 psi source of medical air and oxygen.

The pneumatic drive mechanism (Figure 8-38) consists of two servo control valves, one for air and the other for oxygen. Oxygen and air may enter the servo valves between 29 and 94 psi (2–6.5 bar). However, the valves are designed to operate the most efficiently

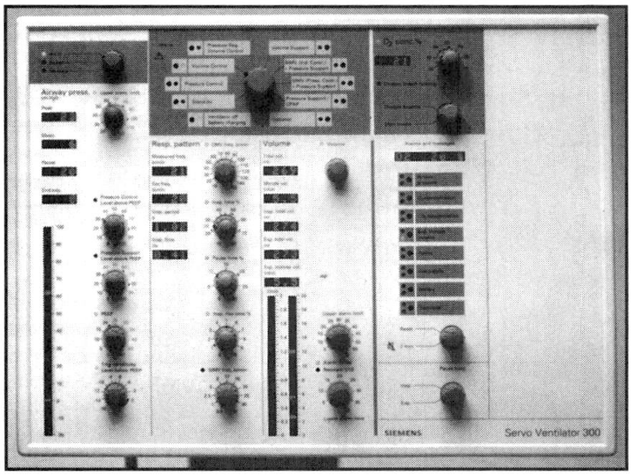

Figure 8-37 *A photograph of the Siemens Medical Systems, Inc., Servo 300 control panel. (Courtesy Siemens Medical Systems, Electromedical Group, Danvers, MA)*

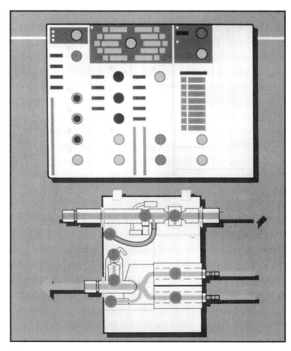

Figure 8-38 *A schematic diagram showing the Servo 300 ventilator's pneumatic system. (Courtesy Siemens Medical Systems, Electromedical Group, Danvers, MA)*

and accurately at the standard line pressures of 50 psi.

Control Circuit

The Servo 300 utilizes six microprocessors, two servo control valves, two differential pressure transducers and a flow transducer to regulate the output from the ventilator. These components are all contained within the gas control modules (one each for air and oxygen). The ventilator determines flow output from the servo valves based upon valve position (how far it has opened), control settings, and signals from the two differential pressure transducers. Valve position is determined by an optical sensor contained within each gas control module. The two servo valves regulate flow, pressure, volume (flow multiplied by time), and F_IO_2.

Control Variables

The control variable for the Servo 300 is both flow and pressure. Inspiratory flow is measured by the flow transducer and differential pressure transducers contained within the gas control modules. Flow is used as a control variable during control, and the mandatory portions of SIMV. In these modes volume becomes a derivative of flow (flow multiplied by inspiratory time).

Pressure is used as the control variable during PEEP/CPAP, pressure support, and pressure control delivery and pressure regulated volume control and volume support. Pressure is monitored by two pressure transducers, one on the inspiratory side and one on the expiratory side. Flow output from the gas control modules is adjusted by the feedback control system to maintain the desired pressure levels.

Phase Variables
Trigger Variables

The trigger variables of the Servo 300 include pressure, flow, time and manual. Pressure becomes a trigger variable when the patient inhales, reducing pressure in the circuit below the reference level set on the trigger sensitivity control. Trigger sensitivity may be adjusted between 0.0 and 17 cmH_2O below baseline pressure. Pressure operates as a trigger variable in all modes.

Flow becomes a trigger variable when the trigger sensitivity control has been adjusted into the area marked in "green" or "red." Flow

triggering may be set for the following types of patients; adult (0.7 to 2.0 L/min), pediatric (0.3 to 1.0 L/min), and infant (0.17 to 0.5 L/min). Once the established flow threshold (flow sensitivity) has been sensed by the microprocessor, the flow control valves open delivering flow to the patient circuit. Flow triggering may be used in all breath types and all modes.

Time is a trigger variable during volume control, pressure regulated volume control, pressure control, and SIMV when no spontaneous breaths occur. Breath delivery is based upon the respiratory rate setting (time).

The ventilator may also be manually triggered by rotating the start breath control. When rotated into this position, the ventilator initiates a controlled breath at the tidal volume, inspiratory time percent, pause time, rise time percent and F_IO_2 set on the control panel.

Limit Variables

The limit variables include pressure, volume and flow. Pressure becomes the limit variable during the spontaneous breaths when in SIMV (with PEEP/CPAP added), CPAP, pressure control, and pressure support modes. The pneumatic system will maintain the desired pressure control, and pressure support modes. The pneumatic system will maintain the desired pressure in the patient circuit as adjusted by the practitioner. PEEP/CPAP is adjustable between 0.0 and 50 cmH_2O, pressure support may be adjusted between 0.0 and 100 cmH_2O above PEEP, and pressure control may be set between 0.0 and 100 cmH_2O above PEEP.

Volume becomes a limit variable when inspiratory pause time percent has been selected by the practitioner. When selected, inspiratory pause time percent may be adjusted between 0 and 30% of the ventilatory cycle. The ventilator will deliver a breath and it will be held following breath delivery until the set time interval has elapsed.

Flow is the limit variable during volume controlled ventilation. The flow delivery is limited to the values set on the tidal volume and inspiratory time percent controls. Inspiratory flow is equal to the minute volume divided by the inspiratory time fraction. This is only true in the volume control, volume control + SIMV and pressure support modes.

Cycle Variables

The cycle variables include pressure, flow and time. Pressure becomes the cycle variable when inspiratory pressure reaches the pressure set on the upper pressure limit control. The upper pressure limit is adjustable between 16 and 120 cmH$_2$O. When the pressure limit is reached, inspiratory flow is stopped and both audible and visual alarms are activated and the patient is allowed to exhale.

Flow becomes the cycle variable during pressure support. When inspiratory flow decays to 5% of the peak inspiratory flow or 80% of the patient breath cycle time has been reached, breath delivery stops.

Time becomes the cycle variable during mandatory breath delivery. The microprocessor determines volume as a function of flow and inspiratory time percent. Once the appropriate inspiratory time has been reached, breath delivery ceases.

Baseline Variable

PEEP/CPAP pressures may be adjusted between 0.0 and 50 cmH$_2$O. The Servo 300 ventilator creates PEEP/CPAP pressure by partially closing the exhalation valve.

Output Waveforms
Pressure

The pressure output of the Servo 300 ventilator may be rectangular, exponential or adjustable. The rectangular waveform output occurs when the ventilator is operated with the inspiratory rise time percent control set at the zero position. In this setting, pressure rises sharply to the level set on the pressure support/insp pressure control. Pressure is maintained until the criteria for breath termination has been met.

Pressure output becomes exponential when the flow output is rectangular. When the flow output is rectangular, pressure output becomes exponential.

Pressure output becomes adjustable when the ventilator is operated in pressure regulated volume control. The basic waveform morphology, however, remains rectangular with the rise time set at zero. The pressure output is variable, depending upon the patient's compliance and resistance. Each delivered breath is compared to the previous breath, and pressure is adjusted between 0 and 3 cmH$_2$O, until the tidal volume delivery corresponds to the settings on the control panel when it becomes constant. If excess volume is delivered, pressure decreases in incremental values until the desired volume delivery has been met.

Volume

Volume output is an ascending ramp when the ventilator is operated with the inspiratory rise time percent control set at zero. Under these conditions, the volume gradually increases in a linear fashion as pressure increases.

Flow

The flow output of the Servo 300 is rectangular. The flow waveform may be modified by use of the inspiratory rise time percent control. This control determines how quickly the flow rises to its limit value. The rise time percent is adjustable between 0 and 10% of the ventilatory cycle.

Alarms
Input Power Alarms

The input power alarms include loss of electrical and loss of pneumatic power. In the event of a loss of electrical power, an audible and visual alarm will be activated. The ventilator will automatically switch to internal battery operation. If sufficient capacity is left in the battery, the alarm can be silenced and a visual caution indicator will be illuminated.

If the oxygen or air lines become disconnected, or if either gas control module becomes disconnected, an audible and visual alarm will be activated.

Control Circuit Alarms

The control circuit alarms are included in the technical alarms section of the control panel. Some of these alarms may be corrected by the practitioner, while others require the attention of a qualified biomedical service technician. The alarm conditions that can be checked by the practitioner include: circuit leakage; check tubings (internal pressure transducer tubing on the inspiratory and expiratory sides); and over range (control settings out of range for the maximum flow or volume capability for the patient range).

Output Alarms
Pressure

The pressure output alarm is the upper pressure limit control. The upper pressure limit is adjustable between 16 and 120 cmH$_2$O. There is also a high continuous pressure alarm which will be activated if the airway pressure

ASSEMBLY AND TROUBLESHOOTING

Assembly—Servo 300

To assemble the Siemens Medical Systems Servo 300 for use, complete this suggested assembly guide.

1. Assemble the humidifier and attach it to the side of the ventilator using the supplied rail system. Fill it with water and connect the inlet of the humidifier to the ventilator outlet. Since many humidifiers may be adapted to this ventilator, assembly instructions will not be included here.

2. Assemble the patient circuit and attach the inspiratory limb to the humidifier outlet and the expiratory limb to the expiration channel.

3. Connect the ventilator supply lines to 50 psi air and oxygen sources.

4. Connect the power cord to a 120 volt, 60 Hz outlet.

5. Perform a leak test using the inspiratory pause hold control.

Troubleshooting

The comprehensive monitors and alarms simplify ventilator troubleshooting. Careful assembly and pressure testing will readily identify leaks in the patient circuit.

Refer to the troubleshooting algorithms found at the end of this chapter for further troubleshooting assistance.

---

exceeds the PEEP/CPAP level by 15 cmH$_2$O for greater than 15 seconds.

Flow

The Servo 300 incorporates both high and low minute ventilation alarms which rely on the expiratory flow transducer signal to the microprocessor. Lower limits range from 0.06 to 60 L/min (adult) or 0.0 to 0.6 L/min (neonatal), while the upper limits range from 0.3 to 40 L/min (adult) or 0.06 to 4 L/min (neonatal).

Time

An apnea alarm may be set between 10 and 20 seconds. If a breath has not been detected within this time window, both audible and visual alarms will be activated.

Inspired Gas

The Servo 300 has a built-in oxygen analyzer. Alarm limits are set at 6% above and below the desired F$_I$O$_2$. If those parameters are exceeded, the alarm will be activated.

Table 8-29 summarizes the Servo 300 alarms, and Table 8-30 summarizes its capabilities.

TABLE 8-29: Servo 300 Ventilator Alarm Systems

ALARM	CONDITION/SETTINGS
Input Power	
Gas Supply	Loss of air or oxygen supply or disconnection of gas control modules
Electric Power	Loss of 120 volt, 60 Hz power or insufficient internal battery power
Output Alarms	
High Pressure Limit	16.0–120 cmH$_2$O
Low Exhaled Minute Vol.	0.06–40 L/min
High Minute Volume	0.0–60 L/min
Apnea	No pressure trigger for 10–20 seconds
Inspired Gas	
Oxygen Percentage	20–100% oxygen

TABLE 8-30:	Servo 300 Ventilator Capabilities
Modes	Volume Control, Pressure Control, Pressure Regulated Volume Control, Volume Support, SIMV (Volume Control) + Pressure Support, SIMV (Pressure Control) + Pressure Support, Pressure Support/CPAP
Volume	0.0–4,000 mL
PEEP/CPAP	0.0–50 cmH$_2$O
Press. Support	0.0–100 cmH$_2$O above PEEP
Press. Control	0.0–100 cmH$_2$O above PEEP
Rate (control)	5–150 BPM
Rate (SIMV)	0.5 to 40 BPM
Insp. Time %	10 to 80%
Pause Time %	0.0 to 30%
PEEP/CPAP	0.0–50 cmH$_2$O
Sensitivity	0.0–17 cmH$_2$O below baseline pressure
Flow Triggering	0.7–2.0 L/min (adult); 0.3–1.0 L/min (pediatric); 0.17–0.5 L/min (neonatal)
F$_I$O$_2$	0.21–1.0

Chapter Summary

Several ventilators have been presented in this chapter which are classified as flow and pressure controllers. These ventilators all have a common characteristic in that flow or pressure is measured and used as a feedback control signal to regulate the ventilator's output. Table 8-31 may help you to learn the similarities and differences between the ventilators presented in this chapter.

To assist you in troubleshooting refer to the algorithms found in ALG 8-1, 8-2, and 8-3.

TABLE 8-31: Flow and Pressure Controllers Classified

VENTILATOR	INPUT POWER	CIRCUIT	DRIVE MECHANISM	CONTROL VARIABLE	TRIGGER VARIABLE	LIMIT VARIABLE	CYCLING VARIABLE	ALARMS
BEAR I/II	Electric	Single	Pneumatic	F/P	P/T/M	P/V/F	P/T	I/CC/P/V/T
BEAR III	Electric	Single	Pneumatic	F/P	P/T/M	P/V/F	P/F/T	I/CC/P/V/T
BEAR 1000	Electric	Single	Pneumatic	F/P	P/T/M	P/V/F	P/V/F/T	I/CC/P/F/T
Bird 8400ST®i	Electric	Single	Pneumatic	F/P	P/F/T/M	P/V/F	P/F/T	I/CC/P/F/T
Bird TBird® AVS	Electric	Single	Pneumatic	P	F/T/M	P/VF	P/F/T	I/CC/P/F/T
Dräger Evita 4	Electric	Single	Pneumatic	F/P	F/T/M	P/F	P/F/T	I/CC/P/V/F/T/IG
Nellcor Puritan Bennett 840	Electric	Single	Pneumatic	F/P	P/F/T/M	P/V/F	P/F/T	I/CC/P/V/F/T
Hamilton Veolar	Electric	Single	Pneumatic	F/P	P/T/M	P/V/F	P/F/T	I/CC/P/F/T/IG
Infrasonics Adult Star	Electric	Single	Pneumatic	F/P	P/T/M	P/V/F	P/F/T	I/CC/P/V/F/T
Newport Wave	Electric	Single	Pneumatic	F/P	P/T/M	P/F	P/F/T	I/CC/P/F
P-B 7200ae	Electric	Single	Pneumatic	F/P	P/F/T/M	P/V/F	P/F/T	I/CC/P/V/F/T
Siemens Servo 900C	Electric	Single	Pneumatic	F/P	P/T/M	P/V/F	P/F/T	I/P/F/T/IG
Servo 300	Electric	Single	Pneumatic	F/P	P/F/T/M	P/V/F	P/F/T	I/CC/P/F/T/IG

Key:^{TM}*P–Pressure, T–Time, F–Flow, CC–Control Circuit, IG–Inspired Gas, V–Volume, M–Manual, I–Input Power*

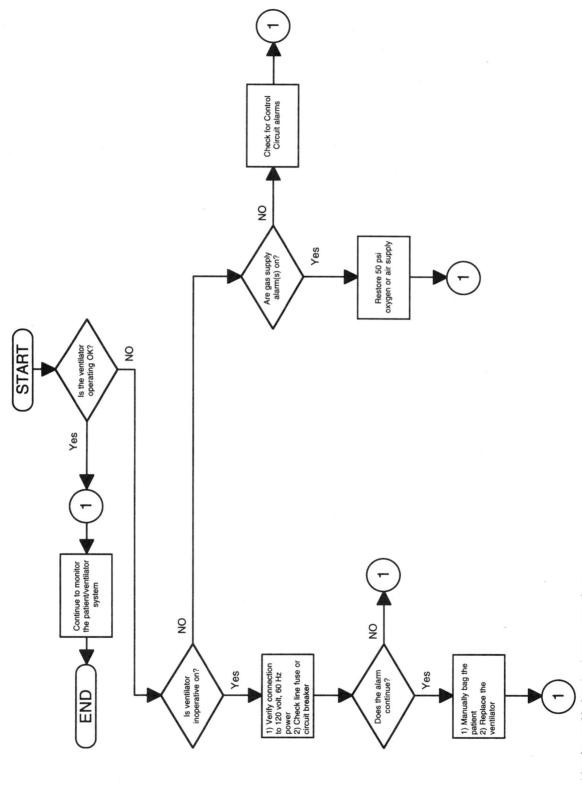

ALG 8-1 *An algorithm for troubleshooting input power alarms.*

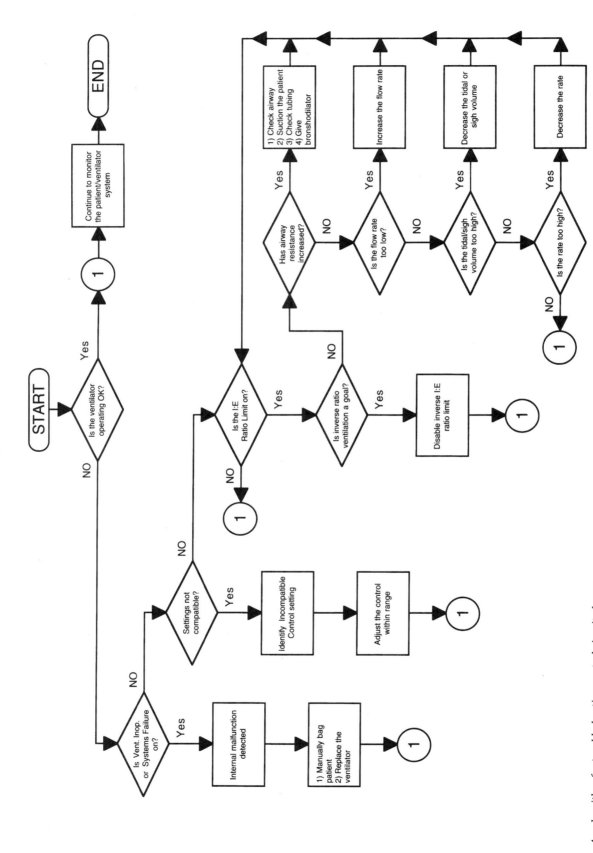

ALG 8-2 *An algorithm for troubleshooting control circuit alarms.*

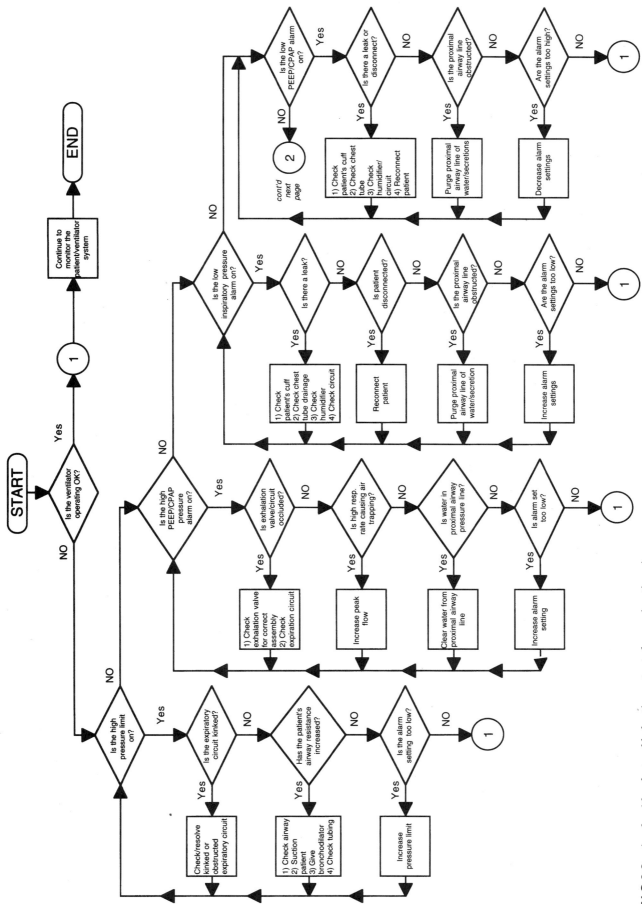

ALG 8-3 *An algorithm for troubleshooting output alarms. (continues)*

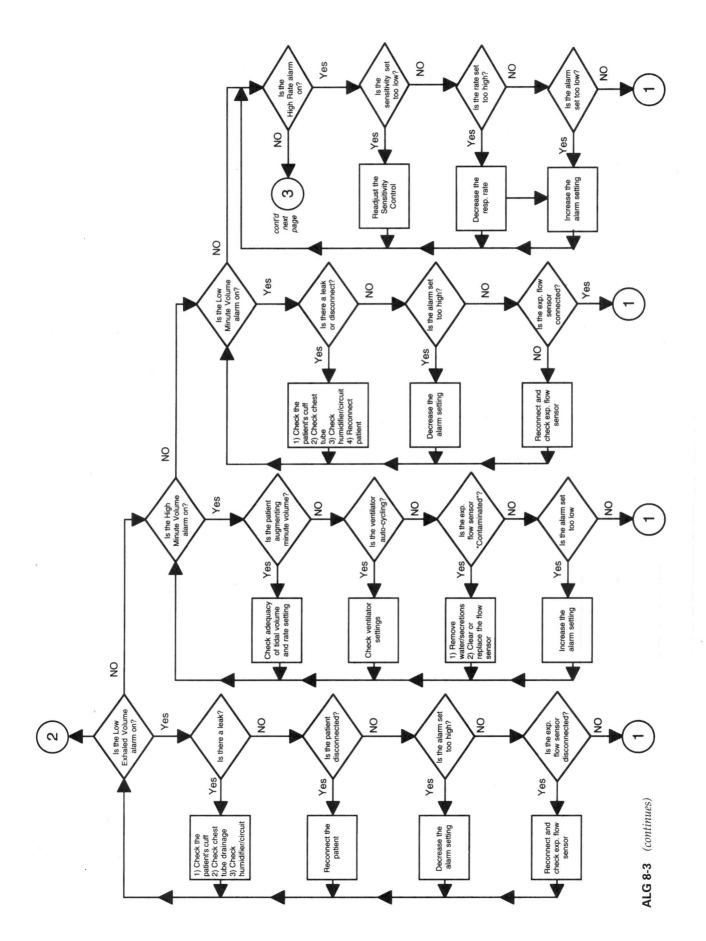

ALG 8-3 *(continues)*

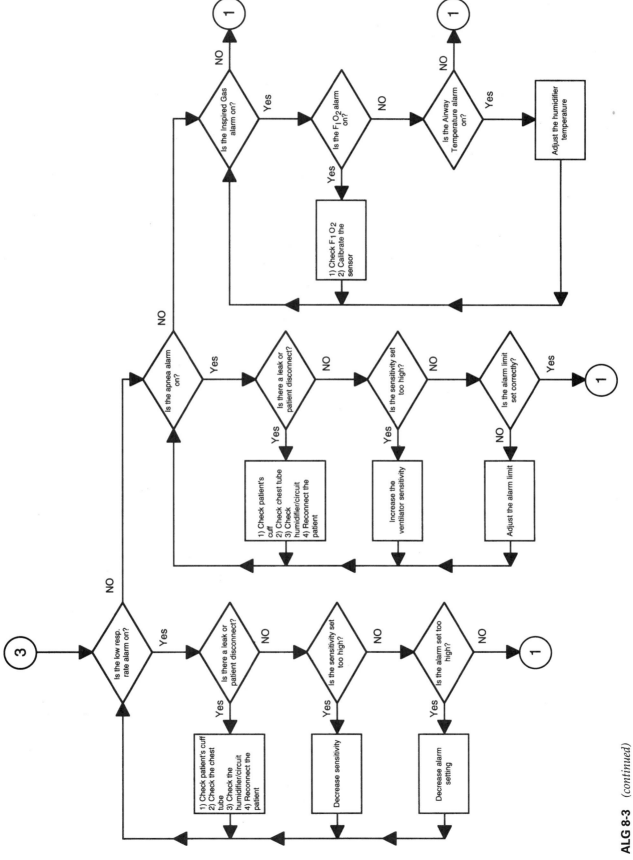

ALG 8-3 (continued)

CLINICAL CORNER

BEAR 1000 ventilator

1. You are adjusting the flow triggering for a patient who is on SIMV (volume controlled ventilation) with pressure support of 10 cmH$_2$O. Describe how you can assess whether your flow sensitivity adjustment is appropriate.
2. A physician wants you to correct for tubing compliance. In spite of your best efforts, you cannot locate the compliance factor for a clean circuit by looking at the package insert. How can you determine the tubing compliance for your patient's circuit?

Bird Products Corporation 8400ST®*i* ventilator

1. You are asked to evaluate a patient who is being ventilated by a Bird 8400ST®*i*. The High Pressure alarm is sounding when you enter the room. Describe in sequence what you would do.
2. You are adjusting the alarms for a patient being ventilated by a Bird 8400ST®*i* ventilator. The patient is on pressure control (assist/control), with a rate of 10, pressure of 32 cmH$_2$O, and PEEP of 8 cmH$_2$O. Describe in detail how you would set your alarm limits.

Nellcor Puritan Bennett 7200ae ventilator

1. You are establishing flow triggering for a patient who is on a 7200ae ventilator and is being ventilated in pressure control mode. Describe in detail the key stroke sequence you would follow to change from pressure to flow triggering.
2. You place an in-line nebulizer with 2.5 mg Albuterol in 2.5 mL of normal saline on the circuit of a 7200ae ventilator. The patient is currently on volume control (tidal volume of 700 mL, rate of 12/min, PEEP of 5 cmH$_2$O, F$_I$O$_2$ of 0.40, and flow-by of 8/3 L/min). What must you remember to do when turning off the ventilator's nebulizer control?

Self-Assessment Quiz

1. Under which of the following conditions is pressure a control variable?
   I. Mandatory volume breath delivery.
   II. CPAP.
   III. Sigh breath delivery.
   IV. Pressure support.
   a. I and II
   b. I and III
   c. II and III
   d. II and IV
2. Under which of the following situations is flow a control variable?
   I. Mandatory volume breath delivery.
   II. PEEP/CPAP.
   III. Sigh breath delivery.
   IV. Pressure support.
   a. I and II
   b. I and III
   c. II and III
   d. II and IV

3. Which of the following ventilators have the capability of flow triggering?
   I. Bird 8400ST®*i*.
   II. Siemens Servo 900C.
   III. Puritan Bennett 7200ae.
   IV. BEAR 1000.
   a. I and II
   b. I and III
   c. II and III
   d. II and IV

4. Which of the following methods can be used to measure flow?
   a. Differential pressure.
   b. Vortex sensing.
   c. Strain gauge technology.
   d. All of the above.

5. Which of the following are limit variables for the BEAR 1000 ventilator?
   I. Pressure.
   II. Volume.
   III. Flow.
   IV. Time.
   a. I
   b. I and II
   c. I, II and III
   d. I, II, III, and IV

6. If a ventilator is a flow controller, how is inspiratory volume delivery during mandatory breaths controlled?
   a. By measuring volume.
   b. By integrating volume.
   c. By measuring pressure.
   d. By controlling inspiratory time.

7. A ventilator becomes flow limited when:
   a. Inspiratory flow reaches a maximum value.
   b. Inspiratory flow no longer increases but remains constant.
   c. Inspiratory flow reaches a maximum value then decreases.
   d. Inspiratory flow starts at a maximum value then rapidly tapers.

8. A ventilator becomes volume limited when:
   a. Inspiratory pause is used.
   b. Sigh volume delivery is used.
   c. A preset volume has been reached and inspiration is terminated.
   d. When inspiration terminates prior to the delivery of the complete volume.

9. Which of the following ventilators are *not* volume limited?
   a. BEAR 1000.
   b. Bird 8400ST®*i*.
   c. Newport Wave.
   d. Puritan Bennett 7200ae.

10. Which of the following ventilators can be volume cycled?
    a. BEAR 1000.
    b. Bird 8400ST®*i*.
    c. Infrasonics Adult Star.
    d. Puritan Bennett 7200ae.

11. Which of the following would be examples of a control circuit alarm?
    I. Peak pressure.
    II. I:E ratio.
    III. Low tidal volume.

IV. Incompatible settings.
   a. I and II
   b. II and III
   c. II and IV
   d. III and IV

12. Which of the following are examples of output alarms?
   I. Peak pressure.
   II. I:E ratio.
   III. Low tidal volume.
   IV. Incompatible settings.
   a. I and II
   b. I and III
   c. II and III
   d. II and IV

13. Which of the following is an example of a flow output alarm?
   a. High respiratory rate.
   b. Low minute volume.
   c. Low tidal volume.
   d. Low PEEP/CPAP.

14. The limit variables for the Infrasonics Adult Star ventilator are:
   I. Pressure.
   II. Volume.
   III. Flow.
   IV. Time.
   a. I
   b. I and II
   c. I, II and III
   d. I, II, III and IV

15. The Newport Wave is capable of delivering up to 45 cmH$_2$O PEEP/CPAP; this variable is termed the:
   a. Control variable.
   b. Limit variable.
   c. Cycling variable.
   d. Baseline variable.

16. When the Hamilton Veolar is operating as a flow controller:
   a. Flow is measured and used as a feedback signal.
   b. Flow is a trigger variable.
   c. Flow is regulated by a reducing valve.
   d. Flow becomes independent of volume.

17. Which of the following ventilators require an external blender?
   I. BEAR 1000.
   II. Bird 8400ST®i.
   III. Newport Wave.
   IV. Siemens Servo 900C.
   a. I and II
   b. I and III
   c. II and III
   d. I and IV

18. Which of the following ventilators have a sinusoidal flow output?
   I. BEAR 1000.
   II. Bird 8400ST®i.
   III. Newport Wave.
   IV. Siemens Servo 900C.
   a. I and II
   b. I and III

    c. II and III
    d. II and IV

19. Which of the following ventilators have pressure control capability?
    I. Newport Wave.
    II. Bird 8400ST®*i*.
    III. Hamilton Veolar.
    IV. BEAR III.
    a. I and II
    b. I and III
    c. II and III
    d. II and IV

20. Which of the following ventilators have pressure support capability?
    I. Newport Wave.
    II. Bird 8400ST®*i*.
    III. Hamilton Veolar.
    IV. BEAR III.
    a. I
    b. I and II
    c. I, II and III
    d. I, II, III and IV

21. Which of the following ventilators rely on an independent exhalation valve on the patient circuit?
    I. BEAR I/II.
    II. BEAR 1000.
    III. Newport Wave.
    IV. Siemens Servo 300.
    a. I
    b. I and II
    c. I, II and III
    d. I, II, III and IV

22. Which of the following ventilators utilizes an electromagnetic exhalation valve?
    a. BEAR 1000.
    b. Bird 8400ST®*i*.
    c. Hamilton Veolar.
    d. Newport Wave.

23. Inspiration ends and exhalation begins when a preset pressure has been reached best describes:
    a. Pressure control.
    b. Pressure support.
    c. Pressure limiting.
    d. Pressure cycling.

24. Inspiration begins when the expiratory flow drops to a preset value best describes:
    a. Flow triggering.
    b. Flow limiting.
    c. Flow cycling.
    d. Flow controlling.

25. Inspiration begins when the baseline pressure drops to a preset value best describes:
    a. Pressure limiting.
    b. Pressure support.
    c. Pressure triggering.
    d. Pressure control.

26. An example of an inspired gas alarm is:
    a. Peak pressure.
    b. Low PEEP/CPAP pressure.

   c. F_1O_2.
   d. Oxygen gas supply disconnect.

27. An example of an input power alarm would be:
   a. Peak pressure.
   b. Low PEEP/CPAP pressure.
   c. F_1O_2.
   d. Oxygen gas supply disconnect.

28. Delivery of a breath to a preset pressure for a specific inspiratory time best describes:
   a. Pressure support.
   b. Pressure control.
   c. Pressure limiting.
   d. Pressure cycling.

29. Termination of a breath when peak flow drops to 25% of the peak inspiratory flow level best describes:
   a. Pressure support.
   b. Pressure control.
   c. Pressure limiting.
   d. Flow cycling.

30. Which of the following ventilators has an internal battery that can power it for a short time period following termination of the 115 volt, 60 Hz power supply?
   a. BEAR 1000.
   b. Bird 8400ST®*i*.
   c. Siemens Servo 300.

Selected Bibliography

Barnes, Thomas A., et al., *Core Textbook of Respiratory Care Practice*, 2nd Ed., Mosby-Yearbook, 1994.

BEAR Medical Systems, Inc., *BEAR I Ventilator Instruction Manual*, Riverside, CA, 1977.

BEAR Medical Systems, Inc., *BEAR II Ventilator Instruction Manual*, Riverside, CA, 1981.

BEAR Medical Systems, Inc., *BEAR 1000 Ventilator Instruction Manual*, Riverside, CA, 1992.

BEAR Medical Systems, Inc., *BEAR 5 Ventilator Instruction Manual*, Riverside, CA, 1987.

BEAR Medical Systems, Inc., *BEAR 3 Ventilator Instruction Manual*, Riverside, CA, 1991.

Bird Products Corporation, *8400ST®i Volume Ventilator Instruction Manual*, Palm Springs, CA, 1990.

Bird Products Corporation, *TBird® Ventilator Series Service Manual L1314*, Palm Springs, CA, 1997.

Branson, Richard D., and Robert L. Chatburn, "Technical Description and Classification of Modes of Ventilator Operation," *Respiratory Care*, Vol. 37, No. 9, pp. 1026–1044, 1992.

Chatburn, Robert L., "A New System for Understanding Mechanical Ventilators," *Respiratory Care*, Vol. 36, No. 10, pp. 1123–1155, 1991.

Chatburn, Robert L., "Classification of Mechanical Ventilators," *Respiratory Care*, Vol. 37, No. 9, pp. 1009–1025, 1992.

Dräger, Inc., *Evita 4 Intensive Care Ventilator Operating Instructions*, Telford, PA, 1996.

Dupis, Yvon, *Ventilators: Theory and Clinical Application*, 2nd Ed., Mosby-Yearbook, 1992.

Hamilton Medical, *Veolar Operator's Manual*, 1988.

Infrasonics, Inc., *Adult Star Ventilator Operating Instructions*, San Diego, CA, 1991.

Newport Medical Instruments, Inc., *Newport Wave Ventilator Operational Instructions*, Newport Beach, CA, 1991.

Puritan Bennett Corporation, *7200 Series Ventilator Operator's Manual*, Carlsbad, CA, 1990.

Siemens Medical Systems, *Servo Ventilator 900C Operating Manual*, Danvers, MA, 1984.

Siemens Medical Systems, *Servo Ventilator 300 Operating Manual*, Danvers, MA, 1993.

CHAPTER 9

PEDIATRIC AND NEONATAL VENTILATORS

INTRODUCTION

This chapter describes the many unique characteristics of pediatric and neonatal ventilators which merit the separation of this content into its own chapter. Chapters 7 and 8 described the adult acute care ventilators having volume, flow and pressure as control variables. Like the ventilators described in Chapter 8, pediatric and neonatal ventilators utilize flow and pressure as control variables.

As discussed in Chapter 6, for a variable (pressure, volume, flow or time) to be classified as a control variable, certain conditions must be met. Those conditions are that: 1) the variable must be measured and 2) the variable must be used as a feedback signal to control the ventilator's output. Chatburn's ventilator classification system will be applied to classify the ventilators in this chapter.

OBJECTIVES

After completing this chapter, the student will accomplish the following objectives.
- Explain what is meant by the term *control variable* and how a specific ventilator may be classified as having flow or pressure as a control variable.
- For the ventilators described in this chapter, apply Chatburn's classification system and classify them according to:
  — Input power
  — Drive mechanism
  — Control scheme
  — Alarm systems
- Describe how to assemble and troubleshoot the following ventilators:
  — Bear Medical Systems, BP-200 and BEAR CUB
  — Bird Products Corporation, Babybird and VIP Bird®
  — Dräger Babylog 8000
  — Infrasonics, Inc., Infant Star
  — Newport Medical Instruments, Inc., Breeze
  — Sechrist Industries, Model IV-100B and IV-200

THE CONTROL VARIABLE

During a ventilator-supported breath, a mechanical ventilator can control one of the following variables: pressure, volume, flow, or time. In order for a ventilator to be classified as controlling one of these variables, two conditions must be met. First, that variable must be measured, and second, it must be used as feedback to control the ventilator's output. Therefore, for a ventilator to be classified as a flow or pressure controller, flow or pressure must be measured and used as a signal to control the output from the ventilator. The ventilators discussed in this chapter meet these criteria and are classified as either flow or pressure controllers.

BEAR MEDICAL SYSTEMS BP-200 AND BEAR CUB

The BP-200 and the BEAR CUB are similar in that they are pressure or flow controllers that can be time or manually triggered and time cycled (Figures 9-1A and 9-1B). In both ventilators, gas flows continuously through the circuit, unless interrupted by the exhalation valve. Since many similarities exist between the ventilators, they will be considered together. When differences occur, they will be discussed on an individual basis.

POWER INPUT

The BP-200 and the BEAR CUB are both pneumatically powered and electronically

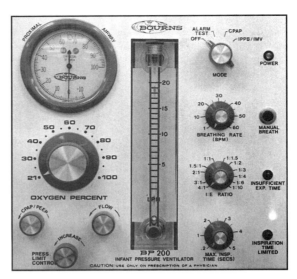

Figure 9-1B *Bear Medical Systems BP-200 ventilator.*

controlled. The drive mechanism is pneumatically powered, while the control circuit is electronically controlled. Both air and oxygen at 50 psi enter the ventilator through fittings on the rear panel. A power cord for 120 volts, 60 Hz electrical power is also connected to the rear of both ventilators.

DRIVE MECHANISM

Air and oxygen, at 50 psi after entering the ventilators, flow past pressure switches, which will activate an alarm if pressure falls below 22.5 psi (30 psi O_2 and 15 psi air for the BP-200). The gas supplies then pass through check valves (one-way valves), which prevent gas from leaving the ventilator and going back into the supply system (Figures 9-2 and 9-3).

Both the air and oxygen are then conducted to a single-stage reducing valve, which reduces the line pressure to 17 psi (about 10 psi in the BP-200). From the regulators, the gases are mixed in a blender that operates using a proportioning valve. Figures 9-2 and 9-3 illustrate the pneumatic systems for the BP-200 and BEAR CUB ventilators.

CONTROL CIRCUIT

Both the BP-200 and the BEAR CUB utilize pneumatic and electronic components in their respective control circuits. The electronic components consist of electronic timers and popet valves.

The ventilatory rate and I:E ratios are con-

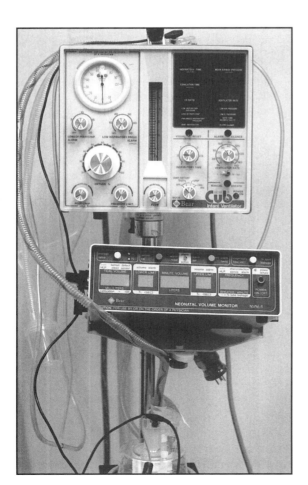

Figure 9-1A *The BEAR CUB BP-2001 ventilator.*

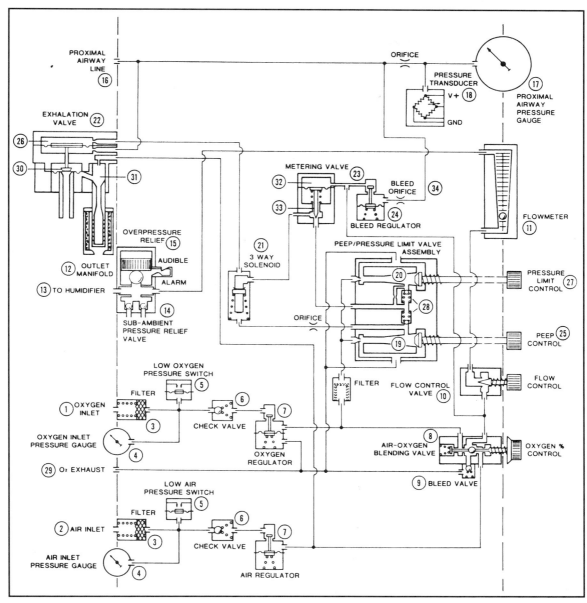

Figure 9-2 *A schematic of the Bear Medical Systems BEAR CUB BP-2001 ventilator pneumatic system. (Courtesy of Bear Medical Systems, Inc., Riverside, CA)*

trolled by an electronic timer. The rate control establishes the ventilatory rates of between 1 and 150 breaths per minute. The inspiratory time control sets the length of the inspiratory time to between 0.1 and 3.0 seconds. The inspiratory time control is also an electronic timer; however, it functions independently from the rate control.

For the BEAR CUB, the ventilator rate combined with the inspiratory time determines the I:E ratio. Once these controls are set, expiratory time is the duration left between end inspiration and the next breath. The I:E ratio is displayed on an LED display on the monitor panel.

The BP-200 has an I:E ratio control. The value set on this control determines the I:E ratio during IPPB/IMV mode. The control electronically divides the ventilatory cycle into inspiratory and expiratory times.

The pneumatic components include a flow control valve, PEEP/CPAP and inspiratory pressure limit control, three-way solenoid (BEAR CUB), a metering valve (BEAR CUB), and the exhalation valve.

The flow control valve on these ventilators

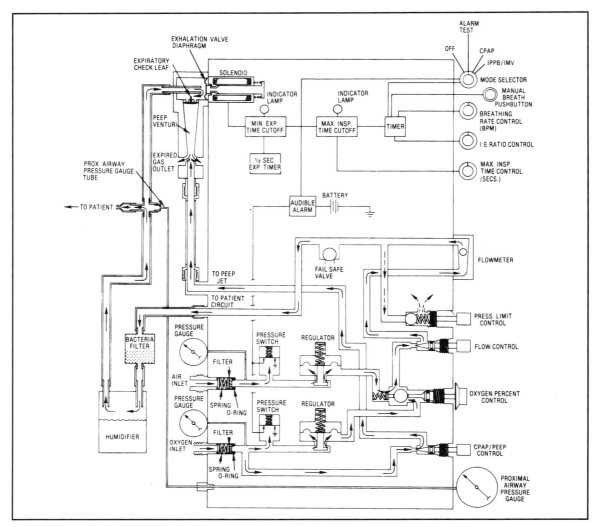

Figure 9-3 *A schematic of the Bear Medical Systems BP-200 pneumatic systems. (Courtesy of Bear Medical Systems, Inc., Riverside, CA)*

consists of an uncompensated Thorpe tube flowmeter (the needle valve is positioned upstream from the Thorpe tube). Low resistance humidifiers should be used to reduce the effects of back pressure on the flowmeter. Flows of between 3 and 30 L/min are available (0.0 to 20 L/min on the BP-200). The operation of Thorpe tube flowmeters was discussed in Chapter 1.

The PEEP/CPAP system provides elevated baseline pressures during CPAP and CMV/IMV modes. The levels of positive pressures are adjustable between 0.0 and 20 cmH₂O. Adjustment of the control varies flow sent to a venturi. The venturi provides the driving pressure of the PEEP/CPAP system. Adjustment of the control either restricts or opens the outlet of the venturi. In the BEAR CUB, gas pressure

from the venturi is conducted to a three-way solenoid that directs flow to the exhalation valve, partially closing it. The partially closed exhalation valve allows PEEP/CPAP pressure to build within the circuit. The BP-200 conducts the gas from the venturi directly to the exhalation valve, which allows PEEP/CPAP pressures to build.

The pressure limit control establishes the maximum pressure that can occur during inspiration. Pressure limits are available between 10 and 80 cmH₂O.

The CUB's pressure limit control uses a venturi system very similar to the PEEP/CPAP system. Adjustment of the control varies the pressure output from the venturi. Gas pressure from the venturi is applied through the three-way solenoid during inspiration to the exhalation valve. Once the pressure level in the circuit equals the value established by the pressure limit control (applied to the exhalation valve), excess flow is vented past the exhalation valve to the atmosphere until the inspiratory time limit is reached.

The BP-200's pressure limit system consists of an adjustable, spring-loaded valve exposed to the inspiratory side of the circuit (rather than the expiratory side). If the inspiratory pressure equals the limit set, gas is vented to the atmosphere.

The exhalation valve in the BP-200 is an electronic solenoid valve, while the exhalation valve in the BEAR CUB is pneumatically driven.

The subambient pressure relief valve opens in the event that line pressure (gas source) fails when the circuit pressure drops approximately 2 cmH_2O below ambient pressure. This would allow the patient to obtain gas from the atmosphere in the event of line pressure failure.

The metering valve (BEAR CUB) shapes the inspiratory pressure waveform. At low flows, the inspiratory pressure waveform is nearly exponential. At high flows, the inspiratory waveform is more rectangular.

CONTROL VARIABLES

The BP-200 and BEAR CUB (BP-2001) ventilators both are designed to control pressure. Pressure is limited by the adjustment made on the pressure limit control. The control is not calibrated; therefore, the pressure limit is set by observing the pressure manometer during inspiration. The pressure limit is adjustable between 10 and 80 cmH_2O (BP-200) or 0.0 and 72 cmH_2O (BEAR CUB).

Flow is a control variable in that inspiratory flow will not exceed the value established by the flow control. Flow is indicated by the Thorpe tube flowmeter, and is adjusted with the flow control knob. Depending upon inspiratory time, a given flow may not be sufficient to achieve the set pressure limit, and the ventilator therefore becomes a flow controller.

PHASE VARIABLES

Trigger Variables

The trigger variables of the BP-200 and BEAR CUB include time and manual triggering. Time is a trigger variable that is established by the rate control. The rate control is an electronic timer that divides 1 minute by the set ventilatory rate. The rate may be adjusted between 1 and 60 breaths (older BP-200 ventilators) or 1 and 150 breaths per minute, for the newer BP-200 ventilators (since 1981) as well as the BEAR CUB.

The ventilators may be manually triggered by depressing the manual breath button, delivering a ventilator supported breath.

Limit Variables

The limit variables for the BP-200 and BEAR CUB include pressure and flow. Pressure limit is established using the pressure limit control. As already described, the control is not calibrated and the pressure manometer must be used when setting the control.

The ventilators may also be flow limited. Inspiratory flow will not exceed the value established using the flow control valve and is indicated on the Thorpe tube flowmeter. Tidal volume delivery may be estimated, during flow limited ventilation, by multiplying the inspiratory flow by the inspiratory time and correcting for the compressible volume in the patient circuit.

Cycle Variable

The cycle variable for both ventilators is time. The inspiratory time control determines the length of inspiration and, therefore, when expiration begins. Inspiratory time is adjustable between 0.1 and 3 seconds (BEAR CUB). Inspiratory time set on the BP-200 is variable and determined by the rate and I:E ratio controls. The inspiratory time may be calculated using the following formula.

$$Insp.\ Time = \frac{60 \div f}{I + E}$$

f = Respiratory Rate

I = Numerator of the I:E ratio

E = Denominator of the I:E ratio

Baseline Variable

The baseline variable for the BEAR ventilators is pressure. PEEP/CPAP pressure may be adjusted between 0 and 20 cmH_2O for both ventilators.

OUTPUT WAVEFORMS

The output waveform characteristics of the BP-200 and BEAR CUB include pressure and flow waveforms. The pressure waveform may be almost square or exponential. The exponential waveform becomes a function of the pres-

ASSEMBLY AND TROUBLESHOOTING

Assembly—BEAR CUB, BP-200

To assemble the BEAR CUB and BP-200, follow the suggested assembly guide which follows.

1. Connect the high-pressure hoses to 50 psi sources of air and oxygen.

2. Connect the electrical power cord to a suitable 120 volt, 60 Hz, source.

3. Assemble the humidifier and attach it to the ventilator. Since many different humidifiers may be used, specific instructions are not included here.

4. Connect the inspiratory limb of the circuit to the humidifier. Attach the expiratory limb to the exhalation valve (fitting labeled "from patient").

5. Connect the proximal airway pressure line between the patient wye and the pressure monitor fitting.

6. Attach a short piece of tubing between the humidifier inlet and the ventilator outlet.

Troubleshooting

Refer to the troubleshooting algorithms found at the end of this chapter.

---

sure limit and flow settings. When the pressure limit is set for a maximum value, the pressure waveform rises exponentially. Simultaneously, the flow waveform is square.

When the ventilator is pressure limited and time cycled, with flow being the control variable, the pressure waveform assumes a nearly square-shaped morphology. The front portion of the square wave is rounded somewhat, so it is not truly a square wave pattern. Simultaneously, the flow waveform is nearly square, with a decelerating portion prior to exhalation.

ALARM SYSTEMS

Input Power

The input power alarms for the BP-200 and BEAR CUB include loss of electrical power and loss of gas pressure. Should 120 volts, 60 Hz power become lost or disconnected, an audible alarm will alert the practitioner to the event. Both ventilators incorporate pressure switches that will activate if the gas pressure drops below 22.5 psi (BEAR CUB) or 15 psi air and 30 psi oxygen (BP-200).

Control Circuit Alarms
Inspiratory Time / I:E Ratio

Both ventilators incorporate some form of inspiratory time or I:E ratio alarm. The BP-200 utilizes an inspiration time–limited indicator lamp. When the inspiratory time exceeds the maximum inspiratory time allotted for the breath (maximum inspiratory time control),

inspiration is terminated and the I:E control is overridden.

The BEAR CUB will activate the I:E ratio alarm if the controls are set such that the I:E ratio is greater than 3:1. When the I:E ratio reaches this setting, both audible and visual alarms will be activated.

Rate/Time Incompatibility

The BEAR CUB has an alarm that will alert the practitioner to rate and inspiratory time settings that result in an expiratory time less than 0.25 seconds. When this occurs, expiratory time will not be less than 0.25 seconds, and the displayed inspiratory time will be less than that set on the inspiratory time control. The Rate/Time incompatibility indicator will be illuminated, alerting the practitioner to the settings incompatibility.

Ventilator Inoperative

The BEAR CUB incorporates a ventilator inoperative alarm that alerts the practitioner to the following conditions: failure to cycle, electric power failure, panel control malfunction, prolonged solenoid "on" time, high/low inspiratory time and timing circuit failure.

Output Alarms

The BP-200 does not have any output alarms incorporated into the ventilator design. Therefore, when this ventilator is used, it is important to use it in conjunction with an external alarm/monitoring system.

TABLE 9-1: BP-200 and BEAR CUB (BP-2001) Capabilities

	BP-200	**BEAR CUB**
Rate	1–60 BPM	1–150 BPM
	1–150 BPM (since 1981)	
Inspiratory Time	0.5–5.0 seconds	0.1–3.0 seconds
	0.2–5.0 (since 1981)	
I:E Ratio	4:1 to 1:10	
Pres. Limit	10–80 cmH$_2$O	0–72 cmH$_2$O
PEEP/CPAP	0–20 cmH$_2$O	0–20 cmH$_2$O
Flow	0–20 L/min	3–30 L/min
F$_I$O$_2$	0.21–1.0	0.21–1.0

Pressure

The BEAR CUB incorporates both low baseline and low inspiratory pressure alarms. The low baseline pressure is adjustable from 0.0 to 20 H$_2$O. The low inspiratory pressure is adjustable between 0.0 and 50 H$_2$O.

Tables 9-1 and 9-2 highlight the capabilities and alarms systems of the BP-200 and the BEAR CUB (BP-2001).

TABLE 9-2: BP-200 and BEAR CUB (BP-2001) Alarms

	BP-200	**BEAR CUB (BP-2001)**
Input Power		
Electric Power	X	X
Air Pressure	< 15 psi	< 22.5 psi
Oxygen	< 30 psi	< 22.5 psi
Control Circuit		
Insp. Time	X	
I:E Ratio		X
Rate/Time Incompatible		X
Ventilator Inoperative		X
Output Alarms		
Low Inspiratory Pres.		X
Low Baseline Pres.		X

BIRD PRODUCTS CORPORATION, BABYBIRD VENTILATOR

The Bird Products Corporation Babybird ventilator is a pressure or flow controller that can be time or manually triggered and time cycled (Figure 9-4). Gas flows continuously through the circuit, unless interrupted by the exhalation valve. The ventilator is pneumatically powered and controlled.

POWER INPUT

The Babybird ventilator does not have a blender incorporated into its design. An external blender (proportioning valve) must be attached between the air and oxygen supply sources and the gas inlet to the ventilator.

DRIVE MECHANISM

Once gas passes through the blender, it is conducted to the inlet manifold, as shown in Figure 9-5. The manifold provides a gas source to several components including the Mark 2 cartridge, the low-pressure alarm, the flow regulator, the nebulizer control and the compound lockout cartridge.

CONTROL CIRCUIT

The Babybird uses the time cycling mechanism of the Bird Mark 2. This provides the timing mechanism that controls the inflation of the exhalation valve. The only variation

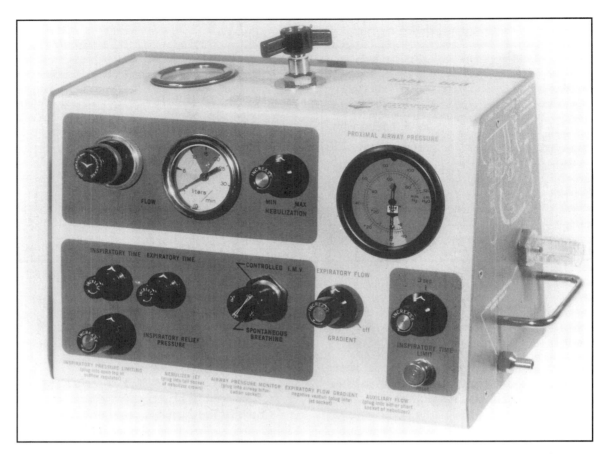

Figure 9-4 *The Bird Products Corporation Babybird ventilator. (Courtesy of Bird Products Corporation, Palm Springs, CA)*

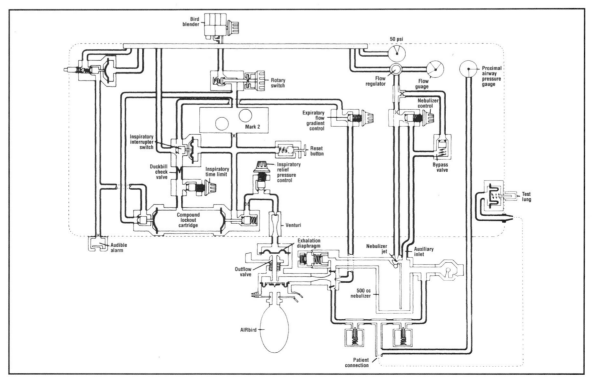

Figure 9-5 *A schematic diagram of the Bird Products Corporation Babybird ventilator. (Courtesy of Bird Products Corporation, Palm Springs, CA)*

from the original Mark 2 ventilator is the deletion of the inspiratory flow control.

Bird Mark 2.   The Bird Mark 2 controls the closure of the exhalation valve by working with the compound lockout cartridge and a venturi. Gas flows through the lockout cartridge to the venturi, which supplies gas pressure to the exhalation diaphragm. The amount of pressure applied to the diaphragm is determined by the inspiratory pressure relief control.

Inspiratory Pressure Relief Control.   The inspiratory pressure relief control determines the maximum pressure that is allowed to develop in the patient circuit. The control consists of a needle valve that allows pressure from the venturi to vent into the atmosphere. If the leak is high, low pressures will be applied to the exhalation valve, and vice versa. Since continuous flow is passing through the patient circuit, occlusion of the exhalation valve establishes inspiration. Pressure above that set by the inspiratory pressure control is ventilated to the atmosphere. Inspiratory pressure limits may be adjusted between 13 and 81 cmH$_2$O.

Inspiratory Time Control.   An inspiratory time control sets the length of inspiration from about 0.4 seconds to 2.5 seconds. The control is uncalibrated and the practitioner should adjust it based upon clinical observation and the use of a watch. The inspiratory time control determines the duration of output from the Mark 2, which powers the exhalation valve diaphragm, as already described.

Inspiratory Time Limit Control.   This control serves as a backup in the event that the Mark 2 fails to limit the inspiratory phase. It also is an uncalibrated control, having only a 3-second calibrated position.

The control functions by using the compound lockout cartridge. During inhalation, gas is allowed to leak out of the cartridge through the inspiratory time limit control (a needle valve). Springs on opposite sides of the cartridge compress two diaphragms at each end. The right-hand diaphragm is displaced due to the reduced volume as gas leaks from the cartridge. Attached to the diaphragm is a control valve that interrupts flow to the venturi, which is pressurizing the exhalation diaphragm. If the cartridge depressurizes before the Mark 2 ends inspiration, inspiration will be terminated and gas will be conducted to trigger an audible alarm.

Flow Regulator.   The flow regulator determines the amount of continuous flow through the patient circuit. The flow regulator operates in a way similar to a Bourdon gauge regulator. Adjustment of the control varies the pressure against a fixed orifice. The flowmeter on the front of the ventilator is a pressure gauge that is calibrated in liters per minute. Flow rates are adjustable between 0.0 and 30 L/min, with the normal operating range being between 10 and 20 L/min.

Expiratory Flow Gradient Control.   The expiratory gradient control is used to reduce inadvertent PEEP/CPAP due to resistance in the patient circuit. This control helps to evacuate gas from the patient circuit, thereby reducing pressure. The control operates only in the CPAP mode and during the expiratory phase of controlled IMV mode. Pressures within the circuit may be reduced to zero, or even become subambient.

PEEP/CPAP Control.   The PEEP/CPAP control determines the level of positive pressure applied to the circuit. Pressures from 0.0 to 20 cmH$_2$O are available. Functionally, the control moves the exhalation port closer to the diaphragm, increasing expiratory resistance.

Overpressure Governor.   The overpressure governor is a spring-loaded safety valve that is preset to 88 cmH$_2$O. If the valve opens, pressure is vented to the atmosphere and to an audible alarm.

Nebulizer Control.   The nebulizer control determines how much gas flows to the jet powering the 500-cc in-line nebulizer. The control is a needle valve that channels gas from the inlet manifold to the nebulizer.

Some gas bypasses the nebulizer jet through the bypass valve to the auxiliary port of the nebulizer. If a high flow is desired, the nebulizer jet may cause too much resistance and limit total flow delivery. Under these circumstances, some of the gas will vent through the bypass valve and be directed into the nebulizer, through the auxiliary port, to maintain the high desired flow.

CONTROL VARIABLES

The control variables for the Babybird are pressure and flow. Pressure is limited by the adjustment made on the inspiratory pressure relief control. The control is not calibrated, therefore, the pressure limit is set by observing the pressure manometer during inspiration. Pressure limit may be adjusted between 13 and 81 cmH$_2$O.

Flow is a control variable in that inspiratory flow will not exceed the value established by the flow control. Flow is indicated by the Bour-

ASSEMBLY AND TROUBLESHOOTING

Assembly—Babybird Ventilator

The following is a suggested assembly guide for the Babybird ventilator. Refer to Figure 9-6 when reviewing these instructions.

1. Connect the high-pressure hoses from the blender to an air and oxygen source.

2. Assemble and fill the 500-cc mainstream nebulizer and attach it to the overpressure governor.

3. Attach one limb of the patient circuit to the outlet of the nebulizer and the other to the inlet of the overpressure governor (shuttle assembly).

4. Attach the inspiratory limb of the patient circuit to the nebulizer outlet and the expiratory limb to the base of the shuttle valve assembly.

5. Connect the 500-cc nebulizer to its nipple under the ventilator and attach the bypass tubing from the nebulizer to the auxiliary flow outlet.

6. Connect the proximal airway pressure line to the airway pressure monitor outlet.

7. Connect the small-diameter red tubing between the shuttle valve assembly and the expiratory flow gradient outlet on the bottom of the ventilator.

Troubleshooting

Refer to the troubleshooting algorithms found at the end of this chapter.

---

don gauge flowmeter, and is adjusted with the flow control knob. Depending upon inspiratory time, a given flow may not be sufficient to achieve the set pressure limit, and the ventilator, therefore, becomes a flow controller.

PHASE VARIABLES

Trigger Variables

The trigger variables for the Babybird include time and manual triggering. Time is a trigger variable, which is established by the inspiratory time and expiratory time controls. The rate is the sum of the inspiratory time and expiratory time in seconds, divided into 60 seconds per minute. The rate may be adjusted between 1 and 100 breaths per minute.

The ventilator may be manually triggered by manually compressing the Airbird bag, delivering gas into the patient circuit.

Limit Variables

The limit variables for the Babybird include pressure and flow. The pressure limit is established using the inspiratory pressure relief control. As already described, the control is not calibrated and the pressure manometer must be used when setting the control. Pressure limits are adjustable between 13 and 81 cmH_2O.

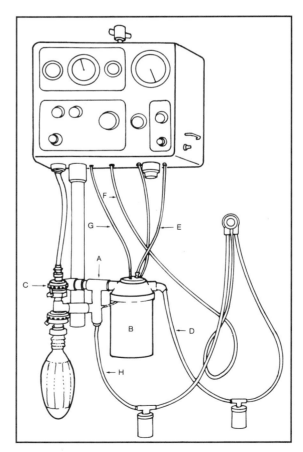

Figure 9-6 *The assembly of the Babybird ventilator: (A) Overpressure governor (shuttle valve assembly), (B) 500-cc mainstream nebulizer, (C) outflow valve, (D) inspiratory limb, (E) bypass tubing, (F) proximal airway pressure line, (G) nebulizer drive line, and (H) expiratory limb.*

The ventilators may also be flow limited. Inspiratory flow will not exceed the value established using the flow control valve, and is indicated on the Bourdon gauge flowmeter. Tidal volume delivery may be estimated during flow-limited ventilation by multiplying the inspiratory flow by the inspiratory time and correcting for the compressible volume in the patient circuit.

Cycle Variable

The cycle variable for the ventilator is time. The inspiratory time control determines the length of inspiration and, therefore, when expiration begins. Inspiratory time is adjustable between 0.4 and 2.5 seconds.

Baseline Variables

The baseline variable for the Babybird is pressure. PEEP/CPAP may be adjusted between 0 and 20 cmH$_2$O.

OUTPUT WAVEFORMS

The output waveform characteristics of the Babybird include pressure and flow waveforms. The pressure waveform is an ascending ramp and a function of the pressure limit and flow settings. The waveform assumes this shape when the ventilators are operated in pressure-limited modes.

The flow waveform is rectangular. This shape is achieved when the ventilator is operated such that the inspiratory pressure is set high enough so that the ventilator becomes a flow controller.

ALARM SYSTEMS

Input Power

The input power alarm in the Babybird alerts the practitioner to loss of gas pressure. A pressure switch will activate if the gas pres-

TABLE 9-4: Babybird Alarms

Input Power

Gas Pressure	< 43 psi at the manifold

Control Circuit

Inspiratory Time Limit

Output Alarms

None

sure drops below 43 psi in the manifold. The alarm is a pneumatic, reed-type alarm.

Control Circuit Alarms
Inspiratory Time Limit

The operation of the inspiratory time limit control was already described, in the section discussing the control circuit. When the Mark 2 fails to limit inspiration, inspiration is terminated and the ventilator resorts to the spontaneous breathing mode. An audible alarm alerts the practitioner that the ventilator has switched from IMV to CPAP modes.

To switch the ventilator back to IMV mode, the reset button must be depressed, releasing the gas pressure between the Mark 2 and the compound lockout cartridge.

Output Alarms

The Babybird does not have any output alarms incorporated into the ventilator design. Therefore, when this ventilator is used, it is important to use it in conjunction with an external alarm/monitoring system.

Tables 9-3 and 9-4 summarize the Babybird capabilities and alarm systems.

Table 9-3: Babybird Capabilities

Rate	1–100 BPM
Inspiratory Time	0.4–2.5 seconds
Pres. Limit	13–81 cmH$_2$O
PEEP/CPAP	0–20 cmH$_2$O
Flow	0–30 L/min
F$_I$O$_2$	0.21–1.0 (external blender)

BIRD PRODUCTS CORPORATION, V.I.P. BIRD®

The Bird Products Corporation V.I.P. BIRD® is a microprocessor controlled, pneumatically actuated ventilator designed for neonatal, infant and pediatric use (Figures 9-7 and 9-8). It is a pressure and flow controller that can be pressure, time, flow or manually triggered. It

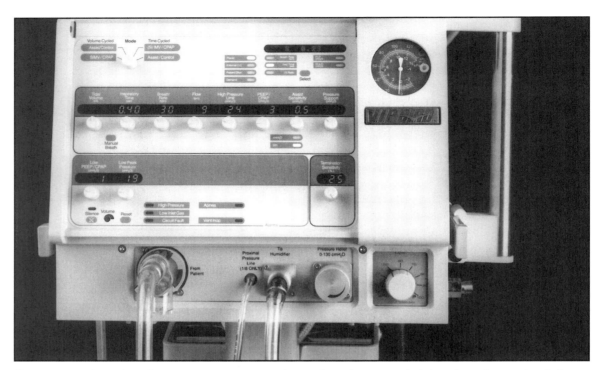

Figure 9-7 *The Bird Products Corporation V.I.P. Bird® Ventilator. (Courtesy of Bird Products Corporation, Palm Springs, CA)*

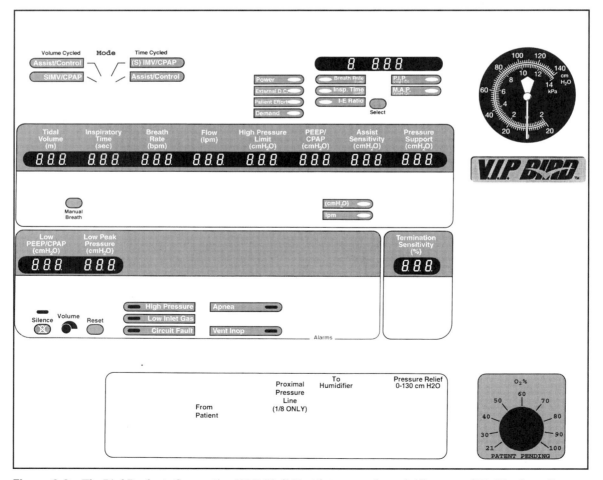

Figure 9-8 *The Bird Products Corporation V.I.P. Bird® Ventilator control panel. (Courtesy of Bird Products Corporation, Palm Springs, CA)*

is capable of operating in a time cycled continuous flow mode (IMV/CPAP), Assist/Control, IMV, SIMV, CPAP, volume cycled mode, or pressure support.

POWER INPUT

Electric power at 120 volts, 60 Hz provides power to run the microprocessor, control systems and alarm systems.

Two gas supply lines (oxygen and air) at 50 psi enter the rear of the ventilator and pass through check valves and an inlet filter (Figure 9-9). The two gas lines continue to an oxygen proportioning valve (blender), where they are mixed to the desired F_IO_2. From the blender, the gas is conducted to a 1.1 liter accumulator.

DRIVE MECHANISM

The accumulator provides additional flow during peak demands to augment the output from the blender. The 1.1 liter volume is sufficient to handle most patient care situations. The accumulator is a rigid structure; therefore, when it empties, large fluctuations in pressure could

occur. However the 200 mL pulsation dampener prevents this from affecting gas delivery.

From the accumulator, gas enters a reducing valve, where the line pressure is reduced to 25 psi. The reducing valve is a single-stage reducing valve similar to those discussed in Chapter 1.

Gas flow from the reducing valve outlet goes to the blender bleed system, the pulsation dampener and the flow control valve. The blender bleed system provides a continuous bleed rate of approximately 6 liters per minute during low flow demands. This assures a continuous flow of gas through the accumulator, which facilitates a more rapid change in F_IO_2, when required. The pulsation dampener is another rigid reservoir, of approximately 200 mL volume. The pulsation dampener minimizes pressure changes caused by the rapid movement of the flow control valve and from the accumulator.

CONTROL CIRCUIT

The flow control valve is a linear, electromechanical valve controlled by a stepper

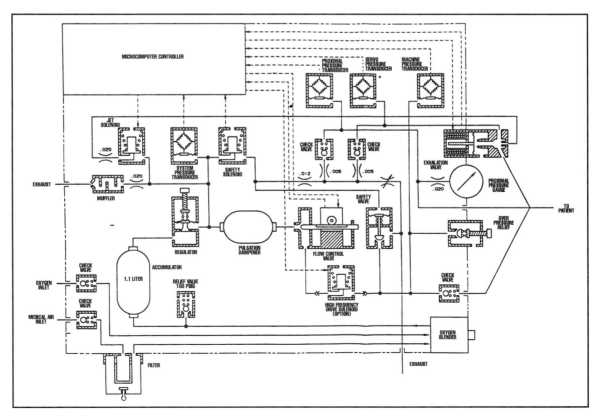

Figure 9-9 *A schematic diagram of the the Bird Products Corporation V.I.P. Bird® Ventilator. (Courtesy of Bird Products Corporation, Palm Springs, CA)*

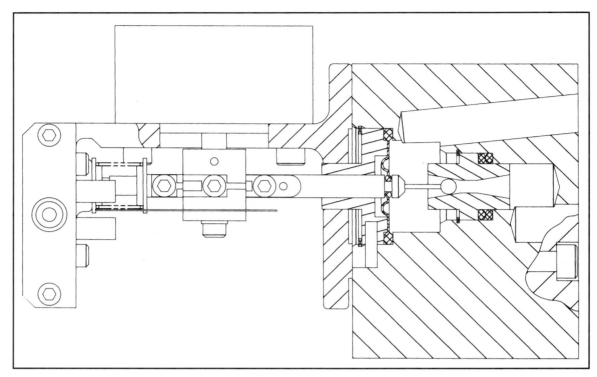

Figure 9-10 *The V.I.P. Bird® flow control valve. (Courtesy of Bird Products Corporation, Palm Springs, CA)*

motor (Figure 9-10). This valve has a rapid response through a relatively short travel. The rapid opening and closing of the valve would place excessive demands on the reducing valve if the pulsation dampener were not incorporated into the design. Gas flow through the valve is sonic up to a system back-pressure of 5 psi (350 cmH$_2$O). Flow rate range through the valve is between 0.0 and 120 liters per minute. From the flow control valve, the gas exits the ventilator to the patient circuit.

The exhalation valve is an electromechanical, linear actuator. Signals to the valve from the microprocessor control the opening and closing of the valve. PEEP/CPAP pressures are regulated by pressure feedback signals to the microprocessor, causing the microprocessor to partially close the exhalation valve.

CONTROL VARIABLES

The control variables for the V.I.P. BIRD® are pressure and flow. Pressure is limited by the adjustment made on the high pressure limit control. The control is adjustable between 3.0 and 80 cmH$_2$O during time-cycled, pressure-limited ventilation.

Flow is a control variable during time-cycled, pressure-limited ventilation, in that inspiratory flow will not exceed the value estab-lished by the flow control. Flow is adjustable between 3.0 and 40 liters per minute, using the flow control. Depending upon inspiratory time, a given flow may not be sufficient to achieve the set pressure limit, and the ventilator therefore becomes a flow controller.

During volume ventilation, the V.I.P. BIRD® also operates as a flow controller. Flow from the flow control valve is based upon valve position. An optical sensor detects the valve's position. Gas flow exiting the valve is sonic up to a back-pressure of 350 cmH$_2$O. Mass flow from the flow control valve is unchanged up to the 350 cmH$_2$O maximum back-pressure. Therefore, flow from the valve is directly proportional to how far the valve has opened. The microprocessor uses an algorithm to determine flow based upon the feedback from the optical sensor, which senses valve position. Although flow is not directly measured, valve position is directly proportional to flow. Tidal volume delivery then becomes a function of flow and inspiratory time.

PHASE VARIABLES

Trigger Variables

The trigger variables for the V.I.P. BIRD® include flow, pressure, time and manual triggering. With the addition of the Partner Volume Monitor, mechanical breaths can also be flow triggered in the pressure-limited, time-cycled mode. The patient must exceed the flow sensitivity setting to trigger a breath. Flow sensitivity is adjustable between 0.2 and 5 L/min.

In the volume-controlled mode, mechanical breaths can be pressure triggered. The patient must exceed the pressure trigger threshold to obtain a mechanical breath. Sensitivity may be set between 1 and 20 cmH$_2$O below baseline pressure.

Time is a trigger variable, which is established by the breath rate control. The rate is adjustable from 0.0 to 150 breaths per minute. The rate control sets a reference for the microprocessor, which controls the opening and closing of the exhalation valve. The exhalation valve servos to the high-pressure limit setting in the time-cycled mode.

Manual triggering occurs when the practitioner depresses the manual breath button. When pressed, the ventilator delivers a mandatory breath. The breath is given at the tidal volume, peak flow and F$_I$O$_2$ set on the control panel.

Limit Variables

The limit variables for the V.I.P. BIRD® ventilator include pressure and flow. The pressure limit is established during time-cycled ventilation using the high-pressure limit control. Pressure limits are adjustable between 3 and 80 cmH$_2$O.

The ventilator may also be flow limited. Inspiratory flow will not exceed the value established on the flow rate control. During time-cycled ventilation, flows are adjustable between 3 and 40 liters per minute. In the volume controlled mode, peak flow can be set from 3 to 100 L/min, with 120 L/min available for spontaneous breaths.

Cycle Variable

The cycle variables for the V.I.P. BIRD® are pressure, volume, flow and time. Pressure becomes a cycle variable when the V.I.P. is operated as a volume ventilator. The high-pressure limit control establishes the pressure at which a volume-cycled breath will be terminated. This control is adjustable between 3.0 and 120 cmH$_2$O. Once the pressure limit is reached, inspiration is terminated and both audible and visual alarms will be activated.

The ventilator is volume cycled during volume-controlled ventilation. In this mode, the flow control valve's position and inspiratory time are used to determine delivered volume. Technically, flow and time are measured, and volume is derived from the two measurements.

Flow becomes a cycle variable during pressure support. Inspiration is terminated when the inspiratory flow rate falls to a range of 5 to 25% of the peak inspiratory flow rate for that breath. Once flow decays to this point, inspiration is terminated and the ventilator cycles into exhalation. Pressure support may be adjusted between 1.0 and 50 cmH$_2$O.

Time is a cycle variable during pressure-limited, time-cycled ventilation. Inspiratory time is determined by the inspiratory time control. Inspiratory time may be adjusted to between 0.1 and 3.0 seconds.

Baseline Variables

The baseline variable for the V.I.P. BIRD® ventilator is pressure. PEEP/CPAP pressure may be adjusted between 0 and 24 cmH$_2$O.

OUTPUT WAVEFORMS
Pressure

The output pressure waveform characteristic of the V.I.P. BIRD® is rectangular. The rectangular waveform is characteristic during time-cycled, pressure-limited ventilation, and in volume-cycled SIMV/CPAP mode with the addition of pressure support.

Flow

The flow output waveform is rectangular. This waveform occurs when the ventilator is operated in the volume control modes, and it functions as a flow controller.

ALARM SYSTEMS
Input Power

The input power alarms for the V.I.P. BIRD® include loss of gas pressure and loss of electrical power. The low gas pressure alarm will be activated if the system pressure (distal to the reducing valve) falls below 22.5 psi or increases to greater than 27.5 psi. Both audible and visual alarms will result if these conditions are met.

In the event of a loss of electrical power, the

ASSEMBLY AND TROUBLESHOOTING

Assembly—V.I.P. BIRD® Ventilator

To assemble the ventilator for use, complete the suggested assembly guide. Since this ventilator is designed for neonatal, infant and pediatric patients, different circuits are required depending upon the ventilator's application. The circuits are similar as far as connections, but differ in size. Therefore, one set of circuit assembly instructions are provided.

1. Connect the ventilator to a 120 volt, 60 Hz grounded power source. If used in the emergency or transport setting where A/C current is not available, use a 12 volt, 5 amp, power supply.

2. Connect both air and oxygen supplies providing 50 psi to the fittings on the rear of the ventilator.

3. Assemble the patient circuit:
   a. Attach a bacteria filter to the ventilator outlet.
   b. Connect a sufficient length of 22-mm diameter tubing between the bacteria filter and a heated, high-efficiency humidifier.
   c. Install water traps onto the inspiratory and expiratory limbs of the circuit.
   d. Attach the expiratory limb of the circuit to the exhalation valve assembly.
   e. Pressure-test the circuit.

Troubleshooting

Refer to the troubleshooting algorithms found at the end of this chapter.

---

ventilator inoperative alarm will be activated (audible and visual), and the safety and exhalation valves will be automatically opened.

Control Circuit Alarms

The control circuit alarms for the V.I.P. BIRD® include ventilator inoperative and circuit fault. The ventilator inoperative alarm will be activated if the gas system pressure is less than 20 or greater than 30 psi for more than 1 second. It will also sound if an internal malfunction has been detected. The circuit fault alarm will be activated if a problem is detected in the patient circuit or with the pressure transducer.

Output Alarms
Pressure

Pressure alarms are available for high pressure limit, low peak pressure, low PEEP/CPAP and high/prolonged pressure. The pressure limit alarm is adjustable between 3 and 120 cmH₂O. The alarm is active in assist/control and SIMV/CPAP modes.

The low peak pressure alarm is adjustable

between 3 and 120 cmH₂O. This alarm is available in all modes of operation.

The low PEEP/CPAP alarm is adjustable between 9 and 24 cmH₂O. This alarm is available in all modes of ventilation.

The high/prolonged pressure alarm works during pressure-controlled, time-cycled ventilation. This alarm is activated if the proximal pressure exceeds the high peak pressure limit setting by 10 cmH₂O. Once the alarm is activated, the flow control valve closes and the exhalation valve and safety valve are both opened, venting excess pressure in the circuit.

Time

The V.I.P. BIRD® has an apnea alarm. This alarm is activated if the ventilator does not detect any inspiratory effort over a set time period. The range for the alarm is 20, 40 or 60 seconds. Once activated, both audible and visual alarms result.

Table 9-5 and 9-6 summarize the V.I.P. BIRD® ventilator's capabilities and alarm systems.

TABLE 9-5: V.I.P. BIRD® Ventilator Capabilities

Modes	Time cycled (IMV/CPAP)
	Volume (Assist/control, SIMV/CPAP), Assist/Control/SIMV (with Partner Volume Monitor)
Tidal volume	20–995 ml
Rate	0.0–150 BPM
Inspiratory Time	0.10–3.0 seconds
Peak Flow	Time cycled (3–40 L/min)
	Volume cycled (3–100 L/min), with 120 L/min for all spontaneous breaths
Pres. Limit	3–80 cmH$_2$O
PEEP/CPAP	0.0–24 cmH$_2$O
Sensitivity	1–20 cmH$_2$O (Below baseline)
	0.2 to 5 L/min with Partner Volume Monitor
Pressure support	1–50 cmH$_2$O
Pressure relief	0.0–130 cmH$_2$O
F$_i$O$_2$	0.21–1.0

TABLE 9-6: V.I.P. BIRD® Ventilator Alarm Systems

Input Power

Low Gas Pressure	System pressure < 22.5 psi
	System pressure > 27.5 psi
Electrical Power	

Control Circuit

Ventilator Inoperative	Loss of electrical power
	System pressure < 20 psi or system pressure > 30 psi for more than 1 second
	Internal system fault detected
Circuit Fault	Patient circuit fault detected
	Pressure transducer fault

Output Alarms

High Pressure Limit	3–120 cmH$_2$O
Low Peak Pressure	3–120 cmH$_2$O
Low PEEP/CPAP	-9 to 24 cmH$_2$O
High Pressure	Pressure Limit Setting + 10 cmH$_2$O
Apnea	No inspiratory effort for 20, 40 or 60 seconds

DRÄGER BABYLOG 8000

The Dräger Babylog 8000 ventilator is designed for infant and pediatric use (Figure 9-11, A and B). The ventilator is a pneumatically powered, microprocessor-controlled flow controller, which is pressure, time or manually triggered; pressure limited; and time cycled. It is capable of operating in assist/control, SIMV, and CPAP modes.

Power Input

Gas supplies are connected using DISS fittings on the rear of the ventilator. Medical grade air and oxygen are required at between 45 and 90 psi. Gases pass through a filter and check valves before pressure is reduced by means of two regulators (one for air and the other for oxygen). From the regulators, air and oxygen are taken through a solenoid valve blender system, which mixes them together to the desired F_IO_2.

Standard AC current provides the electrical power required to run the microprocessor control system and monitoring systems of the ventilator, 120/240 VAC, 50/60 Hz power is required.

Control Circuit

Blended gas flows through a pneumatic control valve and a flow rate control before entering the patient circuit (Figure 9-12). During inspiration, the exhalation valve closes and gas flows to the patient's lungs. Airway pressure is monitored by two pressure transducers, and pressure during inspiration is controlled by the exhalation valve.

PEEP/CPAP pressure is generated by the PEEP control valve applying partial pressure to the exhalation valve, partially closing it. PEEP/CPAP pressure may be adjusted between 0 and 15 cmH_2O.

Control Variable

The control variable of the Dräger Babylog 8000 is flow, which is controlled by the flow control valve and adjustable between 1 and 30 L/min. Flow is a control variable during pressure-limited, time-cycled ventilation.

Phase Variables
Trigger Variables

The trigger variables for the ventilator include flow, time and manual triggering. Flow triggering is established by first calibrating the flow sensor, which is attached to the patient's airway. Once calibrated, flow triggering may be adjusted from a range of 1 to 10, which corresponds to flows of between 0 and 3 L/min. Once the patient exceeds the trigger threshold, a mandatory breath is delivered.

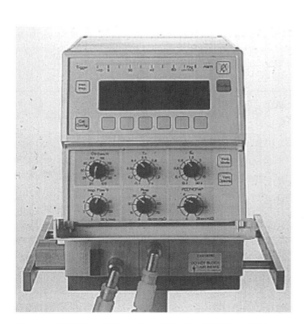

Figure 9-11A *Dräger, Inc. Babylog 8000 ventilator*

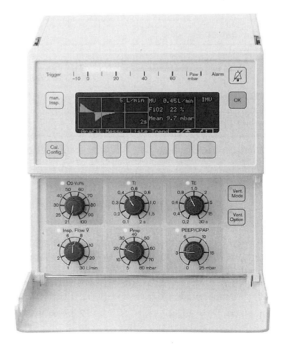

Figure 9-11B *Dräger, Inc. Babylog 8000 control panel.*

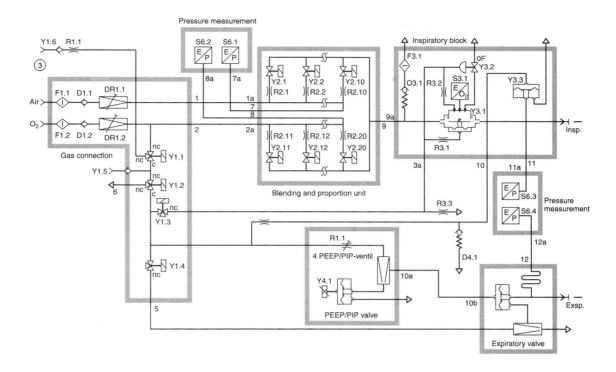

Figure 9-12 *Babylog 8000 pneumatic system.*

Time triggering occurs in the absence of the patient's spontaneous effort and is a function of the inspiratory and expiratory time settings. Frequencies of between 0 and 150 breaths per minute may be set. The frequency may be determined by dividing 60 by the sum of the inspiratory and expiratory times.

Manual triggering occurs when the practitioner depresses the manual inspiration button. When depressed, a manual breath is delivered up to the set inspiratory pressure limit. Inspiration is terminated when the button is released or 5 seconds have elapsed.

Limit Variables

The limit variables for the Dräger Babylog 8000 ventilator include pressure and flow. Pressure is a limit variable during pressure-limited, time-cycled ventilation. The pressure limit is set using the inspiratory pressure control and is adjustable between 10 and 80 cmH_2O. Once the pressure limit is reached, inspiration continues until the inspiratory time has lapsed.

Flow becomes a limit if, during inspiration, inspiratory flow reaches the setting established on the flow rate control. Inspiratory flows may be adjusted between 1 and 30 L/min.

Cycle Variables

The cycle variables of the ventilator include pressure and time. Pressure becomes a cycle variable when the airway pressure exceeds that of the automatically set upper pressure limit value. The high airway pressure limit is automatically set to the peak pressure plus 10 cmH_2O or the PEEP/CPAP pressure plus 4 cmH_2O for spontaneous ventilation. When this threshold is exceeded, inspiration is terminated and audio and visual alarms result.

Time is a cycle variable during pressure-limited, time-cycled ventilation. Inspiratory time is adjusted by using the inspiratory time control and is adjustable between 0.1 and 2.0 seconds. Once the inspiratory time value has been met, inspiration ends and exhalation begins.

Baseline Variable

The baseline variable for the ventilator is pressure. PEEP/CPAP pressures may be adjusted from 0 to 15 cmH_2O. The PEEP control valve adjusts pressure against the exhalation valve, partially closing it and creating the PEEP/CPAP pressure.

ASSEMBLY AND TROUBLESHOOTING

Assembly—Dräger Babylog 8000 Ventilator

To assemble the ventilator in use, complete the suggested assembly guide. Since this ventilator is designed for neonatal, infant and pediatric patients, different circuits are required depending upon what application is desired. All circuits are similar as far as connections and components, but they differ in size.

1. Connect the ventilator to a suitable 120/240 VAC, 50/60 Hz, power source.

2. Connect air and oxygen supplies at 50 psi to the rear of the ventilator using the DISS fittings.

3. Assemble the patient circuit:

   a. From the ventilator outlet, attach a short length of tubing between the outlet and a heated humidifier.

   b. Connect the inspiratory limb of the circuit to the outlet of the humidifier, making sure the temperature probe is placed close to the proximal airway. The use of condensation traps is recommended in both the inspiratory and expiratory limbs of the circuit.

   c. Connect the flow sensor to the patient airway connection and connect the sensing cable to the ventilator.

   d. Connect the expiratory limb of the circuit to the exhalation port on the ventilator.

Troubleshooting

Refer to the troubleshooting algorithms found at the end of this chapter.

Output Waveforms
Pressure

The output pressure waveform of the Dräger Babylog 8000 is rectangular. This is characteristic of most pressure-limited, time-cycled ventilators during mandatory breaths. Pressure rises to the pressure limit value and is held until inspiration ends.

Flow

The flow waveform is also rectangular. Flow rate is limited by the setting on the inspiratory flow control. Flow rises to the value established (0 to 30 L/min) and is held at that value until inspiration is terminated.

Alarm Systems
Input Power

Input power alarms include loss of gas pressure and loss of electrical power. In the event either air or oxygen pressure falls below 43 psi, audible and visual alarms will alert the practitioner to the event. If electrical power is lost, a battery-powered alarm will sound.

Control Circuit

The control circuit alarms include flow measurement inoperative, pressure measurement inoperative, loss of stored data, ventilator malfunction, and I:E ratio. In the event signals from the flow sensor cannot be interpreted by the ventilator, an alarm will alert the clinician to this event. It is possible to continue using the ventilator;, however, the clinician must maintain adequate minute ventilation and other parameters within safe levels without the information provided by the flow-sensing system. A qualified service technician should be contacted and the problem corrected as soon as possible.

If a fault in the pressure-monitoring system is detected, an alarm will alert the practitioner to the event. Some conditions that may cause this may be corrected by the practitioner, such as condensation in the circuit, liquid in the measuring system, or a circuit that is too small or offers too high a resistance. If a circuit fault is detected by the microprocessor, the ventilator should be removed from service and alternate ventilation provided for the patient.

The loss of stored data alarm will occur if the ventilator experiences a power failure. The clinician may enter the previous values and continue to use the ventilator. If the ventilator will not accept the new values after the initial power-up time, a qualified service technician should be contacted and the ventilator removed from service.

If the microprocessor detects a malfunction in the control or logic circuitry, an error code of *xxx* will be displayed. The ventilator should be removed from service and an alternate means of ventilation should be provided for the patient.

The I:E ratio alarm limits the I:E ratio to a maximum of 3:1. If the clinician attempts to exceed this ratio, an alarm will sound and ventilation will be limited to a ratio of 3:1. Settings should then be changed to maintain an acceptable I:E ratio.

Output Alarms
Pressure

Automatically set high-pressure and PEEP/CPAP pressure alarms alert the practitioner to these events. The high pressure limit is automatically set to the peak pressure plus 10 cmH$_2$O or CPAP pressure plus 4 cmH$_2$O. The PEEP/CPAP alarm is automatically set to the PEEP/CPAP pressure level minus 4 cmH$_2$O.

Flow

The Dräger Babylog 8000 ventilator incorporates both high and low minute ventilation

TABLE 9-8: Dräger Babylog 8000 Ventilator Alarm Systems

Input Power
    Loss of air pressure
    Loss of oxygen pressure
    Loss of electrical power
Control Circuit
    Flow measurement inoperative
    Pressure measurement inoperative
    Loss of stored data
    Ventilator malfunction
    I:E ratio
Output
    High airway pressure
    Low PEEP/CPAP pressure
    High and low minute volume
Inspired Gas
    High and low oxygen concentrations

alarms. The high minute ventilation alarm may be set between 0.13 and 15 L/min, while the low minute ventilation alarm may be set between 0.03 and 14 L/min.

Inspired Gas Alarms

The inspired gas alarm available on the ventilator is oxygen concentration. The alarm is automatically adjusted to ±4% of the set value on the oxygen percentage control.

Tables 9-7 and 9-8 summarize the Dräger Babylog 8000 ventilator capabilities and alarm systems.

INFRASONICS, INC., INFANT STAR AND INFANT STAR 500

The Infrasonics, Inc., Infant Star ventilators are pneumatically powered, microprocessor controlled infant ventilators (Figures 9-13, 9-14), manufactured from 1985 to 1992. The Infant Star 500 is similar to the original Infant Star and was released for sale and distribution in 1993. Since many similarities exist between the ventilators, they will be considered to-

TABLE 9-7: Dräger Babylog 8000 Ventilator Capabilities

Modes	Assist/control, time cycled SIMV/CPAP, CPAP
Tidal volumes	0–999 ml
Inspiratory time	0.1–2.0 seconds
Expiratory time	0.2–30 seconds
Frequency	0–150 breaths/minute
Inspiratory flow	1–30 L/min
Pressure limit	10–80 cmH$_2$O
PEEP/CPAP	0–15 cmH$_2$O
Flow sensitivity	0–3 L/min
F$_1$O$_2$	0.21–1.0

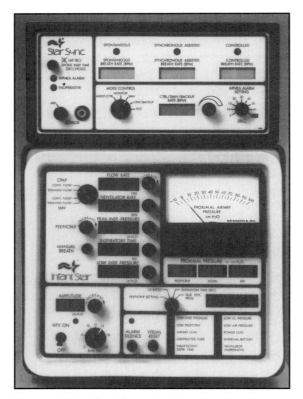

Figure 9-13 *The Infrasonics Infant Star Ventilator. (Courtesy of Infrasonics, Inc., San Diego, CA)*

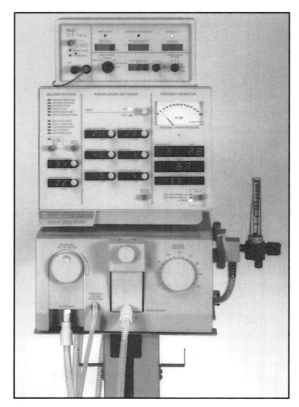

Figure 9-14 *The Infrasonics Infant Star Ventilator control panel. (Courtesy of Infrasonics, Inc., San Diego, CA)*

gether. When differences occur, they will be discussed on an individual basis.

Both ventilators are pressure or flow controllers that are time triggered, pressure limited and time cycled. They are capable of operating in continuous flow CPAP, continuous flow IMV, demand flow CPAP, and demand flow IMV (Infant Star). With the addition of the Star Sync patient-triggered interface, the Infant Star can provide patient-triggered breaths in Assist/Control, SIMV and CPAP. The triggering mechanism used by the Star Sync is based on abdominal movement which is detected by a change in pressure within an abdominal sensor (capsule). The Infant Star 500 is capable of operating in CPAP and IMV modes.

POWER INPUT

A 120 volt, 60 Hz electrical power connection is provided on the rear of the upper electronic modules of the ventilators. Direct current from a 12 volt gell cell battery (120 volt, 60 Hz power charges the battery) is used to operate the dual 8085 microprocessors (Infant Star), the 8085 and 80C31 (Infant Star 500) and other components of the control and alarm systems in the ventilators. The battery power system offers both an uninterruptable power supply and protection from power surges.

Air and oxygen at 50 psi enter the rear of the lower pneumatics module through individual water traps and filters prior to entering the ventilators (Figure 9-15). Gases (air and oxygen) are conducted past pressure switches and to reducing valves, where line pressure is reduced to 38 psi, after which the gases enter the internal blender. The mixed gas exiting the blender passes through a snap-acting regulator and into a 30 cubic inch accumulator. (The snap-acting regulator closes when pressure rises to 36 psi and opens when pressure falls to 26 psi.) The gases are then conducted to another reducing valve, which reduces the pressure to 18 psi, whereupon the gases enter the proportional solenoid valve manifold.

CONTROL CIRCUIT

The proportional solenoid manifold consists of six proportional solenoid valves, 2 L/min, 4 L/min, 8 L/min, 16 L/min, 16 L/min and 16 L/min. These valves open in combinations to provide flow rates for 4 to 40 L/min. When the desired flow rate is set on the electronic module, a control signal is sent to the microprocessor, activating one or more solenoid valves to produce the desired flow rate.

During mandatory breaths, a solenoid valve (SV10, Figure 9-15) sends pressurized gas to the exhalation valve diaphragm, closing it. Once the exhalation valve has closed, gas flow is directed into the patient circuit.

PEEP/CPAP pressure is also controlled through the exhalation valve diaphragm. When the practitioner adjusts the PEEP/CPAP control on the electronic module, a signal is sent to the microprocessor. The microprocessor opens a solenoid valve (SV8, Figure 9-15), which regulates output from the PEEP regulator. Pressure from the PEEP regulator is applied to the exhalation valve diaphragm, creating resistance to gas flow through the exhalation valve and PEEP/CPAP pressure in the circuit. PEEP/CPAP pressures are adjustable between 0.0 and 24 cmH$_2$O.

The Infant Star 500 has a heated exhalation block assembly. The heated exhalation block reduces water buildup in the exhalation block, which helps to minimize baseline pressure fluctuations.

CONTROL VARIABLES

The control variables for the ventilators include pressure and flow. Pressure becomes a control variable during pressure-controlled, time-cycled ventilation. The pressure limit is set using the peak inspiratory pressure control. The pressure limit is adjustable at 5 to 90 cmH$_2$O. During the first 75% of inspiration, gas flow matches the level set on the flow rate control. When 75% of the inspiratory phase has passed, the Infant Star's microprocessor predicts when peak inspiratory pressure will be reached and gradually reduces flow from the solenoid manifold to prevent overshoot of the desired pressure limit. If the pressure limit is met prior to the end of inspiration, the 2 L/min solenoid valve may cycle on and off, to compensate for leaks around the uncuffed endotracheal tube and to maintain the desired pressure limit. As with other infant ventilators, unless sufficient inspiratory time has been allowed, the pressure limit may not be always reached. Proximal (actual) pressure may be less than set if there is a significant leak.

Flow becomes a control variable for these ventilators in that inspiratory flow is set by the operator using the flow rate control. Flow is adjustable between 4 and 40 L/min. If the in-

spiratory time is not sufficient for the pressure limit to be reached, the ventilator becomes a flow controller.

The ventilators also have the ability to provide additional flow to meet the patient's instantaneous demands during spontaneous breathing. In the demand flow mode (Infant Star), a base flow of 4 L/min is established through the patient circuit to eliminate the possibility of rebreathing. In the continuous flow mode (Infant Star), the base flow matches the set IMV flow. The Infant Star 500 has an adjustable background (base flow), which can be set between 2 and 30 L/min. However, the background flow may not be set to a level greater than the flow rate setting. If the inspiratory pressure drops by 1 cmH$_2$O, the microprocessor progressively opens solenoid valves on the manifold to provide the flow needed to maintain the baseline pressure. Using this system, one flow can be set to meet the needs of mandatory ventilation, while the ventilator allows the patient to establish his or her inspiratory flow needs during spontaneous ventilation.

PHASE VARIABLES

Trigger Variables

Trigger variables for the ventilators include pressure (Star Sync), time and manual triggering.

When the Star Sync Patient Triggered Interface is used with either of the ventilators, pressure triggering can be used. The Star Sync senses inspiration using a pressure sensor that detects abdominal movement. Abdominal movement causes pressure changes to occur in the abdominal sensor, triggering a ventilator breath. Using the Star Sync, additional modes of Assist/Control, SIMV, and CPAP/Backup can be provided. The CPAP/Backup mode allows the patient to breathe spontaneously. However, if an apneic period occurs, the ventilator will revert to backup ventilation and deliver mechanical breaths, thus attempting to maintain an adequate minute ventilation.

Time is established using the ventilator's rate control on the electronic module. Respiratory rates may be set between 1 and 150 breaths per minute. The rate control setting establishes a reference for the microprocessor to control the output from the proportional solenoid manifold and the exhalation valve servo (SV10).

The ventilators becomes manually triggered when the practitioner depresses the

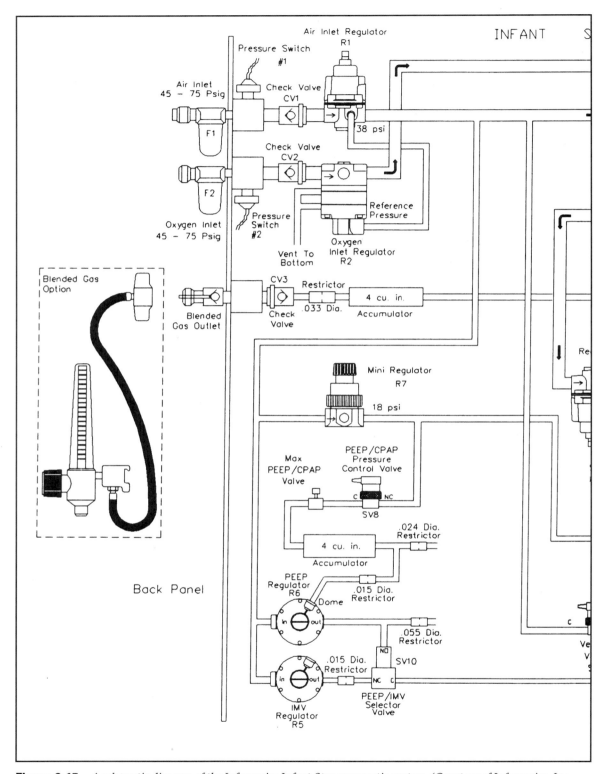

Figure 9-15 *A schematic diagram of the Infrasonics Infant Star pneumatic system. (Courtesy of Infrasonics, Inc., San Diego, CA) (continues)*

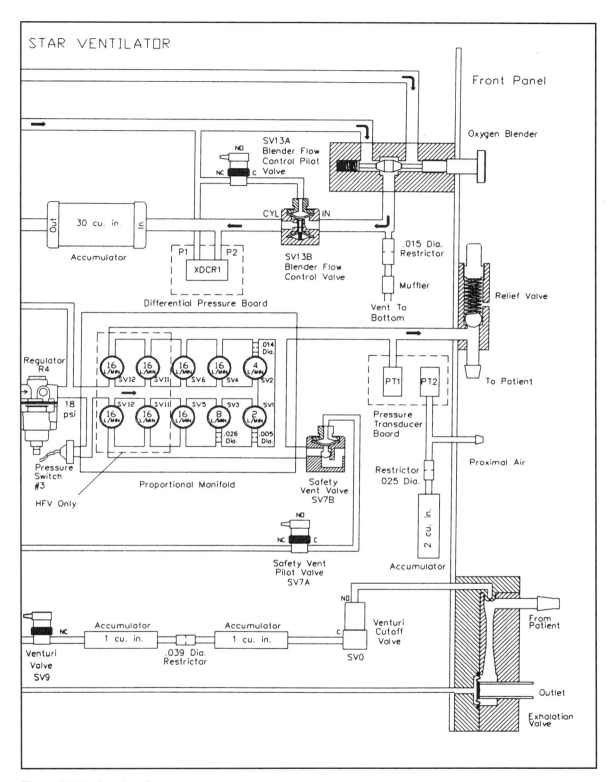

Figure 9-15 *(continued)*

manual breath button on the electronic control panel. Once depressed, a breath is delivered based upon the settings on the peak inspiratory pressure and inspiratory time controls.

Limit Variables

The limit variables for the ventilators include pressure and flow. The pressure limit is set using the peak inspiratory pressure control. Pressure limits may be adjusted between 5 and 90 cmH$_2$O. Pressures may also be limited by adjustment of the mechanical pop-off valve located on the front of the pneumatics module. If the pressure is limited by using the mechanical pop-off valve, many of the alarm and monitoring systems, which are based on proximal and internal pressure, may not be activated due to the limiting effect of the pop-off valve. The mechanical pop-off valve is adjustable between 5 and 90 cmH$_2$O (Infant Star) and 5 and 105 cmH$_2$O (Infant Star 500).

Flow becomes a limit variable when the pressure limit is not reached during inspiration. Under these conditions, flow is limited by the setting on the flow rate control. Flow rates may be adjusted between 4 and 40 L/min.

Cycle Variables

The cycle variables for the ventilators include pressure and time. If inspiratory pressure on the Infant Star reaches a level 5 cmH$_2$O greater than the peak inspiratory pressure setting, the exhalation valve opens, or both the exhalation valve and the safety valve may be opened to relieve circuit pressure. In either case, both an audible and visual alarm will result. The Infant Star 500 incorporates a high inspiratory pressure alarm. This alarm is adjustable between 5 and 105 cmH$_2$O. If the alarm threshold is exceeded, the ventilator will open the exhalation valve and stop all inspiratory flow delivery. This alarm system allows the clinician to adjust pressures up to 15 cmH$_2$O above the peak inspiratory pressure setting.

The ventilators are normally time cycled. Inspiratory time is adjusted using the inspiratory time control. Inspiratory times may be adjusted between 0.1 to 3.0 seconds. Once the set inspiratory time has been reached, flow through the proportional solenoid manifold ceases and the exhalation valve opens.

Baseline Variables

The baseline variable for the Infrasonics Infant Star and Infant Star 500 is pressure.

PEEP/CPAP pressures may be adjusted between 0 and 24 cmH$_2$O.

OUTPUT WAVEFORMS

Pressure

The output pressure waveform characteristic of the Infant Star is a rectangular waveform, which is characteristic during time-cycled, pressure-limited ventilation. This waveform may be modified by using lower flow rates, whereupon it will assume a more sinusoidal shape.

Flow

The flow output waveform is rectangular. This waveform occurs when the peak inspiratory pressure control is set high enough that it is not reached during inspiration. Under these circumstances, the ventilator is operating as a flow controller.

ALARM SYSTEMS

Input Power Alarms

The input power alarms include loss of electrical power and gas pressure. In the event that 120 volts, 60 Hz electrical power is lost, a lamp will illuminate, indicating the loss of power. The internal battery can provide up to 30 minutes of power minimum, and usually 45–50 minutes when fully charged. When 5 to 10 minutes of battery time remains, both an audible and a visual alarm will be activated to alert the practitioner. Once the internal battery is fully discharged, reconnection to 120 volts, 60 Hz power will fully charge the battery in about 1 hour.

If either air or oxygen inlet pressures fall below 45 psi, both audible and visual alarms will be activated. If the oxygen pressure falls but air pressure remains unaffected, the ventilator will continue to operate at 21% oxygen (Infant Star). The Infant Star 500 is capable of operating on either air or oxygen if one gas source is lost. If pressure in both gases is lost, both the internal safety valve and the exhalation valve are opened, permitting ambient gas flow to the patient circuit.

Control Circuit Alarms

The control circuit alarms for the ventilators include ventilator inoperative and insufficient expiratory time alarms. If the microprocessor detects a fault in the electronics or the exhalation valve operation, the ven-

ASSEMBLY AND TROUBLESHOOTING

Assembly—Infant Star Ventilator

To assemble the ventilator for use, complete the suggested assembly guide. Since this ventilator may be used with several different humidifiers, assembly instructions for these are not included.

1. Select an appropriate low compressible volume humidifier and mount it to the pedestal directly below the ventilator.

2. Connect the high pressure air and oxygen supply lines to an appropriate 50 psi gas source for each.

3. Connect the electrical power cord to a 120 volts, 60 Hz, electrical outlet.

4. Connect the inspiratory limb of the patient circuit to the ventilator outlet on the front of the pneumatics module. The use of water traps in the patient circuit is recommended.

5. Connect the expiratory limb of the patient circuit to the exhalation valve block on the front of the pneumatics module.

Troubleshooting

Refer to the troubleshooting algorithms found at the end of this chapter.

tilator stops cycling. All gas flow from the proportional solenoid manifold ceases and the safety valve and the exhalation valve are both opened, allowing gas to flow through the patient circuit. The ventilator inoperative alarm is both audible and visual, and codes will be displayed on the multiple display window on the electronics module to assist the practitioner in troubleshooting it.

The insufficient expiratory time alarm is activated when the rate and inspiratory time controls are incompatible. This occurs when the expiratory time is shorter than the minimum allowed for a given breath rate. For respiratory rates of up to 100 breaths per minute, the minimum expiratory time is 0.3 seconds. For respiratory rates greater than 100 breaths per minute, the minimum expiratory time is 0.2 seconds. When this alarm is activated, the respiratory rate is automatically decreased to ensure the minimum expiratory time. Simultaneously, a flashing rate indicator alerts the practitioner to the incompatibility of the settings.

Output Alarms
Pressure

Pressure alarms are available for peak and baseline pressures. A low peak pressure alarm is adjustable between the baseline pressure (PEEP/CPAP setting) and 60 cmH$_2$O.

The low baseline pressure alarm setting varies depending upon the PEEP/CPAP level set. Table 9-9 lists the pressures required to activate this alarm.

The alarm parameters are automatically established by the microprocessor. These variances in alarm threshold pressures allow for the normal fluctuations in baseline pressure which occur during PEEP/CPAP. The pressure difference (setting vs. proximal pressure) must be maintained below the threshold for 25 seconds to trigger an alarm.

The ventilators also include an obstructed tube alarm. This alarm will be activated under several circumstances.

If proximal pressure rises to 5 cmH$_2$O greater than the peak inspiratory pressure setting (adjustable on the Infant Star 500), all gas flow will cease and the exhalation valve will be opened. The alarm code *HI-PP-A01* will be displayed in the multiple display window. If proximal pressures exceed the peak inspiratory pressure setting by 10 cmH$_2$O (the Infant Star 500 is adjustable based upon the High In-

TABLE 9-9: PEEP/CPAP Alarm Pressures

PEEP/CPAP Setting	Pressure Difference (Setting vs. Proximal Airway)
0 - 5 cmH$_2$O	2 cmH$_2$O
6 - 8 cmH$_2$O	3 cmH$_2$O
9 - 12 cmH$_2$O	4 cmH$_2$O
13 - 24 cmH$_2$O	5 cmH$_2$O

spiratory Pressure alarm), all gas flow will cease, the safety valve and exhalation valve will be opened, and the alarm code *HI-PP-A02* will be displayed in the multiple display window.

If the expiratory limb of the circuit becomes partially blocked, the obstructed tube alarm will also be activated. This condition is detected by the pressure failing to drop by 50% of the difference between the peak inspiratory and the baseline pressure within 0.2 seconds after the end of inspiration. The alarm code *HI-PP-A03* will be displayed in the multiple display window. If the baseline pressure exceeds the PEEP/CPAP pressure setting by 6 cmH₂O for more than 5 seconds, the occluded airway alarm is activated and the error code *HI-CP-A04* will be displayed in the multiple display window.

If the machine (internal pressure) exceeds the proximal airway pressure by 15 cmH₂O (adjustable on the Infant Star 500), the obstructed tube alarm will also be activated and the alarm code *HI-PP-A05* will be displayed in the multiple display window.

Table 9-10 and 9-11 summarize the Infant Star ventilator's capabilities and alarm systems.

NEWPORT MEDICAL INSTRUMENTS, INC., BREEZE (E150) VENTILATOR

The Newport Medical Instruments, Inc., Breeze is a microprocessor-controlled, pneumatically powered ventilator designed for neonatal, infant, pediatric and adult use (Figures 9-16 and 9-17). It is a pressure and flow controller that can be pressure, time or manually triggered. It is capable of operating in time-cycled, pressure-controlled modes (Assist/Control, SIMV or Spontaneous) and volume-controlled modes (Assist/Control + Sigh, Assist/Control, SIMV, or spontaneous).

Power Input

Electric power at 120 V AC, 60 Hz (220–240 V AC, 50-60 Hz switchable), provides power to run the microprocessor, control systems and alarm systems. An internal battery provides a minimum of 1 hour of power in case of AC power failure.

Two gas supply lines (oxygen and air) at 50 psi enter the blender from the rear of the ventilator.

Control Circuit

The blender mixes the incoming air and oxygen to the desired oxygen concentration. Gas exiting the blender passes through a check valve assembly (CVA300, Figure 9-18) prior to entering the pneumatic interface valve. The Humphry interface (SOL200P) is an air-piloted valve. When opened, gas flows through the main flow control valve, which establishes the

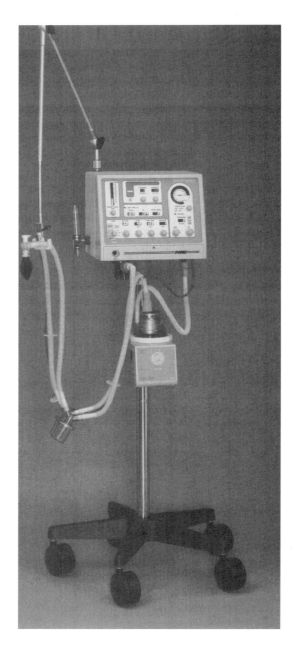

Figure 9-16 *The Newport Breeze Ventilator (Model E150). (Courtesy of Newport Medical Instruments, Inc. New port Beach, CA)*

TABLE 9-10: Infrasonics, Inc., Infant Star Ventilator Capabilities

Modes (Infant Star)	Continuous Flow (IMV, CPAP)
	Demand Flow (IMV, CPAP)
Modes (Infant Star 500)	IMV and CPAP
Rate	1–150 BPM
Inspiratory Time	0.10–3.0 seconds
Flow Rate	4–40 L/min
Pres. Limit	5–90 cmH$_2$O
PEEP/CPAP	0.0–24 cmH$_2$O
Sensitivity	1 cmH$_2$O below baseline
With the Star Sync	
Mech. Pressure Pop-Off	5–90 cmH$_2$O (Infant Star)
	5–105 cmH$_2$O (Infant Star 500)
F$_I$O$_2$	0.21–1.0

TABLE 9-11: Infrasonics, Inc., Infant Star Alarm Systems

Input Power

Low Gas Pressure	Air Pressure < 45 psi
	Oxygen Pressure < 45 psi
Electrical Power	Loss of 115 v 60 Hz (Battery power for 30 minutes is available if fully charged.)

Control Circuit

Ventilator Inoperative	Internal electronics fault
	Exhalation valve malfunction
Incompatible Settings	Expiratory time too short for the set respiratory rate

Output Alarms

Pressure Limit	5–90 cmH$_2$O (Infant Star)
	5–105 cmH$_2$O (Infant Star 500)
Low Insp. Pressure	3–60 cmH$_2$O
Low PEEP/CPAP	Variable (refer to Table 9-10.)
Obstructed Tube (Infant Star)	Prox. Press > PIP by 5 cmH$_2$O (HI-PP-AO1)
	Prox. Press > PIP by 10 cmH$_2$O (HI-PP-AO2)
	Prolonged exhalation (HI-PP-AO3)
	Baseline Pres > PEEP/CPAP Setting by 5 cmH$_2$O (HI-CP-AO4)
	Internal Pres > Proximal Pres by 15 cmH$_2$O (HI-PP-AO5)
Obstructed Tube (Infant Star 500)	Adjustable High Inspiratory Pressure range of 5–105 cmH$_2$O, limited to a maximum of 15 cmH$_2$O above the set peak inspiratory pressure

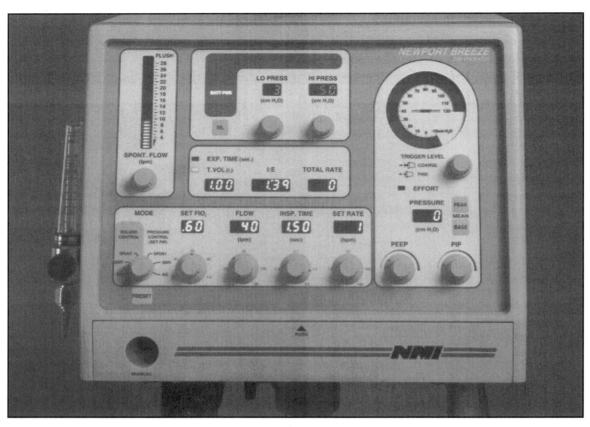

Figure 9-17 *The Newport Breeze Ventilator control panel. (Courtesy of Newport Medical Instruments, Inc. Newport Beach, CA)*

flow of gas into the patient circuit during mandatory breaths. A pilot control solenoid valve (PLV150P, Figure 9-18) prevents gas flow from the spontaneous flow pneumatic interface valve from entering the circuit during a mandatory breath. During expiration, the pilot control solenoid allows the spontaneous pneumatic interface valve to open so that gas can flow to the reservoir bag and through the patient circuit. Two independent flow rates may be established, one for mandatory breaths and the other for spontaneous breathing.

The expiratory drive line outlet delivers pressure to the diaphragm on the permanent exhalation valve. The PEEP and plateau actuators (VLV150A, Figure 9-18) provide pressure to the exhalation valve diaphragm to maintain PEEP/CPAP pressures and to control pressure delivery during time-cycled ventilation. During volume-controlled ventilation, the exhalation valve diaphragm is controlled by the PEEP actuator during exhalation; it is controlled by main flow outlet pressure during mandatory breath inspiration.

Control Variables

The control variables for the Breeze are pressure and flow. During pressure-controlled ventilation, the peak inspiratory pressure control (PIP) is activated and controls the peak pressure during mandatory breaths. The peak inspiratory pressure level may be adjusted between 0.0 and 60 cmH$_2$O. A pressure relief level should be set using the pressure relief valve located on the upper left corner on the rear panel of the ventilator. The control is adjustable between 0.0 and 120 cmH$_2$O, the relief valve is functional during all modes of ventilation. The relief valve should always be set to a value greater than the high pressure alarm setting to act as a safety pop-off.

Flow is a control variable during volume-controlled ventilation, in that inspiratory flow will not exceed the value established by the flow control. Flow is adjustable between 1 and 120 liters per minute using the flow control (mandatory breaths). Flow output is controlled by the combination of the main flow pneumatic interface valve and precision needle valve. Tidal volume delivery then becomes a function of flow rate and inspiratory time. The Breeze is unique in that two flow rates may be set, one for spontaneous ventilation and the other for mandatory breaths. Spontaneous flow is adjusted using the spontaneous flow control, while mandatory flow is adjusted using the flow control knob found at the bottom center of the control panel.

Phase Variables
Trigger Variables

The trigger variables for the Newport Breeze include pressure, time and manual triggering. Pressure triggering may be established by adjusting the trigger level control. Each time the proximal airway pressure drops below the set trigger level on the face of the manometer, a patient effort is recognized. Since the sensitivity trigger setting on the Breeze is an actual rather than a delta pressure setting, it is important to carefully adjust the trigger level so that each patient effort can be detected. If PEEP/CPAP is changed, the trigger level must be readjusted to be relative to the new baseline pressure.

If patient efforts do not exceed the trigger level setting during volume- or pressure-controlled, assist/control or SIMV ventilation, time becomes the trigger variable. The rate control, which is adjustable between 1 and 150 breaths per minute, determines the ventilatory rate.

The ventilator may be manually triggered by depressing the manual inflation button located behind the fold-down door at the bottom face of the control panel. When the manual inflation button is depressed, gas is delivered to the patient at the mandatory flow setting until the manual inflation button is released, 2 seconds elapses, or the high pressure alarm is activated, whichever comes first.

Limit Variables

The limit variables for the Breeze include pressure and flow. As already described, during pressure-controlled ventilation, pressure is limited to the setting on the peak inspiratory pressure control (PIP). Pressure limits are adjustable from 0.0 to 60 cmH$_2$O.

Flow is a limit variable, both during pressure-controlled, time-cycled ventilation and during volume-controlled ventilation. Flow is adjusted using the spontaneous flow control valve (spontaneous breathing) and the flow control (mandatory breaths). During volume-controlled ventilation, mandatory inspiratory flow, which is adjustable between 1 and 120 L/min, will be delivered at the value set on the flow control. Spontaneous flow may be adjusted with the Spont flow control between 0 and 50 L/min. During pressure-controlled ventilation, mandatory inspiratory flow, which is adjustable between 1 and 120 L/min, will be delivered at the value set on the flow control; but when airway pressure equals exhalation valve diaphragm pressure (PIP control), gas exits the exhalation valve rather than entering the patient airway. As in volume control, spontaneous flow may be adjusted with the Spont flow control between 0 and 50 L/min.

Cycle Variables

The cycle variables for the Breeze ventilator include pressure and time. Pressure becomes a cycle variable if the value set on the high-pressure alarm is reached during mandatory breaths. If the pressure is reached, the Breeze cycles to exhalation, mandatory and nebulizer flows stop and the spontaneous flow turns on.

Inspiratory time is set using the inspiratory time control. Inspiratory times are adjustable between 0.1 and 3.0 seconds. When the inspiratory time has been reached, the inspiratory phase will end and exhalation will begin.

Baseline Variables

The baseline variables for the Newport Medical Instruments Breeze (E150) is pressure. PEEP/CPAP pressures may be adjusted between 0 and 60 cmH$_2$O.

Output Waveforms
Pressure

The output pressure waveform characteristic of the Breeze during pressure-controlled ventilation is rectangular.

Flow

The flow output waveform is rectangular. This waveform occurs when the peak inspiratory pressure control is set high enough that it is not reached during inspiration. Under these circumstances, the ventilator is operating as a flow controller.

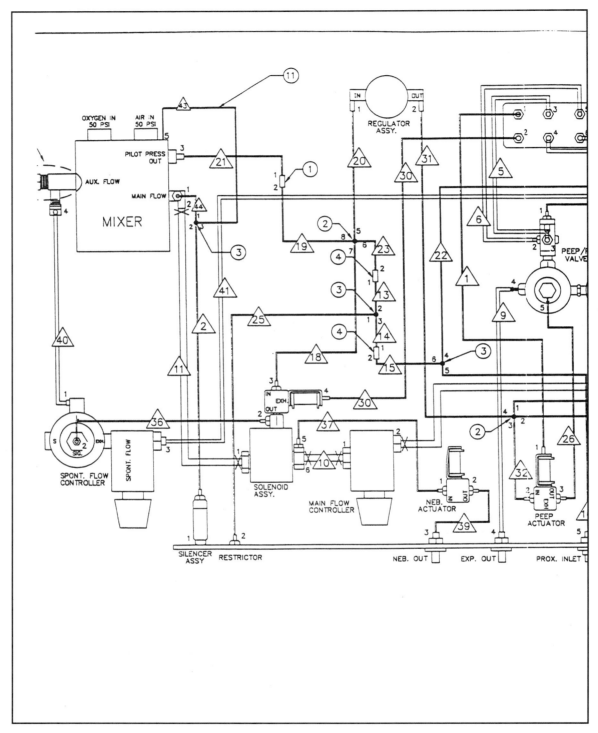

Figure 9-18 *A schematic of the Newport Breeze pneumatic system. (Courtesy of Newport Medical Instruments, Newport Beach, CA)*

Alarm Systems
Input Power

Input power alarms include loss of pneumatic pressure and loss of electrical power. If pressure falls below 35 psi, an audible alarm will alert the practitioner to the event.

If electrical power is lost, the ventilator will automatically operate on an internal battery, which, when fully charged, can operate the ventilator for a minimum of 1 hour. A periodic audible alert reminds the practitioner that the battery is in use. An audible and visual low-

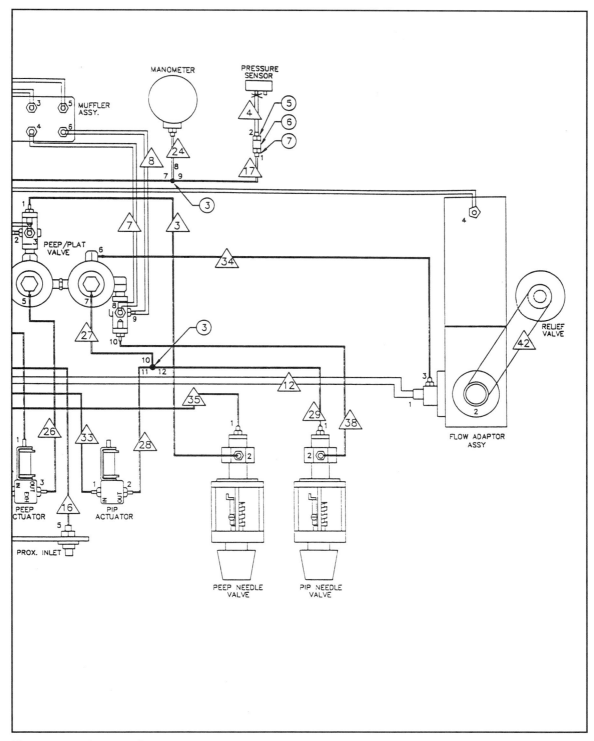

Figure 9-18 *(continued)*

battery alarm will alert the practitioner to a low-battery condition. When this alarm has been activated, less than 15 minutes of battery operation time remain.

Control Circuit

The control circuit has a system failure

alarm. If all the LEDs on the front panel remain on for longer than 2 seconds during the power-on self-test, an internal problem has been detected on the microprocessor board. In the event this alarm has occurred, contact an authorized service representative and use a different ventilator.

ASSEMBLY AND TROUBLESHOOTING

Assembly—Breeze Ventilator

To assemble the ventilator for use, complete the suggested assembly guide. Since this ventilator may be used with several different humidifiers, assembly instructions for these are not included.

1. Select an appropriate low compressible volume humidifier and mount it to the pedestal or cart directly below the ventilator.

2. Connect the high pressure air and oxygen supply lines to an appropriate 50 psi gas source for each.

3. Connect the electrical power cord to a 115 v, 60 Hz electrical outlet (220–230 v, 50-60 Hz, international).

4. Connect the inspiratory limb of the patient circuit to the ventilator outlet beneath the right-hand side of the face panel. The use of water traps or a heated wire system in the patient circuit is recommended.

5. Connect the expiratory limb of the patient circuit to the exhalation permanent exhalation valve and secure it to the exhalation valve on the mounting block beneath the ventilator on the lower left.

6. Connect the proximal airway line to the proximal airway nipple beneath the ventilator on the lower right.

7. Connect a reservoir bag to the large-bore outlet beneath the ventilator at the right rear of the ventilator or use the reservoir bag cap if ventilating neonates.

Troubleshooting

Refer to the troubleshooting algorithms found at the end of this chapter.

Output Alarms

Pressure

The Newport Breeze includes both high and low inspiratory pressure alarms and a low CPAP alarm. The high pressure alarm is set using the HI PRESS alarm control. It is adjustable between 10 and 120 cmH₂O. The low pressure alarm is set using the LO PRESS alarm control. It is adjustable between 3 and 99 cmH₂O. Both pressures are sensed using the proximal airway line and a transducer located inside the ventilator. Both alarms function in all modes except the spontaneous modes. In spontaneous modes, the low inspiratory pressure alarm setting display goes dark (unless the low CPAP alarm is in use).

The low CPAP alarm is available only in the spontaneous modes of ventilation. In these modes, the apnea alarm control may be set to the first, left-most position, thus deactivating the apnea alarm and activating the low CPAP

alarm. When you choose to use the low CPAP alarm in place of the apnea alarm, the total rate display on the panel will display "OFF" and the LO PRESS display will display the low CPAP alarm pressure setting. The low CPAP alarm is adjusted using the LO PRESS alarm control. The low CPAP pressure alarm is adjustable between 0 and 99 cmH₂O. The alarm is activated if the baseline pressure falls below the alarm limit for longer than 4 seconds.

Time

An apnea alarm alerts the practitioner to periods of apnea. The interval is adjustable between 5 and 60 seconds in 5-second increments. Once the detection delay has been set, if no breaths (spontaneous or mandatory) have been sensed by the sensitivity trigger control in that time interval, the apnea alarm will be activated and both audible and visual alarms will be triggered.

TABLE 9-12: Newport Medical Instruments, Inc., Breeze Ventilator Capabilities

Modes	
Pressure Controlled	Spontaneous, SIMV, Assist/Control
Volume Controlled	Spontaneous, SIMV, Assist/Control, Assist/Control + Sigh
Rate	1–150 BPM
Inspiratory Time	0.10–3.0 seconds
Flow Rate	3–120 L/min (mechanical) 0.0–50 L/min (spontaneous)
Pres. Limit	0–60 cmH$_2$O
Maximum Inverse I:E	4:1
Tidal Volume	10–2500 mL
PEEP/CPAP	0.0–60 cmH$_2$O
Sensitivity	0.0–60 cmH$_2$O (actual pressure, not delta pressure)
Mech. Pressure Pop-Off	0–120 cmH$_2$O
F$_I$O$_2$	0.21–1.0

The I:E ratio alarm is activated if the inspiratory time and rate controls are set such that an inverse I:E ratio of greater than 4:1 has been set. If this occurs, the inspiratory time and I:E ratio display flashes and alerts the practitioner to the excessive inverse ratio. The flashing inspiratory time will indicate the actual inspiratory time for the set ventilatory rate. The ventilator will not allow an I:E ratio of greater than 4:1. Once this ratio is reached, the inspiratory time will automatically decrease.

Tables 9-12 and 9-13 summarize the Newport Breeze ventilator's capabilities and alarm systems.

TABLE 9-13: Newport Medical Instruments, Inc., Breeze Ventilator Alarm Systems

Input Power	
Inlet Gas Pressure	< 35 psi
Electrical Power	Loss of 115 v, 60 Hz (battery power for 60 minutes is available if fully charged.) Also, if operated on 220–240 v, 50-60 Hz, similar loss of electrical power alarms function.
Low Battery	Less than 15 minutes of battery time remaining.
Control Circuit	
Systems Failure	Fault detected on the microprocessor board
Output Alarms	
Pressure Limit	10–120 cmH$_2$O
Low Insp. Pressure	3–99 cmH$_2$O
Low PEEP/CPAP	0–99 cmH$_2$O
Time	
I:E Ratio	Inspiratory time and rate exceed an inverse ratio of 4:1
Apnea	No breaths detected for 5, 10, 15, 20 or 25 seconds

SECHRIST INDUSTRIES, MODEL IV-100B AND IV-200

Sechrist Industries, Inc., markets two infant ventilators, the IV-100B and the IV-200. Both ventilators are pneumatically powered, microprocessor and fluidically controlled ventilators (Figure 9-19 and 9-20). They are capable of operating as pressure or flow controllers; pressure, time or manually triggered, pressure or flow limited; and pressure or time cycled ventilators. Both ventilators may be patient triggered with the addition of the SAVI (for Synchronized Assisted Ventilation of Infants) module. Being continuous flow ventilators, mechanical breaths are delivered when the exhalation valve has closed. Since many similarities exist between the ventilators, they will be considered together. When differences occur, they will be discussed on an individual basis.

INPUT POWER

The electronic control circuitry is configured to operate on either AC input (120 volt or 220 volt) or 12 volt DC input. Both the alarm system and electronic manometer have a battery backup. Electrical power enters the rear of the ventilator via a standard AC electric cord

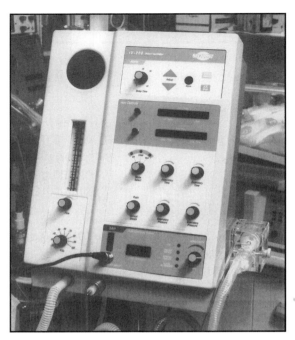

Figure 9-20 *The Sechrist Industries IV-200 ventilator. (Courtesy of Sechrist Industries, Inc., Anaheim, CA)*

and plug or via the supplied DC input cord and plug.

Both ventilators rely on 50 psi air and oxygen for their respective drive mechanisms. The IV-100B uses an external blender to mix the supply gases to the desired output concentration. On the IV-100B, the blender is mounted as an integral part of the ventilator on the left side. A gas flowmeter is used to adjust the continuous flow through the patient circuit.

The IV-200's blender and flowmeter are internal and have been integrated into the design of the front panel (Figure 9-20). For both ventilators, blended gas passes through a 7 micron filter and then to a regulator, which then reduces the 50 psi line pressure to 20 psi to power the internal fluidic system.

CONTROL CIRCUIT

The control circuit of both ventilators consists of both electronic and fluidic elements (Figure 9-21). To initiate inspiration, the microprocessor sends signals to a solenoid valve which, when closed, sends a reference signal to a back-pressure switch and an OR/NOR gate. The back-pressure switch serves as an on-off control, determining whether the ventilator is in the inspiratory phase (mandatory breath) or expiratory phase.

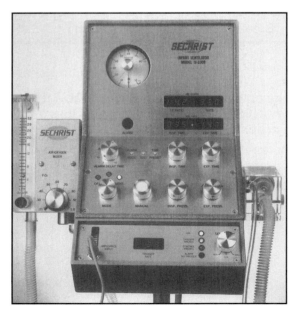

Figure 9-19 *The Sechrist Industries IV-100B ventilator. (Courtesy of Sechrist Industries, Inc., Anaheim, CA)*

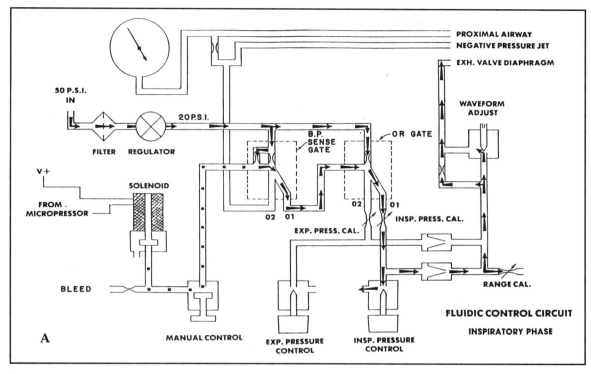

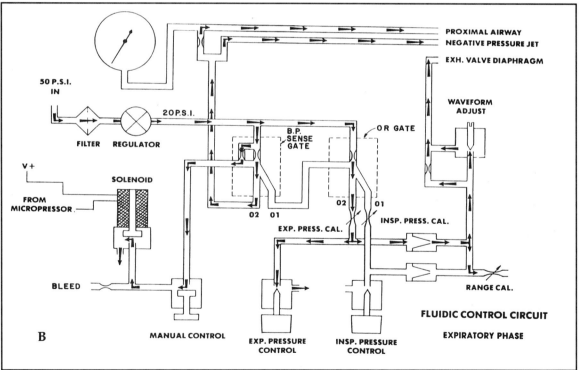

Figure 9-21 *A schematic diagram of the pneumatic system of the Sechrist Industries IV-100B ventilator. (A) Inspiration, (B) Exhalation. (Courtesy Sechrist Industries, Inc., Anaheim, CA)*

In the output 02 state (stable state), the ventilator is in the expiratory phase. Gas flows from 02 on the back-pressure sense gate, and then to a negative pressure jet and the proximal airway pressure line. The negative pressure jet is a venturi that supplies subambient pressure at the exhalation valve. This reduces resistance to flow in the expiratory limb of the circuit from the continuous flow (refer to the exhalation valve in Figure 9-21). Gas supplied to the proximal airway pressure line helps to keep it clear from condensate. A restriction in the line minimizes flow through it.

Either a control signal from the microprocessor, depression of the manual breath control or a signal from the SAVI patient synchronizer module closes the solenoid valve and causes the S control port to be blocked on the back-pressure switch. This causes beam deflection, and the output changes to 01. Output from 01 results in the removal of pressure from the negative pressure jet and proximal airway line. Additionally, a control signal is sent from the back pressure switch to the OR/NOR gate.

The OR/NOR gate controls pressure when inspiratory or expiratory pressure is applied to the exhalation valve diaphragm. The control signal from the back-pressure switch (or absence of one) determines whether the ventilator is in the inspiratory or expiratory phase.

In the expiratory phase, output from the OR/NOR gate is directed to the expiratory pressure control, through a check valve to the waveform adjust control and on to the exhalation valve.

When a control signal from the back-pressure switch is applied to the control port, C3, the OR/NOR gate switches from the stable state, 02, to 01. Output from 01 flows through the inspiratory pressure control, through a check valve, to the waveform adjust control and the exhalation valve.

PEEP/CPAP pressure is controlled by the expiratory pressure control. PEEP/CPAP levels may be adjusted between –2 and 20 cmH$_2$O. The expiratory pressure control is a needle valve that reduces gas pressure from the 20 psi regulator and applies it to the exhalation valve. The needle valve creates a back pressure (expiratory pressure); the excess flow is vented to the atmosphere. Pressure from this control is applied through a check valve to the waveform adjust control and then to the exhalation valve diaphragm, partially closing it. The partially closed diaphragm acts as a threshold resistor, creating the PEEP/CPAP pressure.

CONTROL VARIABLES

The control variables for both ventilators are pressure and flow. During pressure-limited ventilation, the peak inspiratory pressure is controlled by the inspiratory pressure control. This control determines the pressure applied to the exhalation valve diaphragm during the inspiratory phase. Inspiratory pressure may be adjusted between -5 and 70 cmH$_2$O.

A pressure relief level should be set, using the pressure relief valve located on the rear panel of the ventilator above the DISS air and oxygen inlets (IV-100B) or at the lower left on the front (IV-200). The mechanical relief valve is adjustable between 5 and 80 cmH$_2$O, with the relief valve being functional during all modes of ventilation. The relief valve should always be set to a value greater than the expiratory pressure setting in order to act as a safety pop-off.

Flow is a control variable during time cycled, pressure-limited ventilation, in that inspiratory flow will not exceed the value established using the flow meter. Flow is adjustable between 0.0 and 32 liters per minute using the flow meter. Depending on inspiratory time, a given flow may not be sufficient to achieve the set pressure limit, and the ventilator therefore becomes a flow controller.

PHASE VARIABLES

Trigger Variables

The trigger variables for the ventilators include time, manual and electronic triggering. Time triggering is established by the inspiratory and expiratory time control. Inspiratory time is adjustable between 0.1 and 2.9 seconds. An oscillating quartz timer is used to accurately establish inspiratory time. The inspiratory time is displayed using LEDs in the "Insp. Time" display window. Setting the control determines how long the microprocessor will hold the exhalation valve closed through the fluidic control circuit. The expiratory time control sets the time limit for expiration. The same quartz oscillator is used to accurately establish expiratory time. The expiratory time is displayed by LEDs in the "Exp Time" display window. Expiratory times may be set between 0.3 and 60 seconds. The ventilatory rate is 60 divided by the sum of the inspiratory and expiratory time in seconds. The rate and I:E ratio are calculated and displayed above the "Insp." and "Exp." time displays.

ASSEMBLY AND TROUBLESHOOTING

Assembly—IV-100B, IV-200 Ventilators

To prepare the IV-100B and the IV-200 for use, complete the suggested assembly guide. Since the ventilators are very similar, one set of instructions will suffice for both.

1. Assemble and fill a low compressible volume humidifier and attach it to the mounting pole of the ventilator (Figure 9-22). Since a variety of humidifiers may be used, assembly instructions are not included here.

2. Connect the large-bore circuit tubing between the flowmeter outlet and the humidifier inlet.

3. Connect the patient circuit's inspiratory limb to the humidifier outlet and the expiratory limb to the exhalation valve.

4. Connect the proximal airway pressure line to the proximal airway nipple on the exhalation valve block.

5. Connect the temperature probe to the patient wye for the humidifier servo controller.

6. Connect the air and oxygen supply lines to 50 psi gas sources.

7. Connect the power cord to an appropriate AC outlet.

8. If electronic triggering is desired, interface an external impedance, plethysmographic cardiorespiratory monitor to the SAVI Synchronizing Module, using the supplied cable.

Troubleshooting

Refer to the troubleshooting algorithms found at the end of this chapter.

Manual triggering occurs when the practitioner depresses the manual breath button. When depressed, the S control port of the back-pressure switch becomes occluded. This causes the control signal to be sent to the OR/NOR gate, changing its output and closing the exhalation valve. Inspiration will occur as long as the button is depressed and will not be synchronized with the electronic timing circuit.

With the addition of the SAVI monitor, the IV-100B and IV-200 are capable of electronic, patient-triggered ventilation. The ventilator may be servoed to an external impedance, plethysmographic cardiorespiratory monitor. The analog output signal from the cardiorespiratory monitor provides a triggering signal to the SAVI system. By adjusting the sensitivity control, the trigger point may be moved to early or late in the inspiratory phase. Furthermore, the ventilator is able to analyze the impedance of the signal and detect the onset of exhalation. Once exhalation has been detected, the inspiratory phase is terminated and the patient is allowed to exhale. Signals from the respiratory monitor override the normal electronic control and timing mechanism. However, in the absence of any inspiratory effort, the normal timing mechanism acts as a backup system.

Limit Variables

The limit variables for the ventilators include pressure and flow. As already described, pressure is limited to the setting on the inspiratory pressure control. Pressure limits are adjustable from 0 to 70 cmH$_2$O. The inspiratory pressure control is a needle valve that obtains gas from the main, 20 psi regulator. The needle valve creates a back pressure (inspiratory pressure), and excess flow is vented to the atmosphere. Pressure from this control is applied through a check valve to the waveform adjust control and then to the exhalation valve diaphragm, partially closing it.

Flow is a limit variable if the inspiratory pressure is not met during the inspiratory phase. Under these conditions, the ventilator becomes flow limited. Flow is adjusted using the flow meter, and is adjustable from 0.0 to 32 L/min.

Cycle Variable

The cycle variable for the IV-100B and IV-200 is time. Once the time established on the

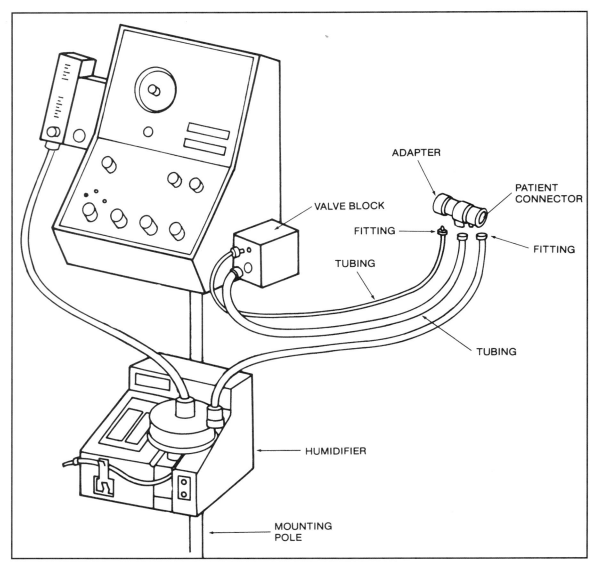

Figure 9-22 *The Sechrist IV-100 and IV-200 circuit.*

inspiratory time control has elapsed, exhalation begins.

Besides time cycling, the IV-100B and IV-200 may be electronically cycled with the addition of the SAVI module. Using the analog output from an external plethysmographic cardiorespiratory monitor, spontaneous patient ventilatory effort can be traced and the ventilator can be synchronized to the patient's breathing efforts. Once the microprocessor has detected the onset of exhalation by analyzing the electronic impedance signal, inspiration is terminated and exhalation begins.

Baseline Variable

The baseline variable for the Sechrist Industries IV-100B and IV-200 is pressure.

PEEP/CPAP pressure may be adjusted between -2 and 20 cmH$_2$O.

OUTPUT WAVEFORMS

Pressure

The output pressure waveform characteristic of the Sechrist IV-100B and IV-200 is rectangular. The rectangular waveform is characteristic during time-cycled, pressure-limited ventilation.

The waveform control can be adjusted such that the output approaches a sinusoidal waveform. The waveform adjust control determines the proximal airway pressure waveform by controlling the rate of the exhalation valve closure and opening. If flow is unimpeded, the valve operation rate is rapid and is essentially a square wave. If the valve impedes flow (sending it through a fixed resistance), the valve operation rate is slowed. This mimics a sine wave flow pattern.

Flow

The flow output waveform for the ventilators is rectangular. This waveform occurs when the peak inspiratory pressure control is set high enough that it is not reached during inspiration. Under these circumstances, the ventilator is operating as a flow controller.

ALARM SYSTEMS

Input Power

Both ventilators have alarms for low gas pressure and loss of electrical power. If either the air or oxygen inlet pressure falls below 25 psi, an audible alarm results. If both source gases fail simultaneously, the ventilator low inspiratory pressure alarm will sound.

If electrical power is lost, audible and visual alarms will result; these are powered by a backup battery supply.

Control Circuit

The IV-100B and IV-200 incorporate a self-test circuit, which checks the microprocessor function. In the event a malfunction has been detected, an audible and visual alarm will alert the practitioner to the failure.

Output Alarms
Pressure

The IV-100B, when supplied with an analog manometer, incorporates a low inspiratory pressure alarm. This alarm consists of a movable needle which is set at a pressure 1 to 2 cmH_2O below the peak inspiratory pressure. The alarm incorporates an infrared sensor into the manometer. The manometer needle must pass the set point within the detection delay time or it will cause the alarm to sound. Primarily, it serves to alert the practitioner to leaks in IMV and disconnects in the CPAP mode.

The detection delay sets the time delay before the alarm is activated. It delay is adjustable between 3 and 60 seconds.

The IV-100B, when used with the an electronic manometer, and the IV-200 incorporate a high-pressure alarm in addition to the low-pressure alarm system.

Tables 9-14 and 9-15 summarize the Sechrist Industries IV-100B and IV-200 ventilator capabilities and alarm systems.

TABLE 9-14: Ventilator Capabilities

IV-100B

Modes	VENT (CMV or IMV)
Rate	1–150 BPM
Inspiratory Time	0.10–2.9 seconds
Expiratory Time	0.3–60 seconds
Expiratory pressure	-2 to 20 cmH_2O
Flow Rate	0.0–32 L/min
Pres. Limit	-5–70 cmH_2O
Mechanical Pop-Off	5–85 cmH_2O
F_IO_2	0.21–1.0

IV-200 and IV-100B
(with an Electronic Manometer)

Modes	VENT (CMV or IMV)
Rate	1–150 BPM
Inspiratory Time	0.10–2.9 seconds
Expiratory Time	0.3–60 seconds
Expiratory pressure	-2–20 cmH_2O
Flow Rate	0.0–32 L/min
Pres. Limit	-5 to 70 cmH_2O
Mechanical Pop-Off	5–85 cmH_2O
F_IO_2	.21–1.0

TABLE 9-15: Sechrist Ventilators Alarm Capabilities

	IV-100B	IV-200
Input Power		
Low Gas Pressure	X	X
Electrical Power	X	X
Control Circuit		
Systems Failure	X	X
Output Alarms		
Pressure:		
High Pressure Limit		X
Low Insp. Pressure	X	X

CHAPTER SUMMARY

Several ventilators have been presented in this chapter that are designed for the pediatric and neonatal patient. These ventilators all have a common characteristic in that flow or pressure is measured and used as a control variable. Table 9-16 may help you to learn the similarities and differences between the ventilators presented in this chapter.

To assist you in troubleshooting refer to the algorithms found in ALG 9-1 and 9-2.

CLINICAL CORNER

BEAR CUB ventilator

1. You have set an inspiratory time of 0.25 seconds and a flow of 9 L/min. What is your approximate tidal volume delivery at these settings?
2. The infant you are assigned to is on a BEAR CUB ventilator. The pressure alarm has been going off about every 5 minutes. What should you check and do to correct the situation?

V.I.P. Bird® Ventilator

1. You have a pediatric patient being ventilated with a V.I.P. Bird® ventilator. Her settings are as follows: rate, 20/min; tidal volume, 125 mL; flow, 60 L/min; pressure, 22 cmH₂O, F₁O₂, 0.45. How would you set your alarm limits?
2. The low inlet gas alarm is sounding—what does this mean?

Sechrist IV-100B and IV-200 Ventilators

1. You have set an inspiratory time of 0.20 seconds and an expiratory time of 1.8 seconds. What are the rate and I:E ratio?
2. In order to use the SAVI triggering capability of the IV-200, what equipment must you have on hand?

TABLE 9-16: Pediatric/Neonatal Ventilators Classifications

Ventilator	Input Power	Circuit	Control Mechanism	Trigger Variable	Limit Variable	Cycling Variable	Alarms
Bear BP-200	Electric	Single	Pneumatic	T/M	P/F	T	I/CC
BEAR CUB	Electric	Single	Pneumatic	T/M	P/F	T	I/CC/P
Babybird	Pneumatic		Pneumatic	T/M	P/F	T	I/CC
Bird® V.I.P.	Electric	Single	Pneumatic	P/T/F/M	P/F	P/V/F/T	I/CC/P/T
Dräger Babylog 8000	Electric	Single	Pneumatic	F/T/M	P/F	P/T	I/CC/P/F/IG
Infrasonics							
Infant Star	Electric	Single	Pneumatic	T/M	P/F	P/T	I/CC/P
Newport Breeze	Electric	Single	Pneumatic	P/T/M	P/F	P/T	I/P/T
Sechrist							
IV-100B	Electric	Single	Fluidic	T/M	P/F	T	I/P
IV-200	Electric	Single	Fluidic	T/M/E	P/F	T/E	I/CC/P

Key: P—Pressure, T—Time, F—Flow, CC—Control Circuit, V—Volume, M—Manual, I—Input Power, E—Electronic, IG—Inspired Gas.

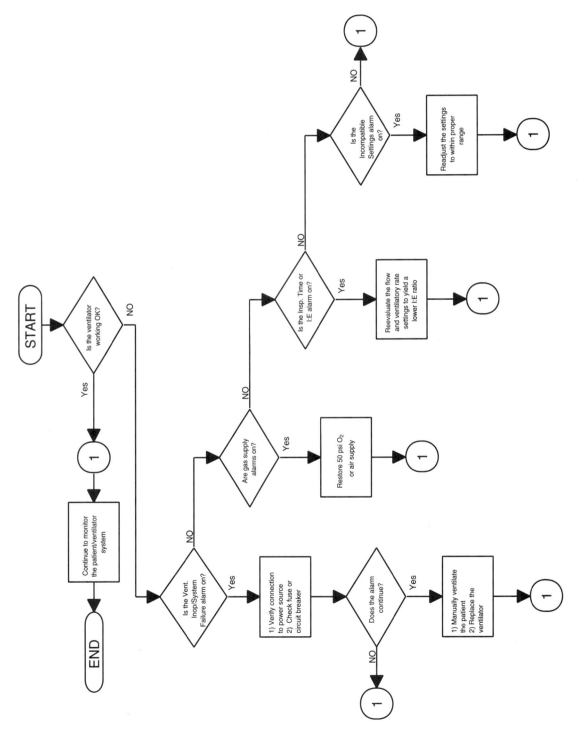

ALG 9-1 *A troubleshooting algorithm for input power and control circuit alarms.*

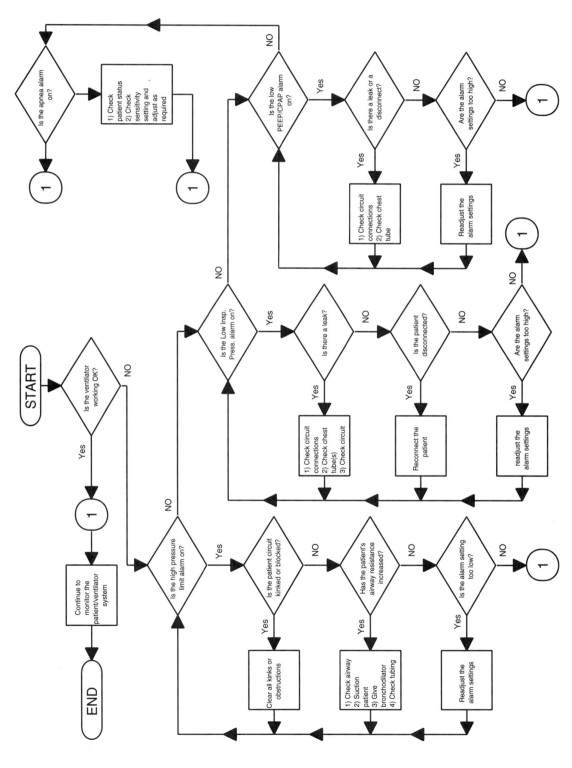

ALG 9-2 *A troubleshooting algorithm for output alarms.*

Self-Assessment Quiz

1. An infant ventilator is operating in pressure-limited, time-cycled ventilation. The inspiratory time is insufficient to allow for the pressure to reach the pressure limit. Under these conditions, which of the following is the control variable?
   a. Pressure.
   b. Volume.
   c. Flow.
   d. Time.

2. An infant ventilator is operating in pressure-limited, time-cycled ventilation. The pressure limit is reached early in the inspiratory phase and is held for the duration of inspiration. Which of the following is the control variable?
   a. Pressure.
   b. Volume.
   c. Flow.
   d. Time.

3. Which of the following infant/pediatric ventilators is (are) capable of pressure support ventilation?
   I. V.I.P. Bird®.
   II. Newport Breeze.
   III. Infrasonics Infant Star.
   IV. Sechrist IV-200.
   a. I
   b. I and II
   c. II and III
   d. I, II, III and IV

4. Which of the following infant/pediatric ventilators must be used with an external monitoring/alarm system?
   a. Bear BP-200.
   b. BEAR CUB.
   c. Sechrist IV-100B.
   d. Newport Breeze.

5. What fluidic element do the Sechrist ventilators use to initiate inspiration?
   a. A back-pressure switch.
   b. A flip-flop.
   c. An OR/NOR gate.
   d. An AND/NAND gate.

6. Which of the following infant/pediatric ventilators are pressure triggered?
   I. V.I.P. Bird®.
   II. Newport Breeze.
   III. Infrasonics Infant Star.
   IV. Sechrist IV-200.
   a. I and II
   b. I and III
   c. II and III
   d. III and IV

7. Which of the following ventilators are time cycled **only**?
   I. BEAR CUB.
   II. Infrasonics Infant Star.
   III. Newport Breeze.
   IV. Sechrist IV-100B.
   a. I and II
   b. I and IV
   c. II and III
   d. II and IV

8. What is the purpose of the mechanical pressure pop-off valve on an infant/pediatric ventilator?
   a. It acts as the pressure limit control.
   b. It determines when inspiration ends.
   c. It is a safety pop-off.
   d. It controls the PEEP/CPAP.

9. Which of the following infant/pediatric ventilators utilizes a manifold of solenoid valves providing flow rates between 4 and 40 L/min?
   a. V.I.P. Bird®.
   b. Newport Breeze.
   c. Infrasonics Infant Star.
   d. Sechrist IV-200.

10. Which of the following infant/pediatric ventilators allows the operator to set one flow rate for spontaneous breaths and another for mechanical breaths?
    a. V.I.P. Bird®.
    b. Newport Breeze.
    c. Infrasonics Infant Star.
    d. Sechrist IV-200.

11. Which of the following infant/pediatric ventilators can be interfaced with an external respiratory monitor for triggering?
    a. V.I.P. Bird®.
    b. Newport Breeze.
    c. Infrasonics Infant Star.
    d. Sechrist IV-200.

12. Which of the following are limit variables for infant/pediatric ventilators?
    I. Pressure.
    II. Volume.
    III. Flow.
    IV. Time.
    a. I and II
    b. I and III
    c. I, II and III
    d. I, II, III and IV

13. Which of the following infant/pediatric ventilators utilize flow as a cycle variable?
    a. V.I.P. Bird®.
    b. Newport Breeze.
    c. Infrasonics Infant Star.
    d. Sechrist IV-200.

14. Which of the following would be examples of a control circuit alarm?
    I. Peak pressure.
    II. I:E ratio.
    III. Low inspiratory pressure.
    IV. Incompatible settings.
    a. I and II
    b. II and III
    c. II and IV
    d. III and IV

15. Which of the following are examples of output alarms?
    I. Peak pressure.
    II. I:E ratio.
    III. Low inspiratory pressure.
    IV. Incompatible settings.
    a. I and II
    b. I and III

   c. II and III

   d. II and IV

16. The Newport Breeze is capable of delivering up to 60 cmH$_2$O PEEP/CPAP. This variable is termed the:

   a. Control variable.

   b. Limit variable.

   c. Cycling variable.

   d. Baseline variable.

17. Which of the following ventilators can deliver a sinusoidal like wave form?

   a. BEAR CUB.

   b. Infrasonics Infant Star.

   c. Newport Breeze.

   d. Sechrist IV-100B.

18. Which of the following ventilators require an exhalation valve as a part of the patient circuit?

   a. BEAR CUB.

   b. Infrasonics Infant Star.

   c. Newport Breeze.

   d. Sechrist IV-100B.

19. An infant/pediatric ventilator is pressure cycled when:

   a. Pressure reaches a preset level and is held for the duration of inspiration.

   b. Pressure reaches a preset level and inspiration is terminated.

   c. Inspiration begins when a preset pressure level is reached.

   d. When the inspiratory pressure falls to baseline.

20. Which of the following is an example of an input power alarm?

   a. Peak pressure.

   b. Low PEEP/CPAP pressure.

   c. F$_I$O$_2$.

   d. Oxygen gas supply disconnect.

21. Exhalation begins when the inspiratory flow drops to a preset value best describes:

   a. Flow triggering.

   b. Flow limiting.

   c. Flow cycling.

   d. Flow controlling.

22. Inspiration begins when the baseline pressure drops to a preset value best describes:

   a. Pressure limiting.

   b. Pressure support.

   c. Pressure triggering.

   d. Pressure controlling.

23. Delivery of a breath to a preset pressure for a specific inspiratory time best describes:

   a. Pressure support.

   b. Pressure control.

   c. Pressure limiting.

   d. Pressure cycling.

24. Which of the following ventilators have an internal battery which can power them if the main electrical power fails?

   I. V.I.P. BIRD®.

   II. Newport Breeze.

   III. Infrasonics Infant Star.

   IV. Sechrist IV-200.

   a. I and II

   b. II and III

   c. I and IV

   d. II and IV

25. Which of the following ventilators have a control circuit alarm?
    I. BEAR CUB.
    II. V.I.P. Bird®.
    III. Infrasonics Infant Star.
    IV. Sechrist IV-200.
    a. I
    b. I and II
    c. I, II, and III
    d. I, II, III and IV

26. When calculating tidal volume delivery when using an infant/pediatric ventilator operating in pressure-limited, time-cycled ventilation, which of the following must be known?
    I. Inspiratory time.
    II. Pressure limit.
    III. Flow.
    IV. Expiratory time.
    a. I and II
    b. I and III
    c. II and III
    d. I and IV

27. You are using a Sechrist IV-100B ventilator. The inspiratory time is 0.2 seconds and the expiratory time is 0.8 seconds. What is the ventilatory rate?
    a. 120 BPM.
    b. 90 BPM.
    c. 60 BPM.
    d. 30 BPM.

28. What is the most common output waveform when the inspiratory pressure limit is set such that flow becomes a control variable?
    a. Rectangular.
    b. Ascending ramp.
    c. Descending ramp.
    d. Sinusoidal.

29. You are using a Bear CUB with the following settings:
    Inspiratory Time   0.6 seconds.
    Pressure Limit   20 cmH$_2$O.
    Ventilator Rate   60 BPM.
    Flow Rate   20 L/min.
    What is the delivered tidal volume (neglecting loss in the ventilator circuit)?
    a. 20 ml.
    b. 60 ml.
    c. 120 ml.
    d. 200 ml.

30. The Babybird ventilator utilizes which of the following in its control circuit?
    a. Electric components.
    b. Electronic components.
    c. Pneumatic components.
    d. Fluidic components.

Selected Bibliography

Barnes, Thomas A., et al., *Core Textbook of Respiratory Care Practice*, 2nd Ed., Mosby-Yearbook, 1994.

Bear Medical Systems, *BEAR CUB Infant Ventilator Model BP 2001, Part # 2937*, Riverside, CA, 1982.

Bird Products Corporation, *Bird® V.I.P. Infant-Pediatric Ventilator Instruction Manual, Part # L1194,* Palm Springs, CA, 1991.

Bourns Life Systems Division, *Bourns Infant Pressure Ventilator Instruction Manual Model BP 200 Part # 500000-10200,* Riverside, CA.

Chatburn, Robert L., "A New System for Understanding Mechanical Ventilators," *Respiratory Care,* Vol. 36, No. 10, pp. 1123–1152, 1991.

Chatburn, Robert L., "Classification of Mechanical Ventilators," *Respiratory Care,* Vol. 37, No. 9, pp. 1009–1025, 1992.

Dupuis, Yvon, *Ventilators: Theory and Clinical Application,* 2nd Ed., Mosby-Yearbook, 1992.

Infrasonics, Inc., *Infant Star Neonatal Ventilator Operating Instructions, Form 9910005,* San Diego, CA, 1989.

Infrasonics, Inc., *Infant Star Ventilator Service and Repair Instructions, Form 9910103,* San Diego, CA, 1992.

Newport Medical Instruments, Inc., *Newport Breeze Ventilator Operating Manual,* Newport Beach, CA, 1991.

Sechrist Industries, Inc., *Operational Instructions and Routine Maintenance Infant Ventilator Model IV-100B, Part Number 1000006,* Anaheim, CA.

CHAPTER 10

HOMECARE AND TRANSPORT VENTILATORS

INTRODUCTION

Homecare and extended care are two of the most rapidly growing segments of the health care environment. Maintenance of mechanically ventilated patients in the home and in extended care and skilled nursing facilities is very common. It is important to understand the unique characteristics of these ventilators and how their capabilities differ from one another.

Transport ventilators are commonly used for ground, airborne and intrahospital patient transports. The use of these ventilators for such special applications is becoming more common. As a practitioner, you should understand how these ventilators operate, how the controls function and how the ventilators differ in their capabilities and operation.

OBJECTIVES

After completing this chapter, the student will accomplish the following objectives:
- For the homecare ventilators described in this chapter, apply Chatburn's classification system and classify them according to:
  — Input power
  — Drive mechanism
  — Control scheme
  — Alarm systems

- For the transport ventilators described in this chapter, apply Chatburn's classification system and classify them according to:
  — Input power
  — Drive mechanism
  — Control scheme
  — Alarm systems

HOMECARE VENTILATORS

NELLCOR PURITAN BENNETT LP20 VENTILATOR

The Nellcor Puritan Bennett LP20 volume ventilator is designed to meet the needs of the homecare and sub–acute care patient (Figure 10-1). The ventilator is electrically powered and microprocessor controlled. It is a volume controller and is either time or pressure triggered. It may be pressure limited and pressure, volume or time cycled. The ventilator may be powered by AC current (120 or 220 volts) or by an external 12 VDC battery. The ventilator may be operated in assist/control, SIMV, or pressure cycled modes.

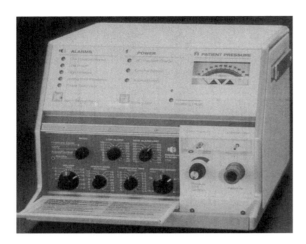

Figure 10-1 *A photograph of the Aequitron Medical, Inc., LP20 ventilator. (Courtesy Aequitron Medical, Inc, Minneapolis, MN)*

Input Power

The LP20 ventilator is electrically powered. The practitioner may choose between 120 volt, 60 Hz, or 220–230 volt, 50-60 Hz, AC power; external, 12 VDC battery; or if charged, an internal battery. If fully charged and in good condition, the internal battery can power the ventilator for 30 to 60 minutes.

If supplemental oxygen is desired, an oxygen elbow may be attached to the ventilator outlet. When so configured, approximately 40% oxygen may be delivered. Alternatively, an oxygen source may be connected to the rear of the ventilator, and when using an external reservoir (3 L anesthesia bag), up to 100% oxygen delivery may be achieved.

Drive Mechanism

The ventilator's drive mechanism consists of an electrically powered, rotary driven piston. Gas enters the piston during its backstroke through a one-way valve and an inlet filter. During the forward stroke, gas is compressed and delivered to the ventilator outlet through another one-way valve. A secondary port adjacent to the ventilator outlet powers the exhalation valve on the patient circuit.

If desired, PEEP can be accommodated by adding an external threshold resistor to the patient circuit. The PEEP valve should be placed proximally to the exhalation valve to minimize volume loss through the latter. Volume loss may be more of a concern when using disposable circuits.

Control Variable

The control variables of the LP20 ventilator are volume and pressure. Volume is a control variable during mandatory breath delivery. Adjustment of the tidal volume control varies the stroke of the piston drive mechanism. Tidal volumes are adjustable between 100 and 2,200 mL.

Pressure becomes a control variable when the pressure limit control is set to a level lower than the high alarm limit control that would normally be reached during a mandatory breath. When the pressure limit is adjusted in this way, excess pressure is vented to the atmosphere and the set pressure limit is maintained. The pressure limit is adjustable between 15 and 50 cmH₂O.

Phase Variables
Trigger Variables

The trigger variables of the LP20 ventilator include pressure and time. Pressure triggering is accomplished by adjusting the breathing effort (sensitivity) control, which may be adjusted between 15 and 50 cmH₂O below baseline pressure. When the trigger pressure has been reached, the ventilator will deliver a mandatory breath (assist/control mode), or if in the SIMV mode, the breathing effort lamp will be illuminated.

Time is a trigger variable in the absence of spontaneous breathing efforts. The rate control establishes the length of time for the ventilatory cycle (inspiration and expiration). Ventilatory rates are adjustable between 22 and 38 breaths per minute in increments of 2 breaths per minute.

Limit Variable

The limit variable for the LP20 is pressure. As already described, if the pressure limit is set lower than the normal peak pressure for a given tidal volume, the pressure will rise to that level and be held constant. Excess pressure during inspiration will be vented to the atmosphere.

Cycle Variables

The cycle variables for the LP20 include pressure, volume and time. Pressure becomes a cycle variable when the peak inspiratory pressure exceeds the value set on the high-pressure alarm. When this condition is met, inspiration is terminated and both audible and

ASSEMBLY AND TROUBLESHOOTING

Assembly—Nellcor Puritan Bennett LP20 Ventilator

To assemble the Nellcor Puritan Bennett LP20 ventilator for use, follow the suggested assembly guide.

1. Select a power source:
   a. Connect the ventilator to an appropriate AC power source.
   b. Connect the ventilator to an external 12 VDC, deep-cycle battery using the supplied cables and observing the correct polarity (red = positive, and black = negative)
   c. If the internal battery is charged, the ventilatory may be operated for up to 30 to 60 minutes.

2. Assemble the patient circuit
   a. Attach one end of the 16-inch, 22-mm diameter tubing to the ventilator outlet and the other end to a heated humidifier.
   b. Connect one end of the 60-inch, 22-mm diameter tubing to the humidifier outlet and the other to the exhalation manifold.
   c. Attach the proximal line and the exhalation valve drive line to the exhalation manifold.
   d. Attach a 4- or 6-inch tracheostomy flex tube to the exhalation manifold and the appropriate patient interface to the other end.
   e. Connect the exhalation valve to the exhalation valve port fitting on the ventilator, using 1/8-inch, small-diameter tubing.
   f. Connect the proximal pressure line to the patient pressure fitting on the ventilator using 1/4-inch tubing.

Troubleshooting

To assist you in troubleshooting the ventilator, refer to the algorithms at the end of this chapter.

---

visual alarms are activated. High-pressure alarm limits may be set between 15 and 90 cmH$_2$O in increments of 5 cmH$_2$O.

Volume is a cycle variable during mandatory breath delivery if neither the high-pressure limit nor the pressure limit setting is met. Under these circumstances, gas delivery ceases when the piston reaches the end of its stroke. Tidal volumes are adjustable between 100 and 2,200 mL.

Time becomes a cycle variable if the pressure limit has been reached before the end of inspiration. Under these circumstances, the breath will be time cycled (determined by the inspiratory time). Inspiratory times are adjustable between 0.5 and 1.0 second in increments of 0.1 and 1.2 seconds. Inspiratory times may also be adjusted between 1.5 and 5.5 seconds in increments of 0.5 seconds.

Output Waveforms

The flow output of the ventilator is a sinusoidal waveform. This results from the ventilator having a rotary-driven, piston drive mechanism (refer to Chapter 6). Although the flow waveform is sinusoidal, the pressure assumes a sigmoidal shape, with peak pressures occurring at differing times from the peak flow values.

Alarm Systems
Input Power

When operating on an external battery, the ventilator will indicate this condition by the illumination of the amber-colored, external battery LED.

When the ventilator is operating on the internal battery, a flashing amber LED and an audible tone, which sounds every 5 minutes, will alert the clinician that the ventilator is operating on the internal battery. If fully charged and in good condition, the internal battery can power the ventilator up to 10 hours.

If the ventilator switches from a higher power source to a lower one (i.e., from AC to

DC power source), a pulsating tone will signify the event. No alarm sounds will occur when switching from a lower power source to a higher one, however.

Control Circuit Alarm

Microprocessor Failure

In the event that a microprocessor malfunction is detected, a steady-tone (audible) alarm will result. In this event, the clinician should provide an alternate means of ventilation for the patient and remove the ventilator from service.

Settings Error

If the clinician establishes settings beyond the capabilities of the ventilator, a audible and a flashing setting error/presilence LED will be illuminated. Control settings must be within range for the alarm to silence.

Output Alarms

Pressure

The LP20 ventilator has both high and low airway pressure alarms. Both alarms incorporate LEDs and an audible, pulsating tone. The low-pressure alarm is adjustable between 2 and 32 cmH₂O in 2-cmH₂O increments. The high-pressure alarm is adjustable between 15 and 90 cmH₂O in 5-cmH₂O increments. (The high-pressure alarm was already described, in the "cycling variables" section.) The low-pressure alarm helps alert the clinician to patient disconnects and leaks and is activated following two ventilator breaths.

Tables 10-1 and 10-2 summarize the LP20 ventilator's alarms and capabilities.

TABLE 10-1: Nellcor Puritan Bennett LP20 Alarm Systems

Input power

Low Battery

Power Switch-over

Control circuit

Microprocessor Failure

Settings Error

Output alarms

High Pressure	15 to 90 cmH₂O
Low Pressure	2 to 32 cmH₂O

TABLE 10-2: Nellcor Puritan Bennett LP20 Ventilator Capabilities

Modes	Assist/control, SIMV, pressure cycle
Volume	100 to 2200 ml
Breath rate	1 to 20 breaths/min in 1 breath/min increments; 22 to 38 breaths/min in 2 breath/min increments
Pressure limit	15 to 50 cmH₂O
Inspiratory time	0.5 to 1.0 seconds in 0.1 and 1.2 second increments; 1.5 to 5.5 seconds in 0.5 second increments
Sensitivity	-10 to +10 cmH₂O
F₁O₂	0.40 to 1.0

AEQUITRON MEDICAL, INC., LP6 PLUS AND LP10

The Aequitron Medical's LP6 PLUS volume ventilator is designed to meet the needs of homecare patients (Figure 10-2). The LP10 volume ventilator differs from the LP6 PLUS in that a pressure limit control is provided for pressure-limited ventilation (Figure 10-3). The

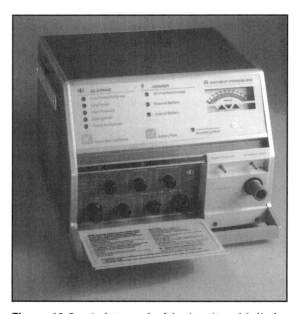

Figure 10-2 *A photograph of the Aequitron Medical, Inc., LP6 PLUS Volume Ventilator (Courtesy Aequitron Medical, Inc.)*

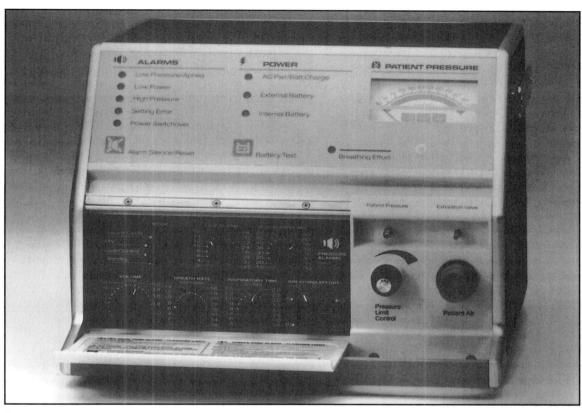

Figure 10-3 *A photograph of the Aequitron Medical, Inc., LP10 Volume Ventilator (Courtesy Aequitron Medical, Inc.)*

LP10 ventilator is intended to meet the needs of those patients requiring volume and/or pressure ventilation modalities. Both ventilators are microprocessor-controlled volume controllers which can be time or pressure triggered. The ventilators may be pressure limited and pressure, volume or time cycled. The ventilators may be operated from 120 or 220 volt electrical power or operated by an internal or external 12 volt DC battery. Since so many features are common between the two ventilators, they will be presented together. When differences occur, they will be presented and compared.

INPUT POWER

The ventilators are electrically powered, and the practitioner has several choices regarding the power source. Standard electrical power of 120 volt, 60 Hz (United States) or 220–230 volt, 50–60 Hz (international) may be selected. Additionally, the ventilators may be powered for up to 1 hour using the internal 12 volt DC battery, if fully charged. Alternatively, an external, deep-cycle, 12 volt DC bat-

tery may be used to power the ventilators.

If supplemental oxygen is required, an oxygen elbow may be added to the outlet of the ventilators, which can provide an F_IO_2 of up to 0.4. Oxygen concentration is increased by bleeding in oxygen at the elbow to achieve the desired F_IO_2. If a higher oxygen concentration is required, an oxygen enrichment kit may be added to the filter port on the rear of the ventilator to increase the oxygen concentration delivered to the patient. Through the use of this kit, the F_IO_2 may be increased to 1.0.

DRIVE MECHANISM

Both ventilators utilize an electrically powered, rotary driven, 2.2 liter piston. Gas enters the piston during its backstroke through a one-way valve and an inlet filter (Figure 10-4, A and B). During the forward stroke, gas is compressed and delivered to the patient air port through another one-way valve. A port adjacent to the patient air port powers the exhalation valve, closing it.

If desired, an optional PEEP valve may be

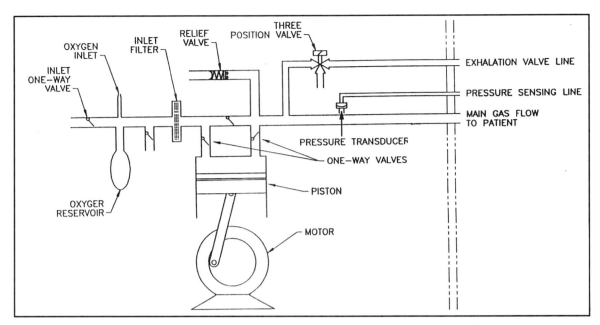

Figure 10-4A *A schematic diagram of the Aequitron Medical, Inc., LP6 PLUS Volume Ventilator pneumatic system (Courtesy Aequitron Medical, Inc.)*

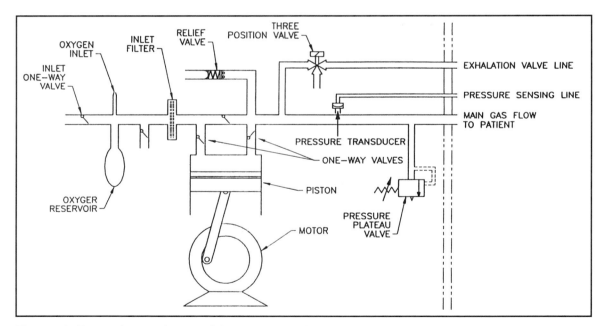

Figure 10-4B *A schematic diagram of the Aequitron Medical, Inc., LP10 Volume Ventilator pneumatic system (Courtesy Aequitron Medical, Inc.)*

added to the patient circuit's exhalation valve. This valve should be added proximally to the exhalation valve to minimize any potential volume losses through the latter. If the PEEP valve is located distal to the exhalation valve, a pressure gradient may develop between the PEEP valve and the exhalation valve diaphragm, preventing it from completely sealing under some circumstances and resulting in a loss of delivered volume. This effect may be more prominent when using disposable circuits.

CONTROL VARIABLES

The control variable for the LP6 PLUS ventilator is volume, while the control variables for the LP10 ventilator are both pressure and volume.

Pressure is a control variable for the LP10

when the pressure limit control is set to a level that is lower than the high alarm limit control and the peak pressure that would normally be reached during a mechanical breath. When the pressure limit is adjusted in this way and the pressure limit has been reached, excess pressure is vented to the atmosphere and the set pressure limit is maintained. When operated in this way the ventilator becomes a pressure controller. The pressure limit is adjustable between 15 and 50 cmH$_2$O.

The volume control determines the tidal volume delivered with each breath. Adjustment of this control varies the stroke of the piston, and therefore the tidal volume. Tidal volumes may be adjusted between 100 and 2200 mL. Volume is adjusted at a rate of 100 mL per machine cycle (piston stroke) until the desired volume has been reached.

PHASE VARIABLES

Trigger Variables

The trigger variables for the ventilators include pressure and time. The ventilators may be pressure triggered by adjusting the breathing effort control. This control sets the trigger sensitivity level and is adjustable from −10 to +10 cmH$_2$O. When the pressure in the patient circuit (measured at the proximal airway) falls to the adjusted level, a ventilator assisted breath is triggered (Assist/Control), or if in the spontaneous portion of SIMV, the breathing effort lamp will be illuminated.

The ventilators are time triggered in the absence of any spontaneous ventilatory efforts. The breath rate control establishes the length of time for the ventilatory cycle (inspiration and expiration). Ventilatory rates are adjustable between 1 and 20 breaths per minute (in 1 breath per minute increments), and 22 to 38 breaths per minute (in 2 breath per minute increments).

Limit Variables

As already described, if the mechanical pressure limit valve (LP10) is adjusted to less than the high alarm limit control and less than the peak inspiratory pressure, airway pressure will not exceed that level of adjustment. Under these circumstances, the ventilator is a pressure controller. Excess pressure is vented through the pressure limit valve to the atmosphere, maintaining the set pressure limit for the remaining tidal volume delivery.

Cycle Variables

The cycle variables for the ventilators include pressure, volume and time. The ventilators are pressure cycled when the peak inspiratory pressure exceeds the pressure level set on the high alarm limit control. When this condition is met, inspiration is terminated and both audible and visual alarms are activated. High alarm limits are adjustable between 15 and 90 cmH$_2$O in 5 cmH$_2$O increments.

The ventilators are volume cycled during mechanical breath delivery if both the high alarm limit and pressure limit settings are not reached. Under these circumstances gas delivery ceases when the piston reaches the end of its travel. Tidal volumes are adjustable between 100 and 2,200 mL.

If the pressure limit has been reached prior to the end of inspiration, the breath will be time cycled and will be terminated after the set inspiratory time has elapsed. Inspiratory times are adjustable between 0.5 and 1.0 seconds in 0.1 second increments, 1.0 and 1.2 seconds in 0.2 second increments, and 1.5 and 5.5 seconds in 0.5 second increments. The inspiratory time control adjusts the motor speed and determines the time required to deliver the selected tidal volume. The inspiratory time control, in conjunction with the tidal volume control, determines the inspiratory flow. Inspiratory flow is equal to the tidal volume divided by the inspiratory time.

OUTPUT WAVEFORMS

The output flow waveforms for the ventilators are sinusoidal. This results from the fact that the piston accelerates at different rates depending upon the wheel and connecting rod positions (refer to Chapter 6). Although the flow waveform is sinusoidal, the pressure waveform assumes a sigmoidal shape, with the peak values occurring at differing times.

ALARM SYSTEMS

Input Alarms

When operating on an external battery, the ventilators will indicate it by the illumination of the amber colored external battery LED.

When the ventilators are operating on the internal battery, an amber LED will flash and an audible tone will sound every 5 minutes, alerting the practitioner that the ventilator is operating on the internal battery. If the internal battery fails to charge or if its charge is

ASSEMBLY AND TROUBLESHOOTING

Assembly—Aequitron Volume Ventilators

To assemble the Aequitron Medical, Inc. volume ventilators for use, follow the suggested assembly guide.

1. Select a power source:
   a. Connect the ventilator to an external power source (120 volt, 60 Hz, or 220–230 volt, 50–60 Hz) outlet and select the appropriate power source on the rear of the ventilator.
   b. Connect the ventilator to an external, 12VDC deep-cycle battery using the supplied cables and observing the correct polarity (red is "+" and black is "–").
   c. If the internal battery is charged, the ventilator may be operated for 45 to 60 minutes on the internal battery.
2. Assemble the patient circuit:
   a. Attach one end of the 16-inch, 22-mm diameter tubing to the ventilator outlet and the other to a heated humidifier. Suitable humidifiers include the Bird Wick, Fisher Paykel MR 410 or MR 480, Puritan Bennett Cascade, or any other high-efficiency, heated humidifiers.
   b. Connect one end of the 60-inch, 22-mm diameter tubing to the humidifier outlet and the other to the exhalation manifold.
   c. Attach the proximal line and the exhalation valve drive line to the exhalation manifold.
   d. Attach a 4- or 6-inch tracheostomy flextube to the exhalation manifold and an appropriate patient interface to the other end.
   e. Connect the exhalation valve to the exhalation valve port fitting on the ventilator.
   f. Connect the proximal pressure line to the patient pressure fitting on the ventilator.

Troubleshooting

To assist you in troubleshooting the ventilators, refer to the algorithms at the end of this chapter.

low, both audible and visual (Low Power LED) alarms will alert the practitioner to the event.

If the ventilators switch from a higher power source to a lower one, a pulsating tone will signify the event (i.e., from an AC to a DC power source). No alarm sounds will occur when switching from a low power source to a higher one (i.e., DC power source to AC; internal battery to external battery).

Control Circuit Alarm
General Systems Failure

In the event that a microprocessor malfunction is detected, a steady-tone audible alarm will result. In the event this occurs, ensure that the patient is being ventilated by other means and remove the ventilator from service.

Settings Error

The setting error alarm is activated when the practitioner sets control settings that are out of the range the ventilators can achieve. Control settings must be within range for the alarm to silence. The alarm consists of a pulsating audible tone.

Output Alarms
Pressure

The ventilators incorporate high- and low-pressure alarms. Both alarms incorporate LEDs and an audible, pulsating tone. The low pressure alarm is adjustable between 2 and 32 cmH_2O in 2 cmH_2O increments. The high alarm limit is adjustable between 15 and 90 cmH_2O in 5 cmH_2O increments. (The function of the high-pressure alarm was described in the "cycling variables" section.) The low pressure alarm is helpful in alerting the practitioner to patient disconnects and leaks, and is activated following two ventilator breaths.

Tables 10-3 and 10-4 summarize the Aequitron Medical, Inc., LP6 PLUS and LP10 ventilators' capabilities and alarm systems.

TABLE 10-3: Aequitron Medical Inc., Volume Ventilator Capabilities

Modes	Assist/Control, SIMV, Pressure Control
Volume	100 to 2200 mL
Breath Rate	1 to 20 (1 breath per minute increments)
	22 to 38 (2 breaths per minute increments)
Press. Limit	15 to 50 cmH$_2$O (LP10 only)
Insp. Time	0.5 to 1.0 second (0.1 second increments)
	1.0 to 1.2 seconds (0.2 second increments)
	1.5 to 5.5 seconds (0.5 second increments)
Sensitivity	-10 to 10 cmH$_2$O
F$_I$O$_2$	.21 to .40 (Oxygen elbow attachment)
	.40 to 1.0 (Oxygen enrichment kit attachment)

BEAR MEDICAL SYSTEMS, INC., BEAR 33

The BEAR 33 volume ventilator is a microprocessor controlled, rotary driven, piston ventilator capable of control, assist/control and SIMV modes (Figure 10-5). It is a volume controller, which may be flow limited and may be pressure, volume, or time cycled.

INPUT POWER

The BEAR 33 ventilator may be powered by AC power (120 volt, 60 Hz or 220-230 volt, 50-60 Hz), an internal 12 VDC battery or an external, deep-cycle 12 VDC battery.

If supplemental oxygen is required, an oxygen source may be connected to the oxygen accumulator nipple on the front of the ventilator. A 9-inch-long section of 22-mm, large-bore tubing is then connected between the accumulator outlet and the gas inlet port directly above it. The percentage of oxygen delivered to the patient varies depending upon the tidal volume and respiratory rate.

TABLE 10-4: Aequitron Medical, Inc., Volume Ventilator Alarm Systems

Input Power

Low Battery

Power Switch-over

Control Circuit

Microprocessor Failure

Settings Error

Output Alarms

High Pressure 15 to 90 cmH$_2$O

Low Pressure 2 to 32 cmH$_2$O

DRIVE MECHANISM

On the reverse stroke of the piston, gas is drawn into the cylinder from the oxygen accumulator through a filter and a check valve (Figure 10-6). As already described, if oxygen-enriched gas is desired, the oxygen accumulator may be connected to an oxygen source.

During the inspiratory phase (forward piston stroke), gas flows through a check valve into the patient circuit (Figure 10-6). Two other gas lines originate near the output of the cylinder. These include a line that powers the exhalation valve and a line that purges the proximal airway line.

The line powering the exhalation valve is attached to the overpressure relief valve, the pressure limit valve and the sigh solenoid. Should excessive pressure build within the circuit, two relief valves ensure that excessive pressure is not delivered to the patient. The sigh solenoid delivers 1.5 times the tidal volume (up to 80 cmH$_2$O) when the sigh system is on.

The proximal airway purge line reduces the condensate in the proximal airway line by purging it with a small volume of gas during inspiration. The inspiratory pressure transducer and other electronic components inside the ventilator could be harmed if excessive moisture were to enter the ventilator.

PEEP may be accomplished by adding an external threshold resistor valve to the patient circuit. This valve should be added proximal

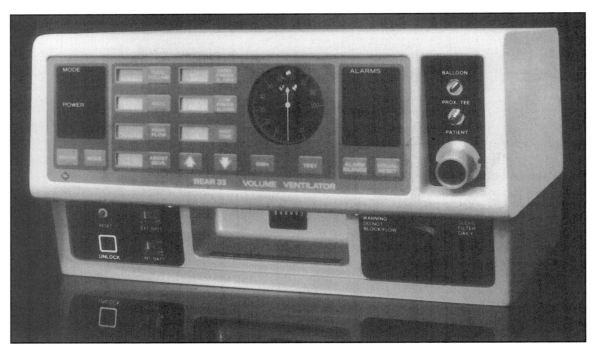

Figure 10-5 *A photograph of the Bear Medical Systems, Inc., BEAR 33 Volume Ventilator. (Courtesy of Bear Medical Systems, Inc., Riverside, CA)*

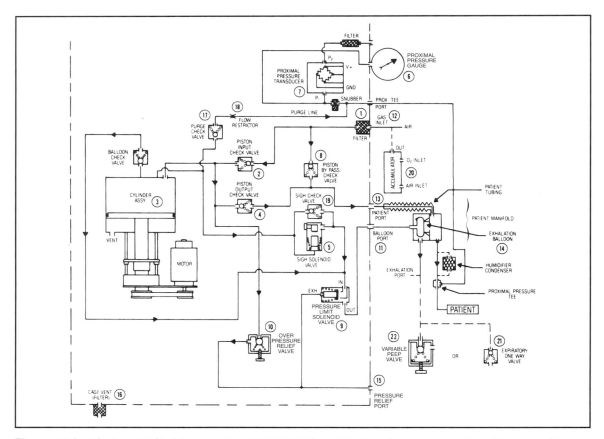

Figure 10-6 *The Bear Medical Systems, Inc., BEAR 33 Volume Ventilator's pneumatic system. (Courtesy of Bear Medical Systems, Inc.)*

to the exhalation valve to minimize any potential volume losses through the exhalation valve. If the PEEP valve is located distal to the exhalation valve, a pressure gradient may develop between the PEEP valve and the exhalation valve diaphragm, preventing it from completely sealing and, under some circumstances, resulting in a loss of delivered volume. This effect may be more prominent when using disposable circuits.

CONTROL VARIABLE

The control variable for the BEAR 33 ventilator is volume. The tidal volume control allows adjustment of the tidal volumes between 100 mL and 2,200 mL, with incremental adjustments of 10 mL. The tidal volume control determines the stroke of the piston, and therefore, the volume of gas contained within the cylinder.

PHASE VARIABLES

Trigger Variables

The trigger variables for the BEAR 33 ventilator are pressure and time. The trigger variable is adjusted using the assist sensitivity control. Sensitivity is adjustable between -9 and 19 cmH$_2$O in increments of 1 cmH$_2$O. Adjustment of the control establishes a reference value that the microprocessor uses to compare with what the proximal pressure transducer measures. When the values equal one another, a ventilator assisted breath is delivered. When operated in Control mode, the sensitivity control is inactive and inspiratory efforts will not be recognized by the microprocessor.

The ventilator is time triggered in the absence of any spontaneous ventilatory efforts. The rate control establishes the length of time for the ventilatory cycle (inspiration and expiration). Ventilatory rates are adjustable between 2 and 40 breaths per minute. Between the rates of 2 and 20 breaths per minute, the rate may be adjusted in increments of 0.5 breaths per minute. Between the rates of 10 and 40 breaths per minute, the rate may be adjusted in increments of 1 breath per minute.

Limit Variable

Flow is the limit variable for the BEAR 33 ventilator. Flow becomes a limit variable if the peak flow control is set such that the flow rate value is met early during inspiration and is held for the remainder of the inspiratory time. Peak flow rates are adjustable between 20 and 120 L/min in 1 L/min increments. The peak flow control changes the speed of the electric drive motor during the forward stroke of the piston, adjusting the flow rate.

Cycle Variables

The cycle variables for the BEAR 33 ventilator include pressure, volume and time. Pressure becomes a cycle variable when the inspiratory pressure exceeds the value set on the high pressure alarm. The high pressure alarm is adjustable between 10 and 80 cmH$_2$O. Once the alarm limit is reached, the piston stops its forward travel (terminating the breath), the alarm indicator illuminates, the pressure limit solenoid valve opens and the exhalation valve on the circuit depressurizes. If two consecutive breaths exceed the pressure limit, an audible alarm will sound as well.

Volume becomes a cycle variable if the ventilator-assisted breath is not terminated before either the pressure limit or inspiratory time has been met. Under these circumstances, inspiration ends following delivery of the volume contained within the piston.

Volume is also a cycle variable when sighs have been selected. Under these circumstances, a volume of 1.5 times the set tidal volume or 3,300 mL (whichever is less), will be delivered 6 times per hour. Both the high-pressure alarm and the expiratory time are automatically lengthened by 50% whenever sigh mode is selected. This precludes the delivery of stacked breaths.

Time may be a cycle variable if the inspiratory time control is adjusted so that inspiration is terminated prior to the delivery of the volume contained within the piston. Inspiratory time is adjustable between 0.25 and 4.99 seconds. Under these circumstances, the inspiratory time LCD will flash *0.25* and another parameter (tidal volume or peak flow) will also flash, indicating that the limiting factor is insufficient inspiratory time.

OUTPUT WAVEFORMS

Pressure, Volume and Flow

The flow output waveform for the ventilator is sinusoidal. This results from the fact that the piston accelerates at different rates, depending upon the wheel and connecting rod positions (refer to Chapter 6). Although the flow waveform is sinusoidal, the pressure

ASSEMBLY AND TROUBLESHOOTING

Assembly—BEAR 33

To assemble the BEAR Medical Systems, Inc., BEAR 33 volume ventilator, follow the suggested assembly guide.

1. Connect the ventilator to an appropriate power source:
   a. External, deep-cycle 12 VDC battery.
   b. AC wall electrical supply (120 volt, 60 Hz, or 220–230 volt, 50-60 Hz).
   c. Internal battery if fully charged

2. Assemble the patient circuit:
   a. Attach one end of the 18-inch, 22-mm diameter tubing to the ventilator outlet and the other end to a heated humidifier. Suitable humidifiers would include the BEAR VH-820, Bird Wick, Fisher

Paykel or other high efficiency humidifiers.
   b. Connect one end of the 60-inch, 22-mm diameter tubing to the humidifier outlet and the other to the patient manifold.
   c. Attach the proximal pressure tee to the patient manifold and a 4- or 6-inch tracheostomy flextube to its outlet.
   d. Connect the exhalation valve to the balloon fitting on the ventilator.
   e. Connect the proximal pressure line to the Prox. Tee fitting on the ventilator.

Troubleshooting

To assist you in troubleshooting the ventilators, refer to the algorithms at the end of this chapter.

---

waveform assumes a sigmoidal shape, with the peak values occuring at different times.

Alarm Systems
Input Alarms
Input Power

The BEAR 33 ventilator low-battery alarm will be triggered if the internal battery falls below 25% of its operating capacity. This represents approximately 15 minutes of operation. The alarm is a continuous, audible alarm accompanied by a flashing alarm indication. This alarm may not be reset. If the ventilator is being powered by the internal battery and the alarm sounds, an alternative power source must be provided (wall AC or an external battery).

The power change alarm will activate when the ventilator switches power sources. For example, if an external, deep-cycle battery becomes discharged or the AC power cord becomes disconnected, the ventilator will automatically switch to internal battery power. Under these circumstances, the visual and audible power change alarm will alert the practitioner to the event. This alarm may be reset using the visual reset control.

Control Circuit Alarms

In the event that a microprocessor error or problem has been detected, the BEAR 33 ventilator will default to the parameters listed in Table 10-5.

Under these circumstances, make sure the patient is receiving alternative ventilation and turn the power switch off and then back on. If the ventilator enters the default condition again, remove it from service and contact a qualified biomedical repair facility.

TABLE 10-5: Default Parameters

Rate	16 BPM
Volume	500 mL
Flow	35 L/min
Hi Press.	40 cmH$_2$O
Lo Press.	10 cmH$_2$O
Mode	Assist/Control
Sensitivity	−1.0 cmH$_2$O

Output Alarms
Pressure

As already described ("cycle variables" section), the BEAR 33 ventilator has a high-pressure alarm, which is adjustable between 10 and 80 cmH₂O. The BEAR's low-pressure alarm is adjustable between 3 and 70 cmH₂O. During inspiration, if the inspiratory pressure fails to reach the alarm threshold, the low pressure alarm will flash. If on a second breath the same event occurs, an audible alarm will sound and the flashing display will change to a steady illumination. If, on the second breath, inspiratory pressure exceeds the threshold value, the visual indicator will automatically reset to the off condition.

Time

An apnea alarm will be triggered if a breath has not occurred for 20 seconds during mechanical or spontaneous breathing. Both audible and visual alarms will trigger after this time interval. If a breath occurs after the alarm condition has been met, the audible alarm will cancel and the visual display will continue to be illuminated until it is reset.

Tables 10-6 and 10-7 summarize the BEAR 33 volume ventilator's capabilities and alarms systems.

TABLE 10-7: BEAR 33 Ventilator Alarm Systems

Input Power	
Low Battery	
Power Switch-over	

Control Circuit	
Ventilator Inoperative	

Output Alarms	
Pressure	
High Pressure	10 to 80 cmH₂O
Low Pressure	3 to 70 cmH₂O

Time	
Apnea	

LIFECARE PLV-100 AND PLV-102

The Lifecare PLV-100 and PLV-102 volume ventilators are electrically powered, linearly driven piston ventilators. The PLV-100 (Figure 10-7) is capable of operating in control, assist/control and SIMV modes. The PLV-102 (Figure 10-8) is capable of operating in control, assist/control and SIMV modes and providing sighs in control and assist control modes. Both ven-

TABLE 10-6: BEAR 33 Capabilities

Modes	Control, Assist/Control, SIMV, Sigh
Volume	100 to 2,200 mL
Breath Rate	2 to 10 (0.5 breath per minute increments)
	10 to 40 (1 breath per minute increments)
Insp. Time	0.25 to 3.99 seconds
Peak Flow	20 to 120 L/min
Sigh Volume	150% of tidal volume at 6 sighs per hour
Sensitivity	–9 to 19 cmH₂O
F₁O₂	.21 to 1.0

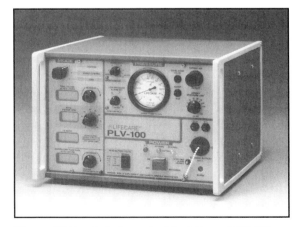

Figure 10-7 *A photograph of the Lifecare PLV-100 Volume Ventilator. (Courtesy of Lifecare, Inc. Lafayette, CO)*

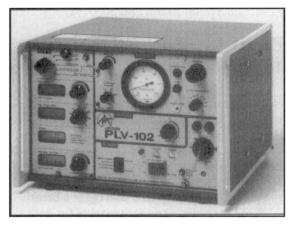

Figure 10-8 *A photograph of the Lifecare PLV-102 Volume Ventilator. (Courtesy of Lifecare, Inc.)*

tilators are volume controllers that are pressure or time triggered and volume or pressure cycled.

INPUT POWER

The ventilators may be powered from three power sources: AC electrical current, 12 VDC,

deep-cycle, external batteries and a 12 VDC internal battery. When powered by AC current, either 120 volt, 60 Hz (U.S. model) or 220 volt, 60 Hz (international model) may be used.

If supplemental oxygen is required, a 50 psi medical oxygen source must be connected to the DISS fitting on the rear of the ventilator (PLV-102). To provide supplemental oxygen for the PLV-100, an oxygen inlet adaptor must be added between the ventilator outlet and the humidifier (Figure 10-9), and oxygen must be bled in to provide the desired F_iO_2.

DRIVE MECHANISM

Both ventilators utilize a linearly driven piston. During the backstroke of the piston, gas is drawn through a check valve and an intake filter to the piston (Figure 10-9, PLV-100; Figure 10-10, PLV-102). The piston compresses the gas during the forward stroke (inspiration), causing gas to flow to the patient circuit exhalation valve, safety pop-off (mechanical), solenoid dump valve and a pressure transducer.

PEEP may be accomplished by adding an

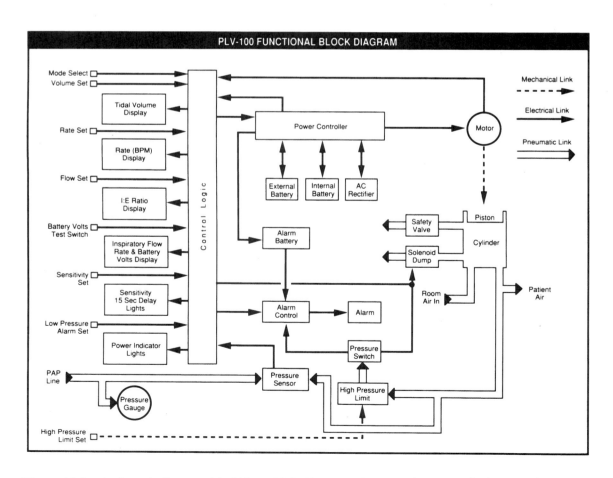

Figure 10-9 *A schematic diagram of the Lifecare PLV-100 pneumatic system. (Courtesy of Lifecare, Inc.)*

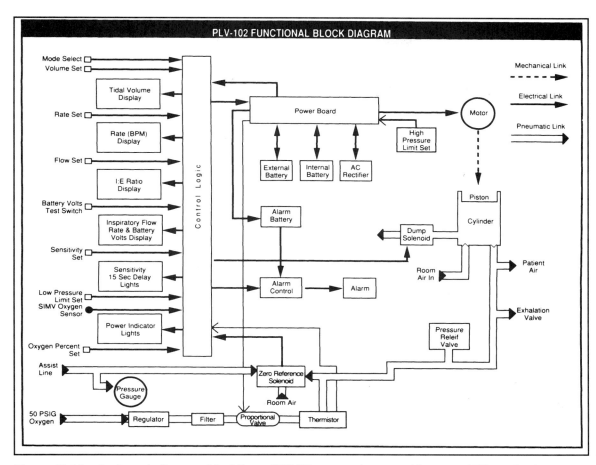

PLV-102 FUNCTIONAL BLOCK DIAGRAM

Figure 10-10 *A schematic diagram of the Lifecare PLV-102 pneumatic system. (Courtesy of Lifecare, Inc.)*

external threshold resistor valve to the patient circuit. This valve should be added proximal to the exhalation valve to minimize any potential volume losses through the exhalation valve. If the PEEP valve is located distal to the exhalation valve, a pressure gradient may develop between the PEEP valve and the exhalation valve diaphragm, preventing it from completely sealing under some circumstances and resulting in a loss of delivered volume. This effect may be more prominent when using disposable circuits.

CONTROL VARIABLE

The control variable for both ventilators is volume. The tidal volume control determines the length of the piston's backward stroke and, therefore, the volume within the cylinder. During the forward stroke (inspiration), the volume in the cylinder (tidal volume) is delivered to the patient. Tidal volumes are adjustable between 50 mL and 3,000 mL.

PHASE VARIABLES

Trigger Variables

The trigger variables for the ventilators include pressure and time. Pressure is a trigger variable during assist/control ventilation. Pressure triggering is adjusted using the sensitivity control. The sensitivity may be adjusted between –6 and 3 cmH_2O (PLV-100) and –5 and 18 cmH_2O (PLV-102). This control determines the patient effort required to trigger a breath.

Time becomes a trigger variable for both ventilators in the absence of any spontaneous patient effort. This trigger variable is adjusted using the rate control. Respiratory rates may be adjusted between 2 and 40 breaths per minute.

Limit Variables

The limit variable for the ventilators is pressure. Pressure limit is adjustable between 5 and 89 cmH_2O (PLV-100) and 10 and 100 cmH$_2$O (PLV-102). When the pressure limit is reached, excess pressure is vented to the atmosphere and the piston continues its forward stroke. Thus inspiration does not end when the pressure limit is met.

Cycle Variables

The cycle variable for the PLV-100 and PLV-102 is volume. Volume is a cycle variable during mechanical breath delivery. Under these circumstances, the delivery of the full tidal volume determines the end of inspiration. Volume is also a cycle variable during sigh delivery (PLV-102). When sigh delivery is selected, a volume equal to 150% of the set tidal volume is delivered every 100 breaths.

OUTPUT WAVEFORMS

Pressure, Volume and Flow

The flow output waveform for the ventilators are sinusoidal. This results from the fact that the piston accelerates at different rates. Even though the piston is linearly driven, the microprocessor alters its acceleration to mimic a rotary driven piston's flow pattern. Thus, although the flow waveform is sinusoidal, the pressure waveform is sigmoid in shape. The peak values of the flow and pressure waveforms occur at different times.

ALARM SYSTEMS

Input Alarms
Loss of Electrical Power

In the event that the ventilators are turned on and no power is connected (no AC or external 12 VDC battery or a deeply discharged, internal battery), an alarm will sound.

An audible alarm will be activated if the practitioner attempts to attach a battery with the leads reversed (positive lead connected to the negative battery terminal and vice versa). This alarm will activate even when the ventilators are in the "off" position. The circuitry of the ventilators has been designed such that improper connection will not cause any internal damage. The ventilators should be turned off, the battery terminal connections reversed, and normal operation then resumed.

If the ventilators automatically switch power sources (AC to internal battery or external battery to internal battery), an alarm will be activated. When operated on the internal battery, a maximum of 60 minutes' operation time is provided.

Oxygen System (PLV-102)

If the oxygen flow is inadequate or if the medical source gas pressure falls below 35 psi, the oxygen system alarm will be activated. The alarm code "A-4" will appear in the flow LCD window, alerting the practitioner to this event.

Control Circuit Alarms
Ventilator Malfunction (PLV-100), Internal Failure (PLV-102)

This alarm condition will be activated if a fault is found in the pressure transducer, if the piston has stalled, if an internal battery circuit has failed or if a microprocessor failure has been detected. A fast-beeping (audible) alarm will result and the code A-5 (PLV-102) will be displayed in the flow LCD window.

Incompatible Settings

If the practitioner has set an insufficient inspiratory flow rate for the tidal volume and rate settings, the increase inspiratory flow LED will flash and the ventilator will automatically increase the inspiratory flow up to the maximum flow of 120 L/min. The ventilators will also alert the practitioner to inverse I:E ratio conditions by flashing the I:E ratio LCD display off and on.

Output Alarms
Pressure

Both ventilators incorporate high and low pressure alarms. The high pressure alarm was discussed earlier in the cycling variables section, and it is the pressure limit control. The low pressure alarm is adjustable between 2 and 50 cmH$_2$O. This alarm is helpful in detecting leaks and patient disconnect conditions.

Time

Both ventilators incorporate a 15 second delay alarm. If a breath (mechanical or spontaneous) has not been detected for 15 seconds, the low pressure alarm will be activated. If a spontaneous effort or mechanical breath occurs, a green LED illuminates, alerting the practitioner to the patient's ventilatory condition.

Tables 10-8 and 10-9 summarize the Lifecare PLV-100 and PLV-102 capabilities and alarm systems.

ASSEMBLY AND TROUBLESHOOTING

Assembly—PLV-100, PLV-102

To assemble the Lifecare PLV-100 and PLV-102, follow the suggested assembly guide.

1. Connect the ventilator to a power source:
   a. AC current 120 volt, 60 Hz (U.S. model) or 220-230 volt, 50-60 Hz (international model).
   b. External, deep-cycle 12 VDC battery.
   c. Fully charged internal battery (good for approximately 1 hour).

2. Assemble the patient circuit:
   a. Attach one end of the 18-inch, 22-mm diameter tubing to the ventilator outlet and the other to a heated humidifier. Suitable humidifiers would include all that are capable of body humidity at high flow rates.
   b. Connect one end of the 60-inch, 22-mm diameter tubing to the humidifier outlet and the other to the exhalation valve assembly.
   c. Attach the proximal pressure adapter to the patient manifold and a 4- or 6-inch tracheostomy flextube to its outlet.
   d. Attach an appropriate patient interface to the tracheostomy flextube to mate to the patient's airway.
   e. Connect the exhalation valve drive line to the exhalation valve and the exhalation valve fitting on the ventilator.
   f. Connect the proximal pressure line to the proximal airway adapter and to the PAP fitting on the ventilator.
   g. If supplemental oxygen is desired:
      [1.] Attach the oxygen adapter between the ventilator outlet and the humidifier inlet and bleed in oxygen to the desired F_IO_2 (PLV-100).
      [2.] Attach a 50 psi oxygen source to the DISS fitting on the rear of the ventilator and adjust the oxygen percent control to the desired level, verifying it with an oxygen analyzer.

Troubleshooting

To assist you in troubleshooting the ventilators, refer to the algorithms at the end of this chapter.

TABLE 10-8: Lifecare PLV-100 and PLV-102 Ventilator Capabilities

	PLV-100	PLV-102
Modes	Cont., Asst./Cont.,SIMV	Cont., Asst./Cont., SIMV Sigh (Cont., Asst./Cont.)
Volume	50 to 3,000 mL	50 to 3,000 mL
Breath Rate	2 to 50 BPM	2 to 40 BPM
Peak Flow	20 to 120 L/min	20 to 120 L/min
Sigh Volume		150% of tidal volume every 100th breath
Sensitivity	−6 to 3 cmH$_2$O	−5 to 18 cmH$_2$O
F$_I$O$_2$	.21 to 1.00	.21 to 1.0

TABLE 10-9: Lifecare PLV-100 and PLV-102 Alarm Systems

	PLV-100	PLV-102
Input Power		
Loss of Electrical Power	X	X
Low Battery	X	X
Power Switch-over	X	X
Control Circuit		
General Systems Failure	X	X
Incompatible Settings	X	X
Inverse I:E Ratio	X	X
Output		
High Pressure	5 to 95 cmH₂O	10 to 100 cmH₂O
Low Pressure	2 to 50 cmH₂O	2 to 50 cmH₂O
Time		
Apnea	15 second delay	15 second delay

NONCONTINUOUS VENTILATORY AUGMENTATION

Two of the primary treatments for obstructive and mixed sleep apnea syndromes include CPAP and bi-level positive airway pressure systems. These noninvasive ventilatory support systems may also be used to augment the ventilation of patients unable to adequately maintain normal blood gases spontaneously but not acutely ill enough to require continuous mechanical ventilatory support. There are several advantages to augmenting a patient's ventilation using these devices. These include lack of complications from an artificial airway, patient who may communicate effectively and patients who have control of their ventilatory rate and tidal volumes.

Both CPAP and bi-level positive airway pressure systems are effective in the management of obstructive sleep apnea syndromes by acting as a pneumatic splint and preventing the upper airway from closing. The positive pressure created in the nasopharynx forces the tongue anteriorly, maintaining an open airway and preventing the airway from collapsing during inspiration. (The airway collapses during obstructive sleep apnea due to the loss of muscle tone in the upper airway and the pressure gradient between the airway and atmospheric pressure.)

PURITAN BENNETT COMPANION 318 NASAL CPAP SYSTEM

The Puritan Bennett Companion 318 CPAP system is a continuous flow pressure controller that is designed to provide intermittent CPAP ventilatory support for patients with obstructive sleep apnea (Figure 10-11). The CPAP system may operate in the normal (on) or delay setting. Some patients experience difficulty adjusting to their prescribed pressures when initially falling asleep. The delay feature allows up to 20 minutes to elapse prior to delivery of the full prescribed CPAP pressure (explained in more detail under "control variables").

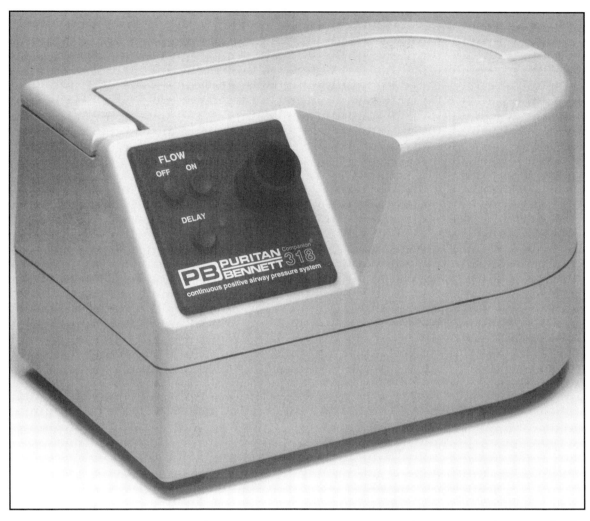

Figure 10-11 *A schematic diagram of the Puritan Bennett Companion 318 Nasal CPAP System. (Courtesy of Nellcor Puritan Bennett Inc., Lenexa, KS)*

POWER INPUT

The Companion 318 CPAP system is electrically powered. It is powered by standard AC current. A selector switch on the bottom of the unit allows usage of 120 volt, 60 Hz (domestic) or 220-230 volt, 50-60 Hz (international) electric power. If the use of international (220-230 volt, 50-60 Hz) power is required, the fuse (part number 290492-01) must also be changed and the selector switch must be repositioned.

CONTROL CIRCUIT

The control circuit of the Companion 318 consists of a electronically controlled fan, a pressure regulator and a flow transducer. Signals from the pressure regulator and flow transducer are monitored by the microprocessor, and the fan's output is adjusted to maintain the desired pressure. CPAP pressure is adjusted using a control on the bottom of the unit and is adjustable between 3 and 20 cmH_2O.

If supplemental oxygen is desired, oxygen may be bled in to the desired concentration by using an oxygen adapter between the CPAP system outlet and the patient tubing. Oxygen flow from the oxygen source is then adjusted until the desired concentration is verified using an oxygen analyzer.

CONTROL VARIABLE

The control variable for the Companion 318 CPAP system is pressure. Pressure is controlled using CPAP control on the base of the

ASSEMBLY AND TROUBLESHOOTING

Assembly—Companion 318 CPAP

To prepare the Companion 318 CPAP system for use, complete the suggested assembly guide.

1. Connect the CPAP system to a suitable AC power source. Either 120 volt, 60 Hz or 220-230 volt, 50-60 Hz electrical power may be used.

2. Connect the patient tubing to the outlet of the CPAP system.

3. Attach either nasal pillows or a nasal mask to the outlet of the patient tubing.

4. Adjust the CPAP pressure to the prescribed level using the CPAP adjustment control on the bottom of the

unit. CPAP pressures should be titrated for each individual patient based upon the results of a polsomnographic sleep study.

5. Turn the unit on:
   a. Depress the "on" button on the control panel.
   b. If a ramp pressure delay is desired, select the delay time using the four-position switch on the bottom of the unit. Press the delay button on the front control panel.

Troubleshooting

Use the troubleshooting algorithm at the end of this chapter to assist you with troubleshooting problems associated with intermittent CPAP systems.

---

unit. Adjustment of the control results in a change in gas flow through the control valve causing a higher or lower pressure to be delivered.

The delay feature allows the inspiratory pressure to be ramped over a period of time. Many patients find it difficult to go to sleep with the CPAP system set at the prescribed pressure. The delay control may be set between 5 and 20 minutes, in 5 minute increments. Once the delay time has passed (presumably the patient has reached stage II sleep), the unit will automatically increase the pressure to the set pressure level at a rate of 2 cmH_2O per minute. Many patients are more comfortable as the pressure gradually ramps to the set level. The delay feature is activated by setting the delay time (four-position switch on the bottom of the unit) and then depressing the delay button on the front control panel.

PHASE VARIABLES

Baseline Variable

The baseline variable for the Companion 318 is pressure. As already described, pressure is adjusted using the inspiratory pressure con-

trol valve. CPAP pressures may be adjusted between 3 and 20 cmH_2O.

RESPIRONICS, INC., REMSTAR CHOICE® NASAL CPAP SYSTEM

The Respironics Inc. REMstar Choice® is an electrically powered intermittent CPAP system designed to be used for patients with obstructive sleep apnea (Figure 10-12). It is a pressure controller that is capable of delivering CPAP pressures between 3 and 20 cmH_2O. The pressure may be ramped or delayed for up to 45 minutes before the REMstar Choice® reaches the prescribed pressure setting. The REMstar Choice® includes a battery-powered, infrared remote control to activate the unit and initiate the ramp feature.

INPUT POWER

The input power for the SleepEasy III CPAP system is either 120 volt, 60 Hz (Domestic) or 220-230 volt, 50-60 Hz (international) AC electrical power. A selector switch on the

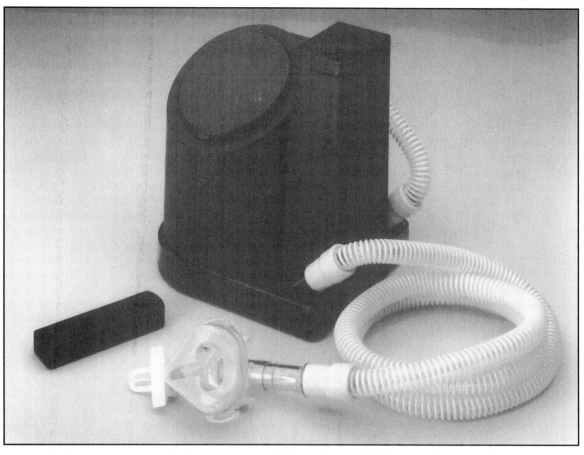

Figure 10-12 *A photograph of the Respironics, Inc., REMstar Choice® CPAP system. (Courtesy of Respironics, Inc.)*

ASSEMBLY AND TROUBLESHOOTING

Assembly—REMstar Choice

To assemble the REMstar Choice for use, follow the suggested assembly guide (Figure 10-13).

1. Connect the CPAP system to a suitable AC power source. Either 120 volt, 60 Hz, or 220-230 volt, 50-60 Hz electrical power may be used.

2. Assemble the patient circuit:
   a. Connect a Sanders' CPAP valve to the patient circuit. Alternatively, the Whisper swivel may be used.
   b. Connect the opposite end of the patient tubing to the outlet of the REMstar Choice®.
   d. Connect either nasal pillows or a nasal mask to the outlet of the NRV-2 valve.
   e. Connect a spacer to the top of the mask and adjust the spacer/mask

assembly to fit the patient using the headgear.

3. Adjust the CPAP pressure to the prescribed level using the CPAP adjustment control on the rear of the unit. CPAP pressures should be titrated for each individual patient based upon the results of a polsomnographic sleep study.

4. Turn the unit on by pressing the on/off switch on the right front of the control panel.

Troubleshooting

Use the troubleshooting algorithm at the end of this chapter to assist you with troubleshooting problems associated with intermittent CPAP systems.

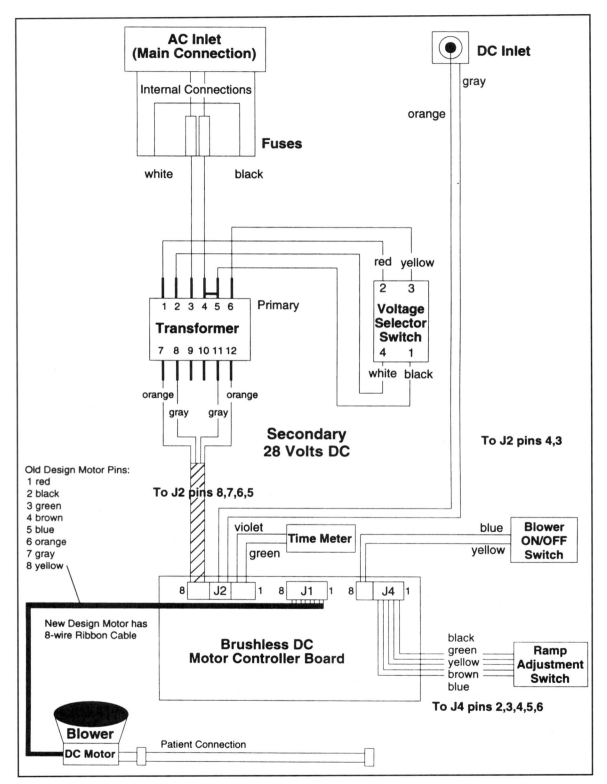

Figure 10-13 *A schematic diagram of the Respironics, Inc., REMstar Choice® Nasal CPAP system. (Courtesy of Respironics, Inc.)*

rear of the unit allows the selection of either power source.

CONTROL CIRCUIT

The control circuit consists of an electrically powered fan (flow generator) and an electronic controlling circuit. Adjustment of the CPAP pressure control on the rear of the unit causes the speed of the fan to change, changing the delivered pressure. A pressure manometer is used to verify the desired pressure. Once the desired pressure is reached, the electric motor speed powering the fan remains constant.

CONTROL VARIABLE

The control variable for the REMstar Choice® is pressure. As already described, pressure is varied using the CPAP control and results in changes in the motor speed. CPAP pressures may be adjusted between 3 and 20 cmH$_2$O by making the adjustments on the rear of the unit.

The ramp feature allows the inspiratory pressure to be delayed over a period of time. Many patients find it difficult to go to sleep with the CPAP system set at the prescribed pressure. The ramp control may be set between 5 and 45 minutes, in 5 minute increments. By setting the delay period, the REMstar Choice® calculates a linear pressure slope to achieve the desired pressure setting. The pressure increases gradually until the set pressure is reached at the end of the delay period. Many patients are more comfortable as the pressure gradually ramps to the set level. The ramp feature is activated by setting the delay time (10-position switch on the rear of the unit) and then depressing the ramp switch.

PHASE VARIABLE

Baseline Variable

The baseline variable for the REMstar Choice is pressure.

BI-LEVEL POSITIVE AIRWAY PRESSURE SYSTEMS

Bi-level positive airway pressure systems are similar to CPAP systems except that two pressure levels are delivered. One pressure is delivered during inspiration (inspiratory positive airway pressure, or IPAP), which is greater; and the other during exhalation (expiratory positive airway pressure, or EPAP), which is less. By applying a lower pressure during exhalation (EPAP), the patient exhales against a lower resistance, which many find more comfortable. Bi-level positive airway pressure ventilators sense inspiration and expiration by monitoring flow, and therefore are flow triggered and flow cycled.

PURITAN BENNETT COMPANION 320I/E BI-LEVEL RESPIRATORY SYSTEM

The Puritan Bennett Companion 320I/E Bi-Level system is a bi-level positive airway pressure ventilator system (Figure 10-14). As described earlier, a practitioner may adjust two independent pressures IPAP (inspiratory) and EPAP (expiratory). The bi-level positive airway pressure ventilator is an electrically powered pressure controller, which is flow triggered and flow cycled. The 320I/E also in-

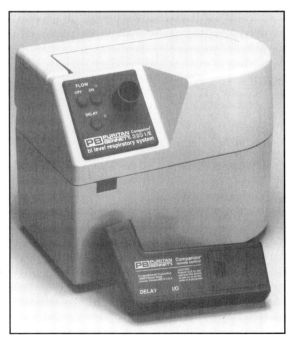

Figure 10-14 *A photograph of the Puritan Bennett Companion 320I/E Bi-Level Respiratory System. (Courtesy of Puritan Bennett Corporation)*

ASSEMBLY AND TROUBLESHOOTING

Assembly—320I/E Bi-Level Respiratory System

1. Connect the CPAP system to a suitable AC power source. Either 120 volt, 60 Hz or 220–230 volt, 50-60 Hz electrical power may be used.

2. Connect the patient tubing to the outlet of the CPAP system.

3. Attach either nasal pillows or a nasal mask to the outlet of the patient tubing.

4. Adjust the pressure levels:
   a. IPAP pressure is adjustable between 3 and 30 cmH$_2$O using the IPAP control on the rear of the ventilator.
   b. Set the EPAP pressure (3 to 30 cmH$_2$O) using the EPAP control on the rear of the ventilator.

5. Turn the unit on:
   a. Depress the on button on the control panel.
   b. If a ramp pressure delay is desired:
      [1.] Set the delay time using the delay control on the rear of the ventilator (5 to 30 minutes).
      [2.] Set the ramp rate (1, 2, or 3 cmH$_2$O/minute).
      [3.] Activate the delay feature by depressing the delay control on the front control panel.

Troubleshooting

Use the troubleshooting algorithm at the end of this chapter to assist you with troubleshooting problems associated with intermittent bi-level positive airway pressure systems.

---

corporates a delay feature similar to the Companion 318 CPAP system, allowing a gradual ramping of pressure to the preset level for patient comfort.

INPUT POWER

The input power for the Companion 320I/E is AC electrical power. The unit may be operated from 120 volt, 60 Hz (domestic) or 220-230 volt, 50-60 Hz (international) AC power by adjusting a selector switch on the rear of the ventilator.

CONTROL CIRCUIT

The control circuit of the Companion 320I/E consists of a electrically powered fan and an adjustable pressure controlling valve. As IPAP and EPAP pressures are adjusted using controls on the bottom of the ventilator, the pressure controlling valve opens or closes, creating the threshold resistance required against the fan to create the desired pressure

levels. A flow transducer senses changes in flow to the patient.

When inspiration begins, flow is high, signaling the beginning of a breath. When flow tapers to a level lower than the leak threshold, IPAP delivery ceases and inspiration ends.

If supplemental oxygen is desired, it may be bled in to the desired concentration by using an oxygen adapter between the CPAP system outlet and the patient tubing. Oxygen flow from the oxygen source is then adjusted until the desired concentration is verified using an oxygen analyzer.

CONTROL VARIABLE

The control variable for the Companion 320I/E is pressure. Pressures are adjusted using the IPAP and exhale EPAP pressure controls on the bottom of the ventilator. Both pressures are adjustable between 3 and 20 cmH$_2$O. The EPAP control must always be set to a lower pressure than the IPAP control. Adjustment of the pressure control causes the pressure control valve to open or close changing the threshold resistance.

The delay feature allows the inspiratory pressure to be ramped over a period of time. Many patients find it difficult to go to sleep with the bi-level positive airway pressure system set with IPAP at the prescribed pressure. The delay control may be set between 5 and 30 minutes, in 5 minute increments. Once the delay time has passed (presumably the patient has reached stage II sleep), the unit will automatically increase the pressure to the set pressure level at a rate of 1, 2, or 3 cmH$_2$O per minute. Many patients are more comfortable as the pressure gradually ramps to the set level. The delay feature is activated by setting the delay time (four-position switch at the rear of the ventilator) and then depressing the delay button on the front control panel.

PHASE VARIABLES

Trigger Variable

As already described, the trigger variable is flow. Changes in flow sensed by the flow transducer signal the start and end of inspiration. The trigger sensitivity may be adjusted using two controls located on the back of the unit. Both inspiratory and expiratory sensitivity may be adjusted to better match the patient's spontaneous ventilatory efforts. These controls are labeled inhale and exhale.

Limit Variable

The limit variable is pressure. Once inspiration begins, pressure rises to a preset level and is maintained at that level until the end of inspiration. The pressure level reached is established using the IPAP control on the rear of the ventilator.

Cycle Variable

The cycle variable is flow. Once inspiratory flow decays to a level less than the leak threshold, pressure falls from the IPAP level to the EPAP level.

Baseline Variable

The baseline variable is pressure and is set using the EPAP control on the rear of the ventilator. Once inspiration ends, the delivered pressure falls to the EPAP level and is maintained at that level until the next breath is sensed.

RESPIRONICS, INC.,[1] BIPAP® S/T

The Respironics BiPAP® S/T Ventilatory Support System (Figure 10-15) is an electrically powered, noncontinuous, ventilatory augmentation system designed to support a patient's ventilatory efforts with inspiratory (IPAP) and expiratory (EPAP) pressures. The BiPAP® S/T system is a pressure controller that is flow or time triggered, pressure limited, and flow or time cycled. The BiPAP® S/T may operate in spontaneous, spontaneous/time cycled, time cycled, and CPAP modes.

INPUT POWER

The input power for the BiPAP® S/T ventilatory support system is AC electrical power. Either 120 volt, 60 Hz (domestic) or 220–230 volt, 50-60 Hz (international) AC current may be used. Either may be selected by rotating the voltage selector switch on the rear of the ventilator to the right of the power cord receptacle.

CONTROL CIRCUIT

The control circuit consists of an electrically powered fan (flow generator) and an electrodynamic pressure control valve. Adjustment of the IPAP and EPAP pressure controls on the rear of the unit causes electrical current to the coils in the valve to vary, increasing or decreasing magnetic attraction between the valve core and the permanent magnet housing (Figure 10-16). The magnetic attraction between the valve core and the valve disc causes pressure to build within the pressure chamber. As magnetic attraction increases, so does the pressure. Once pressure exceeds the magnetic attraction, excess pressure is vented through the exhaust valve.

Inspiration and expiration is determined by flow sensing logic in the ventilator. Flow is detected by a flow transducer. When the total flow increases above the leak threshold by 40 cc/second for 0.03 seconds, inspiration is triggered and pressure rises to the IPAP level. When flow tapers below the estimated leak threshold, inspiration is terminated and pressure falls to the EPAP level.

If supplemental oxygen is desired, it may

---

[1] *BIPAP is a registered trademark of Respironics, Inc.*

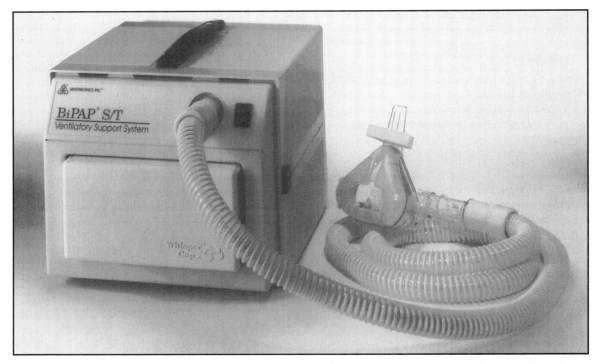

Figure 10-15 *A photograph of the Respironics, Inc., BiPAP® S/T Ventilator Support System (Courtesy of Respironics, Inc.)*

be bled in by placing the oxygen enrichment attachment between the ventilator outlet and the patient circuit. Oxygen is bled in until the desired oxygen concentration is reached and verified with an oxygen analyzer.

CONTROL VARIABLE

The control variable for the BiPAP® S/T is pressure. IPAP and EPAP levels are adjustable between –4 and 20 cmH$_2$O. As already described, the pressure control valve (Figure 10-16), determines the delivered pressure.

PHASE VARIABLES

Trigger Variables

The trigger variables for the BiPAP® S/T system include flow and time. When operated in the spontaneous mode, flow is the trigger

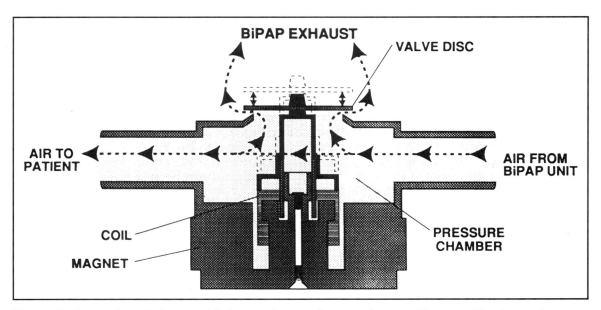

Figure 10-16 *A schematic diagram of the Respironics, Inc., flow control system. (Courtesy of Respironics, Inc.)*

ASSEMBLY AND TROUBLESHOOTING

Assembly—BiPAP® S/T

To assemble the BiPAP® S/T system for use, follow the suggested assembly guide.

1. Connect the ventilator to a suitable AC power source. Either 120 volt, 60 Hz or 220–230 volt, 50-60 Hz electrical power may be used:
   a. Rotate the voltage selector switch to the correct current setting.

2. Assemble the patient circuit:
   a. Connect the patient tubing to the outlet of the ventilator.
      [1.] If supplemental oxygen is desired, attach the oxygen enrichment fitting between the ventilator outlet and the patient circuit.
   b. Connect the whisper swivel to the distal end of the patient circuit.
   c. Connect either nasal pillows or a nasal mask to the outlet of the whisper swivel.
   d. Connect a spacer to the top of the mask and adjust the spacer/mask assembly to fit the patient using the headgear.

3. Adjust the pressure levels:
   a. Adjust the IPAP pressure using the IPAP control on the rear of the ventilator.
   b. Adjust the EPAP pressure using the EPAP control on the rear of the ventilator.

4. Select the mode of operation:
   a. CPAP: Select either the IPAP or EPAP position. Whichever position is selected, the ventilator will operate in CPAP mode delivering either IPAP or EPAP pressure to the circuit.
   b. Spontaneous: The ventilator will cycle between the IPAP and EPAP pressure based upon its flow sensing logic.
   c. Spontaneous/Timed: This setting allows spontaneous ventilation with a backup ventilatory rate in the absence of spontaneous efforts.
   d. Timed: This mode delivers augmented ventilation at the set ventilatory rate and percent IPAP time.

5. Turn the unit on by pressing the on/off switch on the right front of the control ventilator.

Troubleshooting

Use the troubleshooting algorithm at the end of this chapter to assist you with troubleshooting problems associated with intermittent bi-level positive airway pressure systems.

---

variable. As already described, the flow sensing logic determines when inspiration begins and ends, cycling the ventilator into and out of IPAP.

When the ventilator is operated in the spontaneous/timed mode, the ventilator may be flow or time triggered. If the patient has spontaneous efforts that are detected by the flow sensing logic at a rate equal to or greater than the breath per minute control setting (respiratory rate), the BiPAP® S/T system functions using flow as a cycle variable. If the patient's spontaneous rate falls below the set respiratory rate, the ventilator becomes time

triggered, delivering pressure augmented breaths at the set rate (breaths per minute).

If the ventilator is operated in the timed mode, the BiPAP® S/T system delivers pressure augmented breaths at the set ventilator rate (breaths per minute) and percent IPAP time. Rates may be adjusted between 4 and 30 breaths per minute. Percent IPAP times may be adjusted between 10 and 90%.

Limit Variable

The limit variable is pressure. Pressure increases during inspiration to the IPAP pressure setting. IPAP is adjustable between –4 and 20 cmH$_2$O. Once inspiration begins, pressure increases to the IPAP level and plateaus until exhalation begins.

Cycle Variables

The cycle variables include flow and time. Flow cycling occurs when inspiratory flow falls to a level less than the estimated leak flow. When this flow threshold is reached, inspiratory assistance is terminated and pressure falls to the EPAP level.

Time cycling occurs when the BiPAP® S/T system is operated in the timed mode. Inspiration is terminated when the percent IPAP time has been reached. The percent IPAP time may be adjusted between 10 and 90%.

Baseline Variable

The baseline variable is pressure. EPAP pressures may be adjusted between –4 and 20 cmH$_2$O. It is important to adjust the EPAP pressure to a lower value than the IPAP pressure.

TRANSPORT VENTILATORS

Transport ventilators are commonly used for ground, airborne and intrahospital patient transports. Examples of intrahospital transports include moving the patient from the emergency room to ICU or transporting the patient from ICU to CT scan, MRI scan, or fleuroscopy for special procedures. As a practitioner, you should understand how these ventilators operate, how controls function and how these ventilators differ in their capabilities and operation from conventional critical care adult and pediatric ventilators.

AMBU, INC., TRANSCARE 2

Ambu, Inc., markets the TransCARE 2 portable, pneumatically powered, transport ventilator, which incorporates an electronic monitoring system (Figure 10-17). The TransCARE 2 ventilator is produced by Omni-Tech Medical, Inc., and has many similarities to the Omni-Vent ventilator (described later in this

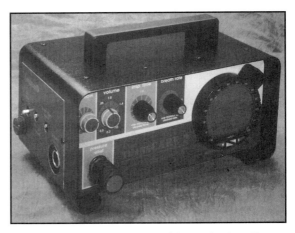

Figure 10-17 *A photograph of the Ambu, Inc., TransCARE 2 Ventilator (Courtesy of Ambu, Inc.)*

chapter.) The ventilator is pneumatically powered and controlled. It is a flow controller that is pressure or time triggered, pressure or flow limited and time cycled. It may be operated in volume control, pressure control, IMV (volume or pressure controlled modes), and CPAP modes.

INPUT POWER

The TransCARE 2 is pneumatically powered and controlled. A medical gas source of between 25 and 140 psi may be used to power the ventilator. A 50 psi source is the recommended pressure. However, if desired, the ventilator may be calibrated to run at lower pressures (25 psi) to utilize liquid systems, which may be desirable in some situations, or higher pressure sources (140 psi), which may be used for the TransCARE 1-HB for hyperbaric clinical applications.

The electronic monitoring system may be powered by an internal "AAA" battery pack (350 hours), or an external 12 to 24 VDC power source. Additionally, an optional AC power adapter may be purchased to utilize commercial AC power.

CONTROL CIRCUIT

Gas to power the ventilator enters through a filter in the gas inlet assembly (Figure 10-18). It then passes through an on/off valve in the same assembly and on to the inspiratory-and-expiratory valve block. From the inspiratory/expiratory valve block the gas is

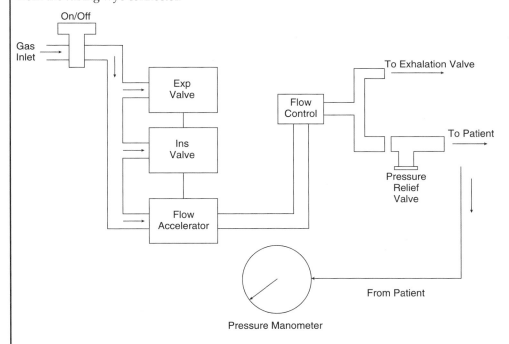

INSPIRATORY PHASE

Source gas is introduced through a filter in the gas inlet assembly; then gas flows to the pneumatic valve supply inlet. The gas flows to the flow control, then to the tee assembly which directs gas simultaneously to the exhalation valve and pressure relief valve to the patient.

As gas pressure increases in the lung, it is transmitted to the manometer through a tubing independent from the tubing wye connector.

EXPIRATORY PHASE

Source gas follows the identical path of the inspiratory phase to the pneumatic valves and is then held until the inspiratory phase begins.

Figure 10-18 *A schematic diagram of the Ambu, Inc., TransCARE 2 ventilator during inspiration and expiration. (Courtesy of Ambu, Inc.)*

conducted to a flow accelerator and then to a flow control valve. From the flow control valve the gas flow is split, with one path flowing to a pressure relief valve and patient circuit and the other path flowing to the exhalation valve diaphragm.

PEEP/CPAP may be added using an external threshold resistor valve attached to the patient circuit. PEEP/CPAP pressures of between 0 and 20 cmH₂O may be added using the external valve.

CONTROL VARIABLE

The control variable for the TransCARE 2 ventilator is flow, which is determined by the flow control valve. Flow rates may be adjusted between 0 and 85 L/min. The flow control valve is a variable orifice needle valve. Opening or closing the valve regulates the flow of gas through it. Since flow is constant, volume delivery becomes a function of inspiratory flow and inspiratory time (volume is equal to flow multiplied by time).

PHASE VARIABLES

Trigger Variables

The trigger variables include pressure and time. Pressure is a trigger variable during IMV ventilation. When inspiratory effort is sufficient to open a one-way valve in the IMV reservoir, gas is delivered to the patient. An IMV flow rate may be adjusted from 0 to 60 L/min by using the IMV flow knob (needle valve) on the left front of the control panel. IMV gas flows out of the ventilator via the nipple on the left side of the ventilator.

Time is the control variable for volume- and pressure-controlled ventilation, as well as the mandatory portion of IMV. The expiratory time control acts as a rate control. The expiratory valve is a needle valve, which controls the rate of gas leakage through a timing cartridge. If gas flow leaking from the cartridge is high, expiratory time is less. Conversely, if gas leakage is slow, expiratory time is longer. Respiratory rates are adjustable between 0 and 150 breaths per minute.

Limit Variables

The limit variables for the TransCARE 2 include pressure and flow. Pressure becomes a

limit variable if the pressure relief valve is set lower than the peak inspiratory pressure for a given inspiratory time and flow rate. Under these circumstances, pressure will rise to the pressure limit setting and plateau until the inspiratory time has elapsed with the ventilator operating in pressure control mode. The pressure limit may be adjusted between 0 and 120 cmH₂O.

The ventilator may also be flow limited. If the flow rate is set at a lower setting and inspiratory time is set such that flow increases and plateaus, the ventilator is then flow limited.

Cycle Variable

The cycle variable for the ventilator is time. Inspiratory time is determined by the inspiratory time needle valve. The control, like the expiratory time control, is a pneumatic timing cartridge. Adjustment of the needle valve controls the rate of gas leakage from the cartridge, which either lengthens or shortens inspiratory time. Inspiratory times may be adjusted between 0.2 and 2.0 seconds.

ALARM/MONITORING SYSTEMS

Monitoring System

The TransCARE 2 incorporates a compact electronic monitoring and alarm package into its design. The monitoring/alarm system measures pressure in the patient circuit and can integrate that electronic pressure signal over time. All data is displayed on a back-lit LCD displaying both a circular bar graph and alphanumeric data. The monitoring capability is summarized in Table 10-10.

Control Circuit Alarms

The TransCARE 2 incorporates a failure-to-cycle alarm into its alarm system. If the ventilator fails to cycle, the alarm will be activated.

Output Alarms
Pressure

Both high- and low-pressure alarms are incorporated in the alarm system. The high-pressure alarm alerts the practitioner to pressures that exceed the alarm setting. The alarm may be set between –10 and 120 cmH₂O. The low pressure alarm may be set between the same range (–0 and 120 cmH₂O.) The low-

ASSEMBLY AND TROUBLESHOOTING

Assembly—TransCARE 2

To prepare the Ambu, Inc., Trans-CARE 2 for use, follow the suggested assembly guide.

1. Select a power source for the monitoring/alarm system:
   a. Internal "AAA" battery pack
   b. External 12 to 24 VDC source
   c. AC power adapter

2. Connect the ventilator to a medical gas source (25 to 140 psi). If an F_1O_2 of less than 1.0 is desired, the ventilator may be powered from a blender operating from independent sources of medical air and oxygen.

3. Assemble the patient circuit:
   a. Connect one end of the 22-mm diameter patient circuit to the ventilator outlet.
   b. Connect the patient manifold assembly to the distal end of the 22-mm diameter patient circuit.
   c. Connect one end of the 1/8-inch diameter line to the exhalation valve nipple on the side of the ventilator and the other end to the exhalation valve on the patient manifold assembly.
   d. Connect the other 1/8-inch diameter line between the airway pressure nipple on the ventilator and the proximal airway tap on the patient manifold.

e. Connect a 6-inch flex tube to the patient manifold assembly and attach a mask adapter or tracheostomy adapter to the distal end to interface with the patient airway.

4. Turn on the gas supply and calibrate the ventilator by depressing the blue "*" switch on the side of the ventilator. Next press and hold the two gray up/down keys on the monitor simultaneously to calibrate the ventilator and set the zero. Once the word "calibrate" and "0000.00" appear on the display, the ventilator has been calibrated.

5. Confirm the ventilator's operation:
   a. Connect the patient circuit to a test lung and rotate the on/off switch to the on position.
   b. Adjust flow, inspiratory and expiratory time to the desired settings.
   c. Confirm rate and volume delivery using a Wright respirometer or other volume-measuring device and a watch.
   d. Occlude the patient circuit and adjust the pressure relief valve to the desired pressure.

Troubleshooting

To assist you in troubleshooting the TransCARE 2 ventilator, refer to the troubleshooting algorithm at the end of this chapter.

pressure alarm is helpful in detecting leaks and patient disconnect situations.

A leak detection alarm may also be used in addition to the low-pressure alarm. The leak detection alarm is an adjustable pressure alarm that may be set between 0 and 10 cmH_2O below the high-pressure alarm, independent of the low-pressure alarm.

Tables 10-11 and 10-12 summarize the TransCARE 2 ventilator's capabilities and alarm systems.

TABLE 10-10: Ambu, Inc., TransCARE 2 Monitoring System

Pressure	-10 to 120 cmH_2O
Respiratory Rate	4 to 400 BPM
Inspiratory Time	0.01 to 10 seconds
Expiratory Time	0.01 to 60 seconds
I:E Ratio	2:1 to 1:99

TABLE 10-11: TransCARE 2 Ventilator Capabilities

Modes	Volume and Pressure Control, IMV, CPAP
Tidal Volume	0 to 2000 mL
Respiratory Rate	0 to 150 BPM
Inspiratory Time	0.2 to 2 seconds
Expiratory Time	0.2 to 60 seconds
Flow Rate	0 to 85 L/min
IMV Flow Rate	0 to 60 L/min
Pressure Relief	0 to 120 cmH$_2$O
PEEP/CPAP	0 to 20 cmH$_2$O (external threshold resistor)

TABLE 10-12: TransCARE 2 Alarm Systems

Control Circuit

Failure to Cycle

Output

High Pressure	-10 to 120 cmH$_2$O
Low Pressure	-10 to 120 cmH$_2$O
Leak Detection	0 to 10 cmH$_2$O below high pressure

BIO-MED DEVICES CROSSVENT 4

The Bio-Med Devices Crossvent 4 is a electronically controlled, electrically powered (battery or AC) ventilator (Figure 10-19). It may be operated in control, assist/control, SIMV, CPAP, pressure support and pressure-limited, time-cycled ventilation modes. The ventilator is a flow controller that is pressure, time or manually triggered, pressure or flow limited and pressure, volume or time cycled.

Input Power

The electronic control circuit is powered by either an internal battery (up to 11 hours' operation when the LCD back-light is used for approximately 1 of the 11 hours), external battery or AC power source (120 or 220 volts). When using external power sources, the electrical power should be connected to the left side of the ventilator, utilizing the factory supplied plug.

The pneumatic systems of the ventilator require a compressed gas source of between 44 and 66 psi (55 psi average). An external blender may be used to mix air and oxygen to the desired F$_1$O$_2$.

Control Circuit

Gas enters the ventilator through a DISS inlet fitting via a 40 micron inlet filter and on to an internal pressure regulator. The pressure regulator drops the inlet pressure to approximately 20 psi (Figure 10-20). From the regulator, the gas flows to a solenoid-controlled, two-way pilot valve. From the pilot valve, gas flows to an electronically controlled solenoid valve. The solenoid valve position is controlled by a needle valve. Since inlet pressure is constant (20 psi) and outlet pressure is negligible (patient pressure), the flow rate through the valve is solely a function of the size of the valve's orifice. Maximum flow from the ventilator is dependent upon the gas supply pressure (from 120 L/min at 55 psi to 100 L/min at 45 psi). Gas is delivered from the flow control valve to the patient circuit.

During gas delivery to the patient through the flow control valve, gas flows through another solenoid valve to pressurize the diaphragm of the exhalation valve. During exhalation, gas pressure may be partially removed from the exhalation valve, creating PEEP/CPAP pressure.

Control Variable

The control variable of the Crossvent 4 is flow, which is controlled by the orifice size of the flow control valve. The position of flow

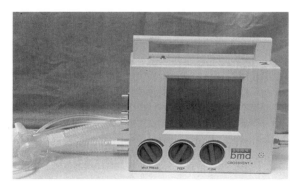

Figure 10-19 *A photograph of the Bio-Med Devices, Inc., Crossvent 4 Ventilator.*

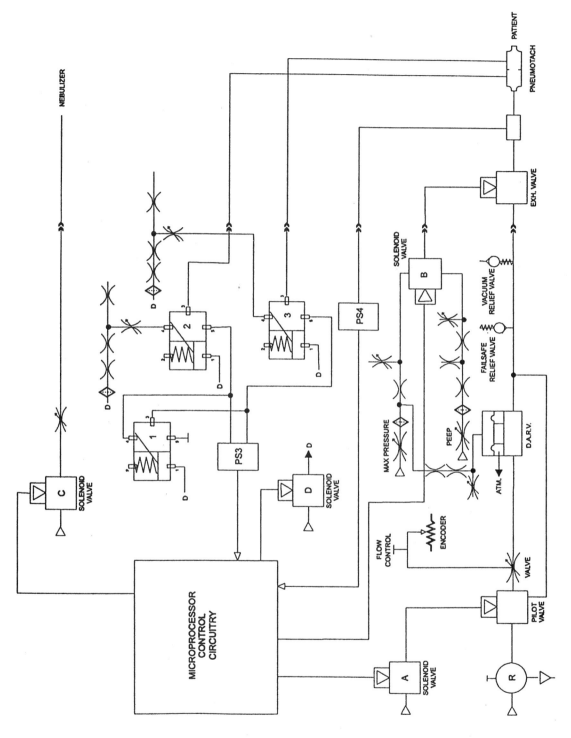

Figure 10-20 A schematic diagram of the Bio-Med Devices, Inc., Crossvent-4 pneumatic system. (Courtesy Bio-Med Devices, Inc., Guilford, CT)

control valve (orifice size) is relayed to the electronic control circuit by a precision potentiometer connected to the flow rate's needle valve. Volume delivery is a function of flow (L/sec) multiplied by inspiratory time.

Phase Variables
Trigger Variables

The trigger variables of the Crossvent 4 include pressure, time and manual triggering. Pressure triggering is adjusted using the inspiratory effort control. Pressure triggering may be adjusted from 0 to 10 cmH$_2$O below baseline pressure (PEEP or atmospheric). Pressure triggering will not function during time cycled pressure limited ventilator or at respiratory rates greater than 60 breaths per minute.

Time triggering is a variable used during assist/control, the mandatory portion of SIMV and time-cycled, pressure-limited ventilation. Time triggering is established by using the rate control. Respiratory rates of between 5 and 150 breaths per minute may be set.

Manual triggering is accomplished by depressing the manual screen button. Doing so delivers a manual breath at the set rate, tidal volume and inspiratory time. This control is only operational in the CPAP mode.

Limit Variables

The Crossvent 4 may be pressure or flow limited. The ventilator is pressure limited in the infant mode (pressure-limited, time-cycled ventilation). The pressure limit is set maximum pressure control. Pressure is adjustable between 0 and 120 cmH$_2$O.

Flow becomes a limit variable when the inspiratory flow rate is adjusted low enough that the ventilator reaches that flow and plateaus during inspiration while in volume control ventilation. Flow is also a limit variable during pressure-limited, time-cycled ventilation.

Cycle Variables

Cycle variables of the Crossvent 4 include pressure, volume and time. Pressure becomes a cycle variable when the pressure exceeds that set by the high-peak pressure alarm limit (adjustable between 1 and 120 cmH$_2$O). When this pressure value is reached, inspiration is terminated and the alarm sounds. This feature is not operative during time-cycled, pressure-limited ventilation.

Volume is a cycle variable during sigh breath delivery (CMV mode). When de-

pressed, a sigh breath of 1.5 times the tidal volume is delivered (up to 2,500 mL) for every 100 mandatory breaths.

Time is a cycle variable during infant ventilation (time-cycled, pressure-limited ventilation). Inspiratory time is adjustable between 0.1 and 1.5 seconds.

Alarm Systems
Input Power

While operating on the ventilator's internal battery, an alarm will sound and the indication "BATT LOW" will be displayed when approximately 20 minutes of battery power remain. Additionally, a bar graph continuously displays battery power remaining, decreasing in 20% increments.

Control Circuit
I:E Ratio Alarm

The Crossvent 4 incorporates an I:E ratio alarm, which will flash and audibly sound when the I:E ratio is greater than 3:1, inspiratory time is greater than 3 seconds or less than 0.1 seconds or expiratory time is less than 0.2 seconds. The alarm can be permanently silenced only by changing the ventilation parameters or correcting the I:E ratio or inspiratory or expiratory time.

Output Alarms
Pressure

The Crossvent 4 has a peak pressure alarm, which is adjustable between 0 and 125 cmH$_2$O. During sigh breath delivery, the peak pressure alarm is automatically increased by 1.5 times the display setting, to a maximum of 125 cmH$_2$O.

A mean airway pressure alarm may be used to alert the practitioner of changes in the mean airway pressure. Pressures may be adjusted between 0 and 125 cmH$_2$O. Both high and low-pressure limits may be established.

The PEEP/CPAP pressure alarm has high and low limits, which may be adjusted between 0 and 99 cmH$_2$O. In the event a of loss of PEEP/CPAP pressure, the alarm will flash and an audible alarm will sound.

Volume Alarm

The Crossvent 4 may be equipped with an optional exhaled tidal volume alarm. The alarm is adjustable between 0 and 2,500 mL. The ventilator must be configured with an ex-

ASSEMBLY AND TROUBLESHOOTING

Assembly—Bio-Med Devices, Inc., Crossvent 4

1. Connect a 50 psi gas source to the ventilator using the DISS fitting on the ventilator's right-hand side.

2. If using an external power source or AC power, connect the external power connector to its receptacle on the left side of the ventilator.

3. Assemble the patient circuit for use:
   a. Attach the exhalation valve manifold to the 22 mm large diameter tubing.
   b. Attach a 6-inch piece of 22-mm, large-diameter tubing to the patient outlet side of the exhalation valve manifold, securing a mask adapter or elbow fitting to interface with the patient's airway.
   c. Attach the exhalation valve drive line to the exhalation valve and the proximal pressure monitoring line to the circuit.
   d. If the optional pneumotachometer is used, use a standard patient wye fitting to interface with the patient's airway and connect the pneumotachometer to the expiratory side of the wye, between the wye and the exhalation valve assembly.
   e. Connect the exhalation valve drive line, proximal airway pressure line and pneumotachometer lines to their respective fittings on the left side of the ventilator.

Troubleshooting

To assist you in troubleshooting the ventilator, follow the troubleshooting algorithm at the conclusion of this chapter.

---

ternal pneumotachometer, which is accurate between 200 and 2,500 mL and at flows from 13 to 140 L/min. Both high and low parameters may be set when using this alarm.

Flow

The Crossvent 4 may be purchased with an optional minute ventilation alarm for use when using the external pneumotachometer. Alarm limits may be adjusted between 0 and 200 L/min. Both upper and lower minute volume limits may be set.

Time

The Crossvent 4 ventilator incorporates a high breath rate alarm, which is adjustable between 0 and 199 breaths per minute.

Inspired Gas

When equipped with the optional oxygen sensor, the Crossvent 4 can alert the practitioner to changes in oxygen delivery. Both high and low alarm limits may be set between 21 and 100%. Tables 10-13 and 10-14 summarize the Crossvent 4 ventilator's capabilities and alarm systems.

TABLE 10-13:	Crossvent 4 Transport Ventilator Capabilities
Modes	Assist/control, SIMV, CPAP, pressure support, and time-cycled, pressure-limited ventilation.
Rate	5 to 150 breaths per minute
Flow	1 to 120 L/min
Pressure Limit	1 to 120 cmH$_2$O
Pressure Support	0 to 50 cmH$_2$O
PEEP/CPAP	0 to 35 cmH$_2$O
Inspiratory Time	0.1 to 1.5 seconds
Tidal Volume	5 to 2500 mL
Sensitivity	-1 to -10 cmH$_2$O
Sigh	1.5 times the tidal volume every 100th breath

Table 10-14:	Crossvent 4 Transport Ventilator Alarm Systems

Input Power

Low Battery

Control Circuit

I:E Ratio

Output Alarms

Pressure

High Pressure	0 to 125 cmH₂O
Low Pressure	0 to 125 cmH₂O
Mean Airway Pressure	0 to 125 cmH₂O
PEEP/CPAP Pressure	0 to 99 cmH₂O

Volume

Exhaled Tidal Volume	0 to 2,500 mL

Flow

Exhaled Minute Volume	0 to 200 L/min

Time

Breath Rate	0 to 199 breaths/ minute

Inspired Gas Alarm

Oxygen percent	21 to 100%

BIRD PRODUCTS CORPORATION, AVIAN™

The Avian™ Transport Ventilator is a microprocessor controlled, battery-powered ventilator (Figure 10-21). It is capable of operating in control, assist/control, SIMV, and CPAP modes. The ventilator is a flow controller, which is pressure or time triggered, pressure or flow limited, and pressure, volume (in sigh mode) or time cycled.

INPUT POWER

The microprocessor control system of the Avian™ Transport Ventilator is powered by an internal, rechargeable, 6 volt DC battery. The ventilator may also be powered by a 120/230 volt AC power source using an external power adaptor supplied with the ventilator. Additionally, the ventilator may be powered from an external 11 to 30 volt DC power source. An automotive-style cigarette lighter power cord is also supplied with the ventilator.

Gas to the pneumatic system must be provided between 40 and 60 psi. A blender may be used to mix air and oxygen to the desired F₁O₂. The ventilator does not have a blender incorporated into its design.

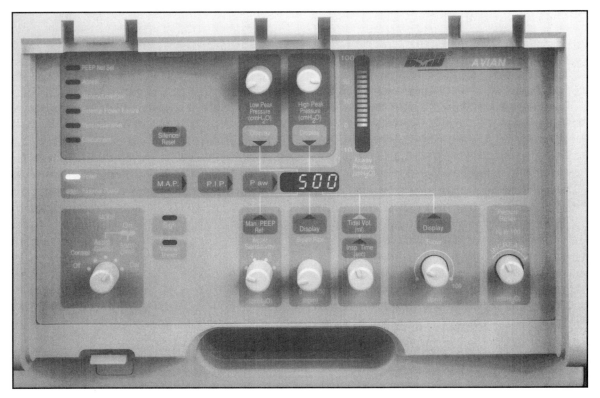

Figure 10-21 *A photograph of the Bird Avian™ transport ventilator. (Courtesy of Bird Products Corporation)*

CONTROL CIRCUIT

Gas enters the ventilator through a DISS gas inlet port. The gas then flows through a pressure regulator, where pressure is reduced to 30 psi (Figure 10-22). From the pressure regulator, gas is conducted to a main and a demand solenoid valve. Gas flow from the main solenoid valve passes through the flow control valve and a check valve to the patient circuit. Gas flow from the demand solenoid passes through a fixed orifice and then to the patient circuit.

A potentiometer is attached to the poppet of the flow control valve to sense the valve's position. Valve position is directly proportional to flow. The mass flow through the valve is unaffected by downstream pressures of up to 3 psig or 210 cmH$_2$O.

PEEP/CPAP pressure is generated by a user adjustable manual PEEP valve. PEEP pressures may be adjusted between 0 and 20 cmH$_2$O.

CONTROL VARIABLE

The control variable for the Avian™ Transport Ventilator is flow. Flow is directly proportional to valve position and is sensed by a potentiometer attached to the flow control valve's poppet. The feedback signal from the potentiometer (valve position) is used by the microprocessor to calculate tidal volume delivery (volume equals flow multiplied by time). Mass flow through the valve is not affected by back pressure in the patient circuit up to a pressure of 3 psig or 210 cmH$_2$O.

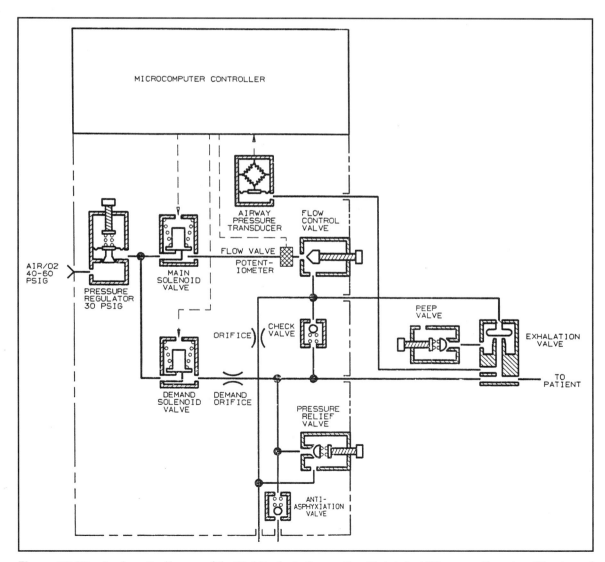

Figure 10-22 *A schematic diagram of the Bird Products Corporation Bird Avian's™ pneumatic system (Courtesy of Bird Products Corporation)*

PHASE VARIABLES

Trigger Variables

The trigger variables for the Avian™ include pressure, time and manual triggering. Pressure is a trigger variable during assist/control, SIMV (spontaneous breaths), and CPAP modes. Inspiratory pressure is sensed in the patient circuit by a pressure transducer. The electronic signal is used as a feedback signal to the microprocessor to initiate a breath or open the demand valve. Trigger sensitivity may be adjusted between –2 and –8 cmH_2O.

Time is a trigger variable during control mode, assist/control mode (in the absence of spontaneous efforts) and during the mandatory portion of SIMV. The breath rate control is used to set the respiratory rate and time triggering. Respiratory rates may be adjusted between 0 and 150 breaths per minute.

The ventilator is manually triggered if the practitioner depresses the manual breath button. When depressed, the ventilator delivers a mandatory breath at the set volume and inspiratory flow rate or at the set inspiratory time and flow rate.

Limit Variables

The limit variables include pressure and flow. Pressure becomes a limit variable if the pressure relief valve is adjusted to a pressure lower than the peak inspiratory pressure for the set tidal volume. Under these conditions, the inspiratory pressure reaches a plateau (pressure relief limit) and is held until the inspiratory time ends. Pressure relief is adjustable between 10 and 100 cmH_2O.

Flow may become a limit variable if the inspiratory flow is adjusted such that the flow reaches the control's set value and plateaus, delivering a square waveflow pattern.

Cycle Variables

The cycle variables for the Avian™ Transport Ventilator include pressure, volume and time. Pressure becomes a cycle variable if the peak inspiratory pressure exceeds the value set on the peak inspiratory pressure control. Peak inspiratory pressure is adjustable between 1 and 100 cmH_2O. If the pressure limit is reached, inspiratory flow is terminated, the exhalation valve opens and an audible and visual alarm will result.

Volume becomes a cycle variable when sigh breath delivery is selected. When sighs are activated, a sigh breath equal to 1.5 times the current tidal volume setting (2000 mL maximum volume), or 1.5 times the current inspiratory time setting (maximum of 3.0 seconds), will be delivered every 100th breath or every 7 minutes, whichever occurs first. The high pressure limit and inspiratory time are automatically increased by 1.5 times when a sigh breath is delivered, up to a maximum value of 100 cmH_2O pressure limit and 3.0 seconds inspiratory time.

Time becomes a cycle variable when the ventilator is in time cycled mode. Under these circumstances, inspiration ends when the inspiratory time has elapsed. Inspiratory time is adjustable between 0.1 and 3.0 seconds or until an I:E ratio of 1:1 is reached.

ALARM SYSTEMS

Input Power
Battery Low/Fail

In the event that no external power is applied and the internal battery is less than 5.6 volts ±0.2 volts the "Battery Low/Fail" LED will be illuminated on the front panel. The alarm may be silenced for 5 minute intervals.

External Power Low/Fail

In the event that an external power source is out of range, the ventilator automatically switches to the internal battery and activates the "External Power Low/Fail" LED on the front control panel. This alarm may be silenced until the internal battery voltage falls to 5.6 volts, activating the Battery Low/Fail alarm.

Control Circuit
Ventilator Inoperative

Ventilator inoperative alarms may be classified into recoverable and non-recoverable conditions. A recoverable alarm will occur if external power is interrupted and the internal battery is low, the mode switch is momentarily set to the off position, or the power supply voltages are out of range. Once the condition has been corrected, the ventilator will return to normal operation.

Nonrecoverable conditions occur if the microprocessor or control system fails a self-check. Under these conditions, the ventilator ceases to operate; however, the antisuffocation valve and exhalation valve are designed to allow a patient to spontaneously breathe from the ambient air.

ASSEMBLY AND TROUBLESHOOTING

Assembly—Avian™ Transport Ventilator

To assemble the Avian™ Transport Ventilator for use, follow the suggested assembly guide.

1. Connect the ventilator to a 50 psi medical gas source. If an F_IO_2 less than 1.0 is desired, operate the ventilator by connecting it to an oxygen blender having separate air and oxygen gas sources at 50 psi.

2. Choose the desired power source:
   a. Internal 6 VDC battery
   b. External 11–30 VDC battery
   c. 120 volt, 60 Hz or 220-230 volt, 50-60 Hz AC power using the AC power adapter

3. Assemble the patient circuit:
   a. Connect one end of the 22-mm, large-bore patient tubing to the ventilator outlet.
   b. Connect the distal end of the 22-mm, large-bore tubing to the patient manifold assembly (exhalation valve assembly).
   c. Connect the exhalation valve drive tubing to the exhalation valve nipple and the opposite end to the exhalation valve drive port on the side of the ventilator.
   d. Connect the proximal airway pressure tubing between the proximal airway pressure nipple on the patient manifold and the airway pressure port on the side of the ventilator.
   e. Connect a six-inch flextube to the outlet of the patient manifold and use a mask adapter or tracheostomy adapter to interface the patient circuit with the patient's airway.

Troubleshooting

To assist you in troubleshooting the Avian™ Transport Ventilator, refer to the troubleshooting algorithm at the end of this chapter.

I:E Ratio

If the inspiratory time exceeds 50% of the total breath period (inspiratory plus expiratory time), the I:E alarm flashes and inspiration is limited to 50% of the total breath time. This alarm alerts the practitioner to inspiratory time and tidal volume, or flow and breath rate control settings, which result in this condition.

Disconnect

If the airway pressure fails to rise at least 2 cmH_2O above the initial inspiratory pressure (baseline) during a breath period (inspiratory plus expiratory time), both audible and visual alarms will result.

Output Alarms
Pressure

As already described, the Avian™ incorporates a high peak pressure alarm. This alarm is adjustable between 1 and 100 cmH_2O and results in the termination of inspiration and an audible and visual alarm condition.

The Avian™ also has a low peak pressure alarm. This alarm has an off position and is adjustable between 2 and 50 cmH_2O. When activated, both an audible and a visual alarm will result. This alarm is helpful in the detection of leaks or patient disconnects.

PEEP Not Set

In the event that the PEEP/CPAP pressure varies more than 5 cmH_2O from the selected reference value, a visual LED indicator will be illuminated. The practitioner may adjust the reference value between 0 and 20 cmH_2O. Once set, this electronic reference value is used to compare the circuit pressure to the desired setting established using the manual PEEP valve on the expiratory port.

Time
Apnea

If no breath (inspiratory start) is detected for a 20 second time window, both audible and visual alarms will result and a backup

TABLE 10-15: Avian™ Transport Ventilator Capabilities

Modes	Control, Assist/Control, SIMV, CPAP
Rate	0 to 150 BPM
Flow	5 to 100 L/min
Insp. Time	0.1 to 3.0 seconds
Tidal Volume	50 to 2000 mL
Sensitivity	-2 to -8 cmH$_2$O
Pressure Limit	1 to 100 cmH$_2$O
PEEP/CPAP	0 to 20 cmH$_2$O
Sigh	1.5 times tidal volume every 100th breath or every 7 minutes

TABLE 10-16: Avian™ Transport Ventilator Alarm Systems

Input Power

Battery Low/Fail	
External Power Low/Fail	

Control Circuit

Ventilator Inoperative	
I:E Ratio	
Ventilator Disconnect	

Output Alarms

Pressure	
High Pressure	1 to 100 cmH$_2$O
Low Pressure	Off, 2 to 50 cmH$_2$O
PEEP Not Set	

Time

Apnea	No trigger for 20 seconds

breath rate of 12 BPM will be initiated. All other ventilator parameters (tidal volume, inspiratory time, etc.) will be as previously set by the practitioner.

Tables 10-15 and 10-16 summarize the Avian™ Transport Ventilator capabilities and alarm systems.

HAMILTON MEDICAL, INC., MAX

Hamilton Medical, Inc., markets and distributes the Max transport ventilator (Figure 10-23). The Max is a pneumatically powered electronically controlled transport ventilator. It is a flow controller which is pressure, time or manually triggered, pressure or flow limited, and time cycled. The ventilator may operate in control and spontaneous (IMV) modes of ventilation.

INPUT POWER

The ventilator is pneumatically powered and requires a medical gas source of between 50 and 90 psi. Once gas enters the ventilator, it is reduced in pressure by a single stage reducing valve to 50 psi.

The electronic control system may be powered by alkaline batteries, rechargeable NiCad batteries, or by an AC adapter. NiCad batteries can operate the ventilator for approximately 8 hours. If alkaline batteries are used, the ventilator may be operated for over 30 hours.

CONTROL CIRCUIT

Gas flows from the single-stage reducing valve to an electronically controlled solenoid valve (Figure 10-24). The solenoid valve when opened allows gas to flow through the flow control valve (tidal volume) and into the patient circuit. Between mandatory breaths, the patient's spontaneous inspiratory effort opens a demand valve, admitting gas to the patient circuit. A manual breath button when depressed allows gas to bypass the solenoid valve and flow directly through the flow control valve to the patient circuit.

PEEP may be provided by adding an external threshold resistor valve to the patient circuit. PEEP pressures may typically range from 0 to 20 cmH$_2$O when using these devices.

CONTROL VARIABLE

The control variable for the MAX ventilator is flow. Flow is adjusted using the tidal volume control. The control is a variable orifice valve which throttles flow from the electronic solenoid. Flow rate is adjustable between 0 and 90 L/min through the flow control valve. Since inspiratory time is fixed at 1 second, vol-

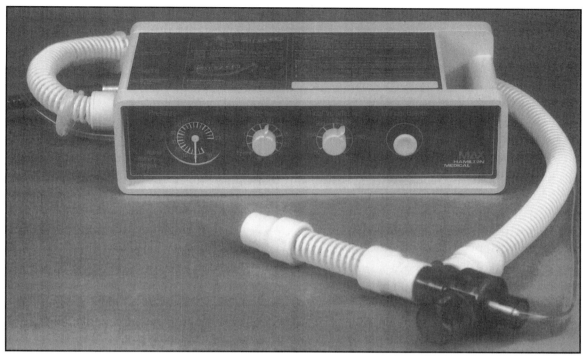

Figure 10-23 *A photograph of the Hamilton MAX ventilator, (Courtesy of Hamilton Medical, Inc.)*

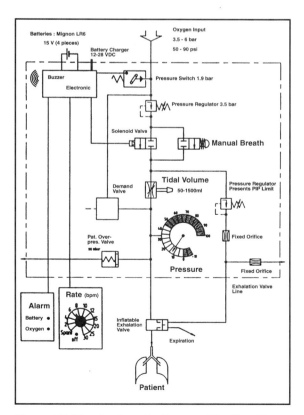

Figure 10-24 *A schematic diagram of the Hamilton Medical, Inc., MAX ventilator's pneumatic system. (Courtesy of Hamilton Medical, Inc.)*

ume becomes a function of flow (valve position) and time.

PHASE VARIABLES

Trigger Variables

The trigger variables for the MAX ventilator include pressure, time, and manual triggering. During spontaneous ventilation, if the patient inspiratory effort (pressure) is sufficient to open the demand valve gas will flow into the patient circuit. The trigger sensitivity is not adjustable, but is preset to -2 cmH$_2$O.

Time is the trigger variable during mandatory breaths. Time triggering is adjusted using the rate control. Respiratory rates of between 0 and 30 breaths per minute may be set. The respiratory rate control is a timer, which determines the cycling rate of the electronic solenoid valve.

The ventilator is manually triggered when the practitioner depresses the manual breath button on the right of the control panel. When depressed, gas flow bypasses the electronic solenoid valve, flows through the flow control valve and on to the patient circuit. Inspiration is terminated once the manual breath button is

ASSEMBLY AND TROUBLESHOOTING

Assembly—MAX Ventilator

To assemble the Hamilton Medical, Inc., MAX ventilator for use, follow this suggested assembly guide.

1. Select an electrical power source:
   a. Internal rechargeable NiCad or alkaline batteries (4 "AA" batteries).
   b. Use 120 volt, 60 Hz power and the AC adapter.

2. Connect the ventilator to a 50 psi medical gas supply using the DISS fitting on the left side of the ventilator.

3. Assemble the patient circuit:
   a. Connect one end of the 22-mm diameter patient circuit to the outlet of the ventilator located on the left side.
   b. Connect the distal end of the 22-mm diameter patient circuit to the patient manifold assembly.
   c. Connect the 1/8-inch diameter exhalation valve drive line between the exhalation valve nipple on the left side of the ventilator and the exhalation valve on the patient manifold assembly.
   d. If PEEP is desired, connect an external PEEP threshold device to the outlet of the patient manifold.
   e. Connect a 6-inch flex tube to the patient connection on the manifold assembly. Attach a mask adapter or a tracheostomy adapter to the flex tube to interface the ventilator to the patient's airway.

4. Check the ventilator for proper operation:
   a. Connect the patient circuit to a test lung.
   b. Set the tidal volume control for 500 mL and the rate control for 10 breaths per minute.
   c. Use a watch to verify the rate and a Wright respirometer or other volume measuring device to verify volume delivery.
   d. Disconnect the test lung and obstruct the patient circuit. Observe the pressure limit setting and adjust as required.

Troubleshooting

To troubleshoot the MAX ventilator, follow the troubleshooting algorithm at the conclusion of this chapter.

---

released. When the manual breath button is depressed, there is no fixed inspiratory time.

Limit Variables

The limit variables for the ventilator are pressure and flow. Pressure in the patient circuit is limited by an internal adjustable pressure relief valve. The pressure relief limit may be adjusted between 10 and 100 cmH$_2$O. To adjust the pressure relief, the ventilator cover must be removed, the patient circuit must be occluded, and the internal pressure regulator adjusted to the desired pressure limit during inspiration. If the pressure limit is set to a level that is lower than the peak inspiratory pressure for a given tidal volume, pressure will rise and plateau at the set pressure limit. When operated in this way, the ventilator is pressure limited. Inspiratory

pressure is displayed on a circular pressure manometer located at the left side of the control panel.

The pressure limit control operates by adjusting the pressure applied to the exhalation valve. Once pressure in the patient circuit exceeds the pressure in the exhalation valve, excess pressure is vented past the exhalation valve to ambient air. When this occurs, a loud noise results as gas flows through the partially closed exhalation valve.

Flow is a limit variable when tidal volume is set at a low setting and flow rises and plateaus during the inspiratory phase. Since inspiratory time is fixed at 1 second, it is possible at low tidal volume settings to be flow limited. The tidal volume control, as discussed earlier, is really a flow rate control, which is calibrated in mL.

TABLE 10-17:	The MAX Ventilator Capabilities
Modes	Control, IMV
Respiratory Rate	2 to 30 BPM
Inspiratory Time	1 second
Tidal Volume	50 to 1,500 mL
Flow Rate	0 to 90 L/min (mandatory)
	0 to 145 L/min (spontaneous)
Pressure Limit	10 to 100 cmH$_2$O
Sensitivity	-2 cmH$_2$O

Cycle Variable

The cycle variable for the ventilator is time. Inspiratory time is not adjustable and is set at 1 second. With a constant inspiratory time, volume delivery is a function of the flow rate through the flow control valve (tidal volume control).

ALARM SYSTEMS

Input Power

When less than 30 minutes of operation remain (when using the internal battery pack), the battery light will illuminate on the front control panel and an audible alarm will sound. The battery pack consists of four "AA" batteries.

A low oxygen alarm will result if the pressure powering the ventilator falls to less than 27 psi. If this occurs, both audible and visual alarms will result.

Tables 10-17 and 10-18 summarize the Hamilton Medical, Inc., MAX ventilator's capabilities and alarm systems.

IMPACT MEDICAL CORPORATION UNI-VENT® MODEL 750

Impact Medical Corporation's Uni-Vent® Model 750 is a microprocessor controlled portable ventilator (Figure 10-25). The ventilator is capable of operating in control, assist/control and SIMV modes. It is a flow controller

TABLE 10-16:	The MAX Ventilator's Alarm Systems
Input Power	
Low Battery	Less than 30 minutes' operation remaining
Low Gas Pressure	Gas supply pressure less than 27 psi

which may be pressure, time or manually triggered, and pressure, volume or time cycled.

INPUT POWER

The ventilator may be powered by internal batteries for up to 9 hours when fully charged. The ventilator may also be operated using a multivoltage power supply (120/230 volt, 50 to 400 Hz) or 11 to 30 volt DC external deep cycle battery. When operated on the multivoltage power supply, the internal batteries are automatically charged.

A medical gas source at 50–90 psi is required to power the pneumatic system of the ventilator. If an F$_I$O$_2$ of less than 1.0 is desired, the ventilator may be operated from an external blender with independent gas sources for air and oxygen at 50–90 psi.

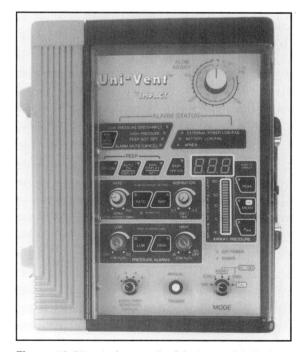

Figure 10-25 *A photograph of the Impact Medical Corporation's Uni-Vent® Model 750 ventilator. (Courtesy Impact Medical Corporation)*

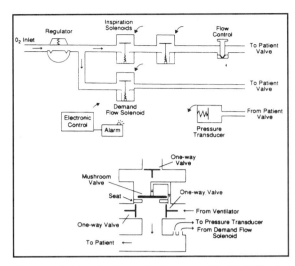

Figure 10-26 *A schematic diagram of the Uni-Vent® Model 750 pneumatic system. (Courtesy of Daedalus Enterprises, Inc.)*

CONTROL CIRCUIT

The gas enters the ventilator through a DISS fitting on the top of the ventilator. Once gas enters the ventilator, it is reduced in pressure to 50 psi by a single-stage reducing valve (Figure 10-26). Gas flow from the reducing valve then flows to two inspiration solenoids and a demand solenoid valve. Duplication of the inspiration solenoid valves provides a safety feature in the event that a solenoid valve should fail. Gas flows from the second inspiration solenoid to a flow control valve and then to the patient circuit. Gas flow from the demand solenoid flows to the patient circuit. Pressure in the patient circuit is measured by a pressure transducer connected to the patient manifold.

PEEP pressure can be provided by using an external PEEP valve. Sensitivity can be PEEP compensated using the auto-PEEP compensation system. When activated, the pressure transducer measures the baseline pressure and uses it as the baseline pressure to reference the sensitivity setting.

CONTROL VARIABLE

The control variable for the ventilator is flow. Flow is controlled by the flow control valve. Flow is adjustable between 0 and 100 L/min. Volume delivery becomes a function of flow and inspiratory time (flow multiplied by inspiratory time).

PHASE VARIABLES

Trigger Variables

The trigger variables for the ventilator include pressure, time and manual triggering. Pressure is a trigger variable during assist/control and SIMV modes. When pressure sensed in the airway by the pressure transducer is less than the trigger threshold, the inspiration solenoid valves open, delivering gas flow to the circuit. During spontaneous ventilation, a drop in circuit pressure results in the demand solenoid opening, providing gas flow to the patient. Sensitivity is adjustable between –2 and –8 cmH$_2$O in 2 cmH$_2$O increments.

Time becomes a trigger variable in control and assist/control modes. Time triggering is adjusted using the ventilation rate control. Respiratory rates are adjustable between 1 and 150 breaths per minute.

The ventilator may be manually triggered by the practitioner depressing the manual trigger button. Once depressed, the ventilator delivers a breath at the set flow and inspiratory time. Manual breaths may be delivered during all modes of ventilation.

Limit Variables

The limit variable for the ventilator is flow. Flow is adjustable between 0 and 100 L/min.

Cycle Variables

The cycle variables include pressure, volume and time. Pressure is a cycling variable when the peak inspiratory pressure exceeds the value set on the high pressure alarm. The high pressure alarm may be adjusted between 15 and 100 cmH$_2$O. Once the set pressure level has been reached, the alarm is activated.

Volume becomes a cycle variable when the sigh mode is activated. When activated, the ventilator delivers a sigh breath equal to 150% of the volume setting every 100th breath, or every seven minutes, whichever occurs first.

Time is a cycling variable during mechanical breath delivery. Inspiratory time is set using the inspiration time control. Inspiratory times are adjustable between 0.1 and 3.0 seconds in 0.1 second increments. Once the inspiratory time has lapsed, inspiration ends.

ALARM SYSTEMS

Input Power Alarms

The ventilator alerts the practitioner to both loss of external power as well as a dis-

ASSEMBLY AND TROUBLESHOOTING

Assembly—Uni-Vent® Model 750

To assemble the Impact Medical Corporation's Uni-Vent® Model 750 for use, follow the suggested assembly guide.

1. Select a power source:
   a. Multivoltage power supply (external battery or 120/230 volt, 60 Hz AC power)
   b. Internal batteries if charged
2. Connect the ventilator to a 50–90 psi medical gas source using the DISS fitting on the top of the ventilator.
3. Assemble the patient circuit:
   a. Connect the 22-mm diameter, large-bore tubing (patient circuit) to the outlet of the ventilator.
   b. Connect the patient manifold to the distal end of the 22-mm diameter patient circuit.
   c. Connect 3/16-inch diameter tubing to the patient manifold and the proximal end to the outlet of the demand flow solenoid.
   d. Connect the 1/8-inch diameter tubing from the patient manifold to the pressure transducer nipple on the top of the ventilator.
   e. Connect a 6-inch flextube to the outlet of the patient manifold and attach a mask adapter or tracheostomy adapter to interface the circuit with the patient's airway.

Troubleshooting

To assist you in troubleshooting the ventilator, follow the troubleshooting algorithm at the conclusion of this chapter.

---

charged internal battery pack. If the external multivoltage power supply becomes disconnected, the ventilator automatically switches to the internal batteries and activates the external power low/fail alarm.

If the internal battery's voltage drops to less than 11 volts, the battery low/fail alarm will be activated. Once the internal batteries reach this voltage, approximately one hour of operation time remains.

Control Circuit Alarms

The control circuit alarm consists of an inverse I:E ratio alarm. When inspiration becomes greater than 50% of the breath cycle time, the alarm is activated. Once activated, inspiration is terminated and the ventilator cycles into exhalation.

Output Alarms
Pressure

As described earlier, the ventilator has a high pressure alarm that is adjustable between 15 and 100 cmH$_2$O. In addition, the ventilator also has a low pressure/disconnect alarm. It is adjustable between 0 and 50 cmH$_2$O. This alarm is helpful in detecting leaks and patient disconnects.

The PEEP not set alarm alerts the practitioner to baseline pressure changes from that set on the manual display setting. Changes in baseline pressure may be caused by leaks or patient disconnects.

Time

The ventilator also incorporates an apnea alarm. If the ventilator does not detect a breath trigger for 20 seconds, the alarm will be activated. This is helpful in detecting disconnects as well as apneic events.

Tables 10-19 and 10-20 summarize the Uni-Vent® capabilities and alarm systems.

LIFE SUPPORT PRODUCTS, INC., AUTOVENT 2000/3000

Life Support Products, Inc., produces two portable transport ventilators, the AutoVent

TABLE 10-19: Uni-Vent® Ventilator Capabilities

Modes	Control, Assist/Control, SIMV, Sigh
Pressure	0 to 100 cmH$_2$O
Flow	0 to 100 L/min
Inspiratory Time	0.1 to 3.0 seconds
Expiratory Time	0.1 to 59.9 seconds
Rate	1 to 150 breaths per minute
Sigh	150% of tidal volume
Sensitivity	-2 to -8 cmH$_2$O
PEEP	0 to 20 cmH$_2$O

TABLE 10-20: Uni-Vent® Alarm Systems

Input Power

External Power Low/Fail

Battery Low/Fail

Control Circuit

Inverse I:E Ratio

Output

High Pressure	15 to 100 cmH$_2$O
Low Pressure	0 to 50 cmH$_2$O
PEEP Not Set	

Time

Apnea	No breath detected for 20 seconds

2000 and AutoVent 3000 (Figure 10-27). Both ventilators are pneumatically powered and controlled. They are flow controllers which are time or pressure triggered, pressure or flow limited, and time cycled. Since many similarities exist between the ventilators, they will be considered together. When differences occur, they will be discussed on an individual basis.

INPUT POWER

Power input for both the AutoVent 2000 and AutoVent 3000 is a medical gas supply between 40 and 90 psi. Since the ventilator is a single circuit ventilator, if an F$_I$O$_2$ different from the source gas is desired, the ventilator may be operated from a blender using a separate air and oxygen supply.

CONTROL CIRCUIT

Gas enters the ventilator through a DISS fitting on the left side of the ventilator. Once gas enters the ventilator, it is filtered and reduced in pressure by a single stage reducing valve to 30 psi.

During the inspiratory phase, gas flow is split (Figure 10-28A) with one path flowing through the timing cartridge and the other path flowing through the tidal volume control (flow control valve). The volume control is a variable orifice flow control valve which regulates the continuous flow of gas through the patient circuit. Gas flow through the timing cartridge is also split, with one path going through a fixed orifice valve (adjustable in the AutoVent 3000) which is the inspiratory time

control and to a volume accumulation chamber. The other gas pathway is to the exhalation valve diaphragm in the patient manifold. Once the volume accumulation chamber is filled, gas pressurizes the right portion of the timing cartridge, sliding it left and cycling the ventilator into exhalation.

During exhalation, pressurized gas in the volume accumulation chamber and inspiratory time control is exhausted to the atmosphere (10-28B). Gas flow from the reducing valve is conducted to the rate control. The rate control has an adjustable orifice which regulates gas flow to its accumulation chamber. Once the accumulation chamber becomes pressurized, the timing cartridge slides to the right, cycling the ventilator into inspiration.

CONTROL VARIABLE

The control variable for both ventilators is flow. Flow is controlled by the tidal volume control. Flow is adjustable between 16 and 48 L/min. Since gas flow through the patient circuit is continuous, volume delivery becomes a function of inspiratory time and flow.

PHASE VARIABLES

Trigger Variables

The trigger variables for both ventilators include pressure and time. Pressure is a trig-

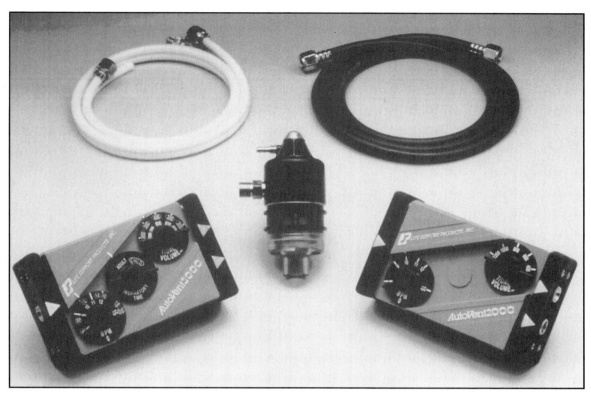

Figure 10-27 *A photograph of the Life Support Products, Inc., AutoVent 2000 and AutoVent 3000. (Courtesy of Life Support Products, Inc.)*

ger variable during spontaneous ventilation. If the patient's inspiratory effort is sufficient, gas can be drawn from the continuous flow through the patient manifold. Sensitivity is not adjustable, but is preset at –2 cmH$_2$O. Gas flow is available up to 48 L/min.

Time is the trigger variable during mandatory ventilation. Time triggering is adjusted using the respiratory rate control (labeled in BPM).

The rate control, as described earlier, is a pneumatic timing cartridge that controls expiratory time. The AutoVent 2000 has ventilatory rates adjustable between 0 and 20 breaths per minute. The AutoVent 3000 may be adjusted between 0 and 28 breaths per minute.

Limit Variables

The limit variable for both ventilators are pressure and flow. Pressure limit is adjusted using the pressure limit alarm incorporated into the patient manifold assembly. Pressure limit is set at 50 cmH$_2$O, ±5 cmH$_2$O. Once the pressure limit is reached, excess pressure is vented to the atmosphere until the inspiratory time has lapsed.

The ventilators may also be flow limited. If the tidal volume is set at a lower setting

and the inspiratory time is such that flow increases and plateaus, the ventilator is then flow limited. Since inspiratory time is fixed (1.5 or 0.75 seconds), this may occur under some circumstances.

Cycle Variable

The cycle variable for both ventilators is time. Inspiratory time for the AutoVent 2000 is fixed at 1.5 seconds. The inspiratory time for the AutoVent 3000 is selectable between 0.75 seconds (child) and 1.5 seconds (adult). As described earlier, the inspiratory time control is a pneumatic timer, controlling the length of inspiration.

ALARM SYSTEMS

Output Alarm

The output alarm for both ventilators is pressure. When the pressure limit is reached, an audible pneumatic reed alarm will also sound. As described earlier, the pressure limit is set at 50 cmH$_2$O, ±5 cmH$_2$O.

Tables 10-21 and 10-22 summarize the Life Support Products, Inc. AutoVent 2000 and 3000 ventilator capabilities and alarm systems.

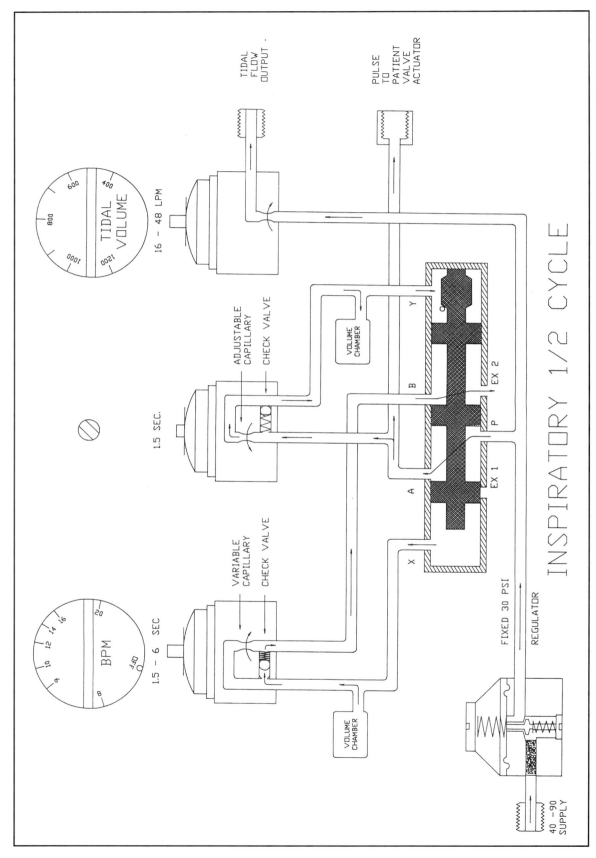

Figure 10-28A *A schematic diagram of the Life Support Products, Inc., AutoVent 2000/3000 pneumatic system during inspiration. (Courtesy of Life Support Products, Inc.)*

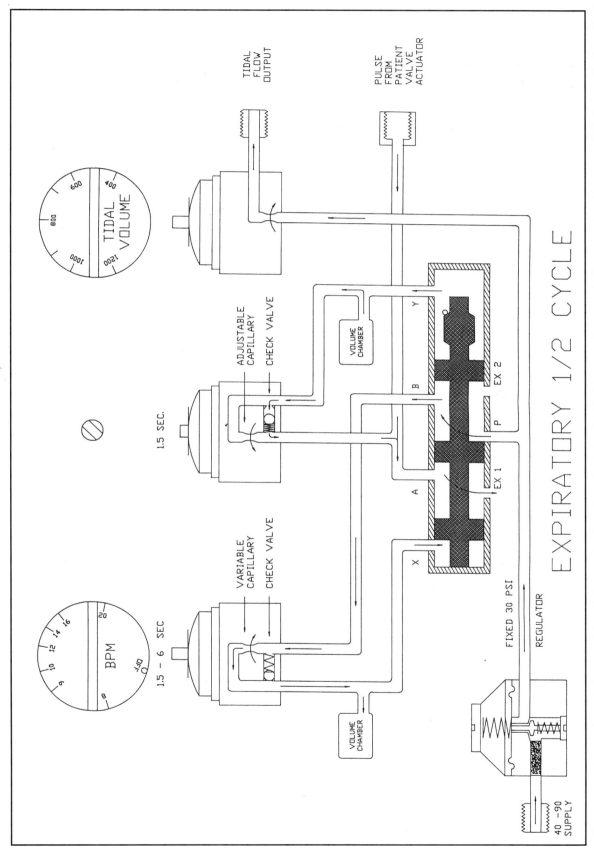

Figure 10-28B *A schematic diagram of the Life Support Products, Inc., AutoVent 2000/3000 pneumatic system during expiration. (Courtesy of Life Support Products, Inc.)*

ASSEMBLY AND TROUBLESHOOTING

Assembly—AutoVent 2000 and 3000

To assemble the AutoVent 2000 or AutoVent 3000 for use, follow the suggested assembly guide.

1. Connect the ventilator to a medical gas source between 40 and 90 psi. The ideal pressure input is 50 psi. If a different F_IO_2 from the source gas is desired, an oxygen blender may be used with separate oxygen and air gas sources.

2. Assemble the patient circuit:
   a. Connect the patient valve supply tubing to the ventilator outlets on the right side of the ventilator. The outlets are indexed with internal and external threads to prevent accidental mismatching.
   b. Connect the patient valve supply tubing to the patient manifold, observing the indexing of the tubing.
   c. Connect a 6-inch flextube to the outlet of the patient manifold and a mask adapter or tracheostomy adapter to its distal end to interface with the patient's airway.

3. Verify the ventilator's operation:
   a. Set the BPM control for 12 breaths per minute.
   b. Set the tidal volume control to 800 mL.
   c. Set the inspiratory time to the adult setting on the AutoVent 3000 (1.5 seconds).
   d. Connect the patient manifold to a test lung.
   e. Use a watch and a Wright respirometer or other volume-measuring device to verify the rate and tidal volume delivery.
   f. Occlude the patient outlet and verify that the pressure limit alarm is operational.

Troubleshooting

To troubleshoot the AutoVent 2000 and AutoVent 3000, refer to the troubleshooting algorithm at the conclusion of this chapter.

TABLE 10-21: AutoVent 2000 and AutoVent 3000 Capabilities

	AUTOVENT 2000	**AUTOVENT 3000**
Flow Rate	16–48 L/min	16–48 L/min
Tidal Volume	400–1,200 mL	200-1,200 mL
Rate	8 – 20 BPM	8–28 BPM
Inspiratory Time	1.5 seconds	0.75 or 1.5 seconds
Expiratory Time	1.5 to 6.0 seconds	1.5 to 6.0 seconds
Pressure Limit	50 cmH$_2$O, ±5 cmH$_2$O	50 cmH$_2$O, ±5 cmH$_2$O
Sensitivity	–2 cmH$_2$O	– 2 cmH$_2$O

TABLE 10-22: AutoVent 2000 and AutoVent 3000 Alarm Systems

	AUTOVENT 2000	**AUTOVENT 3000**
Output Alarm		
Pressure	50 cmH$_2$O, ±5 cmH$_2$O	50 cmH$_2$O, ±5 cmH$_2$O

NEWPORT MEDICAL INSTRU- MENTS, INC., NEWPORT E100M

Newport Medical Instruments, Inc., produces the E100M transport ventilator (Figure 10-29). The E100M is a microprocessor-controlled, pneumatically powered ventilator. It is a flow controller that is time, pressure, or manually triggered, pressure or flow limited and time cycled. The ventilator may operate in assist/control, SIMV, and spontaneous ventilation modes.

Input Power

The Newport E100M incorporates an integral blender into its design. Both air and oxygen are connected to the blender using the DISS fittings located on the rear of the blender. Medical gas sources between 35 and 70 psi may be used, with 50 psi being the recommended input pressure.

The ventilator may be operated from three different electrical power sources. Standard AC current (100/120 VAC or 220/240 VAC,

50/60 Hz), external battery or internal battery. When fully charged, the internal battery can power the ventilator for approximately 6 to 8 hours.

Control Circuit

Gas from the blender is split into three paths (Figure 10-30). One path flows to the spontaneous toggle switch. This switch has two positions: off (no gas flow for spontaneous breathing) and 8 L/min. When toggled to the 8 L/min setting, approximately that amount is delivered to the reservoir bag and then enters the patient circuit during spontaneous ventilation. Gas flow from this toggle switch also provides pneumatic power to the pilot valve, which, in conjunction with the flow control valve, determines inspiration.

Another gas path directs blended gas to the transport toggle switch, which is designed to conserve gas during transport. This is accomplished by blocking the air/oxygen blender bleeds, thus limiting gas consumption to about 15 L/min. This feature may cause the F_IO_2 to vary by more than 0.03; therefore, when using this feature, careful monitoring of oxygen delivery is important.

The third gas path is to the main flow control valve. When the pilot valve is electronically actuated, gas from the pilot valve activates the main flow valve, delivering gas through the flow control valve and a muffler and then into the patient outlet. Bleed gas from the outlet of the main flow valve powers

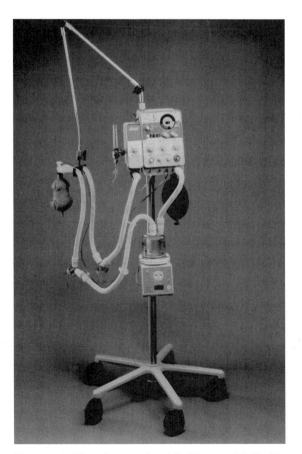

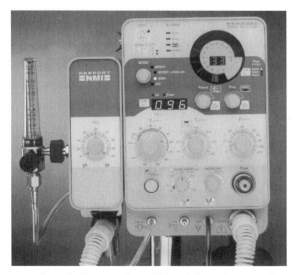

Figure 10-29 *Photographs of the Newport Medical Instruments, Inc., E100M ventilator (A) and the E100M ventilator's control panel (B). (Courtesy Newport Medical Instruments, Inc., Newport Beach, CA)*

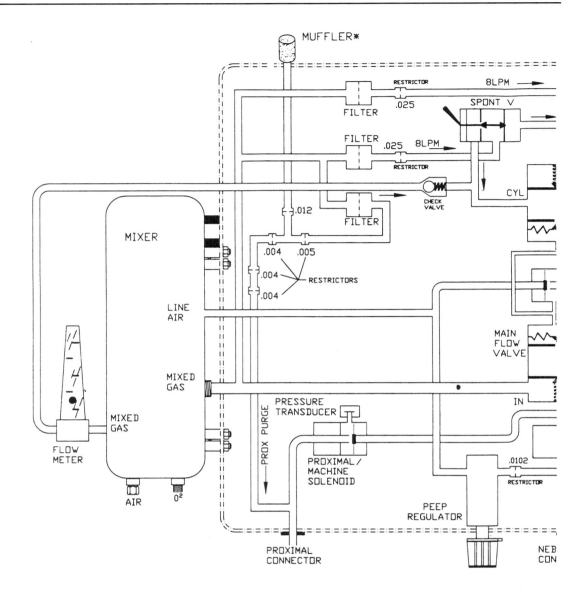

Figure 10-30 *A schematic of the Newport Medical Instruments, Inc., E100M ventilator's pneumatic system. (Courtesy Newport Medical Instrucments, Inc., Newport Beach, CA) (continues)*

the nebulizer and the exhalation solenoid valve.

The exhalation valve is controlled by an exhalation solenoid, which inflates the exhalation valve during inspiration, thus delivering gas to the patient. PEEP/CPAP pressure is generated by bleed gas from the pilot valve. The bleed gas is directed through the PEEP regulator and provides pressure, partially closing the exhalation valve, which acts as a threshold resistor, thus creating PEEP/CPAP pressure in the circuit.

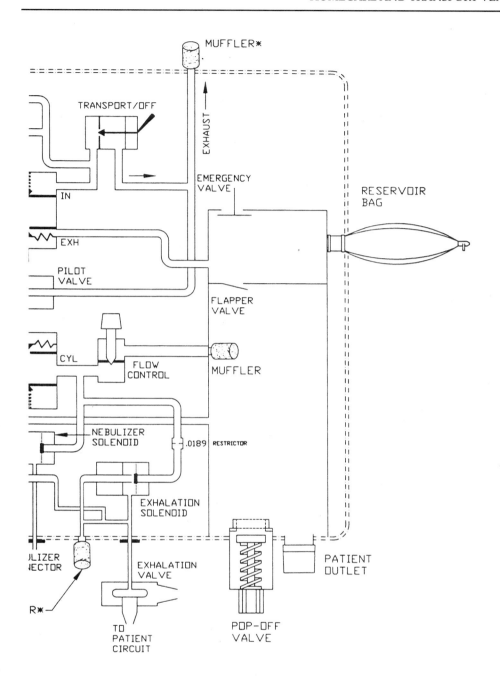

Figure 10-30 *(continued)*

Control Variables

The control variable for the Newport E100M ventilator is flow. Flow is controlled by the flow control valve and is adjustable between 1 and 100 L/min. Volume delivery becomes a function of inspiratory flow and inspiratory time (volume equals flow multiplied by inspiratory time).

Phase Variables
Trigger Variables

The trigger variables of the ventilator include pressure, time and manual triggering.

Pressure triggering occurs when the patient's inspiratory effort exceeds the level set on the pressure trigger control. Pressure triggering may be adjusted between –10 and 25 cmH$_2$O. By depressing the automatic trigger control (ATC) button, a function is activated that maintains the pressure triggering as sensitively as possible within a specified range while preventing artifacts or autotriggering. When using this feature, the ventilator attempts to maintain a trigger threshold of –2 cmH$_2$O below baseline pressure.

Time triggering occurs during assist/control and the mandatory portion of SIMV. Time triggering is set using the respiratory rate control. Respiratory rates are adjustable between 1 and 120 breaths per minute. The rate control functions with the microprocessor control system and determines the opening and closing of the pilot valve.

Manual triggering occurs when the practitioner depresses the manual button. When depressed, gas flow is directed through the flow control valve and into the patient circuit. The breath ends when the button is released, the maximum pressure alarm threshold is met, or 4 seconds have elapsed.

Limit Variables

The limit variables of the Newport E100M include pressure and flow. The pressure limit is adjusted using the pressure limit control, which is a manually adjustable pop-off valve. The pressure limit may be adjusted between 0 and 120 cmH$_2$O. When the pressure limit is reached, pressure is held constant and excess pressure is vented through the relief valve to the atmosphere. Inspiration is terminated once the inspiratory time has passed.

Flow becomes a limit variable if the flow rate is set at a lower setting and inspiratory time is set such that flow increases and plateaus. Under these conditions, the ventilator becomes flow limited. Inspiratory flow rates may be set between 1 and 100 L/min.

Cycle Variables

The cycle variables for the Newport E100M include pressure and time. Pressure becomes a cycle variable if the inspiratory pressure exceeds the setting on the high-pressure alarm. If the high-pressure alarm threshold is met, inspiration is terminated and audible and visual alarms result. The high-pressure alarm is an adjustable pressure sensor. The alarm is set by pushing in the "P" alarm knob, and then rotating it clockwise, to increase, or counterclockwise, to decrease, the setting. The high-pressure alarm settings may be set between 5 and 120 cmH$_2$O.

Time becomes a cycle variable when the microprocessor control system deactivates the pilot valve, thus closing it. Time cycling is adjusted using the inspiratory time control. Inspiratory times are adjustable between 0.1 and 3.0 seconds.

Baseline Variable

The baseline variable for the ventilator is pressure. PEEP/CPAP pressures are adjustable between 0 and 25 cmH$_2$O. The PEEP/CPAP control regulates pressure transmitted against the exhalation valve diaphragm, creating a threshold resistor that generates PEEP/CPAP pressure.

Modes of Ventilation
Assist/control

When operated in this mode, the ventilator delivers breaths at the set rate, flow and inspiratory time. If the patient has spontaneous efforts sufficient enough to be detected by the sensitivity system, a ventilator-supported breath will be delivered.

SIMV

The E100M ventilator SIMV system allows the patient to breathe spontaneously between mandatory breaths. The first patient-triggered breath during a mandatory breath interval will be ventilator assisted. Following the initial assisted breath, any breaths taken during the rest of the time interval are spontaneous breaths. If no spontaneous breaths are taken, the ventilator will deliver mandatory breaths at the rate established by the setting on the frequency control.

Time-Cycled, Pressure-Limited Ventilation (Assist/Control or SIMV)

During this mode of ventilation, the practitioner sets a pressure plateau level using the mechanical pressure relief valve. The ventilator will deliver breaths at the set rate and inspiratory time, but all breaths will be pressure limited at the set plateau level. All pressure in excess of the pressure limit setting will be vented to the atmosphere.

ASSEMBLY AND TROUBLESHOOTING

Assembly—Newport Medical Instruments, Inc., E100M Ventilator

To prepare the Newport Medical Instruments E100M ventilator for use, follow this suggested assembly guide.

1. Select a power source:
   a. 120/230 volt, 60 Hz electrical power
   b. External, 12 VDC battery
   c. Internal battery (if fully charged)

2. Connect the ventilator to 50 psi medical gas supplies (air and oxygen) using the DISS fittings on the rear of the blender.

3. Assemble the patient circuit:
   a. Connect a high-range flowmeter to the DISS fitting on the left of the integral blender.
   b. Connect oxygen supply tubing between the flowmeter and the reservoir bag inlet.
   c. Connect a 2 liter reservoir bag to the reservoir bag adapter fitting.
   d. Connect the inspiratory limb of the patient circuit to the main flow ventilator outlet, the expiratory limb of the patient circuit to the exhalation valve and the proximal pressure sensing line to the proximal connection.
   e. Connect the 1/8-inch diameter exhalation valve drive line to the exhalation valve nipple on the front of the ventilator.
   f. Connect the distal end of the 1/8 inch exhalation valve drive line to the exhalation valve on the patient circuit manifold assembly.

Troubleshooting

To assist you in troubleshooting the Newport Medical Instruments E100M ventilator, refer to the troubleshooting algorithms at the end of this chapter.

Spontaneous

In this mode of ventilation, the E100M ventilator will deliver gas to the patient exclusively through the reservoir system. The constant-flow toggle switch must be opened and/or flow from the auxiliary flowmeter must be added in order to provide gas flow to the reservoir system. All gas flowing through the system is blended gas from the integral blender.

Mandatory and spontaneous flows may be adjusted independently using the DuoFlow system incorporated into the E100M ventilator. The mandatory flow rate control will set the flow delivered during mandatory breaths, while the spontaneous toggle switch and the auxiliary flowmeter may be set to establish an independent flow for the spontaneous breaths.

Flow assist may be used to augment a patient's peak flow needs during spontaneous breathing. During the flow assist time interval, a high flow (the flow setting on the mandatory flow control) is delivered. After the flow assist time has lapsed, the flow rate becomes the combination of the spontaneous toggle switch and auxiliary flow meter settings. The flow assist may be set between 0.0 and 1.0 seconds.

Alarm Systems
Input Power

The input power alarms include loss of electric power, low battery and low gas inlet pressure. If electrical power has been lost, a continuous alarm will result to indicate the loss of electrical power. If the external battery pack has become discharged, the same alarm will result. In addition, in the event that either air or oxygen pressure is lost, a pneumatic reed alarm will sound continuously.

Control Circuit Alarms

The control circuit alarms of the E100M ventilator include I:E ratio and fault system alarms. The I:E ratio alarm is activated if the inspiratory time is longer than the expiratory time. When this occurs, a yellow LED will blink, indicating that the 1:1 ratio has been exceeded.

If the microprocessor detects a function problem with the ventilator or its control system, a continuous audible alarm results and an error code is displayed in the control monitor. In the event this occurs, provide an alternate source of ventilation for the patient and remove the ventilator from service.

Output Alarms
Pressure

The E100M ventilator incorporates both high- and low-pressure alarms and an automatic baseline pressure alarm. The high-pressure alarm is adjustable between 5 and 120 cmH₂O, and the low-pressure alarm is adjustable between 3 and 118 cmH₂O.

The automatic baseline pressure alarm provides for both high and low baseline pressure indications. The high baseline pressure alarm is activated if the airway pressure remains above the minimum pressure alarm setting at the end of exhalation. The minimum baseline pressure alarm is activated if the airway pressure remains below the low baseline alarm setting for greater than 3 seconds.

Time

The ventilator incorporates an apnea alarm. If the ventilator is operated in the spontaneous mode, the apnea alarm will alert the

---

TABLE 10-23: Newport Medical Instruments, Inc., E100M Ventilator Capabilities

Modes	Assist/Control, SIMV, Time-Cycled, Pressure-Limited A/C or SIMV; Spontaneous
Rate	1 to 120 breaths per minute
Pressure	0 to 120 cmH₂O
Pressure limit	0 to 120 cmH₂O
Inspiratory time	0.1 to 3.0 seconds
Tidal volume	5 to 5,000 mL
Sensitivity	−10 to 25 cmH₂O
Flow Rate	1 to 100 L/min
PEEP/CPAP	0.0 to 25 cmH₂O
F₁O₂	0.21 to 1.0

TABLE 10-24: Newport Medical Instruments, Inc., E100M Ventilator Alarm Systems

Input Power
  Loss of electrical power
  Low battery
  Low air/oxygen pressure

Control Circuit
  Inverse I:E ratio
  Fault system

Output
  Pressure
    High pressure
    Low pressure
    High baseline pressure
    Low baseline pressure

Time
  Apnea

---

practitioner to apneic events. The detection delay has three settings: 0, or off; 15 seconds; and 30 seconds. If the sensitivity system fails to detect any spontaneous breaths within the detection delay time period, both audible and visual alarms will result. This alarm is also helpful in detecting patient disconnects.

Tables 10-23 and 10-24 summarize the Newport E100M ventilator capabilities and alarm systems.

OMNI-TECH MEDICAL, INC., OMNI-VENT

Omni-Tech Medical, Inc., produces the Omni-Vent portable pneumatically powered transport ventilator (Figure 10-31). The ventilator is pneumatically powered and controlled. It is a flow controller which is pressure or time triggered, pressure or flow limited and time cycled. It may be operated in volume control, pressure control, IMV (volume- or pressure-controlled modes), and CPAP modes.

INPUT POWER

The Omni-Vent is pneumatically powered and controlled. A medical gas source of be-

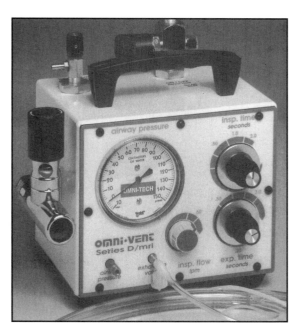

Figure 10-31 *A photograph of the Omni-Tech Medical, Inc., Omni-Vent portable ventilator. (Courtesy Omni-Tech Medical, Inc.)*

tween 25 and 140 psi may be used to power the ventilator. A 50 psi source is the recommended pressure to power the ventilator. However, if desired, the ventilator may be calibrated to run at lower pressures (25 psi) to utilize liquid systems which may be desirable in some situations.

CONTROL CIRCUIT

Gas powering the ventilator enters through a filter in the gas inlet assembly (Figure 10-32). It then passes through an on/off valve in the same assembly and on to the inspiratory and expiratory valve block. From the inspiratory/expiratory valve block, the gas is conducted to a flow accelerator and then to a flow control valve. From the flow control valve the gas flow is split, with one path flowing to a pressure relief valve and patient circuit and the other path flowing to the exhalation valve diaphragm.

IMV may be provided by the addition of an external reservoir and one-way valve assembly. Gas is deverted to the reservoir through a needle valve located on the top of the ventilator.

PEEP/CPAP may be added using an external threshold resistor valve attached to the patient circuit. PEEP/CPAP pressures of between 0 and 20 cmH₂O may be added using the external valve.

CONTROL VARIABLE

The control variable for the Omni-Vent is flow. Flow is determined by the flow control valve. Flow rates may be adjusted between 0 and 98 L/min. The flow control valve is a variable orifice needle valve. Opening or closing the valve regulates the flow of gas through it. Since flow is constant, volume delivery becomes a function of inspiratory flow and inspiratory time (volume is equal to flow multiplied by time).

PHASE VARIABLES

Trigger Variables

The trigger variables include pressure and time. Pressure is a trigger variable during IMV ventilation. When inspiratory effort is sufficient to open a one-way valve in the IMV reservoir, gas is delivered to the patient.

Time is the control variable for volume and pressure controlled ventilation, as well as the mandatory portion of IMV. The expiratory time control acts as a rate control. The expiratory valve is a needle valve which controls the rate of gas leakage through a timing cartridge. If gas flow leaking from the cartridge is high, expiratory time is less. Conversely, if gas leakage is slow, expiratory time is longer. Respiratory rates are adjustable between 0 and 150 breaths per minute.

Limit Variables

The limit variables for the Omni-Vent include pressure and flow. Pressure becomes a limit variable if the pressure relief valve is set lower than the peak inspiratory pressure for a given inspiratory time and flow rate. Under these circumstances, pressure will rise to the pressure limit setting and plateau until the inspiratory time has elapsed, with the ventilator operating in pressure control mode. The pressure limit may be adjusted between 0 and 120 cmH₂O.

The ventilator may also be flow limited. If the flow rate is set at a lower setting and inspiratory time is set such that flow increases and plateaus, the ventilator is then flow limited.

Cycle Variable

The cycle variable for the ventilator is time. Inspiratory time is determined by the inspiratory time needle valve. The inspiratory time like the expiratory time control is a pneumatic

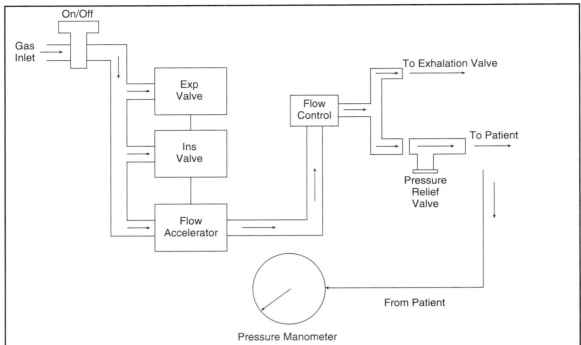

INSPIRATORY PHASE

Source gas is introduced through a filter in the gas inlet assembly; then gas flows to the pneumatic valve supply inlet. The gas flows to the flow control then to the tee assembly which directs gas simultaneously to the exhalation valve and pressure relief valve to the patient.

As gas pressure increases in the lung, it is transmitted to the manometer through a tubing independent from the tubing wye connector.

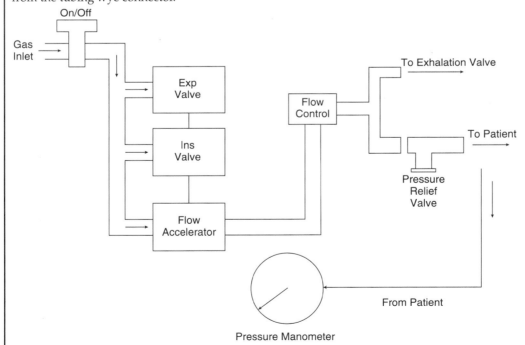

EXPIRATORY PHASE

Source gas follows the identical path of the inspiratory phase to the pneumatic valves and is then held until the inspiratory phase begins.

Figure 10-32 *A schematic diagram of the Omni-Tech Medical, Inc., Omni-Vent pneumatic system. (Courtesy Omni-Tech Medical, Inc.)*

ASSEMBLY AND TROUBLESHOOTING

Assembly—Omni-Vent

To prepare the Omni-Tech Medical, Inc., Omni-Vent for use, follow the suggested assembly guide.

1. Connect the ventilator to a medical gas source (25 to 140 psi). If an F_IO_2 of less than 1.0 is desired, the ventilator may be powered from a blender operating from independent sources of medical air and oxygen.

2. Assemble the patient circuit:
   a. Connect one end of the 22-mm diameter patient circuit to the ventilator outlet.
   b. Connect the patient manifold assembly to the distal end of the 22-mm diameter patient circuit.
   c. Connect one end of the 1/8-inch diameter line to the exhalation valve nipple on the side of the ventilator and the other end to the exhalation valve on the patient manifold assembly.
   d. Connect the other 1/8-inch diameter line between the airway pressure nipple on the ventilator and the proximal airway tap on the patient manifold.
   e. Connect a 6-inch flextube to the patient manifold assembly and attach a mask adapter or tracheostomy adapter to the distal end to interface with the patient airway.

3. Confirm the ventilator's operation:
   a. Connect the patient circuit to a test lung and rotate the on/off switch to the on position.
   b. Adjust flow, inspiratory and expiratory time to the desired settings.
   c. Confirm rate and volume delivery using a Wright respirometer or other volume-measuring device and a watch.
   d. Occlude the patient circuit and adjust the pressure relief valve to the desired pressure.

Troubleshooting

To assist you in troubleshooting the Omni-Vent ventilator, refer to the troubleshooting algorithm at the end of this chapter.

---

timing cartridge. Adjustment of the needle valve controls the rate of gas leakage from the cartridge, which either lengthens or shortens inspiratory time. Inspiratory times may be adjusted between 0.2 and 3.0 seconds.

MONITORING SYSTEMS

Monitoring System

The Omni-Vent monitoring system consists of an analog pressure gauge located on the upper left of the control panel. The gauge is connected to the patient circuit via the proximal airway line and reflects pressures at the proximal airway.

ALARM SYSTEMS

The Omni-Vent has no built-in alarm systems. Table 10-25 summarizes the Omni-Vent's capabilities.

TABLE 10-25: Omni-Vent Ventilator Capabilities

Modes	Volume and Pressure Control, IMV, CPAP
Tidal Volume	30 to 3,000 mL
Respiratory Rate	0 to 150 BPM
Inspiratory Time	0.2 to 3.0 seconds
Expiratory Time	0.2 to 60 seconds
Flow Rate	0 to 98 L/min
Pressure Relief	0 to 120 cmH$_2$O
PEEP/CPAP	0 to 20 cmH$_2$O (external threshold resistor)

CHAPTER SUMMARY

This chapter has covered a diverse group of ventilators and noncontinuous ventilatory support devices. Tables 10-26 and 10-27 will assist you in learning the similarities and differences among the ventilators presented in this chapter.

TABLE 10-26: Home Care Ventilators and Non-Continuous Ventilatory Support Ventilators

VENTILATOR	INPUT POWER	CIRCUIT	CONTROL MECHANISM	TRIGGER VARIABLE	LIMIT VARIABLE	CYCLING VARIABLE	ALARMS
Homecare Ventilators							
Aequitron Medical, Inc.							
LP6 PLUS	Electric	Single	Electronic	P,T		P,V,T	I, CC, P
Aequitron Medical, Inc.							
LP10	Electric	Single	Electronic	P,T	P	P,V,T	I, CC, P
Aequitron Medical, Inc.							
LP20	Electric	Single	Electronic	P,T	P	P,V,T	I, CC, P
BEAR Medical Systems, Inc.							
BEAR 33	Electric	Single	Electronic	P,T	F	P,V,T	I, CC, P, T
Lifecare							
PLV-100	Electric	Single	Electronic	P,T	P	V	I, CC, P, T
PLV-102	Electric	Single	Electronic	P,T	P	V	I, CC, P, T
Puritan Bennett Corporation							
Companion 2801	Electric	Single	Electronic	P,T	P,F	V,T	I, CC, P, T
Non-Continuous Ventilatory Augmentation Ventilators							
Puritan Bennett Corporation							
Companion							
320I/E	Electric	Single	Electronic	F	P	F	
Respironics, Inc.							
BiPAP® S/T	Electric	Single	Electronic	F	P	F,T	

Key: F—Flow, P—Pressure, V—Volume, T—Time, I—Input Power, CC—Control Circuit.

TABLE 10-27: Transport Ventilators

VENTILATOR	INPUT POWER	CIRCUIT	CONTROL MECHANISM	TRIGGER VARIABLE	LIMIT VARIABLE	CYCLING VARIABLE	ALARMS
AMBU, Inc.							
TransCARE 2	Pneumatic	Single	Pneumatic	P,T	P,F	T	CC, P
Bird Products Corporation							
Avian™	Pneumatic	Single	Electronic	P,T,M	P,F	P,V,T	I, CC, P, T
Hamilton Medical, Inc.							
MAX	Pneumatic	Single	Electronic	P,T,M	P,F	T	I
Impact Medical Corporation							
Uni-Vent®	Pneumatic	Single	Electronic	P,T,M	F	P,V,T	I, CC, P, T
Life Support Products, Inc.							
AutoVent 2000/3000	Pneumatic	Single	Pneumatic	P,T	P,F	T	P
Newport Medical Instruments, Inc.							
E 100M	Pneumatic	Single	Electronic	P,T,M	P,F	P,T	I, CC, P, T
Omni-Tech Medical, Inc.							
Omni-Vent	Pneumatic	Single	Pneumatic	P,T	P,F	T	

Key F—Flow, M—Manual, P—Pressure, V—Volume, T—Time, I—Input Power, CC—Control Circuit.

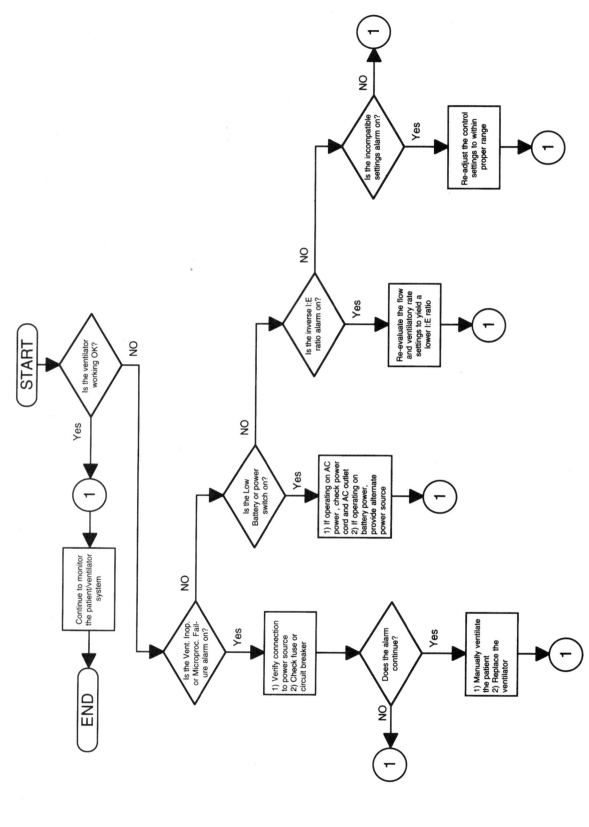

ALG 10-1   *A troubleshooting algorithm for homecare ventilator input power and control circuit alarms.*

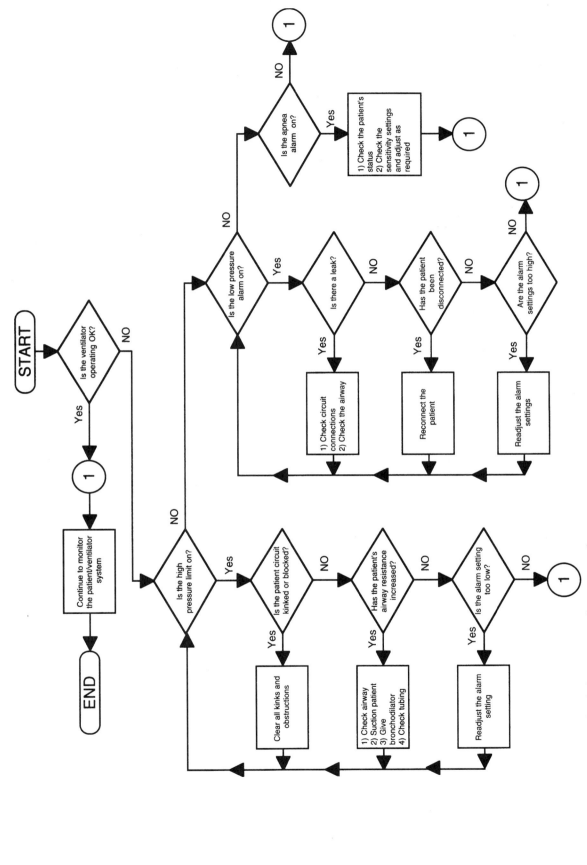

ALG 10-2 *A troubleshooting algorithm for homecare ventilator output alarms.*

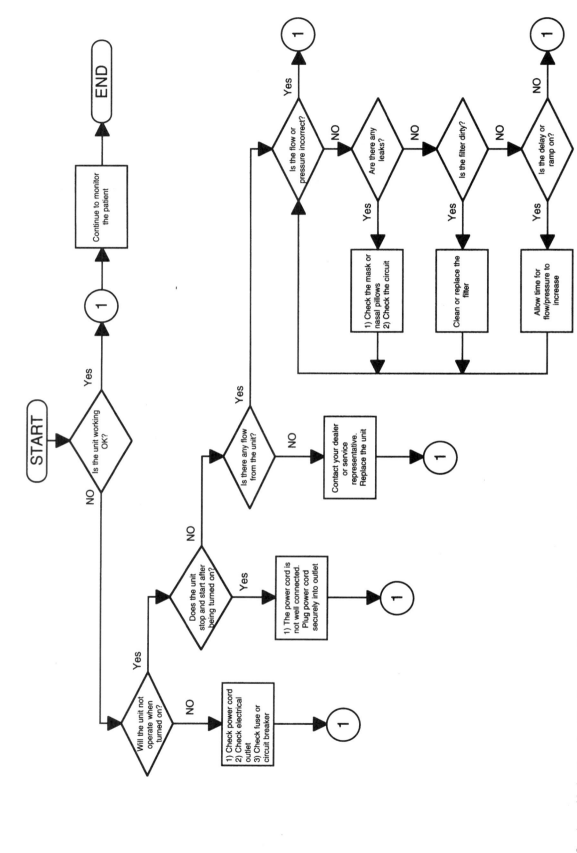

ALG 10-3 *A troubleshooting algorithm for noncontinuous ventilator augmentation devices.*

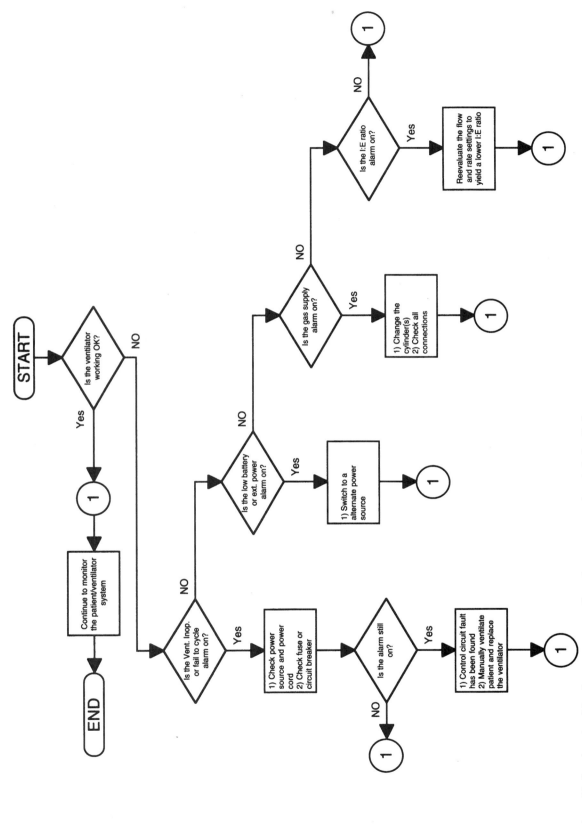

ALG 10-4 *A troubleshooting algorithm for transport ventilator input power and control circuit alarms.*

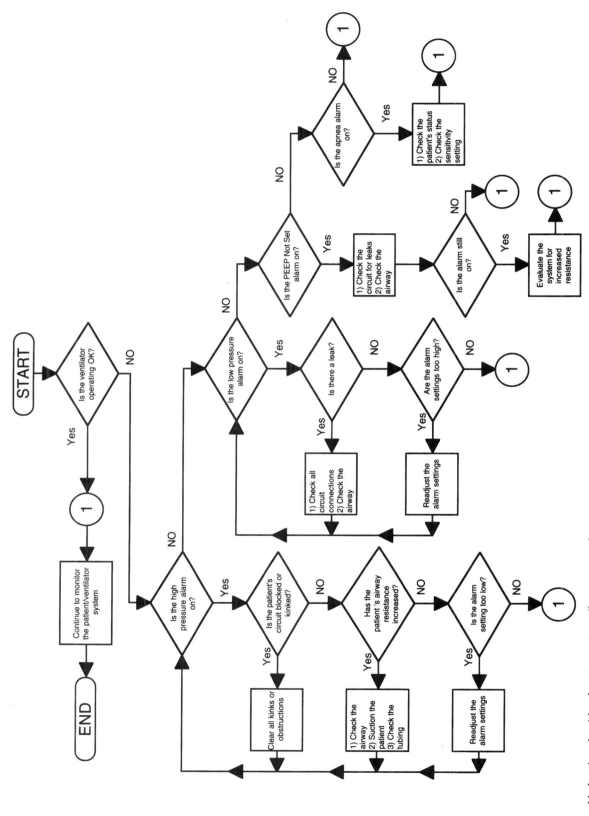

ALG 10-5 *A troubleshooting algorithm for transport ventilator output alarms.*

CLINICAL CORNER

Homecare Ventilators

1. You are making your biweekly visit to a homecare patient who is ventilator dependent. The patient's caregiver expresses concern that the pressure alarm frequently goes off. What should you assess and what might you do?
2. You are helping a caregiver prepare to take a ventilator-dependent patient on a day trip to an art gallery. List the equipment that the caregiver should take along.

Noncontinuous Ventilatory Augmentation Equipment

1. A doctor asks you to explain the difference between a home CPAP and home bi-level positive airway pressure system. What would you say?
2. A patient on a Nellcor Puritan Bennett Companion 320I/E has an order to increase the nocturnal pressure by 10 cmH$_2$O. How can you assist the patient in adjusting to this new pressure level?

Transport Ventilators

1. When maintaining a patient on a transport ventilator during transport, what other equipment should you always have with you (besides the ventilator)?
2. During a helicopter flight a transport ventilator's low-pressure alarm (visual alarm) goes off. What should you check?

Self-Assessment Quiz

1. Which of the following is the common control variable among the homecare ventilators discussed in this chapter?
   a. Pressure.
   b. Flow.
   c. Volume.
   d. Time.

2. Which of the following is a common power source between the homecare ventilators discussed in this chapter?
   a. Electric.
   b. Pneumatic.
   c. Both electric and pneumatic.
   d. None of the above.

3. Which of the following homecare ventilators may be pressure limited?
   I. Aequitron Medical LP10.
   II. BEAR 33.
   III. Lifecare PLV-102.
   IV. Puritan Bennett Companion 2801.
   a. I
   b. I and II
   c. I, II, and III
   d. I, III and IV

4. Pressure rises to a preset value and remains at that level until inspiration is terminated best describes:
   a. Pressure cycling.
   b. Pressure controlling.
   c. Pressure limiting.
   d. Baseline pressure.

5. Which of the following homecare ventilators have an apnea alarm?
   I. Aequitron Medical LP10
   II. BEAR 33.
   III. Lifecare PLV-100.
   IV. Puritan Bennett Companion 2801.
   a. I
   b. I and II
   c. I, II, and III
   d. II, III and IV

6. Which of the following ventilators utilize a rotary-driven piston as the drive mechanism?
   I. Aequitron Medical LP6 PLUS
   II. BEAR 33.
   III. Lifecare PLV-102.
   IV. Puritan Bennett Companion 2801.
   a. I
   b. I and II
   c. I, II and III
   d. I, II, and IV

7. When adding an external PEEP threshold resistor to the circuit, the device should be located:
   a. Proximal to the exhalation valve in the circuit.
   b. Distal to the exhalation valve in the circuit.
   c. At the end of the 6-inch flextube near the patient's airway.
   d. None of the above.

8. Proper location of an external PEEP threshold resister is important because it may cause:
   a. Interference with pressure triggering.
   b. Loss of volume.
   c. Interference with pressure limiting.
   d. Interference with flow limiting.

9. The trigger variables common to the homecare ventilators include:
   I. Pressure.
   II. Flow.
   III. Volume.
   IV. Time.
   a. I and II
   b. I and III
   c. I and IV
   d. III and IV

10. Which of the following homecare ventilators may be flow limited?
    a. Aequitron Medical LP10.
    b. BEAR 33.
    c. Lifecare PLV-100.
    d. Lifecare PLV-102.

11. When a homecare ventilator is operated as a pressure-limited ventilator, the cycle variable is:
    a. Pressure.
    b. Flow.
    c. Volume.
    d. Time.

12. Which of the following are examples of control circuit alarms?
I. Ventilator inoperative.
II. I:E Ratio.
III. Microprocessor error.
IV. Control circuit fault.
a. I
b. I and II
c. I, II, and III
d. I, II, III and IV

13. CPAP is an effective treatment for sleep apnea because:
a. The positive pressure inflates the lungs.
b. The artificial airway keeps the patient's airway patent.
c. The CPAP pressure splints the airway open.
d. Gas exchange is improved.

14. The control variable for CPAP systems is:
a. Pressure.
b. Flow.
c. Volume.
d. Time.

15. The trigger variable for the bi-level positive airway pressure systems discussed in this chapter is:
a. Pressure.
b. Flow.
c. Volume.
d. Time.

16. The limit variable for the bi-level positive airway pressure systems discussed in this chapter is:
a. Pressure.
b. Flow.
c. Volume.
d. Time.

17. Common patient interfaces for both CPAP and bi-level positive airway pressure systems include:
I. Nasal mask.
II. Endotracheal tube.
III. Nasal pillows.
IV. Tracheostomy tube.
a. I and II
b. I and III
c. II and III
d. II and IV

18. Which of the following transport ventilators are **not** pneumatically controlled?
a. Ambu, TransCARE 2.
b. Impact Medical, Uni-Vent®.
c. Omni-Tech Medical, Omni-Vent.
d. Life Support Products, AutoVent 3000.

19. Which of the following transport ventilators may be manually triggered?
I. Ambu, TransCARE 2.
II. Bird Products Corp., Avian™.
III. Impact Medical, Uni-Vent®.
IV. Hamilton Medical, MAX.
a. I and II
b. I and III
c. II and III
d. II, III and IV

20. You are using a transport ventilator which is a flow controller. You set the inspiratory time for 0.3 seconds and the flow rate at 50 L/min. What is the delivered tidal volume?
    a. 150 mL.
    b. 500 mL.
    c. 900 mL.
    d. 1500 mL.

21. Which of the following transport ventilators may be pressure limited?
    I. Ambu, TransCARE 2.
    II. Bird Products Corp., Avian™.
    III. Hamilton Medical, MAX.
    IV. Newport Medical Instruments, E 100M.
    a. I
    b. I and II
    c. I, II and III
    d. I, II, III and IV

22. Which of the following transport ventilators incorporates an integral blender?
    a. Ambu, TransCARE 2.
    b. Bird Products Corp., Avian™.
    c. Hamilton Medical, MAX.
    d. Newport Medical Instruments, E 100M.

23. When a transport ventilator delivers a volume of gas based upon inspiratory time and flow rate, what is the cycle variable?
    a. Pressure.
    b. Flow.
    c. Volume.
    d. Time.

24. If a transport ventilator has inspiratory and expiratory time and flow controls, which control determines time triggering once tidal volume delivery has been determined?
    a. Inspiratory time.
    b. Expiratory time.
    c. Flow rate.
    d. None of the above.

25. Inspiratory pressure rises to a preset level and remains constant until the inspiratory time has lapsed best describes:
    a. Pressure controlling.
    b. Pressure limiting.
    c. Pressure cycling.
    d. None of the above.

26. Which of the following transport ventilators may be operated in IMV or SIMV mode without the addition of an external IMV manifold assembly?
    I. Bird Products Corp., Avian™.
    II. Ambu, TransCARE 2.
    III. Newport Medical Instruments, E 100M.
    IV. Life Support Products, AutoVent 3000.
    a. I and II
    b. I and III
    c. II and III
    d. II and IV

27. Which of the following transport ventilators have PEEP/CPAP incorporated into their design?
    I. Bird Products Corp., Avian™.
    II. Ambu, TransCARE 2.
    III. Newport Medical Instruments, E 100M.
    IV. Life Support Products, AutoVent 3000.
    a. I and II
    b. I and III

c. II and III
d. II and IV

28. Which of the following transport ventilators may be flow limited?
   I. Ambu, TransCARE 2.
   II. Bird Products Corp., Avian™.
   III. Omni-Tech Medical, Omnivent.
   IV. Life Support Products, AutoVent 3000.
   a. I
   b. I and II
   c. I, II, and III
   d. I, II, III and IV

29. Which of the following ventilators can be volume cycled?
   I. Bird Products Corp., Avian™.
   II. Impact Medical, Uni-Vent®.
   III. Omni-Tech Medical, Omni-Vent.
   IV. Newport Medical Instruments, E 100M.
   a. I and II
   b. I and III
   c. II and III
   d. III and IV

30. Inspiration is terminated when a preset pressure is reached best describes:
   a. Pressure controlling.
   b. Pressure limiting.
   c. Pressure cycling.
   d. None of the above.

Selected Bibliography

Aequitron Medical, Inc., *LP6 PLUS Volume Ventilator and LP10 Volume Ventilator with Pressure Limit User's Manual*, Minneapolis, MN, 1994.

Ambu, Inc., *Ambu TransCARE Series Ventilators (TransCARE 1, TransCARE 1-HB, TransCARE 2) Operator's Manual*, Linthicum, MD, 1994.

Bear Medical Systems, Inc., *BEAR 33 Volume Ventilator Clinical Instruction Manual*, Riverside, CA, 1987.

Bio-Med Devices, Inc., *Crossvent 4 Intensive Care/Transport Ventilator Operation and Service Manual*, Guilford, CT, 1996.

Bird Products Corporation, *Bird Avian™ Operators/Service Manual*, Palm Springs, CA, 1994.

Branson, Richard D., "Intrahospital Transport of Critically Ill, Mechanically Ventilated Patients," *Respiratory Care*, Vol. 37, No. 7, pp. 775–795, 1992.

Campbell, Robert S., et al., "Laboratory and Clinical Evaluation of the Impact Uni-Vent 750 Portable Ventilator," *Respiratory Care*, Vol. 37, No. 1, pp. 29–36, 1992.

Chatburn, Robert L., "A New System for Understanding Mechanical Ventilators," *Respiratory Care*, Vol. 36, No. 10, pp. 1123–1152, 1991.

Chatburn, Robert L., "Classification of Mechanical Ventilators," *Respiratory Care*, Vol. 37, No. 9, pp. 1009–1025, 1992.

Gietzen, Jon W., et al., "Effect of PEEP-Valve Placement on Function of a Home-Care Ventilator," *Respiratory Care*, Vol. 36, No. 10, pp. 1093–1098, 1991.

Hamilton Medical, *Operator's Manual MAX*, Reno, NV, 1989.

Lifecare, Inc., *PLV-100 Operating Manual*, Westminster, CO, 1991.

Lifecare, Inc., *PLV-102 Operating Manual*, Westminster, CO, 1991.

Life Support Products, Inc., *AutoVent 2000/3000 Operating Manual,* Irvine, CA, 1991.

McPherson, Steven P., *Respiratory Therapy Equipment,* 4th Ed., Mosby-Yearbook, Inc., 1990.

Newport Medical Instruments, Inc., *The Newport E100M Ventilator Operating Manual,* Newport Beach, CA, 1998.

Newport Medical Instruments, Inc., *The Newport E100M Ventilator Service Manual,* Newport Beach, CA, 1998.

Omni-Tech Medical, Inc., *Omni-Vent Operators/Service Manual,* Topeka, KS, 1994.

Puritan Bennett Corporation, *Companion 2801 Volume Ventilator Operating Instruction Manual,* Lenexa, KS, 1990.

Puritan Bennett Corporation, *Companion 318 Nasal CPAP System Patient Guide,* Lenexa, KS, 1993.

Puritan Bennett Corporation, *Companion 320I/E Bi-Level Respiratory System Patient Guide,* Lenexa, KS, 1993.

Respironics, Inc., *BiPAP® S/T Ventilatory Support System Operators Manual,* Murrysville, PA, 1992.

Respironics, Inc., *BiPAP® Service Manual,* Murrysville, PA, 1993.

Respironics, Inc., *BiPAP® Systems Guidebook: A Discussion of the Systems and Their Applications,* Murrysville, PA, 1992.

Respironics, Inc., *REMstar Choice Nasal CPAP System Patient Pamphlet,* Murrysville, PA, 1994.

Respironics, Inc., *REMstar Choice Service Manual,* Murrysville, PA, 1994.

CHAPTER 11

HIGH-FREQUENCY MECHANICAL VENTILATION

INTRODUCTION

By definition, high-frequency ventilators administer smaller tidal volumes (equal to or less than anatomical dead space) at high frequencies. The U.S. Food and Drug Administration defines a high-frequency ventilator as any ventilator that delivers breaths at a rate greater than 150 breaths per minute or any jet ventilator regardless of its frequency or rate. Today, there are four primary types of high-frequency ventilators: high-frequency positive pressure ventilators, high-frequency flow interrupters, high-frequency jet ventilators, and high-frequency oscillatory ventilators.

High-frequency ventilators are employed in patient care in situations in which the patient has intractable hypoxemia and hypercarbia that is not responsive to conventional positive pressure ventilation. In other circumstances, high-frequency ventilation is used where there is pulmonary insult or damage that results in large air leaks (bronchopulmonary fistulae). Some surgical cases (laser bronchoscopy, laryngoscopy and tracheal surgery) also support the use of high-frequency ventilation, in which it is desirable to maximize the airway caliber while supporting the patient adequately without an airtight seal.

High-frequency ventilation accomplishes the goal of adequately supporting gas exchange without using large tidal breaths at low frequencies. The mechanism of gas exchange with the alveoli is different when compared with bulk convection (as understood with conventional mechanical ventilation). There are several theories of how gas is exchanged during high-frequency ventilation, including asymmetric velocity profiles, pendelluft, Taylor dispersion, cardiogenic mixing and molecular diffusion.

In this chapter you will learn about the different types of high-frequency ventilators, the circumstances when high-frequency ventilation is employed clinically, the different theories of gas exchange and the specifics of some of the high-frequency ventilators currently being marketed.

OBJECTIVES

After completing this chapter, the student will accomplish the following objectives:

- Describe the following types of high-frequency ventilators
  — High-frequency positive pressure ventilator
  — High-frequency flow interrupter
  — High-frequency jet ventilator
  — High-frequency oscillatory ventilator

- Discuss the different mechanisms of gas exchange in the lungs.
  — Bulk convective ventilation
  — Asymmetric velocity profiles
  — Pendelluft
  — Taylor dispersion
  — Cardiogenic mixing
  — Molecular diffusion

- Describe the different clinical situations in which high-frequency ventilators are employed.
  — Refractory hypoxemia and hypercarbia
  — Failure of conventional ventilation
  — Pulmonary insult resulting in air leaks
  — Surgical ventilatory support

- For the ventilators in this chapter, describe the following:
  — Input power
  — Drive mechanism
  — Control scheme
  — Alarm systems
- Describe how to assemble and troubleshoot the following ventilators:
  — Percussionaire® VDR 4
  — SensorMedics Critical Care 3100 Oscillator

TYPES OF HIGH-FREQUENCY VENTILATORS

There are several different types of high-frequency ventilators. These include high-frequency positive pressure ventilators, high-frequency flow interrupters, high-frequency jet ventilators and high-frequency oscillatory ventilators. Each of these ventilator types has the commonality of delivering small tidal breaths at high frequencies; however, some rely on passive exhalation (recoil of the lung tissue and chest wall) while others are active during exhalation (active movement of the gas during exhalation).

HIGH-FREQUENCY POSITIVE PRESSURE VENTILATOR (HFPPV)

The high-frequency positive pressure ventilator (HFPPV) was first described and developed by Swedish investigators Sjöstrand and associates. A *high-frequency positive pressure ventilator (HFPPV)* consists of a conventional mechanical ventilator with a modified circuit employing a low compliance and compressible volume. These modifications allow tidal breath delivery at higher frequencies, which is not possible with the conventional circuit. Fresh gas is introduced into the circuit through a side arm, which functions as a fluidic valve using the Coanda affect (refer to Chapter 6). The exhalation valve on the circuit

permits control of baseline pressures for the application of PEEP/CPAP. Gas delivery is achieved at flows of 175 to 250 L/min and tidal volumes of 3 to 4 mL/kg. Exhalation with this ventilator is passive, relying on the recoil of the lungs and chest wall.

Advantages of this type of ventilator when compared to conventional positive pressure mechanical ventilation include diminished cardiac side effects, including blood pressure fluctuations, and the ability to ventilate through small catheters or cannulas. This type of ventilator is frequently used during laryngoscopy, bronchoscopy and upper airway surgery. The application of the ventilator through a small cannula or catheter allows an improved operative field for the surgeon.

HIGH-FREQUENCY JET VENTILATOR (HFJV)

The *high-frequency jet ventilator (HFJV)* employs high-pressure, short puffs or bursts of gas at high frequencies to accomplish gas exchange. These high-frequency bursts of gas are introduced into the airway through a small catheter at the endotracheal tube port via a special adapter or through a specialized endotracheal tube (High-Lo Jet Tracheal Tube). Through viscous shearing, additional gas flow is entrained around the cannula with each jet pulse, making the tidal volume the sum of the entrained gas and the volume delivered with the pulse, or burst, of gas. Ventilatory rates of 100 to 200 breaths per minute, with I:E ratios of 1:2 to 1:8, are possible. Since tidal volume delivery is a function of the jet pulse and gas entrainment, precise tidal volume measurement is difficult. Exhalation is passive with these ventilators; instead, the elastic recoil of the lungs and chest wall provide the force for exhalation.

HIGH-FREQUENCY FLOW INTERRUPTER (HFFI)

The *high-frequency flow interrupter (HFFI) ventilator* is similar to the HFJV in that small bursts of gas are delivered to the airway by interrupting a high-pressure or high-flow gas source. However, no injector cannula is used. The most common types of HFFI ventilators use a rotating ball with a single orifice or gas pathway (Figure 11-1) to interrupt the gas flow into short bursts. Frequency is determined by

the rate at which the ball is rotating, and volume delivery is controlled by varying the pressure proximal to the rotating ball and through bias flow entrainment (Figure 11-1). Exhalation is passive, relying on the recoil of the lungs and chest wall.

HIGH-FREQUENCY OSCILLATORY VENTILATOR (HFOV)

The *high-frequency oscillatory ventilator (HFOV)* is active both during inspiration and exhalation. Most HFOV ventilators employ a diaphragm, piston or modified acoustic speaker to oscillate the gas into and out of the airway (Figure 11-2). Typically, a bias flow past the airway provides the fresh gas source, while the HFOV provides forward (inspira-

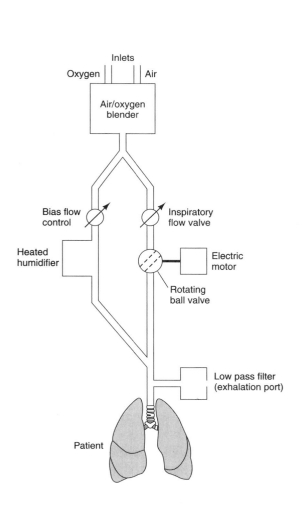

Figure 11-1 *A high-frequency flow interruptor that uses a rotating ball assembly.*

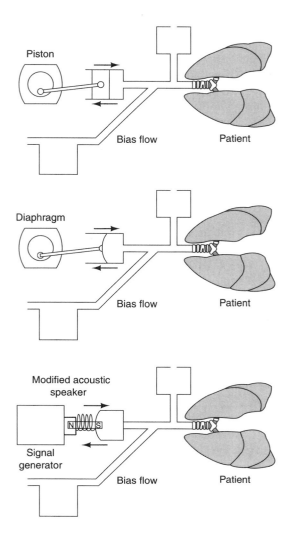

Figure 11-2 *Three types of high-frequency oscillatory ventilators: with piston drive, with diaphragm drive, and with an acoustic speaker drive.*

tion) and backward (exhalation) movement of gas into and out of the artificial airway. The forward and backward motion of the oscillatory device causes a typical sinusoidal flow wave form. HFOV ventilators typically deliver volumes of between 0.8 and 2.0 mL/kg at frequencies of 180 to 1,000 breaths per minute. Tidal breath delivery is dependent on the stroke volume of the oscillator, bias flow, size of the artificial airway and impedance of the low pass filter.

GAS EXCHANGE IN THE LUNGS DURING HIGH-FREQUENCY VENTILATION

High-frequency ventilation relies on small tidal volumes (often equal to or less than dead space) moving at high rates to accomplish gas exchange. Since large volumes of gas are not moving into and out of the lungs by convection, other mechanisms of gas exchange must be at work in order to normalize oxygen and carbon dioxide tensions in the blood. Several mechanisms have been hypothesized besides convective ventilation, including asymmetric velocity profiles, pendelluft, Taylor dispersion, cardiogenic mixing, and molecular diffusion.

CONVECTIVE VENTILATION

Convective ventilation, or the bulk flow of gas into and out of the lungs, is how gas exchange is most readily understood. Large tidal volumes (greater than the anatomic dead space) enter the pulmonary conduction system, with velocity slowing as the airways narrow and the cross-sectional area increasing as the gas moves distally toward the parenchyma. Eventually, the alveoli (comprising the respiratory zone) come into contact with gas that has passed through the conduction zone and oxygen and carbon dioxide are exchanged with the blood.

ASYMMETRIC VELOCITY PROFILES

Asymmetric velocity profiles comprise an attempt to account for differences in the relative shape of the inspiratory and expiratory velocity gradient, or profile. During inspiration, the

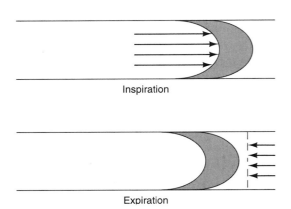

Figure 11-3 *A schematic drawing of asymmetrical velocity profiles. Notice how flow is greatest in the central portion of the airway.*

velocity at the center of the airway is greatest whereas the velocity near the periphery of the airway is less (Figure 11-3). This can be accounted for by the difference in resistance to flow, whereby resistance is greater near the bronchial wall (frictional loss) compared with the central lumen of the airway.

During exhalation, the velocity profile of the exhaled gas is relatively flat when compared with the parabolic inspiratory profile. During oscillatory ventilation, it is hypothesized that the inspiratory gases tend not to decelerate (due to momentum). Therefore, there is a net gas movement during inspiration down the center of the airway, while expiratory gases tend to move out the peripheral portions of the airway. It has been theorized that inspiratory and expiratory flow can occur simultaneously (due to the net inspiratory and expiratory flow gradients).

PENDELLUFT

Pendelluft, a compound word of German origin, means air swinging back and forth freely, or in an oscillatory fashion. Pendelluft occurs due to the fact that different areas of the lung have different time constants, resulting in their filling and emptying at different rates. This results is a net gas flow from one lung region to another which improves the overall uniformity of gas distribution.

TAYLOR DISPERSION

Taylor described a model in which turbulent gas flow in the airways enhances diffusion by augmenting the mixing process caused by the eddies formed in the turbulent flow. Fredberg expanded the work of Taylor and described the flow of gas during high-frequency ventilation as being dependent upon turbulence and dispersion. Fredberg hypothesized that to increase turbulence, flow must be increased, and that at low tidal volumes, the most efficient way to increase flow is to increase frequency. Frequency is optimal in his model when minute ventilation is the greatest at a given pressure, which is dependent on the mechanics of the respiratory system.

CARDIOGENIC MIXING

Cardiogenic mixing is a theory proposed by Slutsky in which the motion of the heart during the cardiac cycle is hypothesized to help with the distribution of gas during high-frequency ventilation. The continuous cardiac motion should help to vibrate the airways, thus further enhancing gas distribution and mixing.

MOLECULAR DIFFUSION

Molecular diffusion theory supports the concept that with the increased frequencies associated with high-frequency ventilation, the kinetic activity of the molecules at the alveolar level should increase. This greater kinetic activity should enhance the transport of gases across the alveolar capillary membrane.

CLINICAL APPLICATION OF HIGH-FREQUENCY VENTILATION

Unlike conventional positive pressure ventilation, high-frequency ventilation can provide adequate gas exchange by using lower tidal volumes at high respiratory rates and lower mean airway pressures. When ventilating patients, there are several potential advantages in the unique aspects of high-frequency ventilation. These advantages, when compared with conventional ventilation, include lower mean airway and intrathoracic pressures; minimum cardiac side effects caused by positive intrathoracic pressure; a stable, motionless operative field; and improvement in gas exchange in some patients.

REDUCED MEAN AIRWAY AND INTRATHORACIC PRESSURE

High-frequency mechanical ventilation accomplishes gas exchange by using small tidal volumes at high respiratory rates. Several investigators have demonstrated that it is possible to maintain adequate gas exchange using high-frequency ventilation at lower mean airway pressures when compared with the pressures required using conventional ventilation. The decrease in mean and peak airway pressures helps to prevent ventilator-induced lung injury and undesirable cardiac side effects associated with elevated intrathoracic pressures. While a reduction in mean and intrathoracic pressures is often a goal of high-frequency ventilation, it is has been shown that it is also important to initially recruit lung volumes while providing adequate pressures to sustain those volumes once those regions have been initially recruited.

HFJV has been used for patients who have a bronchopulmonary fistula, resulting in large air leaks when conventional mechanical ventilation had been employed. The reduced mean airway pressures and minimal chest wall excursion associated with HFJV help with the resolution of such air leaks.

STABLE, MOTIONLESS OPERATIVE FIELD

HFJV has been successfully used for bronchoscopies, tracheal surgery and laryngoscopy to ventilate patients and provide a stable, motionless operative field. Since HFJV can be accomplished through a small cannula (even percutaneously), it offers a large operative field. Furthermore, since ventilation is accomplished using small tidal volumes at lower pressures, it causes minimal chest wall and airway motion.

REFRACTORY HYPOXEMIA AND HYPERCARBIA

Because high-frequency ventilation achieves gas exchange by other mechanisms besides convection, it is often helpful in patients who have refractory hypoxemia and hypercarbia while beings supported by conventional ventilatory methods. Often when these patients are switched to high-frequency ventilation, gas exchange improves, resulting in increases in oxygenation and an improvement in ventilation. The success of high-frequency ventilation has been found, in infants with respiratory failure and patients with adult respiratory distress syndrome (ARDS), using HFPPV, HFJV, and HFOV.

REPRESENTATIVE HIGH-FREQUENCY VENTILATORS

Two high-frequency ventilators currently account for the majority of sales: the Percussionaire® Corporation VDR 4 and the Sensormedics Corporation 3100 Oscillator. In this section the functional characteristics of these ventilators will be explained and you will learn how to assemble and troubleshoot them, in preparation for their clinical application.

PERCUSSIONARE® VDR 4

The Percussionaire® VDR 4 ventilator is a pneumatically powered and controlled, high-frequency ventilator (Figure 11-4, A and B). Some authors have described the VDR 4 as an HFFI, a HFOV, or a HFJV. In reality, the VDR 4 is classified as a pneumatically powered and controlled, time-triggered, time-cycled, pressure-limited ventilator. It is unique in that it has the ability to provide both convective and percussive (high-frequency) ventilation simultaneously.

Power Input

The Percussionaire® VDR 4 is pneumatically powered and requires a 50 psi source of both air and oxygen. DISS fittings are located on the right rear side of the ventilator. The gases enter the ventilator, pass through check valves, and are then conducted to a Bird® air/oxygen blender, where F$_I$O$_2$ levels may be adjusted between 0.21 and 1.00.

Drive Mechanism and Control Circuit

Gas from the air/oxygen blender is reduced from 50 psi to, typically, between 35 and 40 psi before being conducted to the master switch, the drive mechanism, and the control circuits (Figure 11-5). The master switch is an on/off rotary switch, which allow the clinician to select either phasic (percussive, high-frequency) ventilation or demand CPAP and

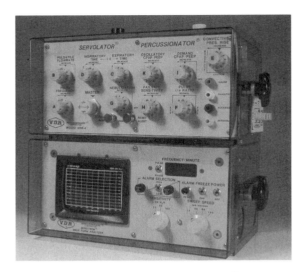

Figure 11-4A *Photo of the Percussionaire® VDR 4 ventilator.*

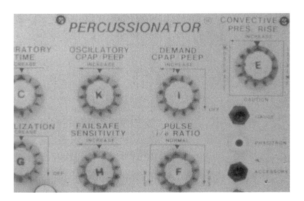

Figure 11-4B *Control panel of the VDR 4 (courtesy Percussionaire Corporation, Sandpoint, ID)*

manual ventilation (spontaneous CPAP breathing or manual breath delivery).

The drive mechanism of the VDR 4 is a high-frequency pulse generator (HFPG). The clinician can program the pulse frequency, pulsatile flow rate and inspiratory and expiratory times. Together, these controls determine the number of subtidal breaths delivered during each oscillatory interval. The pulse frequency control is a needle valve, which controls the breath rate or frequency. It is adjustable from 40 to over 900 breaths per minute. The pulsatile flow rate control determines the inspiratory flow rate of the subtidal volume delivery. Pulsatile flow rates may be adjusted up to 125 liters per minute at an op-

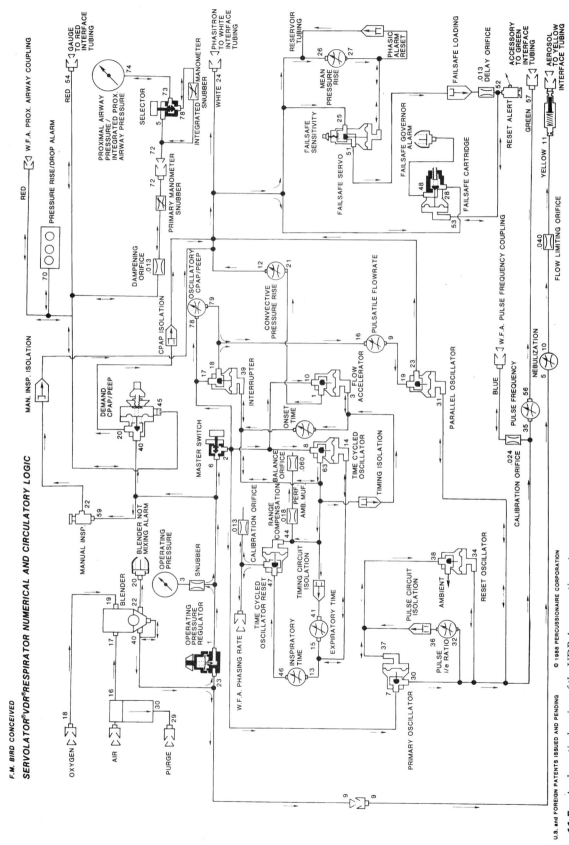

F.M. BIRD CONCEIVED

SERVOLATOR®VDR®RESPIRATOR NUMERICAL AND CIRCULATORY LOGIC

© 1988 PERCUSSIONAIRE CORPORATION

U.S. and FOREIGN PATENTS ISSUED AND PENDING

Figure 11-5 *A schematic drawing of the VDR 4 pneumatic system.*

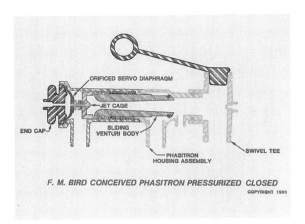

Figure 11-6 *Phasitron® during inspiration*

erating pressure of 40 psi. Peak pressure is controlled by the convective pressure rise control, which is found on the upper right portion of the control panel. The inspiratory and expiratory times determine the duration of the inspiratory and expiratory time intervals, and each may be adjusted independently of the other.

An important component in the overall drive mechanism of the VDR 4 ventilator is the Phasitron®. The Phasitron® is a spring-loaded, sliding venturi, which allows the HFPG to be interfaced with the patient's airway (Figures 11-6 and 11-7). During inspiration, the diaphragm inflates, and

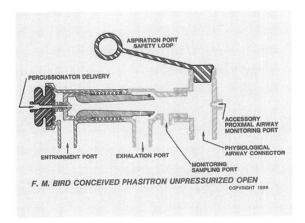

Figure 11-7 *Phasitron® during expiration*

simultaneously, gas is injected into the venturi. Forward displacement of the diaphragm slides the venturi body forward, closing the exhalation port. Simultaneously, humidified gas is entrained through the venturi, augmenting flow to the patient. When gas pressure is removed from the diaphragm (expiratory phase), spring tension opens the exhalation port by sliding the venturi backward and the patient exhales passively.

The output of the nebulizer is adjustable via a needle valve labeled "nebulization." The nebulizer is powered by source gas pressure. Rotation of the control in the counterclockwise direction increases the nebulizer's output.

Control Variable

The control variable for the VDR 4 ventilator is time. The pulse frequency control determines the ventilatory rate, which may be adjusted from 40 to over 900 breaths per minute. Time is a control variable since both pressure and flow vary with changes in resistance and compliance of the pulmonary system.

Phase Variables
Trigger Variable

The trigger variables for the VDR 4 include time and manual triggering. Time triggering is established by setting the pulse frequency control. Manual triggering is accomplished by depressing the manual inspiration button, which delivers a single convective breath up to the pressure set on the operational pressure control.

Cycle Variable

The cycle variable for the VDR 4 is time. The inspiratory time control determines the length of the inspiratory phase before the ventilator cycles into exhalation. The control is adjustable between 0.5 seconds and infinity (breath hold).

Baseline Variable

The baseline variable for the VDR 4 ventilator is pressure. The oscillatory CPAP/PEEP control regulates baseline pressure for the percussive portions of the scheduled breath pattern, and demand CPAP/PEEP regulates the baseline pressure during the static portion of the scheduled breath pattern.

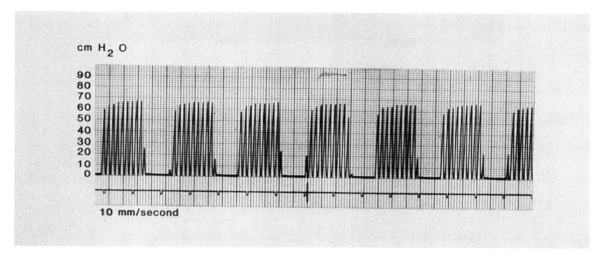

Figure 11-8A *A graphic tracing of diffusive ventilation.*

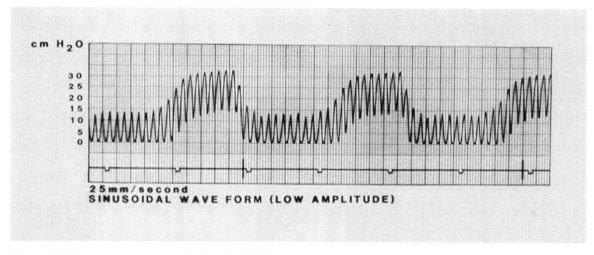

Figure 11-8B *A graphic tracing illustrating diffusive and convective ventilation.*

Conditional Variables

The conditional variable of the VDR 4 is time. Control of convective or diffusive (high-frequency) ventilation is governed by the "pulse i/e ratio" control. In its fully counter-clockwise position, an I:E ratio of 1:1 is delivered. At this ratio, the baseline profile of the waveform remains constant at the set oscillatory CPAP/PEEP level. When the I:E ratio approaches 1:1, the net effect is to improve pulmonary distribution and improve the PaO_2. When the pulse I:E ratio control is rotated clockwise, until the I:E ratio becomes 1:3, the baseline profile will be sinusoidal with the percussive, high-frequency, subtidal breaths superimposed on it (Figure 11-8, A and B). As

the breath delivery becomes more convective, CO_2 elimination is enhanced.

Output Waveforms

The pressure waveform output of the VDR 4 ventilator may be varied from an oscillatory waveform without variation in base pressure to a sinusoidal waveform with oscillatory ventilation superimposed on it (Figure 11-8). As already discussed, the "pulse i/e ratio" control determines the waveform output of the ventilator.

Alarm and Monitoring Systems

The Percussionaire® VDR 4 has several alarm and monitoring features. These include

ASSEMBLY AND TROUBLESHOOTING

Assembly—Percussionaire® VDR 4

1. Assemble the Phasitron® (Figure 11-9):

   a. Connect the green (inspiratory) fail-safe tee to the port closest to the patient outlet of the Phasitron®.

   b. Connect the red (expiratory) fail-safe tee to the port closest to the patient outlet of the Phasitron®.

   c. Install a snap-lock plug onto the small port at the end of the Phasitron®.

   d. Install the rubber-nosed plug into one end of the swivel tee and install the tee onto the outlet of the Phasitron®.

2. Assemble the patient circuit (Figure 11-10).

   a. Assemble the aerosol generator and volume regulator by attaching the volume-regulator cross tee to the nebulizer (Figure 11-11). Before installing it, inspect the three one-way valves for integrity and proper operation (inspiratory valve opens outward, purge valve opens outward, expiratory valve opens inward).

   b. Connect a length of green, 22-mm diameter aerosol tubing to the outlet of the nebulizer.

   c. Install a water trap to the open end of the green aerosol tubing.

   d. Connect another length of green aerosol tubing to the open port of the water trap and connect the remaining end to the inlet of the green (inspiratory) fail-safe tee.

   e. Connect one end of the long red (expiratory) 22-mm diameter tubing to the outlet of the red (expiratory) fail-safe tee and the other end to the expiratory valve of the volume-regulator cross tee.

   f. Attach a 3 liter anesthesia bag to the reservoir bag fitting of the volume-regulator cross tee.

3. Assemble the small-diameter drive and monitoring lines:

   a. Connect the small-diameter red monitoring line to the small port on the swivel tee. Be certain that the check valve points toward the tee. Connect the opposite end to the red gauge fitting on the VDR 4 control panel.

   b. Connect the white small-diameter Phasitron® drive line to the small fitting on the white end cap of the Phasitron®. Attach the opposite end to the white fitting on the VDR ventilator labeled Phasitron®.

   c. Attach the yellow small-diameter nebulizer drive line to the bottom fitting on the nebulizer and attach the opposite end to the yellow fitting labeled aerosol on the VDR 4 ventilator.

   d. Connect the green small-diameter tubing to the remaining port on top of the aerosol generator and its opposite end to the green fitting on the VDR 4 labeled accessory.

Troubleshooting

Refer to the troubleshooting algorithms found at the end of this chapter.

---

pneumatic pressure, a fail-safe sensitivity, pressure-sensing alert/alarm system, and an external oscilloscope/wave form analyzer, which provides real-time graphical analysis of the VDR 4's performance.

Input Power

A pneumatic reed alarm is incorporated into the Bird® blender. In the event that either air or oxygen pressure is lost, the alarm will sound, alerting the practitioner.

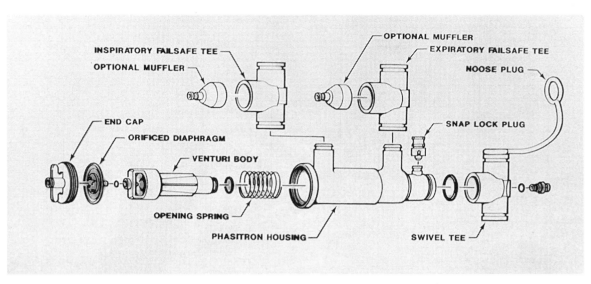

Figure 11-9 *An assembly drawing of the VDR 4 manifold assembly.*

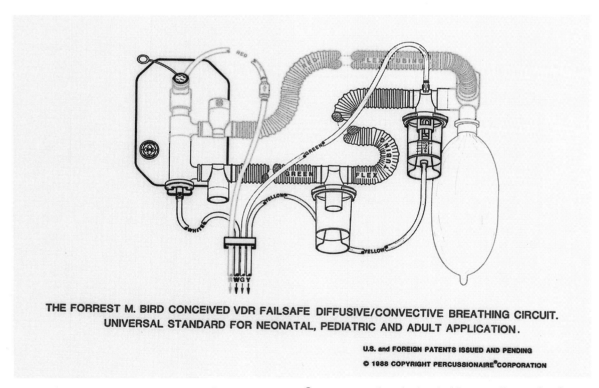

THE FORREST M. BIRD CONCEIVED VDR FAILSAFE DIFFUSIVE/CONVECTIVE BREATHING CIRCUIT.
UNIVERSAL STANDARD FOR NEONATAL, PEDIATRIC AND ADULT APPLICATION.

U.S. and FOREIGN PATENTS ISSUED AND PENDING

© 1988 COPYRIGHT PERCUSSIONAIRE® CORPORATION

Figure 11-10 *An assembly drawing of the Percussionaire® VDR 4 ventilator's circuit. (Courtesy Percussionaire Corporation, Sandpoint, ID)*

Control Circuit

The fail-safe sensitivity monitors the VDR 4 gas delivery through the patient circuit. If the patient circuit were to accidentally become obstructed, the fail-safe sensitivity system opens, allowing the excess pressure in the circuit to be vented. Simultaneously, an audible alarm sounds, alerting the practitioner. The fail-safe sensitivity system may be reset by manually depressing the reset alert thumb-button for several seconds after the obstruction has been cleared or resolved.

It is important to properly adjust the fail-safe sensitivity system to match the pressure delivery required for each patient. If the pulmonary system is very compliant requiring low driving pressures), rotate the fail-safe sensitivity system control counterclockwise. Conversely, if compliance is low and drive pressures are high, rotate the control clockwise.

Output Alarms

The battery-powered, pressure-sensing alert/alarm system is located on the right side of the ventilator. The alert/alarm system provides for clinician alert/alarms for high-pressure (pressure rise) and low-pressure (pressure drop) conditions. The pressure drop delay control allows for the time interval between the time when the pressure drops below the set value on the pressure drop control and the time when the audible alarm is activated. This system provides for the sensing of patient disconnects as well as high-pressure alert conditions.

Oscilloscope Waveform Analyzer

The Oscilloscope/Waveform analyzer (Figure 11-11) provides real-time analysis of the VDR 4 ventilator's performance through a CRT oscilloscope display. The clinician may adjust the pressure scale and sweep speed of the display. A frequency counter is also incorporated into the monitor to assist the clinician with setup and monitoring of the ventilator. The monitor also has high- and low-pressure alarms, which may be clinician adjusted to provide disconnect and high pressure alerts.

SENSORMEDICS CRITICAL CARE 3100A HIGH-FREQUENCY OSCILLATORY VENTILATOR

The SensorMedics Critical Care 3100A high-frequency oscillatory ventilator is an HFOV approved for the ventilatory support of neonates ranging in weight between 0.54 and 4.6 kg and pediatric patients for whom conventional ventilation has failed (Figure 11-12, A and B). The ventilator is a pneumatically powered and electronically controlled, time-triggered, time-cycled, pressure-limited HFOV.

Input Power

Input power for the 3100A HFOV requires two pneumatic gas sources and one electrical source. The DISS connection located at the upper-left rear of the rear control panel must be connected to the outlet of an air/oxygen blender, which must be capable of providing

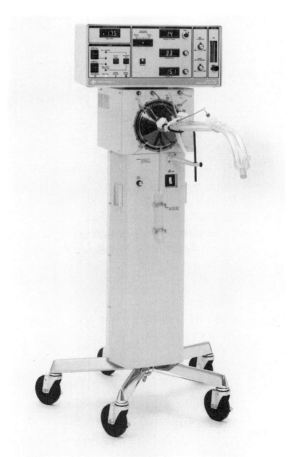

Figure 11-12A *The SensorMedics Critical Care 3100A High-Frequency Oscillatory Ventilator. (Copyright SensorMedics Corporation)*

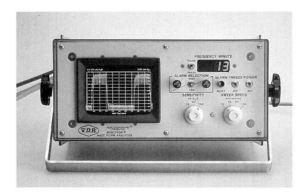

Figure 11-11 *The Oscilloscope Waveform analyzer or monitor.*

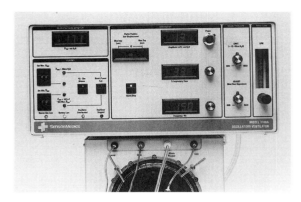

Figure 11-12B *The control panel of the SensorMedics Critical Care 3100A High-Frequency Oscillatory Ventilator. (Copyright SensorMedics Corporation)*

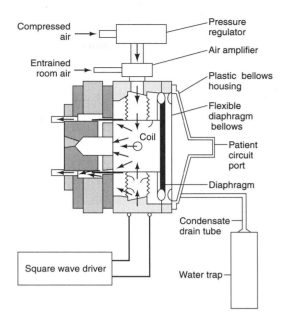

Figure 11-13 *A schematic drawing of the SensorMedics Critical Care 3100A High-Frequency Oscillatory Ventilator's drive mechanism. (Copyright SensorMedics Corporation, Yorba Linda, CA)*

between 30 and 50 psi nominal pressure output. Adjustment of the blender determines the F_IO_2 delivered to the patient. The second pneumatic connection is for cooling air for the oscillator; it is located at the lower right of rear control panel. This pneumatic connection is an air DISS fitting and must be powered by a 50 psi source capable of providing a minimum 15 L/min flow. Electrical power is provided by a standard three-prong electrical cord and plug and is adjustable between 120 v, 60 Hz and 220 v, 50 Hz power supply systems.

Drive Mechanism

The drive mechanism for the 3100A HFOV consists of a square wave driver, which powers an electric linear motor and a piston (Figure 11-13). The electric drive motor consists of a permanent magnet suspended in an electric coil. When alternating square-wave current passes through the coil, positively charged current displaces the piston/diaphragm toward the patient circuit, while negatively charged current displaces the piston/diaphragm away from the patient circuit. The stroke of the piston is determined by the amplitude of the applied current. The piston/diaphragm assembly has a maximum displacement of around 365 mL.

The electric linear motor, when operating at the frequencies required to support a patient's ventilation, requires cooling. Therefore, a 50 psi air source (at 15 L/min) entrains additional air through a venturi, which augments the flow to 60 L/min. Should the temperature of the coil exceed 190°C, the oscillator will

shut down to protect itself. Prior to oscillator shutdown, a yellow caution light will illuminate (at 175°C) to alert the clinician of a potential overtemperature condition.

Amplitude of the square wave drive signal is control by the power/ΔP control. This control is adjustable on a percentage scale of 0 to 100%. Setting the control to a higher percentage results in a greater amplitude of the drive signal, which increases piston displacement. As the piston displacement varies (increases or decreases), the ΔP (inspiration to expiration) also changes.

When operating the ventilator, it is important to center the piston. This is done by using the piston centering control located on the lower-left part of the support column, just opposite the power switch. Rotating this control varies the center position of the piston and is graphically displayed on the centering bar graph on the control panel. Piston centering determines the Paw (limits or increases displacement) and also prevents the piston from striking mechanical stops, which may result in damage to the drive system.

Control Circuit

The control circuit of the 3100A HFOV consists of electronic and microprocessor systems that control the oscillator drive system and the

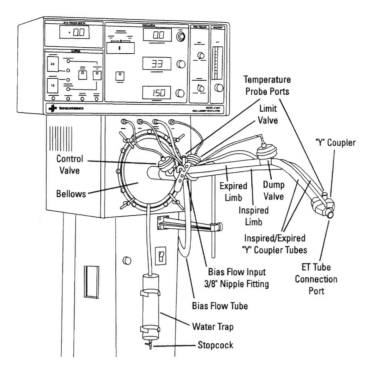

Figure 11-14 *An assembly drawing of the SensorMedics Critical Care 3100A High Frequency Oscillatory Ventilator's Circuit. (Copyright SensorMedics Corporation, Yorba Linda, CA)*

pneumatic logic and control subsystems (Figure 11-14). The oscillator subsystem develops square-wave pulses, resulting in subtidal volume delivery into the patient circuit. Bias flow from the external blender and humidifier into the circuit augments the volume delivered to the patient. Bias flow is adjustable between 0 and 40 L/min and is controlled by a flowmeter located on the upper right of the control panel.

Control Variable

The control variable of the 3100A HFOV is time. The frequency control determines the oscillator frequency, which is calibrated in hertz (cycles per second). Frequencies may be adjusted between 3 and 15 hertz (180 to 900 breaths per minute). A digital LED displays the frequency at which the 3100A HFOV is operating.

Phase Variables
Trigger Variable

The trigger variable for the 3100A HFOV is time. The frequency control determines the

rate at which the oscillator cycles and, therefore, when inspiration occurs.

Limit Variables

The limit variables for the 3100A HFOV are pressure and time. Pressure limit is adjusted using the mean pressure limit control. The mean pressure may be limited between 10 and 45 cmH₂O. The control consists of a needle valve that adjusts a pneumatic valve, limiting mean pressures. The pressure limit may be adjusted below the operating pressure (Paw); however, it is intended as a safety to prevent barotrauma in the event of an overpressure condition and is usually set above the Paw.

Time may be a limit variable and is adjusted using the percent inspiratory time control. This control determines for what percentage of the inspiratory time the piston is displaced at its maximum forward position (closest to the patient circuit). This control is adjustable between 30 and 50%. The inspiratory time percentage is displayed on a digital LED. Changing the percent inspiratory time will have an affect on the Paw and the change in pressure (inspiration to expiration) since it alters the symmetry of the oscillatory waveform.

Cycle Variable

The cycle variable of the 3100A HFOV is time. The cycle variable is not directly set but is a function of the frequency and inspiratory time percentage. Once the allotted inspiratory time has passed, the piston travels away from the patient circuit, initiating exhalation. Exhalation on the 3100A HFOV is active, and gas is withdrawn from the patient circuit and airway by the backward displacement of the piston.

Output Waveforms

The pressure waveform output of the 3100A is square. The oscillator and electronic driver produce a true square wave with each breath or oscillation.

Alarm Systems
Input Power

Input power alarms are included for electrical and source gas power interruptions. In the event of an electrical power failure, a 3 kilohertz, modulated, audible alarm will sound. Once activated, the alarm can only be silenced by depressing the reset button. The power failure alarm is powered by a battery that is independent of the main power supply for the ventilator.

If the line pressure from the external blender falls below 30 psi, a yellow lamp will illuminate to alert the clinician to this condition. This type of alarm is considered a caution alarm, and therefore, no audible condition will result.

Control Circuit Alarms

The control circuit alarm is an oscillator, overheated alarm (already discussed). When the oscillator temperature reaches 175 degrees Celsius, a yellow LED will illuminate to alert the clinician to the condition.

Output Alarms

Output alarms include minimum mean, maximum mean airway pressure, mean airway pressure greater than 50 cmH$_2$O and mean airway pressure less than 20% of set maximum mean airway pressure. The minimum and maximum mean airway pressure alarms are adjustable between 0 and 49 cmH$_2$O. Both are thumbwheel switches located at the lower left portion of the control panel. Adjustment of the alarms can make them serve as high- and low-pressure alarm indicators; they will automatically reset if the condition corrects itself or if the operator depresses the 45-second-silence button.

The mean airway pressure greater than 50 cmH$_2$O alarm will activate if the mean airway pressure exceeds this value. Once the alarm condition is met, a red LED will illuminate; a 3 kilohertz, modulating, audible tone will sound; the oscillator will automatically shut down; a dump valve will open to the atmosphere; and bias flow will continue. The purpose of this alarm is to protect the patient from barotrauma, which may result from the increased pressures. The alarm can be reset only by the clinician correcting the situation and depressing the reset button manually. The oscillator must be started following the startup procedure.

The alarm signalling that mean airway pressure is less than 20% of the set maximum mean airway pressure alarm is another safety alarm. This alarm is indicated by a red LED, a 3 kilohertz modulating tone, shutdown of the oscillator, opening of the dump valve and continuation of the bias flow through the circuit. This alarm occurs when the mean airway pressure drops to this value. The alarm will reset itself if the condition corrects itself. If the clinician must correct the problem, the reset button must be depressed and the oscillator must be started by following the startup procedure.

ASSEMBLY AND TROUBLESHOOTING

Assembly—SensorMedics Critical Care 3100A ventilator

1. Assemble the patient circuit (Figure 11-14):
   a. Attach the patient circuit body to the bellows/water trap assembly (Figure 11-14).
   b. Place the three diaphragms onto their respective seats in the circuit and snap the diaphragm valve caps over them, completing the valve assembly. These components are identical, and therefore are interchangeable.
   c. Attach the bellows/water trap assembly to the front of the ventilator by positioning it correctly and rotating the four T-handles to lock it into place.
   d. Connect the small-diameter control and monitoring tubes to the correct valve caps and connectors:
      (1) Connect the blue tube to the limit valve and limit valve fitting on the ventilator.
      (2) Connect the green tube to the control valve cap and the stop/start fitting on the ventilator.
      (3) Connect the red tube to the dump valve and to the dump valve fitting on the ventilator.
      (4) Connect the clear, 1/8-inch tubing to the pressure port on the patient wye and to the airway pressure fitting on the ventilator.

2. Connect the gas supply lines:
   a. Connect a 50 psi air and oxygen source to an external blender and connect the 50 psi outlet of the blender to the inlet on the ventilator.
   b. Connect a 50 psi air source to the DISS air fitting on the ventilator.

3. Connect an appropriate electrical supply to the ventilator and ensure that the switch is set for the correct voltage.

Troubleshooting

Refer to the troubleshooting algorithms in ALG 11-1 and 11-2.

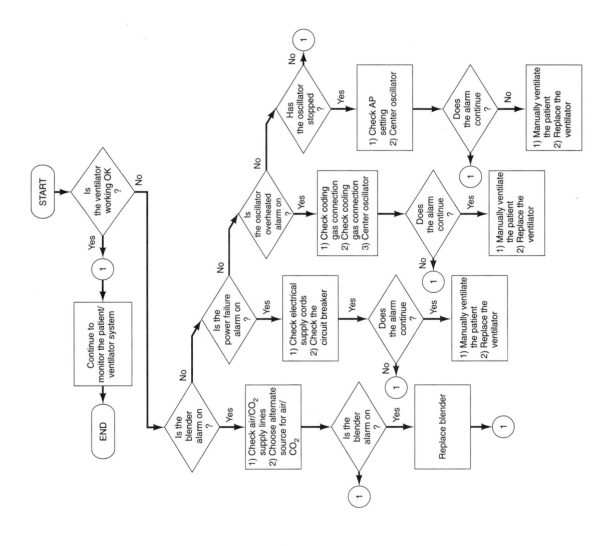

ALG 11-1 *An algorithm for troubleshooting input power and control circuit alarms.*

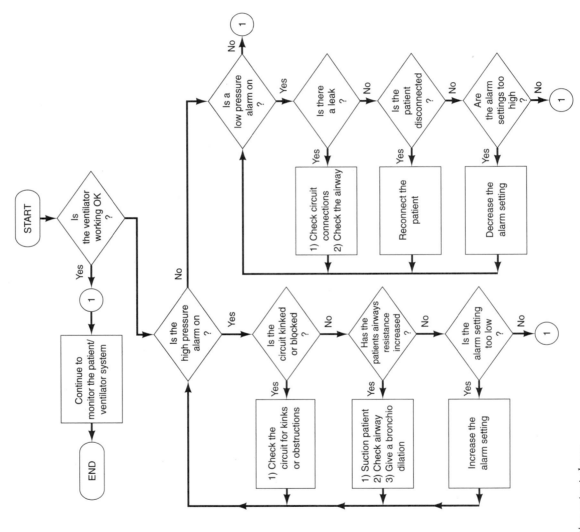

ALG 11-2 *An algorithm for troubleshooting output alarms.*

CLINICAL CORNER

High-Frequency Ventilators

1. Describe two circumstances in which high-frequency ventilators would be used instead of conventional ventilators.
2. Explain why it is important to center the piston of the SensorMedics 3100A ventilator.
3. What control on the Percussionaire® VDR 4 ventilator causes ventilation to become more convective rather than diffusive?
4. Describe what occurs when you depress the manual inspiration button on the Percussionaire® VDR 4 ventilator.

Self-Assessment Quiz

1. Which of the following ventilators depend upon the elastic recoil of the lungs and chest wall for exhalation?
   I. HFPPV.
   II. HFFI.
   III. HFJV.
   IV. HFOV.
   a. I
   b. I and II
   c. I, II, and III
   d. II, III and IV

2. Which of the following ventilators have an active expiratory phase?
   a. HFPPV.
   b. HFFI.
   c. HFJV.
   d. HFOV.

3. Which of the following is a primary application of HFPPV?
   a. Support of neonates in respiratory distress.
   b. Support of adults in respiratory distress.
   c. Ventilation of patients with lung injury.
   d. Surgical cases involving the upper airway.

4. Which of the following ventilators employ a small catheter or a specialized endotracheal tube to interface with the patient's airway?
   a. HFPPV.
   b. HFFI.
   c. HFJV.
   d. HFOV.

5. Which of the following types of high-frequency ventilators employs a rotating-ball valve to determine the respiratory frequency?
   a. HFPPV.
   b. HFFI.
   c. HFJV.
   d. HFOV.

6. Which of the following theories suggests that areas of the lung with a given time constant contribute to gas exchange by emptying into adjacent areas with different time constants?
   a. Taylor dispersion theory.
   b. Pendelluft theory.
   c. Molecular diffusion theory.
   d. Cardiogenic mixing theory.

7. Which of the following theories suggests that gas exchange during high-frequency ventilation is enhanced by turbulent flow within the airways?
   a. Taylor dispersion theory.
   b. Pendelluft theory.
   c. Molecular diffusion theory.
   d. Cardiogenic mixing theory.

8. Which of the following theories suggests that the increased velocities and respiratory rates associated with high-frequency ventilation contributes to a greater molecular kinetic activity, which achieves adequate ventilation at low tidal volumes?
   a. Taylor dispersion theory.
   b. Pendelluft theory.
   c. Molecular diffusion theory.
   d. Cardiogenic mixing theory.

9. Which of the following best describes the asymmetric velocity profile theory of ventilation during high-frequency ventilation?
   a. Increased turbulence resulting in the diffusion and mixing of gases.
   b. Cardiac oscillations, resulting in the agitation of the airways and thus enhancing molecular mixing.
   c. A difference in velocity profiles between inspiration and expiration, causing a greater net flow of gases during inspiration.
   d. Increased kinetic activity of gases caused by the increased frequencies.

10. Which of the following are advantages of high-frequency ventilation?
    I. Low mean airway and intrathoracic pressures.
    II. Minimal cardiac side effects.
    III. Minimal motion of the airways and chest wall.
    IV. Stability of the upper airway structures during ventilation.
    a. I
    b. I and II
    c. I, II, and III
    d. I, II, III and IV

11. Which of the following accounts for the reports of success with high-frequency ventilation being used to ventilate patients with large air leaks?
    I. Low mean airway and intrathoracic pressures.
    II. Minimal cardiac side effects.
    III. Minimal motion of the airways and chest wall.
    IV. Stability of the upper airway structures during ventilation.
    a. I and II
    b. I and III
    c. II and III
    d. III and IV

12. The improvement in cardiovascular side effects of high-frequency ventilation when compared with conventional ventilation is best accounted for by:
    a. Decreased mean airway and intrathoracic pressures.
    b. Decreased expansion of the chest wall.
    c. Decreased motion of the upper airways.
    d. Cardiogenic mixing.

13. Which of the following procedures may benefit from the use of high-frequency ventilation?
    I. Laryngoscopies.
    II. Laser bronchoscopies.

III. Laryngeal surgery.

IV. Tracheal surgery.

a. I

b. I and II

c. I, II, and III

d. I, II, III and IV

14. Which of the following types of high-frequency ventilation may be achieved percutaneously via a small cannula or catheter?

a. HFPPV.

b. HFJV.

c. HFOV.

d. HFFI.

15. High-frequency ventilation has been used successfully in patients who had refractory hypoxemia and hypercarbia while being maintained on conventional ventilation. What best accounts for the success of high-frequency ventilation in these circumstances?

a. The reliance of high-frequency ventilation on convective ventilation.

b. The lower mean airway pressures associated with high-frequency ventilation.

c. The decreased cardiac side effects of high-frequency ventilation.

d. The difference in the way high-frequency ventilation accomplishes gas exchange.

16. What is the drive mechanism of the Percussionaire® VDR 4 ventilator?

a. An electrodynamic motor.

b. A rotating-ball valve.

c. A high-frequency pulse generator.

d. A reducing valve.

17. What is the input power of the Percussionaire® VDR 4 ventilator?

I. 50 psi air.

II. 50 psi oxygen.

III. 120 v, 60 Hz electrical power.

a. I

b. I and II

c. I, II, and III

d. II and III

18. Which of the following are functions of the Percussionaire® VDR 4 ventilator's Phasitron®?

I. Provides an interface to the patient's airway.

II. Acts to entrain additional gas augmenting flow and tidal volumes.

III. Acts as a pneumatic clutch.

a. I

b. I and II

c. II and III

d. I, II, and III

19. How is the control circuit of the Percussionaire® VDR 4 ventilator classified?

a. Electronic.

b. Electric.

c. Pneumatic.

d. Mechanical.

20. Which of the following is the control variable for the Percussionaire® VDR 4 ventilator?

a. Pressure.

b. Volume.

c. Flow.

d. Time.

21. Which of the following is the cycle variable for the Percussionaire® VDR 4 ventilator?

a. Pressure.

b. Volume.

c. Flow.

d. Time.

22. Which of the following is the baseline variable for the Percussionaire® VDR 4 ventilator?
    a. Pressure.
    b. Volume.
    c. Flow.
    d. Time.

23. Which of the following is classified as the input power alarm of the Percussionaire® VDR 4 ventilator?
    a. The fail-safe sensitivity.
    b. The pressure drop alarm.
    c. The blender alarm.
    d. The ventilator inoperative alarm.

24. What is the input power of the SensorMedics Critical Care 3100A ventilator?
    I. 50 psi air.
    II. 50 psi oxygen.
    III. 120 v, 60 Hz electrical power.
    a. I
    b. I and II
    c. I, II, and III
    d. II and III

25. What is the drive mechanism for the SensorMedics Critical Care 3100A ventilator?
    a. An electrodynamic motor.
    b. A rotating-ball valve.
    c. A high-frequency pulse generator.
    d. A reducing valve.

26. What is the control variable for the SensorMedics Critical Care 3100A ventilator?
    a. Pressure.
    b. Volume.
    c. Flow.
    d. Time.

27. What is the cycling variable for the SensorMedics Critical Care 3100A ventilator?
    a. Pressure.
    b. Volume.
    c. Flow.
    d. Time.

28. What determines the tidal volume delivery of the SensorMedics Critical Care 3100A ventilator?
    a. The frequency.
    b. The amplitude of the alternating signal.
    c. Percentage inspiratory time.
    d. The oxygen percentage.

29. What control manipulates time as a phase variable for the SensorMedics 3100A ventilator?
    a. Frequency.
    b. Bias flow.
    c. Percentage inspiratory time.
    d. Mean pressure limit.

30. Which of the following alarms on the SensorMedics 3100A ventilator is powered by an independent battery?
    a. Max. mean airway pressure.
    b. Min. mean airway pressure.
    c. Mean airway pressure greater than 50 cmH$_2$O.
    d. Power failure.

Selected Bibliography

Allen, Julian L., et al., "Alveolar Pressure Magnitude and Asynchrony during High-Frequency Oscillations of Excised Rabbit Lungs," *American Review of Respiratory Diseases*, Vol. 132, pp. 343–349, 1985.

Bird, Forrest M., "The Evolutionary Concept and Functional Logic of the VDR-4 Servolator Percussionator (Ventilator) Conceived and Developed by Forrest M. Bird," Percussionaire® Corporation, Sand Point, ID, 1987.

Bird, Forrest M., "Percussionaire® State of the Art, Universal Mechanical Cardiopulmonary Support for the Nineteen Nineties," Percussionaire® Corporation, Sand Point, ID, 1987.

Bird, Forrest M., "VDR Servator VDR-4 Percussionaire," Percussionaire® Corporation, Sand Point, ID, 1987.

Boynton, Bruce R., "High Frequency Ventilation in Newborn Infants," *Respiratory Care*, Vol. 31, pp. 480–490, 1986.

Cioffi, William G., et al., "High-frequency Percussive Ventilation in Patients with Inhalation Injury," *Journal of Trauma*, Vol. 29, pp. 350–364, 1989.

Coghill, Carl H., et al., "Neonatal and Pediatric High-Frequency Ventilation: Principles and Practice," *Respiratory Care*, Vol. 36, pp. 596–612, 1991.

Cordero, Leandro, et al., "The High-Frequency Pneumatic Flow Interrupter: Effects of Different Ventilatory Strategies," *Respiratory Care*, Vol. 37, pp. 348–356, 1992.

Cordero, Leandro, et al., "High Frequency Ventilation: Comparison of an Electronic Flow Interrupter and a New Pneumatic Oscillator," *Respiratory Care*, Vol. 37, pp. 1241–1249, 1992.

Davis, Kenneth Jr., et al., "High Frequency Percussive Ventilation," *Problems in Respiratory Care*, Vol. 2, pp. 39–47, 1989.

Franz, Ivan D., III, et al., "High-Frequency Ventilation in Premature Infants with Lung Disease: Adequate Gas Exchange at Low Tracheal Pressure," *Pediatrics*, Vo. 71, pp. 483–488, 1983.

Fredberg, Jeffrey J., "Augmented Diffusion in the Airways Can Support Pulmonary Gas Exchange," *Journal of Applied Physiology*, Vol. 49, pp. 232–238, 1980.

Gallagher, James T., "High-Frequency Percussive Ventilation Compared with Conventional Mechanical Ventilation," *Critical Care in Medicine*, Vol. 17, pp. 364–366, 1989.

Herridge, Margaret S., et al., "High-Frequency Ventilation: A Ventilatory Technique That Merits Revisiting," *Respiratory Care*, Vol. 41, pp. 385–396, 1996.

Hurst, James M., et al., "The Role of High-Frequency Ventilation in Post-Traumatic Respiratory Insufficiency," *Journal of Trauma*, Vol. 27, pp. 236–241, 1987.

Lehr, John L., et al., "Photographic Measurement of Pleural Surface Motion during Lung Oscillation," *Journal of Applied Physiology*, Vol. 59, pp. 623–633, 1985.

Rodeberg, D. A., "Decreased Pulmonary Barotrauma with the Use of Volumetric Diffusive Respiration in Pediatric Patients with Burns," *Journal of Burn Care and Rehabilitation*, Vol. 13, pp. 506–511, 1992.

SensorMedics Critical Care, *3100A High Frequency Oscillatory Ventilator Operator's Manual*, Yorba Linda, CA, 1995.

Sjöstrand, Ulf H., et al., "High Rates and Low Volumes in Mechanical Ventilation—Not Just a Matter of Ventilatory Frequency," *Anesthesia and Analgesia*, Vol. 59, pp. 567–576, 1980.

Slutsky, Arthur S., "Mechanisms Affecting Gas Transport during High Frequency Oscillation," *Critical Care in Medicine*, Vol. 12, pp. 713–717, 1984.

Slutsky, Arthur S., "Gas Mixing by Cardiogenic Oscillations: A Theoretical Quantitative Analysis," *Journal of Applied Physiology*, Vol. 51, pp. 1287–1293, 1981.

Weber, Kaye, et al., "Lung-Volume-Dependent Effects of Varying Inspiratory Time during High-Frequency Oscillation of Surfactant-Deficient Rabbits," Respiratory Care, Vol. 37, pp. 973–978, 1994.

ANSWER KEYS TO SELF-ASSEMENT QUESTIONS

Chapter 1 • Oxygen and Mixed-Gas Therapy Equipment

1. b	6. a	11. a	16. c	21. c	26. e
2. c	7. a	12. a	17. e	22. c	27. b
3. c	8. c	13. a	18. d	23. d	28. c
4. d	9. a	14. c	19. c	24. d	29. d
5. c	10. d	15. e	20. c	25. c	30. a

Chapter 2 • Humidity and Aerosol Therapy Equipment

1. d	6. a	11. a	16. a	21. d	26. c
2. b	7. c	12. b	17. b	22. d	27. e
3. c	8. b	13. d	18. d	23. b	28. d
4. d	9. b	14. c	19. b	24. a	29. c
5. b	10. e	15. d	20. b	25. a	30. c

Chapter 3 • Hyperinflation Therapy Equipment

1. b	6. c	11. c	16. c	21. a	26. c
2. a	7. b	12. a	17. e	22. c	27. b
3. c	8. c	13. c	18. a	23. a	28. b
4. a	9. d	14. e	19. e	24. a	29. c
5. c	10. a	15. d	20. c	25. a	30. c

Chapter 4 • Emergency Resuscitation Equipment

1. d	6. e	11. c	16. b	21. a	26. b
2. b	7. d	12. e	17. d	22. b	27. a
3. a	8. e	13. c	18. d	23. d	28. b
4. b	9. d	14. d	19. d	24. b	29. b
5. b	10. d	15. b	20. c	25. d	30. c

Chapter 5 • Physiological Measurement and Monitoring Devices

1. b	6. b	11. a	16. c	21. d	26. b
2. a	7. d	12. b	17. b	22. c	27. d
3. a	8. b	13. b	18. d	23. a	28. a
4. d	9. e	14. a	19. b	24. d	29. d
5. d	10. a	15. c	20. a	25. b	30. c

Chapter 6 • Mechanical Ventilator Theory and Classification

1. e	6. a	11. d	16. c	21. d	26. c
2. e	7. b	12. b	17. a	22. d	27. b
3. d	8. b	13. b	18. d	23. e	28. c
4. e	9. a	14. d	19. b	24. d	29. e
5. b	10. d	15. c	20. c	25. a	30. a

Chapter 7 • Adult Acute Care Ventilators: Ventilators Having Volume as a Control Variable

1. a	6. d	11. b	16. b	21. a	26. d
2. c	7. d	12. a	17. b	22. a	27. b
3. b	8. a	13. d	18. c	23. b	28. d
4. a	9. a	14. b	19. c	24. c	29. c
5. a	10. d	15. c	20. d	25. b	30. c

Chapter 8 • Adult Acute Care Ventilators: Ventilators Having Flow and Pressure Control Variables

1. d	6. d	11. c	16. a	21. a	26. c
2. b	7. b	12. b	17. d	22. b	27. d
3. b	8. b	13. b	18. d	23. b	28. b
4. d	9. c	14. c	19. c	24. a	29. d
5. c	10. a	15. d	20. d	25. c	30. c

Chapter 9 • Pediatric and Neonatal Ventilators

1. c	6. d	11. d	16. d	21. c	26. b
2. a	7. b	12. b	17. d	22. c	27. c
3. a	8. c	13. b	18. c	23. c	28. a
4. a	9. c	14. c	19. b	24. b	29. c
5. a	10. b	15. b	20. d	25. d	30. c

Chapter 10 • Homecare and Transport Ventilators

1. c	6. d	11. d	16. a	21. d	26. b
2. a	7. a	12. d	17. b	22. d	27. b
3. d	8. b	13. c	18. b	23. d	28. d
4. c	9. c	14. a	19. d	24. b	29. a
5. d	10. b	15. b	20. c	25. b	30. c

Chapter 11 • High-Frequency Mechanical Ventilation

1. c	6. b	11. b	16. c	21. d	26. d
2. d	7. a	12. a	17. b	22. a	27. d
3. d	8. c	13. d	18. d	23. c	28. b
4. c	9. c	14. b	19. c	24. c	29. c
5. b	10. d	15. d	20. d	25. a	30. d

GLOSSARY

Absolute Humidity   The amount of water vapor contained in a gas at a given temperature. Absolute humidity is expressed in mg/L.

Accumulator   A rigid reservoir of 1 to 2 liters, used by ventilator manufacturers to help to meet instantaneous flow demands.

A/D Card   An electronic card in a computer that converts analog data to digital data, which can be interpreted by the computer program.

Adsorption   The physical adhesion of a thin layer of molecules to the surface of a porous substance.

Aerosol   Particulate matter suspended in a gas. Aerosols can be solids as well as liquids.

Airway Pressure Release Ventilation (APRV)   A combination of two separate levels of CPAP pressures. The patient may breathe spontaneously from both CPAP levels.

American Standard Safety System (ASSS) A safety system designed by the Compressed Gas Association for large medical gas cylinder valve connections. The system incorporates varying diameters, thread pitches and internal and external threading to prevent the mismatching of regulators or connections with the incorrect cylinder.

Amplitude   The extent of a periodic vibratory motion that reflects the height of the waveform. For ultrasonic nebulizers, amplitude represents the energy transmitted and therefore governs aerosol output or density.

And/Nand Gate   A monostable fluidic element used to control specific functions when interrupted by a control signal. The Monaghan 225/SIMV ventilator uses this element to control the operation of the exhalation valve mushroom.

Aneroid Barometer   A mechanical barometer that employs an evacuated chamber to measure changes in air pressure.

Assisted Mechanical Ventilation   A mode of mechanical ventilation where there is no set respiratory rate. All breaths are patient triggered.

Asymmetric Velocity Profiles   The theory that describes a net flow of gas through the central lumen of the airway during inspiration and expiratory gas simultaneously flowing out the peripheral portion of the airway lumen.

Asynchronous Ventilation   Asynchronous ventilation can be observed when the patient is "fighting the ventilator." An example is if the patient is exhaling while the ventilator is attempting to give a breath. Most often, the sensitivity is improperly adjusted, or the patient is receiving controlled breaths when breathing spontaneously.

Atelectasis   Atelectasis is the collapsing of lung tissue. Atelectasis can include microatelectasis, the collapsing of alveoli and small structures of the lung or it can involve entire lobes.

Atomizer   A jet-type aerosol generator that produces a wide range of particle sizes. An atomizer lacks a baffle, which helps to stabilize particle size in a nebulizer.

Augmented Mandatory Ventilation (AMV) A mode of ventilation in which the respiratory care practitioner sets a minimum minute volume, tidal volume, respiratory, peak flow, assist sensitivity and oxygen percent. If the patient's spontaneous ventilation falls below the minimum minute volume, the ventilator delivers mandatory breaths until that volume is reached.

Babbington Principle   The production of an aerosol using a pressurized glass sphere and a baffle. Water forms a sheet over the sphere which is aerosolized when it encounters a high velocity gas stream exiting the pressurized sphere through a small hole.

Back Pressure Compensated   A device that is designed such that back pressure (pressure distal to the device) will not affect its accuracy. Back pressure compensation is common in Thorpe tube flowmeters.

Bacteria Filter   A low resistance, high efficiency filter capable of removing particles as small as .3 microns in diameter.

Baffle   An object placed in the path of an aerosol flow to remove the larger particles of greater size (mass), by means of inertial impaction.

Beam Deflection The disruption of the coanda effect by a control pressure from one or more control ports on a fluidic element. Once the coanda effect has been disrupted, the beam may be directed to another output port, changing the logic of the output.

Bellows Drive Mechanism A ventilator that uses a bellows to convert its power source to ventilatory work. Examples of these ventilators include the Puritan Bennett MA-1 and MA-2+2 and the Monaghan 225/SIMV.

Bellows Spirometer A spirometer that measures volume displacement using a flexible bellows. The bellows expands and contracts with inspiration and expiration.

Bernoulli's Effect A reduction in pressure which occurs near the walls of a tube as gas flow is increased through the tube. This effect only occurs as long as the gas is contained within a tube and if the flow is laminar.

Bi-Level Positive Airway Pressure A mode of ventilation which combines pressure support with airway pressure release ventilation. Independent airway pressures for inspiration and expiration may be set.

Biofeedback Biofeedback is the application of a monitoring or indicating device to give patient feedback regarding their effort, performance or physiological function. Incentive spirometry is one application of this technique to improve a patient's effort during inspiration.

Body Plethysmography The technique of measuring the residual volume and expiratory reserve volume, indirectly using Boyle's law. A device known as a body plethysmograph is used in the determination of these volumes.

Boeringer Valve A type of PEEP/CPAP valve that depends upon gravity and a weighted ball to generate the expiratory resistance.

Bourdon Flow Meter A type of flowmeter that regulates the flow of a gas using a Bourdon tube and a single-stage reducing valve. The Bourdon gauge is recalibrated to read flow although it measures a change in pressure.

Bourdon Gauge A mechanical pressure gauge that employs a coiled tube to measure gas pressure. As pressure increases the tube straightens, causing a needle to indicate the increased pressure.

Boyle's Law A gas law that relates a change in volume to a change in pressure at a constant temperature. The law states that if pressure increases, volume will decrease provided the temperature remains constant.

Brownian Motion The random motion of small particles, such as smoke observed under a microscope, caused by the kinetic activity of gas molecules.

Calibration The comparison of an instrument to a known physical standard to assess its accuracy and reproducibility.

Capacity Capacity is the maximum amount of water vapor (humidity) that a gas can contain at a given temperature when fully saturated.

Cardiogenic Mixing The motion of the heart during its cycle acting to further agitate the airways, enhancing gas distribution during high-frequency ventilation.

Carrier Gas Carrier gas is the primary gas flow from a device that contains the aerosol generated from the device.

Charles' Law Charles' law relates the volume and the temperature of a gas when the pressure remains constant. The law states that as the temperature of a gas increases, its volume will increase as well.

Chest Physiotherapy A therapeutic technique which involves clapping on a patient's chest wall to promote vibration for secretion removal. Chest physiotherapy may be done manually, using one's hands, or mechanically, using a mechanical percussor.

Choked Flow The phenomenon of choked flow occurs when an increase in the head pressure to a nozzle will no longer increase the gas velocity exiting the nozzle. This velocity is usually close to sonic velocities. Once this maximum velocity is reached, the flow is choked.

Clark Electrode The PO_2 measuring electrode in a blood gas system, oxygen analyzer or transcutaneous electrode.

Coanda Effect The attachment of a high-velocity flow of gas to an adjacent wall by the formation of a separation bubble.

Combined Gas Law A law that relates temperature, pressure and volume of a gas under ideal conditions. This is often referred to as the ideal gas law. The law states that $P_1V_1/T_1 = P_2V_2/T_2$.

Compliance   A change in volume divided by a change in pressure. This measurement is reflective of elastic properties.

Compressible Volume   The volume of gas that is not delivered to a patient but is lost in the ventilator circuit due to compression. Compressible volume may be found by multiplying the peak inspiratory pressure times the tubing compliance.

Compressor   A device that is designed to compress a gas (usually air). Compressors operate using a diaphragm, piston or a centrifugal impeller, to compress the gas entering the device.

Constant Flow Generator   A classification of ventilators that deliver a constant flow during the inspiratory phase. These are often referred to as square wave generators.

Constant Pressure Generator   A classification of ventilators that delivers a constant pressure during the inspiratory phase. The driving pressure may be high (greater than 4,000 cmH$_2$O) or low (less than 45 cmH$_2$O).

Continuous Mandatory Ventilation   A mode of mechanical ventilation where the respiratory care practitioner sets the ventilator to deliver a respiratory rate and tidal volume for the patient. Any spontaneous efforts generated by the patient will be ignored by the ventilator.

Continuous Positive Airway Pressure (CPAP)   A spontaneous mode of ventilation where positive pressure is applied during inspiration and expiration.

Control Circuit   The system that governs or controls the ventilator's drive mechanism. This system may be mechanical, electrical, electronic, fluidic, pneumatic or microprocessor controlled. Both open and closed loop control systems are utilized.

Control Variable   A variable (volume, pressure, flow or time) which is measured and utilized as a feedback signal to control the ventilator's output.

Convective Ventilation   The process of gas exchange whereby gas transport occurs via bulk flow at low respiratory rates. The net result is alveoli coming into contact with the gases, which are directly conducted through the airways.

Corrected Tidal Volume   The actual volume delivered to the patient's lungs by a mechanical ventilator. Corrected tidal volume is calculated by subtracting the compressible volume from the measured volume.

Cuff   A cuff is an inflatable balloon located at the distal tip of some artificial airways (endotracheal tubes, tracheostomy tubes and esophageal obturator airways). The purpose of the cuff is to seal the airway so that positive pressure may be applied to the lungs and to protect the natural airway from aspiration.

Cycle Variable   A variable (pressure, volume, flow or time) which is measured and used to terminate inspiration.

Cylinder Manifold   Two or more gas cylinders connected together, in series, to provide a larger supply of gas.

Dalton's Law   Dalton's law of partial pressures states that the total pressure of a gas mixture is equal to the sum of the partial pressures of the gases that comprise the gas mixture. For example, if a gas mixture is composed of gases A, B and C, the total pressure is equal to the partial pressures of A + B + C.

Demand Flow Pulsed Oxygen Delivery Device   An oxygen delivery device that is designed to deliver a pulsed dose of oxygen during inspiration only. The device senses inspiration and only delivers gas during the inspiratory phase, conserving oxygen.

Demand Valve   A type of mechanical valve that provides gas to a spontaneously breathing patient in response to the pressure gradient developed by the patient's inspiratory effort.

Diameter Index Safety System (DISS)   A safety system designed by the compressed gas association for low pressure (less than 200 psi) applications. The system incorporates varying diameters, thread pitches and internal and external threading to prevent the mismatching of delivery devices with the incorrect gas source.

Differential Pressure Transducer   A type of pressure transducer with two pressure ports separated by a diaphragm. Since two pressures are exerted on the diaphragm, the displacement of it is equal to the pressure difference. These transducers may be strain gauge or variable reluctance transducers.

Direct Acting Cylinder Valve   A cylinder valve that operates by a valve stem opening and closing the valve seat. The stem itself acts directly upon the seat to open or close it.

Double Circuit   A classification of mechanical ventilator circuits in which the gas that drives the ventilator is separate from the gas that is delivered to the patient. The Bennett MA-2+2 and Monaghan 225/SIMV ventilators are examples of double circuit ventilators.

Downs' Valve   A type of PEEP/CPAP valve that operates using a spring and a diaphragm to generate an expiratory resistance.

Drive Mechanism   The system utilized by the ventilator to transmit or convert the input power to useful ventilatory work.

Dry Rolling Seal Spirometer   A type of spirometer that employs a piston in the measurement of lung volumes. The rolling seal term is derived from the fine plastic seals that seal the piston against the cylinder wall.

Ducted Ejector   A device using a nozzle and viscous shearing and vorticity to increase total flow. The nozzle exit is directed into a duct to control gas flow and increase the total flow from the device.

Dysfunctional Hemoglobin   Hemoglobin which is not capable of reversibly binding with oxygen. These hemoglobin variants include carboxyhemoglobin and methemoglobin.

Endotracheal Tube   An endotracheal tube is an artificial airway that is passed through the mouth or nose and advanced into the trachea. Endotracheal tubes may be cuffed or uncuffed, depending upon their size.

End Tidal CO$_2$ Monitor   An infrared monitor that analyzes an exhaled gas sample and displays the partial pressure of carbon dioxide.

Esophageal Gastric Tube Airway (EGTA) An esophageal gastric tube airway is an artificial airway that is designed to intubate the esophagus rather than the trachea. A cuff on the distal end seals the esophagus, helping to prevent aspiration and to allow positive pressure ventilation via a mask. A hollow lumen is provided so that a nasal gastric tube may be used to decompress the stomach.

Esophageal Obturator Airway (EOA)   An esophageal obturator airway is an artificial airway that is designed to intubate the esophagus rather than the trachea. A cuff on the distal

end seals the esophagus, helping to prevent aspiration and to allow positive pressure ventilation via a mask.

Evaporation   The process of liquid water changing to a vapor as a result of molecular kinetic activity. Some molecules in a liquid have sufficient energy to escape the cohesive forces of the liquid and change state to a vapor.

Exhalation Valve   The exhalation valve is a mushroom or diaphragm type valve, located on the patient circuit. During inspiration the valve is pressurized, closing it so that pressure can build in the patient circuit. Many acute care ventilators incorporate the exhalation valve inside the ventilator to more accurately control flows PEEP pressures.

Fenestrated Tracheostomy Tube   A fenestrated tracheostomy tube is a specialized tracheostomy tube with a fenestration (hole) located at the curve of the tube above the cuff, which, when placed correctly, is in the trachea. By removing the inner cannula a patient can be allowed to breathe spontaneously through the natural airway, providing a means of weaning from the tracheostomy tube.

Fick's Law   The rate of diffusion of a gas into another gas is proportional to its concentration. The greater the concentration, the faster the rate of diffusion.

Flip-Flop   A fluidic element that is a bi-stable element; often utilized to control ventilator phasing (inspiration or expiration).

Flow-By   A mode of continuous flow ventilation that functions in CPAP and SIMV modes (Puritan Bennett 7200a only). If flow decreases from the baseline value to the sensitivity level set by the respiratory care practitioner, the microprocessor interprets the change as a patient effort. Flow-by is a flow-activated mode.

Flow Cycling   If inspiration is terminated when a specified flow is reached, the ventilator is said to be flow cycled. An example of a flow-cycled ventilator is the Bennett PR-2.

Flow-Inflating Manual Resuscitator   A flow-inflating manual resuscitator is a type of manual resuscitator that depends upon gas flow to inflate it. It is commonly used in the anesthesia and critical care settings.

Fluidics   Fluidics is the application of specialized pneumatic logic devices to control and regulate a ventilator's operation. All fluidic elements utilize the coanda effect and beam deflection in their operation.

Flutter Valve Therapy A form of hyperinflation therapy that utilizes a threshold resister consisting of a weighted ball resting on a conical seat. As the patient's expiratory flow passes through the valve, the weighted ball rises and falls, creating pressure pulses in the airway. The patient is encouraged to exhale actively to FRC using the device.

Fractional SaO$_2$ The percentage of oxygen saturation when compared to the total of all hemoglobin variants (functional and dysfunctional).

Frequency The frequency refers to the times a periodic function (waveform) repeats in a unit of time. For ultrasonic nebulizers, frequency is expressed in hertz (Hz) or "cycles per second."

Functional Hemoglobin The combination of oxyhemoglobin and deoxyhemoglobin in the blood. This constitutes the portion of hemoglobin capable of reversibly binding with oxygen.

Functional SaO$_2$ The percentage of oxygen saturation when compared to the functional hemoglobin.

Galvanic Oxygen Analyzer An oxygen analyzer that is dependent upon an electrochemical reaction forming free electrons. Electrical current is proportional to oxygen concentration.

Gay Lussac's Law Gay Lussac's law relates the pressure and the temperature of a gas when the volume remains constant. The law states that when temperature increases, the pressure will also increase ($P_1/T_1 = P_2/T_2$).

Graham's Law The rate of gas diffusion through a liquid is proportional to the solubility of the gas and is inversely proportional to the square root of its gram molecular weight.

Heat and Moisture Exchanger A tubular shaped device which contains a hygroscopic element which is placed in-line with the patient's airway. Humidity condenses during exhalation on the hygroscopic element and then evaporates during inspiration, humidifying the inspired gas.

Heated Wire Grid A method used to measure flow. A wire grid placed in a stream of flowing gas is heated to a constant temperature. As gas flow cools the wire grid, more current must be added to maintain a constant temperature. Therefore, gas flow becomes proportional to current.

Hemoglobin A protein-iron compound contained in the red blood cell. Hemoglobin is responsible for the majority of oxygen transport in the blood.

Henry's Law The rate of diffusion of a gas into or out of a liquid is proportional to the partial pressure of that gas at a given temperature. The greater the partial pressure, the faster the rate of diffusion.

Hertz A unit of measure for frequency or rate in cycles per second. Units of frequency were named after German physicist Heinrich Rudolf Hertz (1857–1894).

High Air Flow with Oxygen Entrainment (HAFOE) Devices that employ viscous shearing and vorticity to entrain room air into a stream of high velocity oxygen. These devices precisely mix the air and oxygen to deliver consistent concentrations of oxygen.

High-Frequency Flow Interrupter (HFFI) A type of ventilator that delivers small bursts of gas by interrupting a high-pressure or high-flow gas source. This is most commonly performed by using a rotating ball device that has a single gas port or pathway. These ventilators do not employ an injector cannula or catheter.

High-Frequency Jet Ventilator (HFJV) A high-frequency jet ventilator employs short, high-pressure puffs or bursts of gas at high frequencies to accomplish gas exchange. These high-frequency bursts of gas are introduced into the airway through a small catheter at the endotracheal tube port through a special adapter or through a specialized endotracheal tube (High-Lo Jet Tracheal Tube).

High-Frequency Positive Pressure Ventilator (HPPV) A type of mechanical ventilator with a modified circuit having a low compliance and compressible volume allowing tidal volume delivery at high frequencies.

High-Frequency Oscillatory Ventilators (HFOV) High-frequency oscillatory ventilators (HFOV) are active during both inspiration and exhalation. Most HFOV ventilators employ a diaphragm, piston or modified acoustic speaker to oscillate the gas into and out of the airway.

Humidifier   A device capable of adding water to a gas as water vapor.

Humidity   Water contained in a gas as vapor. Humidity is sometimes referred to as gaseous water.

Humidity Deficit   The humidity deficit is the difference between body humidity and the absolute humidity of the inspired gas expressed in mg/L.

Hygroscopic   A substance that has the ability to absorb water and water vapor. Silica gel is a common compound used in medical equipment to absorb water and is sometimes termed a desiccant.

Hyperbaric Oxygen Therapy   The application of oxygen at pressures greater than atmospheric pressure to treat very specific disease entities. Hyperbaric therapy may employ a multiplace (more than one patient) or monoplace (single patient) chamber.

Hypertonic   A solution having a greater concentration of a solute when compared to another solution. Hypertonic solutions are capable of exerting more osmotic pressure as a result of the higher concentration of solute.

Hypotonic   A solution having a lower concentration of solute when compared to another solution. Hypotonic solutions exert a lower osmotic pressure than solutions which are hypertonic.

I:E Ratio   The I:E ratio is the ratio of inspiratory time to expiratory time. A normal physiological I:E ratio is 1:2. When ventilating a patient, an I:E ratio of 1:2 or greater allows adequate time for the great vessels to fill during expiration, reducing the cardiovascular compromise associated with positive pressure ventilation.

Impedance Plethysmography   The measurement or detection of ventilation by using changes in electrical impedance between two electrodes placed on the chest. As the chest expands and contracts, the electrical impedance changes between the electrodes and can be measured.

Incentive Spirometry   Incentive spirometry is the application of biofeedback devices (incentive spirometers) to coach and encourage patients to take deeper breaths.

Indirect Acting Cylinder Valve   A type of cylinder valve that employs a diaphragm to open and close the valve seat. Turning the valve stem causes the diaphragm to be displaced through a spring, indirectly opening the valve seat.

Inertial Impaction   The process of removing larger aerosol particles from a carrier gas due to their greater inertia (mass × velocity = inertia). The larger particles (greater mass) travel in a straight path and impact against objects placed in the path (baffles).

Input Power   The power source utilized by a ventilator to provide the energy required to support the patient's ventilation. Input power can include pneumatic, electric or combined pneumatic and electric power.

Inspiratory Plateau   Inspiratory plateau, or inspiratory pause, is a brief pause (.5 to 2 seconds) at end inspiration. The purpose of the pause is to improve gas distribution throughout the lungs.

Inspiratory Time   Inspiratory time is the duration of inspiration during mechanical ventilation expressed in seconds. As inspiratory time increases, mean airway pressure increases and the I:E ratio becomes lower.

Intermittent Positive Pressure Breathing (IPPB)   The application of positive pressure for short time intervals (10 to 20 minutes) to hyperinflate the lungs of a spontaneously breathing patient. Positive pressure ventilators (IPPB machines) are employed to deliver the positive pressure.

Intrapulmonary Percussive Ventilation (IPV®)   High-frequency, manually triggered, pressure-limited, time-cycled ventilation combined with aerosol administration. Designed to facilitate the mobilization and removal of pulmonary secretions.

Isotonic   A solution having the same concentration of solutes as another solution. Two solutions that are isotonic exert the same osmotic pressures.

Jackson Tracheostomy Tube   The Jackson tracheostomy tube is a cuffless sterling silver tracheostomy tube. It is intended for long-term application (months or years) and is very durable.

Kinetic Theory   The kinetic theory describes the behavior of an ideal gas. The theory states that 1) molecules are in random motion, 2) any molecular collisions are completely elastic in nature (energy is not lost, only transferred), 3) as temperature increases, kinetic activity also increases and 4) there is no physical attraction between gas molecules.

Kymograph A revolving drum that records a volume tracing providing an x-y plot. The y-axis represents volume while the x-axis represents time. This recorder allows the measurement of expiratory flows.

Laminar Flow Smooth uniform gas flow in one direction. Laminar flow occurs at velocities such that the Reynold's number is less than 2,000.

Levey-Jennings Chart The Levey-Jennings chart is a means of plotting quality control data graphically in relation to the mean and standard deviation. This chart facilitates the identification of out-of-control results, shifts and trends.

Limit Variable A variable (pressure, volume, flow or time) that is allowed to reach a maximum value and is held at that value. Inspiration is not terminated once this value has been met.

Magnetic Valve A PEEP/CPAP generation device that utilizes magnetic attraction to a metal diaphragm to generate PEEP/CPAP pressures.

Mainstream Nebulizer A small-volume nebulizer in which the aerosol is generated in the path of the carrier gas.

Mandatory Minute Ventilation (MMV) A mode of ventilation in which the respiratory care practitioner sets a minimum minute volume, tidal volume, respiratory, peak flow, assist sensitivity and oxygen percentage. If the patient's spontaneous ventilation falls below the minimum minute volume, the ventilator delivers mandatory breaths until that volume is reached.

Mechanical Percussor A mechanical device (electrically or pneumatically powered) that is used for mechanical chest percussion. Use of mechanical percussors is less physically fatiguing and ensures uniformity in administration of chest physiotherapy.

Mercury Barometer A device used to measure air pressure that employs a column of mercury inverted into a mercury reservoir. Gas pressure against the surface of the reservoir causes the mercury column to rise or fall.

Metered Dose Inhaler (MDI) A small, compact, pressurized cartridge containing medication for self-administration. Each time the MDI is squeezed, a metered amount of medication is aerosolized which the patient then inhales.

Molecular Diffusion The theory stating that the increased frequencies associated with high-frequency ventilation will enhance the kinetic activity of gas molecules in the alveoli, increasing their diffusion across the alveolar capillary membrane.

Mouth-to-Mask Ventilation Device A mask and one-way valve or filter assembly, used for cardiopulmonary resuscitiation as a barrier device to protect the caregiver.

Nasopharyngeal Airway The nasopharyngeal airway is an airway that is designed to be inserted through the nose into the posterior pharynx, to relieve upper airway obstruction. The airway separates the tongue from the posterior pharynx.

Nebulizer A device that produces an aerosol. Pneumatic nebulizers contain baffles to help stabilize and reduce particle sizes.

Needle Valve A needle valve is one means of controlling gas flow and pressure. As the valve is opened more, more flow and pressure are allowed past the valve seat. A common application of a needle valve in plumbing is the faucet on a sink.

Negative Pressure Ventilators A classification of ventilators that cause lung expansion by applying a negative pressure outside of the chest. An iron lung is an example of this type of ventilator.

Non–Constant Flow Generator An inspiratory phase classification for a ventilator that produces a sine wave shaped flow pattern during inspiration. These ventilators typically use a rotary-driven piston to produce this flow pattern.

Operator Activation Operator activation occurs when the respiratory care practitioner delivers a manual mandatory (ventilator) breath to the patient by activating the appropriate control.

Or/Nor Gate A monostable, fluidic element with two control ports.

Oropharyngeal Airway The oropharyngeal

airway is an airway designed to be inserted into the mouth, separating the tongue from the posterior pharynx. It is designed specifically to relieve upper airway obstruction by separating the tongue from the posterior pharynx.

Oxygen Concentrator   A device that separates oxygen from room air for delivery of oxygen-rich gas to the patient. Most concentrators operate using molecular sieves, which adsorb the nitrogen from the air and pass the oxygen.

Oxygen Proportioner   A device designed to mix oxygen and air in precise concentrations, using proportioning valves. These devices are sometimes referred to as blenders. An oxygen proportioner provides precise concentrations of gas at 50 psi to operate other equipment.

Paramagnetic Principle   The physical principle that some gases are attracted to the strongest portion of a magnetic field (oxygen is a paramagnetic gas). This principle is employed in the operation of a physical oxygen analyzer.

Pascal's Law   A fluid confined within a container will transmit pressure uniformly in all directions, with the net forces acting perpendicular to the container surface.

Passy-Muir Valve   A tracheostomy valve designed to facilitate the use of the upper airway when the tracheostomy tube cuff is deflated. It is a one-way valve that forces air on exhalation through the upper airway.

Patient Activation   Patient activation occurs when the ventilator sensitivity system detects a patient's spontaneous effort and delivers a mandatory (ventilator) breath.

Peak Flowmeter   A device that is used to measure a patient's peak expiratory flow rate. This is commonly done to assess the effectiveness of bronchodilator therapy.

Pendelluft   A world of German origin which means "air swinging freely." Due to differing time constants, not all areas of the lung fill and empty at the same rates. Therefore, the unequal filling and emptying results in air moving from one lung region to another, making gas distribution more uniform.

Percussionator®   A pneumatically powered pressure controller that is time cycled. The percussionator cycles at a rate of 100 to 250 cycles per minute. It is employed by the Percussionaire Corporation's IPV devices.

Percussors   Percussors are mechanical devices (electric or pneumatic) that produce vibrations when applied to the chest wall. Percussors help to improve the effectiveness of chest physiotherapy by relieving the muscle fatigue experienced by respiratory care practitioners when performing manual percussion.

Pharyngealtracheal Lumen (PTL) Airway
An artificial airway that may be used to intubate the esophagus or the trachea. The airway is used blindly, without the use of a laryngeoscope. It is unique in that two cuffs are used to seal the airway, one in the oropharynx and the other at the distal tip of the airway.

pH Glass   A special type of glass that is permeable to hydrogen ions. This glass is used to develop a potential (voltage) between two solutions of differing pH.

Phase Variable   A variable (pressure, volume, flow or time) that is measured and used to initiate a phase of the ventilatory cycle. For example, a variable used to initiate the change from expiration to inspiration, inspiration, the change from inspiration to expiration or the expiratory phase.

Phasitron®   The phasitron is the mechanical and pneumatic interface between the patient and the percussionator. It is a sliding venturi, which is spring loaded in the closed position. Gas flow during inspiration from the percussionator opens the Phasitron,® delivering a pulsed gas flow to the patient.

Piezoelectric Crystal   A crystal that is capable of converting electrical energy (rf energy) to mechanical energy (vibrations). The crystal resonates at the same frequency as the electrical energy driving it.

Pilot Balloon   The pilot balloon is an inflatable chamber near the distal end of the pilot tube which supplies gas pressure and volume to inflate the cuff of an artificial airway. Inflation of the balloon indicates that the cuff contains air. Cuff pressures should be monitored to help prevent pressure necrosis rather than solely relying on the "feel" of the pilot balloon.

Pilot Tube   The pilot tube is the line that supplies pressure to the cuff of an artificial airway. It is a small-diameter line connected to the artificial airway, and it terminates inside the cuff.

Pin Index Safety System (PISS)   PISS is a safety system designed by the Compressed Gas Association for small cylinders using yoke type valve connections. Two pins are positioned in two of six positions to prevent the mismatching of regulators or cylinder yokes with the incorrect gas cylinder.

Piston Drive Mechanism   A ventilator that uses a piston as the drive mechanism to convert its input power to ventilatory work. The piston may be rotary or linearly driven which determines its waveform characteristics.

Pitt Speaking Tube/Communitrach   The Pitt speaking tube/Communitrach is a specialized tracheostomy tube that facilitates speech when the cuff is inflated. A separate tube supplies a flow of oxygen above the cuff, permitting gas flow through the vocal cords.

Pneumatic Splinting   Maintenance of a patient airway using positive pressure (CPAP or Bi-Level Positive Airway Pressure) to separate the tongue from the soft palate.

Pneumotachometer   A device that is used to measure flow rates. Pneumotachometers typically operate by measuring a pressure difference across a resistance or by creating a pressure difference using a Venturi tube.

Poiseuille's Law   Poiseuille's law describes the relationship between volumetric flow, viscosity, pressure, length and velocity of a gas flowing through a tube. Poiseuille's law only applies for laminar flow. One important relationship of Poiseuille's law is that as the radius of a tube is decreased by 1/2, the resistance to gas flow increases by 16 times.

Polarographic Oxygen Analyzer   An oxygen analyzer that uses a Clark electrode to measure oxygen. Oxygen reacts electrochemically to form free electrons, resulting in current flow being proportional to oxygen concentration. This analyzer differs from a galvanic type by the addition of a battery.

Positive End Expiratory Pressure (PEEP)
The application of positive pressure during the expiratory phase during positive pressure ventilation.

Positive-Expiratory-Pressure (PEP) Therapy
A form of hyperinflation therapy in which the patient exhales actively against a fixed resistance to FRC, which maintains positive pressure in the airways during exhalation. This therapy mechanically splints the airways open during exhalation through the application of pressure.

Potentiometer   A wire-wound variable resister that operates by changing its effective length, altering its total resistance.

Pressure Controlled Ventilation   A form of continuous mandatory ventilation in which all breaths are pressure limited and time cycled. This form of ventilation may also be combined with inverse I:E ratios (4:1 to 1.1:1), which are then termed pressure controlled inverse ratio ventilation (PCIRV).

Pressure Cycling   A means of terminating inspiration when a preset pressure is achieved. The Bird Mark 7 is an example of a pressure cycled ventilator.

Pressure Limited   A pressure limited breath occurs when a volume, flow or time cycled inspiration is terminated when an operator set pressure is reached (pressure limit). A type of breath delivery where pressure rises to a preset value and is maintained at that value until the breath ends.

Pressure Support   A spontaneous mode of ventilation in which a constant pressure is applied during the inspiratory phase. Inspiration is terminated when a specific flow rate is reached.

Pressure Transducer   An electrical component that converts a pressure change into an electrical signal. Two common types of pressure transducers are strain gauge and variable reluctance transducers.

Proportional Solenoid Valve   A type of solenoid valve that is able to open or close in discrete steps or positions. Proportional solenoid valves are typically microprocessor controlled.

Proportioning Valve   A device that mixes oxygen and air in precise concentrations. These devices operate using a proportioning valve. Sometimes proportioning valves are referred to as blenders.

Pulsation Dampener   A small, rigid reservoir (less than 1 liter) used by ventilator manufacturers to reduce pressure changes due to changes in flow.

Pulse Oximeter   A monitoring device that measures oxygen saturation noninvasively using red and infrared light.

Quality Control   The use of statistical analysis in conjunction with known standards to assess an instrument's accuracy, reliability and reproducibility. Quality control programs also identify technical and random errors that may occur in the operation of the instrument.

Reducing Valve A specialized valve that is designed to reduce gas pressure. Reducing valves may reduce pressure in one step (single stage) or many steps (multistage). All reducing valves operate by balancing spring tension and gas pressure across a diaphragm.

Reducing Valve Drive Mechanism A ventilator which employs a reducing valve to convert its input power to ventilatory work. The Bennett PR-2 is an example of a ventilator using a reducing valve drive mechanism.

Regulator A regulator is a combination of a reducing valve and a flowmeter into one device. Regulators may employ Bourdon flowmeters or Thorpe tube flowmeters, depending upon their design.

Relative Humidity Relative humidity is the result of the absolute humidity divided by the capacity multiplied by 100 (absolute / capacity $\times$ 100 = relative humidity). This percentage relates the humidity of a gas to the capacity of that gas at a given temperature.

Reynold's Number The Reynold's number equation is used to predict whether gas flow will be laminar or turbulent. The calculation accounts for the gas' velocity, viscosity density and the diameter of the tube. If the number is less than 2,000, flow will be laminar.

Schmidt Trigger A fluidic element consisting of three proportional amplifiers and two flip-flop elements. This device is often used to detect small pressure changes.

Self-Inflating Manual Resuscitator A self-inflating manual resuscitator is one that does not depend upon gas flow for inflation. The elasticity of the bag causes it to inflate once it is released after applying a breath.

Sensitivity Sensitivity refers to the ventilator's ability to sense a patient's spontaneous breathing effort. Most sensitivity systems employ a pressure sensing device, while others use a flow sensing device. If a ventilator's sensitivity system is adjusted properly, very little patient effort is required to initiate ventilation.

Servo Controlled The application of a closed-loop feedback control system to adjust the output of a heater or valve to regulate temperature, flow, pressure or volume.

Servo Controlled Scissor Valve A type of proportional solenoid valve that is servo controlled and resembles a pair of scissors opening or pinching a gas channel.

Severinghaus Electrode The PCO_2 electrode in a blood gas system or transcutaneous electrode.

Shift A change in quality control values such that all values change from one side of the mean to the other.

Sidestream Nebulizer A small-volume nebulizer in which aerosol is generated adjacent to the flow of carrier gas.

Sigh Mode The periodic delivery of a larger than normal tidal volume to mimic a spontaneous sigh breath.

Single Circuit A classification of ventilator circuits in which the gas that drives the ventilator is the same gas that is delivered to the patient. The Puritan Bennett 7200a is one example of a single circuit ventilator.

Small Particle Aerosol Generator (SPAG) A pneumatically powered nebulizer designed specifically for the administration of Ribaviran for the treatment of respiratory syncytial virus (RSV). The SPAG nebulizer utilizes a secondary gas flow and a drying chamber to further reduce particle size.

Solenoid Valve A type of electromechanical valve that operates using an electromagnet to open the valve. Spring tension usually returns the valve to the closed position.

Spacer A small hollow chamber designed for use with metered dose inhalers (MDI). The spacer enhances medication delivery and helps to alleviate coordination problems for patients using MDIs.

Stepper Motor A type of electric motor that moves in discrete positions or steps in response to an input voltage. The voltage applied to the motor determines how far it will move.

Strain Gauge An electrical device consisting of a thin coil of wire bonded to a paper or plastic substrate. As the gauge is stretched (strained), electrical resistance increases due to the greater length of the wires.

Suction Catheter A suction catheter is a small-diameter tube that is used to aspirate the airway, while removing secretions or foreign material. It may be used with artificial airways as well as with the natural airway.

Suction Regulator   A suction regulator is a device that adjusts the vacuum level applied to another piece of equipment. Suction regulators are employed when performing artificial airway aspiration, using chest tubes and other applications.

Synchronized Intermittent Mandatory Ventilation   A mode of ventilation in which the patient is allowed to breathe spontaneously between mandatory (machine) breaths.

Taylor Dispersion   A model of gas exchange describing that the addition of convective flow to a diffusive process enhances gas distribution. Fredburg expanded upon Taylor's theories and hypothesized that flow and turbulence may be augmented by increasing the ventilatory frequency.

Thermal Anemometer   A type of flow measuring device which operates by gas flow cooling a thermistor bead, wire grid or other electrically heated element. Gas flow is proportional to changes in temperature (electrical current).

Thorpe Tube Flowmeter   A Thorpe tube flowmeter is a type of flowmeter that incorporates a tapered tube and a float to measure gas flow. This type of flowmeter may be uncompensated or compensated for back pressure. Compensation is determined by the placement of the needle valve in relationship to the Thorpe tube.

Tidal Volume   Tidal volume is the amount of gas inhaled or exhaled during a normal spontaneous breath. When mechanically ventilating a patient, tidal volume refers to the volume of gas delivered during the inspiratory phase.

Time Activation   Time activation occurs when inspiration begins following the passage of a specified time.

Time Cycling   Time cycling occurs when inspiration ends following the passage of a specified time.

Tonicity   Tonicity reflects the degree of osmotic pressure between two solutions. A solution may have a greater tonicity (hypertonic), less tonicity (hypotonic) or no tonicity (isotonic).

Tonometry   The equilibration of whole blood with known gas samples for the purpose of quality control. An instrument known as a tonometer is used to mix the whole blood with the known gas samples.

Trach Button   The trach button is a specialized tracheostomy weaning device that is designed to temporarily occlude the tracheostomy stoma. Once it is in place and plugged, the patient must use his or her normal airway to breathe.

Tracheostomy Tube   The tracheostomy tube is an airway that is designed to be surgically placed below the larynx at the second tracheal ring. It will relieve upper airway obstruction and may be cuffed or cuffless.

Transcutaneous Electrode   An electrode that samples PO_2 or PCO_2 transcutaneously or across the skin.

Transducer   A device that converts one form of energy to another. Transducers commonly convert a pressure, flow or temperature to an electrical signal that can be measured.

Trend   A group of six or more quality control results that display an increasing or decreasing pattern from the normal random distribution.

Trigger Variable   A variable (pressure, volume, flow or time) that is measured and used to initiate inspiration.

Tubing/Circuit Compliance   A measure of the distensibility of a ventilator circuit expressed in mL/cmH_2O.

Venturi's Principle   A principle that relates a pressure reduction within a diverging duct to the velocity of the gas flowing through it. As velocity increases, the pressure at the tube's restriction decreases. Venturi's principle applies when the gas flow is noncompressible and is laminar.

Viscous Shearing and Vorticity   A phenomenon by which gas or a liquid may be entrained into a high-velocity gas stream by shear forces and vortices or eddies.

Volume Assisted Pressure Support (VAPS)   A form of pressure support which assures that the patient will receive a specific minimum tidal volume with each pressure supported breath.

Volume-Controlled Ventilation   A form of continuous mandatory ventilation in which all breaths are volume controlled (the ventilator may be a flow controller).

Volume Cycling   The termination of inspiration after a preset volume has been delivered.

Vortex Sensor   A flow measuring device which relies on the vortex shedding principle to detect flow. Struts placed in the gas flow pathway cause turbulence which is detected by ultrasonic energy transmission.

Water Column   A type of PEEP/CPAP device that uses a container of water which generates the expiratory resistance to provide positive pressure. In a water column system the expiratory limb is simply immersed into a container of water.

Water Seal Spirometer   A type of spirometer that employs a bell that is immersed in a water bath to measure lung volumes. As the patient's inhaled and exhaled gases move into and out of the bell, the bell rises or falls, allowing accurate volume determination.

Water-Weighted Diaphragm   A type of PEEP/CPAP device that utilizes a water column pressing on a diaphragm to generate PEEP/CPAP pressures.

Wheatstone Bridge   A sensitive electrical circuit composed of four resisters in series that allows the measurement of small changes in voltage or current. These are used in conjunction with transducers to measure pressure or flow changes.

Wright Respirometer   A portable, vane-type respirometer that measures volumes. The spirometer has a narrow accuracy range of gas flow (10 to 20 L/min) and is easily damaged by excessive flow (greater than 300 L/min).

Zone Valve   A safety valve that is placed in an oxygen piping system such that gas flow may be shut off in the event of a fire or other emergency.

INDEX